# FIRST AID FOR THE®

# USMLE STEP 1 2024

**TAO LE, MD, MHS**

Founder, ScholarRx
Associate Clinical Professor, Department of Medicine
University of Louisville School of Medicine

**VIKAS BHUSHAN, MD**

Founder, *First Aid for the USMLE Step 1*
Boracay, Philippines

**CONNIE QIU, MD, PhD**

Resident, Department of Dermatology
Johns Hopkins Hospital

**ANUP CHALISE, MBBS, MS, MRCSEd**

Registrar, General and Colorectal Surgery
North Middlesex University Hospital, London

**PANAGIOTIS KAPARALIOTIS, MD**

University of Athens Medical School, Greece

**CAROLINE COLEMAN, MD**

Assistant Professor, Department of Medicine
Emory University School of Medicine

**KIMBERLY KALLIANOS, MD**

Assistant Professor, Department of Radiology and Biomedical Imaging
University of California, San Francisco School of Medicine

**SEAN EVANS, MD**

Resident, Department of Medicine
Emory University School of Medicine

New York / Chicago / San Francisco / Athens / London / Madrid / Mexico City
Milan / New Delhi / Singapore / Sydney / Toronto

**First Aid for the® USMLE Step 1 2024: A Student-to-Student Guide**

Photo and line art credits for this book begin on page 755 and are considered an extension of this copyright page.
Portions of this book identified with the symbol ℞ are copyright © USMLE-Rx.com (MedIQ Learning, LLC).
Portions of this book identified with the symbol 🆁🆄 are copyright © Dr. Richard Usatine.
Portions of this book identified with the symbol ✳ are under license from other third parties. Please refer to page 755 for a complete list of those image source attribution notices.

First Aid for the® is a registered trademark of McGraw Hill.

1 2 3 4 5 6 7 8 9  LMN  27 26 25 24

ISBN 978-1-266-07720-3
MHID 1-266-07720-0

---

### Notice

Medicine is an ever-changing science. As new research and clinical experience broaden our knowledge, changes in treatment and drug therapy are required. The authors and the publisher of this work have checked with sources believed to be reliable in their efforts to provide information that is complete and generally in accord with the standards accepted at the time of publication. However, in view of the possibility of human error or changes in medical sciences, neither the authors nor the publisher nor any other party who has been involved in the preparation or publication of this work warrants that the information contained herein is in every respect accurate or complete, and they disclaim all responsibility for any errors or omissions or for the results obtained from use of the information contained in this work. Readers are encouraged to confirm the information contained herein with other sources. For example and in particular, readers are advised to check the product information sheet included in the package of each drug they plan to administer to be certain that the information contained in this work is accurate and that changes have not been made in the recommended dose or in the contraindications for administration. This recommendation is of particular importance in connection with new or infrequently used drugs.

---

This book was set in Electra LT Std by GW Inc.
The editors were Bob Boehringer and Christina M. Thomas.
Project management was provided by GW Inc.
The production supervisor was Jeffrey Herzich.
LSC Communications was printer and binder.

This book is printed on acid-free paper.

McGraw Hill books are available at special quantity discounts to use as premiums and sales promotions, or for use in corporate training programs. To contact a representative please visit the Contact Us pages at www.mhprofessional.com.

## Dedication

To medical students and physicians worldwide for
collaborating to improve medical education and practice.

# Contents

**▶ SECTION I**      **GUIDE TO EFFICIENT EXAM PREPARATION**      **1**

**▶ SECTION I SUPPLEMENT**      **SPECIAL SITUATIONS**      **25**

**▶ SECTION II**      **HIGH-YIELD GENERAL PRINCIPLES**      **27**

# Contributing Authors

**CHRISTIAN FAABORG-ANDERSEN, MD**
Resident, Department of Medicine
Massachusetts General Hospital

**MORGAN BUCHANAN, MPH**
Emory University School of Medicine
Class of 2025

**ANTHONY G. CHESEBRO**
Renaissance School of Medicine, Stony Brook University
MD/PhD candidate

**EMILY HAND**
St. George's University School of Medicine, Grenada
Class of 2024

**KATHERINE LEBLANC, MSc**
University of Washington School of Medicine
MD/PhD Candidate

**ANNA LIGOCKI, MD, MS**
Resident, Department of Medicine
Ascension Saint Agnes Hospital

**FAATEH AHMAD RAUF, MBBS**
Resident, Department of Medicine
ISMMS NYC Health+Hospitals/Queens

**CAROLINA CABAN RIVERA**
Lewis Katz School of Medicine at Temple University
Class of 2025

**JAIMIE LYNN ROGNER, MD, MPH**
Resident, Departments of Medicine and Pediatrics
University of Rochester Medical Center

**GEORGIOS M. STERGIOPOULOS, MD**
Research Fellow, Department of Molecular Medicine
Mayo Clinic, Minnesota

## IMAGE AND ILLUSTRATION TEAM

**YOOREE GRACE CHUNG**
Emory University School of Medicine
MD/PhD Candidate

**TANYA KONDOLAY, MPH**
Aureus University School of Medicine
MD Candidate

**NOAH NEWMAN, MD**
Resident, Department of Internal Medicine
Emory University School of Medicine

# Associate Authors

**MAKENNA ASH**
Emory University School of Medicine
Class of 2025

**MARGARET GINOZA, MD, MPH**
Resident, Internal Medicine–Pediatrics
Baylor College of Medicine

**TALEAH KHAN, MBBS**
CMH Lahore Medical College and Institute of Dentistry, Pakistan

**PRABHAT POUDEL, MBBS**
Nepal Medical College Teaching Hospital, Nepal

**DANUSHA SANCHEZ, MD**
Resident, Department of Emergency Medicine
Poznań University of Medical Sciences, Poland

**ADITYA SINGH, MBBS**
All India Institute of Medical Sciences, Raipur, India

## IMAGE AND ILLUSTRATION TEAM

**ANNABEL LU**
Emory University School of Medicine
Class of 2024

**AUBREY REED**
Emory University School of Medicine
MD/PhD Candidate

# Faculty Advisors

**RITU AMATYA**

FHI 360, Nepal

**MARK A.W. ANDREWS, PhD**

Professor and Founding Chairman, Department of Physiology
Duquesne University College of Osteopathic Medicine

**MARIA ANTONELLI, MD**

Assistant Professor, Division of Rheumatology
Case Western Reserve University at MetroHealth Medical Center, Cleveland

**SAMAN BENTOTA, MD**

Physician and Microbiologist
Sri Lanka

**JOE B. BLUMER, PhD**

Associate Professor, Department of Pharmacology
Medical University of South Carolina College of Medicine

**BRADLEY J. BRUGGEMAN, MD**

Assistant Professor, Obstetrics and Gynecology
University of Florida College of Medicine

**CHRISTOPHER M. BURNS, PhD**

Professor of Basic Medical Sciences
University of Arizona College of Medicine, Phoenix

**BROOKS D. CASH, MD**

Chief, Gastroenterology, Hepatology, and Nutrition
University of Texas Health Science Center at Houston

**DIMITRI CASSIMATIS, MD**

Associate Professor, Department of Medicine
Emory University School of Medicine

**CATHERINE CHILES, MD**

Associate Clinical Professor of Psychiatry
Yale School of Medicine

**BRADLEY COLE, MD**

Assistant Professor of Neurology
Loma Linda University School of Medicine

**CAROLINE COLEMAN, MD**

Assistant Professor, Department of Medicine
Emory University School of Medicine

**MARTHA FANER, PhD**

Associate Professor of Biochemistry and Molecular Biology
Michigan State University College of Osteopathic Medicine

**CONRAD FISCHER, MD**

Associate Professor, Medicine, Physiology, and Pharmacology
Touro College of Medicine

**AYAKO WENDY FUJITA, MD**

Fellow, Division of Infectious Diseases
Emory University School of Medicine

**RAYUDU GOPALAKRISHNA, PhD**

Professor, Department of Integrative Anatomical Sciences
Keck School of Medicine of University of Southern California

**MEREDITH K. GREER, MD**

Assistant Professor, Division of Pulmonary, Allergy, Critical Care, and Sleep
    Medicine
Emory University School of Medicine

**AMBER J. HECK, PhD**

Associate Professor, Department of Microbiology, Immunology, and
    Genetics
University of North Texas Health Science Center, Fort Worth

**VASUDEVA G. KAMATH, MSc, PhD**

Assistant Professor of Biochemistry
The University of Arizona College of Medicine, Phoenix

**CLARK KEBODEAUX, PharmD**

Clinical Associate Professor, Pharmacy Practice and Science
University of Kentucky College of Pharmacy

**MATTHEW KRAYBILL, PhD**

Clinical Neuropsychologist
Cottage Health, Santa Barbara, California

**GERALD LEE, MD**

Associate Professor, Departments of Pediatrics and Medicine
Emory University School of Medicine

**KACHIU C. LEE, MD, MPH**

Assistant Professor (Adjunct), Department of Dermatology
Lewis Katz School of Medicine at Temple University

**JAMES LYONS, MD**

Associate Dean, Professor of Pathology and Family Medicine
Alabama College of Osteopathic Medicine

**NILADRI KUMAR MAHATO, MBBS, MS, PhD**

Assistant Professor of Anatomy
Marian University College of Osteopathic Medicine, Indianapolis

**CARL MARFURT, PhD**

Professor Emeritus, Department of Anatomy, Cell Biology and Physiology
Indiana University School of Medicine–Northwest, Gary

**PETER MARKS, MD, PhD**

Center for Biologics Evaluation and Research
US Food and Drug Administration

**DOUGLAS A. MATA, MD, MPH**

Director of Molecular Pathology
Foundation Medicine, Cambridge, Massachusetts

**SOROUSH RAIS-BAHRAMI, MD, MBA**

Professor of Urology and Radiology
University of Alabama at Birmingham Heersink School of Medicine

**RICHARD P. RAMONELL, MD**

Assistant Professor of Medicine, Division of Pulmonary, Allergy, Critical
    Care, and Sleep Medicine
University of Pittsburgh School of Medicine

**KEISHA RAY, PhD**

Associate Professor, McGovern Center for Humanities and Ethics
University of Texas Health Science Center at Houston

**SASAN SAKIANI, MD**

Assistant Professor of Medicine, Department of Medicine
University of Maryland School of Medicine

**SARAH SCHIMANSKY, MB BCh BAO**

Resident, Department of Ophthalmology
Bristol Eye Hospital

**NATHAN WM. SKELLEY, MD**

Associate Professor, Medical Director of Orthopaedic Surgery
Sanford Health–University of South Dakota School of Medicine

**TONY SLIEMAN, PhD, MSc**

Associate Professor, Department of Basic Sciences
New York Institute of Technology College of Osteopathic Medicine at
    Arkansas State University

**MATTHEW SOCHAT, MD**

Physician, Hematology/Oncology
Southeastern Medical Oncology Center

**HOWARD M. STEINMAN, PhD**

Assistant Dean, Biomedical Science Education
Albert Einstein College of Medicine

**JACQUELINE TRUONG, DPM, MPH**

Associate Professor, College of Podiatric Medicine
Western University of Health Sciences

**RICHARD P. USATINE, MD**

Professor, Dermatology and Cutaneous Surgery
University of Texas Health Science Center San Antonio

**SYLVIA WASSERTHEIL-SMOLLER, PhD**

Professor Emerita, Department of Epidemiology and Population Health
Albert Einstein College of Medicine

**ADAM WEINSTEIN, MD**

Associate Professor of Medical Sciences and Pediatrics
Frank H. Netter MD School of Medicine at Quinnipiac University

**ABHISHEK YADAV, MBBS, MSc**

Associate Professor, Department of Medicine
Rutgers New Jersey Medical School

**KRISTAL YOUNG, MD**

Clinical Instructor, Department of Cardiology
Huntington Hospital, Pasadena, California

# Preface

With the 34th edition of *First Aid for the USMLE Step 1* we continue our commitment to providing students with the most useful and up-to-date preparation guide for this exam. This edition represents an outstanding revision in many ways, including:

- 22 entirely new or heavily revised high-yield topics reflecting evolving trends in the USMLE Step 1.

- Extensive text revisions, new mnemonics, clarifications, and corrections curated by a team of 16 medical student and resident physician authors who excelled on their Step 1 examinations, and verified by a team of expert faculty advisors and nationally recognized USMLE instructors.

- Updated with 81 new and revised diagrams and illustrations as part of our ongoing collaboration with USMLE-Rx and ScholarRx (MedIQ Learning, LLC).

- Updated with 21 new and revised photos to help visualize various disorders, descriptive findings, and basic science concepts. Additionally, revised imaging photos have been labeled and optimized to show both normal anatomy and pathologic findings.

- Updated exam preparation advice, tailored for the current pass/fail scoring system and Step 1 blueprint changes.

- New advice on how to utilize emerging AI tools to increase studying efficiency.

- Updated photos of patients and pathologies to include a variety of skin colors to better depict real-world presentations.

- Improved organization and integration of text, illustrations, clinical images, and tables throughout for focused review of high-yield topics.

- Revised ratings of current, high-yield review resources, with clear explanations of their relevance to USMLE review. Replaced outdated resources with new ones recommended by Step takers.

- Real-time Step 1 updates and corrections can be found exclusively on our blog, www.firstaidteam.com.

We invite students and faculty to share their thoughts and ideas to help us continually improve *First Aid for the USMLE Step 1* through our blog and collaborative editorial platform. (See How to Contribute, p. xv.)

| | |
|---|---|
| *Louisville* | Tao Le |
| *Boracay* | Vikas Bhushan |
| *Baltimore* | Connie Qiu |
| *London* | Anup Chalise |
| *Athens* | Panagiotis Kaparaliotis |
| *Atlanta* | Caroline Coleman |
| *Atlanta* | Sean Evans |
| *San Francisco* | Kimberly Kallianos |

# Special Acknowledgments

This has been a collaborative project from the start. We gratefully acknowledge the thousands of thoughtful comments, corrections, and advice of the many medical students, international medical graduates, and faculty who have supported the authors in our continuing development of *First Aid for the USMLE Step 1*.

We provide special acknowledgment and thanks to the following individuals who made exemplary contributions to this edition through our voting, proofreading, and crowdsourcing platform: Yazmin Allegretti, Athanasios Angistriotis, and Nikitha Crasta.

For support and encouragement throughout the process, we are grateful to Thao Pham, Jinky Flang, and Jonathan Kirsch, Esq. Thanks to Louise Petersen for organizing and supporting the project. Thanks to our publisher, McGraw Hill, for the valuable assistance of its staff, including Bob Boehringer, Jeffrey Herzich, Christina Thomas, Kristian Sanford, and Don Goyette.

We are also very grateful to Dr. Fred Howell and Dr. Robert Cannon of Textensor Ltd for providing us extensive customization and support for their powerful Annotate.co collaborative editing platform (www.annotate.co), which allows us to efficiently manage thousands of contributions. Thanks to Dr. Richard Usatine and Dr. Kristine Krafts for their outstanding image contributions. Thanks also to Jean-Christophe Fournet (www.humpath.com), Dr. Ed Uthman, and Dr. Frank Gaillard (www.radiopaedia.org) for generously allowing us to access some of their striking photographs.

For exceptional editorial leadership, enormous thanks to Megan Chandler. Special thanks to our indexer, Dr. Anne Fifer. We are also grateful to our art manager, Susan Mazik, and illustrators, Stephanie Jones and Rachael Joy, for their creative work on the new and updated illustrations. Lastly, tremendous thanks to our compositor, GW Inc., especially Anne Banning, Gary Clark, Cindy Geiss, Denise Smith, Debra Clark, and Gabby Sullivan.

| | |
|---|---|
| *Louisville* | Tao Le |
| *Boracay* | Vikas Bhushan |
| *Baltimore* | Connie Qiu |
| *London* | Anup Chalise |
| *Athens* | Panagiotis Kaparaliotis |
| *Atlanta* | Caroline Coleman |
| *Atlanta* | Sean Evans |
| *San Francisco* | Kimberly Kallianos |

# General Acknowledgments

Each year we are fortunate to receive the input of thousands of medical students and graduates who provide new material, clarifications, and potential corrections through our website and our collaborative editing platform. This has been a tremendous help in clarifying difficult concepts, correcting errata from the previous edition, and minimizing new errata during the revision of the current edition. This reflects our long-standing vision of a true, student-to-student publication. We have done our best to thank each person individually below, but we recognize that errors and omissions are likely. Therefore, we will post an updated list of acknowledgments at our website, www.firstaidteam.com/bonus/. We will gladly make corrections if they are brought to our attention.

For submitting contributions and corrections, many thanks to Ehsen Abdul-Kabir, Suleiman Jamal Abou Ramadan, Ghaith Abu-Hassan, Raghed Abu Jabeh, Ruby Abu Nassar, Suhaib Abusara, Rochana Acharya, Biplov Adhikari, Sumera Afzal-Tohid, Marium Aisha, Wahid Aloweiwi, Sajjad Altmimi, Mohammad Arabi, Laila Ashkar, Nabil Askar, Emily Babcock, Abdulrahman Bani-Yassin, Angelina Bania, Gabriella Barr, Shreya Bavishi, Heather Beyea, Karun Bhattarai, Pratik Bhattarai, Suzit Bhusal, Iuliia Bochinina, Stephanie Brown, Nicholas Buehler, Jack Carey, Paola Del Cueto, Amy Cunningham, Suyash Dawadi, Molly Dexter, Jeevan Divakaran, Manasa Dutta, Prabin Duwadee, Gian Ferrando, Talia Fradkin, Louna Ftouni, Aaron Goldman-Henley, Priyanka Goswami, Jackson Green, Ishan Gupta, Fariah Asha Haque Haque, Mariam Hassan, Shelly Colleen Heredia, Hung Ho, Rachel Holmes, Kaitlyn Hoyt, Samkit Jain, Subhah Jalil, Abdelrhman Muwafaq Janem, Julia Katcher, Avneet Kaur, Nadim Khutaba, Sourabh Kumar, Nery y Mara Lamothe, Guilherme Leite, Anna Marmalidou, Tanya Mateo, Juliana Maya, Nathan McDermott, Jose Antonio Meade, Shivani Mehta, Muhammed Mikaeel, Dylan Mittauer, Andrew Mohama, Gamble Morrison, Andrew Moya, Alexandra Jan Mrani, Waneeza Mughees, Ziad Nabil, Ezra Nadler, Shamsun Nahar, Sajjad Nazar Majeed, Antony Nemr, Hyder Nizamani, Sophie O'Hare, Charis Osiadi, Fahreddin Palaz, Sharon Pan, Archana Pandey, Abigail Poe, Emily Pompeo, Zoe Pujadas, Yochitha Pulipati, Nicholas Purvis, Denise Qyqja, Parul Rai, Yoshita Rao, Liran Raz, Eva Rest, Carol Sánchez Jiménez, Ridha Saad, Luke Schroeder, Sirous Seifirad, Muhammad Shahzaib, Amir Hossein Shams, Naimatullah Sharifi, Ajay Ajit Pal Singh, Ramzi Skaik, Swati Srivastava, Zargham Abbas Syed, Miranda Teixeira, Grayson Tishko, Hirak Trivedi, Ana Tsiklauri, Luis Vilatuna, Amanjot Virk, Stefani Wren, Richard Wu, and Hsinyu Yin.

# How to Contribute

This edition of *First Aid for the USMLE Step 1* incorporates thousands of contributions and improvements suggested by student and faculty advisors. We invite you to participate in this process. Please send us your suggestions for:

- Study and test-taking strategies for the USMLE Step 1

- New facts, mnemonics, diagrams, and clinical images

- High-yield topics that may appear on future Step 1 exams

- Personal ratings and comments on review books, question banks, apps, videos, and courses

- Pathology and radiology images (high resolution) relevant to the facts in the book

For each new entry incorporated into the next edition, you will receive **up to a $20 Amazon.com gift card** as well as personal acknowledgment in the next edition. Significant contributions will be compensated at the discretion of the authors. Also, let us know about material in this edition that you feel is low yield and should be deleted.

All submissions including potential errata should ideally be supported with hyperlinks to a dynamically updated Web resource such as UpToDate, AccessMedicine, and ClinicalKey.

We welcome potential errata on grammar and style if the change improves readability. Please note that *First Aid* style is somewhat unique; for example, we have fully adopted the *AMA Manual of Style* recommendations on eponyms ("We recommend that the possessive form be omitted in eponymous terms") and on abbreviations (no periods with eg, ie, etc). We also avoid periods in tables unless required for full sentences. Kindly refrain from submitting "style errata" unless you find specific inconsistencies with the *AMA Manual of Style*.

The preferred way to submit new entries, clarifications, mnemonics, or potential corrections with a valid, authoritative reference is via our website: **www.firstaidteam.com**.

This website will be continuously updated with validated errata, new high-yield content, and a new online platform to contribute suggestions, mnemonics, diagrams, clinical images, and potential errata.

Alternatively, you can email us at: **firstaid@scholarrx.com**.

Contributions submitted by **May 15, 2024**, receive priority consideration for the 2025 edition of *First Aid for the USMLE Step 1*. We thank you for taking the time to share your experience and apologize in advance that we cannot individually respond to all contributors as we receive thousands of contributions each year.

## ▶ NOTE TO CONTRIBUTORS

All contributions become property of the authors and are subject to editing and reviewing. Please verify all data and spellings carefully. Contributions should be supported by at least two high-quality references.

Check our website first to avoid duplicate submissions. In the event that similar or duplicate entries are received, only the first complete entry received with valid, authoritative references will be credited. Please follow the style, punctuation, and format of this edition as much as possible.

## ▶ JOIN THE FIRST AID TEAM

The *First Aid*/ScholarRx team is pleased to offer paid editorial and coaching positions. We are looking for passionate, experienced, and dedicated medical students and recent graduates. Participants will have an opportunity to work on a wide variety of projects, including the popular *First Aid* series and the growing line of USMLE-Rx/ScholarRx products, including Rx Bricks. Please use our webform at https://www.usmle-rx.com/join-the-first-aid-team/ to apply, and include a CV and writing examples.

For 2024, we are actively seeking passionate medical students and graduates with a specific interest in improving our medical illustrations, expanding our database of photographs (including clinical images depicting diverse skin types), and developing the software that supports our crowdsourcing platform. We welcome people with prior experience and talent in these areas. Relevant skills include clinical imaging, digital photography, digital asset management, information design, medical illustration, graphic design, tutoring, and software development.

# How to Use This Book

**CONGRATULATIONS:** You now possess the book that has guided nearly two million students to USMLE success for over 30 years. With appropriate care, the binding should last the useful life of the book. Keep in mind that putting excessive flattening pressure on any binding will accelerate its failure. If you purchased a book that you believe is defective, please **immediately** return it to the place of purchase. If you encounter ongoing issues, you can also contact Customer Service at our publisher, McGraw Hill.

**START EARLY:** Use this book as early as possible while learning the basic medical sciences. The first semester of your first year is not too early! Devise a study plan by reading Section I: Guide to Efficient Exam Preparation, and make an early decision on resources to use by checking Section IV: Top-Rated Review Resources. Note that *First Aid* is neither a textbook nor a comprehensive review book, and it is not a panacea for inadequate preparation.

**CONSIDER *FIRST AID* YOUR ANNOTATION HUB:** Annotate this book with material from other resources, such as class notes or comprehensive textbooks. This will keep all the high-yield information you need in one place. Other tips on keeping yourself organized:

- For best results, use fine-tipped ballpoint pens (eg, BIC Pro+, Uni-Ball Jetstream Sports, Pilot Drawing Pen, Zebra F-301). If you like gel pens, try Pentel Slicci, and for markers that dry almost immediately, consider Staedtler Triplus Fineliner, Pilot Drawing Pen, and Sharpies.

- Consider using pens with different colors of ink to indicate different sources of information (eg, blue for USMLE-Rx Step 1 Qmax, green for UWorld Step 1 Qbank, red for Rx Bricks).

- Choose highlighters that are bright and dry quickly to minimize smudging and bleeding through the page (eg, Tombow Kei Coat, Sharpie Gel).

- Many students de-spine their book and get it 3-hole-punched. This will allow you to insert materials from other sources, including curricular materials.

**INTEGRATE STUDY WITH CASES, FLASH CARDS, AND QUESTIONS:** To broaden your learning strategy, consider integrating your *First Aid* study with case-based reviews (eg, *First Aid Cases for the USMLE Step 1*), flash cards (eg, USMLE-Rx Step 1 Flash Facts), and practice questions (eg, the USMLE-Rx Step 1 Qmax). Read the chapter in the book, then test your comprehension by using cases, flash cards, and questions that cover the same topics. Maintain access to more comprehensive resources (eg, ScholarRx Bricks and USMLE-Rx Step 1 Express videos) for deeper review as needed.

**PRIME YOUR MEMORY:** Return to your annotated Sections II and III several days before taking the USMLE Step 1. The book can serve as a useful way of retaining key associations and keeping high-yield facts fresh in your memory just prior to the exam. The Rapid Review section includes high-yield topics to help guide your studying.

**CONTRIBUTE TO FIRST AID:** Reviewing the book immediately after your exam can help us improve the next edition. Decide what was truly high and low yield and send us your comments. Feel free to send us scanned images from your annotated *First Aid* book as additional support. Of course, always remember that **all examinees are under agreement with the NBME to not disclose the specific details of copyrighted test material.**

# Selected USMLE Laboratory Values

\* = Included in the Biochemical Profile (SMA-12)

| Blood, Plasma, Serum | Reference Range | SI Reference Intervals |
|---|---|---|
| \*Alanine aminotransferase (ALT, GPT at 30°C) | 10–40 U/L | 10–40 U/L |
| \*Alkaline phosphatase | 25–100 U/L | 25–100 U/L |
| Amylase, serum | 25–125 U/L | 25–125 U/L |
| \*Aspartate aminotransferase (AST, GOT at 30°C) | 12–38 U/L | 12–38 U/L |
| Bilirubin, serum (adult) Total // Direct | 0.1–1.0 mg/dL  //  0.0–0.3 mg/dL | 2–17 μmol/L  //  0–5 μmol/L |
| \*Calcium, serum (Total) | 8.4–10.2 mg/dL | 2.1–2.6 mmol/L |
| \*Cholesterol, serum (Total) | Rec: < 200 mg/dL | < 5.2 mmol/L |
| \*Creatinine, serum (Total) | 0.6–1.2 mg/dL | 53–106 μmol/L |
| Electrolytes, serum Sodium ($Na^+$) | 136–146 mEq/L | 136–146 mmol/L |
| Chloride ($Cl^-$) | 95–105 mEq/L | 95–105 mmol/L |
| \* Potassium ($K^+$) | 3.5–5.0 mEq/L | 3.5–5.0 mmol/L |
| Bicarbonate ($HCO_3^-$) | 22–28 mEq/L | 22–28 mmol/L |
| Magnesium ($Mg^{2+}$) | 1.5–2 mEq/L | 0.75–1.0 mmol/L |
| Gases, arterial blood (room air) $P_{O_2}$ | 75–105 mm Hg | 10.0–14.0 kPa |
| $P_{CO_2}$ | 33–45 mm Hg | 4.4–5.9 kPa |
| pH | 7.35–7.45 | [$H^+$] 36–44 nmol/L |
| \*Glucose, serum | Fasting: 70–100 mg/dL | 3.8–6.1 mmol/L |
| Growth hormone – arginine stimulation | Fasting: < 5 ng/mL Provocative stimuli: > 7 ng/mL | < 5 μg/L > 7 μg/L |
| Osmolality, serum | 275–295 mOsmol/kg $H_2O$ | 275–295 mOsmol/kg $H_2O$ |
| \*Phosphorus (inorganic), serum | 3.0–4.5 mg/dL | 1.0–1.5 mmol/L |
| Prolactin, serum (hPRL) | Male: < 17 ng/mL Female: < 25 ng/mL | < 17 μg/L < 25 μg/L |
| \*Proteins, serum Total (recumbent) | 6.0–7.8 g/dL | 60–78 g/L |
| Albumin | 3.5–5.5 g/dL | 35–55 g/L |
| Globulins | 2.3–3.5 g/dL | 23–35 g/L |
| Thyroid-stimulating hormone, serum or plasma | 0.4–4.0 μU/mL | 0.4–4.0 mIU/L |
| \*Urea nitrogen, serum (BUN) | 7–18 mg/dL | 25–64 nmol/L |
| \*Uric acid, serum | 3.0–8.2 mg/dL | 0.18–0.48 mmol/L |

*(continues)*

| Cerebrospinal Fluid | Reference Range | SI Reference Intervals |
|---|---|---|
| Cell count | 0–5/mm³ | $0$–$5 \times 10^6$/L |
| Glucose | 40–70 mg/dL | 2.2–3.9 mmol/L |
| Proteins, total | < 40 mg/dL | < 0.40 g/L |
| **Hematologic** | | |
| Erythrocyte count | Male: 4.3–5.9 million/mm³ | $4.3$–$5.9 \times 10^{12}$/L |
| | Female: 3.5–5.5 million/mm³ | $3.5$–$5.5 \times 10^{12}$/L |
| Erythrocyte sedimentation rate (Westergen) | Male: 0–15 mm/hr | 0–15 mm/hr |
| | Female: 0–20 mm/hr | 0–20 mm/hr |
| Hematocrit | Male: 41–53% | 0.41–0.53 |
| | Female: 36–46% | 0.36–0.46 |
| Hemoglobin, blood | Male: 13.5–17.5 g/dL | 135–175 g/L |
| | Female: 12.0–16.0 g/dL | 120–160 g/L |
| Hemoglobin, plasma | < 4 mg/dL | < 0.62 μmol/L |
| Leukocyte count and differential | | |
|   Leukocyte count | 4,500–11,000/mm³ | $4.5$–$11.0 \times 10^9$/L |
|     Segmented neutrophils | 54–62% | 0.54–0.62 |
|     Band forms | 3–5% | 0.03–0.05 |
|     Eosinophils | 1–3% | 0.01–0.03 |
|     Basophils | 0–0.75% | 0–0.0075 |
|     Lymphocytes | 25–33% | 0.25–0.33 |
|     Monocytes | 3–7% | 0.03–0.07 |
| Mean corpuscular hemoglobin | 25–35 pg/cell | 0.39–0.54 fmol/cell |
| Mean corpuscular hemoglobin concentration | 31%–36% Hb/cell | 4.8–5.6 mmol Hb/L |
| Mean corpuscular volume | 80–100 μm³ | 80–100 fL |
| Partial thromboplastin time (activated) | 25–40 sec | 25–40 sec |
| Platelet count | 150,000–400,000/mm³ | $150$–$400 \times 10^9$/L |
| Prothrombin time | 11–15 sec | 11–15 sec |
| Reticulocyte count | 0.5–1.5% of RBCs | 0.005–0.015 |
| **Urine** | | |
| Creatinine clearance | Male: 97–137 mL/min | 97–137 mL/min |
| | Female: 88–128 mL/min | 88–128 mL/min |
| Osmolality | 50–1200 mOsmol/kg $H_2O$ | 50–1200 mOsmol/kg $H_2O$ |
| Proteins, total | < 150 mg/24 hr | < 0.15 g/24 hr |
| **Other** | | |
| Body mass index | Adult: 19–25 kg/m² | 19–25 kg/m² |

# First Aid Checklist for the USMLE Step 1

This is an example of how you might use the information in Section I to prepare for the USMLE Step 1. Refer to corresponding topics in Section I for more details.

**Years Prior**
- ☐ Use top-rated review resources for first-year medical school courses.
- ☐ Ask for advice from those who have recently taken the USMLE Step 1.

**Months Prior**
- ☐ Review computer test format and registration information.
- ☐ Register six months in advance.
- ☐ Carefully verify name and address printed on scheduling permit. Make sure the name on scheduling permit matches the name printed on your photo ID.
- ☐ Go online for test date ASAP.
- ☐ Set up a realistic timeline for study. Cover less crammable subjects first.
- ☐ Evaluate and choose study materials (review books, question banks).
- ☐ Use a question bank to simulate the USMLE Step 1 to pinpoint strengths and weaknesses in knowledge and test-taking skills from early on.

**Weeks Prior**
- ☐ Do test simulations in question banks.
- ☐ Assess how close you are to your goal.
- ☐ Pinpoint remaining weaknesses. Stay healthy (eg, exercise, sleep).
- ☐ Verify information on admission ticket (eg, location, date).

**One Week Prior**
- ☐ Remember comfort measures (eg, loose clothing, earplugs).
- ☐ Work out test site logistics (eg, location, transportation, parking, lunch).
- ☐ Print or download your Scheduling Permit and Scheduling Confirmation to your phone.

**One Day Prior**
- ☐ Relax.
- ☐ Lightly review short-term material if necessary. Skim high-yield facts.
- ☐ Get a good night's sleep.

**Day of Exam**
- ☐ Relax.
- ☐ Eat breakfast.
- ☐ Minimize bathroom breaks during exam by avoiding excessive morning caffeine.

**After Exam**
- ☐ Celebrate, regardless of how well you feel you did.
- ☐ Send feedback to us on our website at **www.firstaidteam.com** or at **firstaid@scholarrx.com**.

# Guide to Efficient Exam Preparation

"One important key to success is self-confidence. An important key to self-confidence is preparation."

—Arthur Ashe

"Wisdom is not a product of schooling but of the lifelong attempt to acquire it."

—Albert Einstein

"Finally, from so little sleeping and so much reading, his brain dried up and he went completely out of his mind."

—Miguel de Cervantes Saavedra, *Don Quixote*

"Sometimes the questions are complicated and the answers are simple."

—Dr. Seuss

"He who knows all the answers has not been asked all the questions."

—Confucius

"The expert in anything was once a beginner."

—Helen Hayes

"It always seems impossible until it's done."

—Nelson Mandela

## ▶ INTRODUCTION

Relax.

This section is intended to make your exam preparation easier, not harder. Our goal is to reduce your level of anxiety and help you make the most of your efforts by helping you understand more about the United States Medical Licensing Examination, Step 1 (USMLE Step 1). As a medical student, you are no doubt familiar with taking standardized examinations and quickly absorbing large amounts of material. When you first confront the USMLE Step 1, however, you may find it all too easy to become sidetracked from your goal of studying with maximal effectiveness. Common mistakes that students make when studying for Step 1 include the following:

- Starting to study (including *First Aid*) too late
- Starting to study intensely too early and burning out
- Starting to prepare for boards before creating a knowledge foundation
- Using inefficient or inappropriate study methods
- Buying the wrong resources or buying too many resources
- Buying only one publisher's review series for all subjects
- Not using practice examinations to maximum benefit
- Not understanding how scoring is performed or what the result means
- Not using review books along with your classes
- Not analyzing and improving your test-taking strategies
- Getting bogged down by reviewing difficult topics excessively
- Studying material that is rarely tested on the USMLE Step 1
- Failing to master certain high-yield subjects owing to overconfidence
- Using *First Aid* as your sole study resource
- Trying to prepare for it all alone

In this section, we offer advice to help you avoid these pitfalls and be more productive in your studies.

## ▶ USMLE STEP 1—THE BASICS

▶ *The test at a glance:*
- *8-hour exam*
- *Up to a total of 280 multiple choice items*
- *7 test blocks (60 min/block)*
- *Up to 40 test items per block*
- *45 minutes of break time, plus another 15 if you skip the tutorial*

The USMLE Step 1 is the first of three examinations that you would normally pass in order to become a licensed physician in the United States. The USMLE is a joint endeavor of the National Board of Medical Examiners (NBME) and the Federation of State Medical Boards (FSMB). The USMLE serves as the single examination system domestically and internationally for those seeking medical licensure in the United States.

The Step 1 exam includes test items that can be grouped by the organizational constructs outlined in Table 1 (in order of tested frequency). In late 2020, the USMLE increased the number of items assessing communication skills. While pharmacology is still tested, they are focusing on drug mechanisms rather than on pharmacotherapy. You will not be required to identify the specific medications indicated for a specific condition. Instead, you will be asked more about drug mechanisms and side effects.

**TABLE 1. Frequency of Various Constructs Tested on the USMLE Step 1.[1,*]**

| Competency | Range, % | System | Range, % |
|---|---|---|---|
| Medical knowledge: applying foundational science concepts | 60–70 | General principles | 12–16 |
| Patient care: diagnosis | 20–25 | Behavioral health & nervous systems/special senses | 9–13 |
| Communication and interpersonal skills | 6–9 | Respiratory & renal/urinary systems | 9–13 |
| Practice-based learning & improvement | 4–6 | Reproductive & endocrine systems | 9–13 |
| **Discipline** | **Range, %** | Blood & lymphoreticular/immune systems | 7–11 |
| Pathology | 44–52 | Multisystem processes & disorders | 6–10 |
| Physiology | 25–35 | Musculoskeletal, skin & subcutaneous tissue | 6–10 |
| Pharmacology | 15–22 | Cardiovascular system | 5–9 |
| Biochemistry & nutrition | 14–24 | Gastrointestinal system | 5–9 |
| Microbiology | 10–15 | Biostatistics & epidemiology/population health | 4–6 |
| Immunology | 6–11 | Social sciences: communication skills/ethics | 6–9 |
| Gross anatomy & embryology | 11–15 | | |
| Histology & cell biology | 8–13 | | |
| Behavioral sciences | 8–13 | | |
| Genetics | 5–9 | | |

*Percentages are subject to change at any time. www.usmle.org

## How Is the Computer-Based Test (CBT) Structured?

The CBT Step 1 exam consists of one "optional" tutorial/simulation block and seven "real" question blocks of up to 40 questions per block with no more than 280 questions in total, timed at 60 minutes per block. A short 11-question survey follows the last question block. The computer begins the survey with a prompt to proceed to the next block of questions.

Once an examinee finishes a particular question block on the CBT, he or she must click on a screen icon to continue to the next block. Examinees **cannot** go back and change their answers to questions from any previously completed block. However, changing answers is allowed **within** a block of questions as long as the block has not been ended and if time permits.

## What Is the CBT Like?

Given the unique environment of the CBT, it's important that you become familiar ahead of time with what your test-day conditions will be like. You can access a 15-minute tutorial and practice blocks at http://orientation. nbme.org/Launch/USMLE/STPF1. This tutorial interface is the same as the one you will use in the exam; learn it now and you can skip taking it during the exam, giving you up to 15 extra minutes of break time. You can gain experience with the CBT format by taking the 120 practice questions (3 blocks with 40 questions each) available online for free (https://www.usmle. org/prepare-your-exam) or by signing up for a practice session at a test center for a fee.

For security reasons, examinees are not allowed to bring any personal electronic equipment into the testing area. This includes both digital and analog watches, cell phones, tablets, and calculators. Examinees are also prohibited from carrying in their books, notes, pens/pencils, and scratch paper (laminated note boards and fine-tip dry erase pens will be provided for use within the testing area). Food and beverages are also prohibited in the testing area. The testing centers are monitored by audio and video surveillance equipment. However, most testing centers allot each examinee a small locker outside the testing area in which he or she can store snacks, beverages, and personal items.

Questions are typically presented in multiple choice format, with 4 or more possible answer options. There is a countdown timer on the lower left corner of the screen as well. There is also a button that allows the examinee to mark a question for review. If a given question happens to be longer than the screen, a scroll bar will appear on the right, allowing the examinee to see the rest of the question. Regardless of whether the examinee clicks on an answer choice or leaves it blank, he or she must click the "Next" button to advance to the next question.

▶ **Keyboard shortcuts:**
 ▪ *A, B, etc—letter choices*
 ▪ *Esc—exit pop-up Calculator and Notes windows*

The USMLE features a small number of media clips in the form of audio and/or video. There may even be a question with a multimedia heart sound simulation. In these questions, a digital image of a torso appears on the screen, and the examinee directs a digital stethoscope to various auscultation points to listen for heart and breath sounds. The USMLE orientation materials include several practice questions in these formats. During the exam tutorial, examinees are given an opportunity to ensure that both the audio headphones and the volume are functioning properly. If you are already familiar with the tutorial and planning on skipping it, first skip ahead to the section where you can test your headphones. After you are sure the headphones are working properly, proceed to the exam.

▶ *Heart sounds are tested via media questions. Make sure you know how different heart diseases sound on auscultation.*

▶ *Be sure to test your headphones during the tutorial.*

The examinee can call up a window displaying normal laboratory values. In order to do so, he or she must click the "Lab" icon on the top part of the screen. Afterward, the examinee will have the option to choose between "Blood," "Cerebrospinal," "Hematologic," or "Sweat and Urine." The normal values screen may obscure the question if it is expanded. The examinee may have to scroll down to search for the needed lab values. You might want to memorize some common lab values so you spend less time on questions that require you to analyze these.

▶ *Familiarize yourself with the commonly tested lab values (eg, Hb, WBC, $Ca^{2+}$, $Na^+$, $K^+$).*

The CBT interface provides a running list of questions on the left part of the screen at all times. The software also permits examinees to highlight or cross out information by using their mouse. There is a "Notes" icon on the top part of the screen that allows students to write notes to themselves for review at a later time. Finally, the USMLE has recently added new functionality including text magnification and reverse color (white text on black background). Being familiar with these features can save time and may help you better view and organize the information you need to answer a question.

▶ *Illustrations on the test include:*
 ▪ *Gross specimen photos*
 ▪ *Histology slides*
 ▪ *Medical imaging (eg, x-ray, CT, MRI)*
 ▪ *Electron micrographs*
 ▪ *Line drawings*

For those who feel they might benefit, the USMLE offers an opportunity to take a simulated test, or "CBT Practice Session" at a Prometric center. Students are eligible to register for this three-and-one-half-hour practice session after they have received their scheduling permit.

The same USMLE Step 1 sample test items (120 questions) available on the USMLE website are used at these sessions. **No new items will be presented.** The practice session is available at a cost of $75 ($155 if taken outside of the US and Canada) and is divided into a short tutorial and three 1-hour blocks of ~40 test items each. Students receive a printed percent-correct score after completing the session. **No explanations of questions are provided.**

▶ *You can take a shortened CBT practice test at a Prometric center.*

You may register for a practice session online at www.usmle.org. A separate scheduling permit is issued for the practice session. Students should allow two weeks for receipt of this permit.

## How Do I Register to Take the Exam?

Prometric test centers offer Step 1 on a year-round basis, except for the first two weeks in January and major holidays. Check with the test center you want to use before making your exam plans.

▶ *The Prometric website will display a calendar with open test dates.*

US students can apply to take Step 1 at the NBME website. This application allows you to select one of 12 overlapping three-month blocks in which to be tested (eg, April–May–June, June–July–August). Choose your three-month eligibility period wisely. If you need to reschedule outside your initial three-month period, you can request a one-time extension of eligibility for the next contiguous three-month period, and pay a rescheduling fee. The application also includes a photo ID form that must be certified by an official at your medical school to verify your enrollment. After the NBME processes your application, it will send you a scheduling permit.

The scheduling permit you receive from the NBME will contain your USMLE identification number, the eligibility period in which you may take the exam, and two additional numbers. The first of these is known as your "scheduling number." You must have this number in order to make your exam appointment with Prometric. The second number is known as the "candidate identification number," or CIN. Examinees must enter their CINs at the Prometric workstation in order to access their exams. However, you will not be allowed to bring your permit into the exam and will be asked to copy your CIN onto your scratch paper. Prometric has no access to the codes. **Make sure to bring a paper or electronic copy of your permit with you to the exam!** Also bring an unexpired, government-issued photo ID that includes your signature (such as a driver's license or passport). Make sure the name on your photo ID exactly matches the name that appears on your scheduling permit.

▶ *Be familiar with Prometric's policies for cancellation and rescheduling due to COVID-19.*

Once you receive your scheduling permit, you may access the Prometric website or call Prometric's toll-free number to arrange a time to take the exam. You may contact Prometric two weeks before the test date if you want to confirm identification requirements. Be aware that your exam may be canceled because of circumstances related to COVID-19 or other unforeseen events. If that were to happen, you should receive an email from Prometric containing notice of the cancellation and instructions on rescheduling.

Although requests for taking the exam may be completed more than six months before the test date, examinees will not receive their scheduling permits earlier than six months before the eligibility period. The eligibility period is the three-month period you have chosen to take the exam. Most US medical students attending a school which uses the two-year preclerkship curriculum choose the April–June or June–August period. Most US medical students attending a school which uses the 18-month preclerkship curriculum choose the December–February or January–March period.

> ▶ Test scheduling is done on a "first-come, first-served" basis. It's important to schedule an exam date as soon as you receive your scheduling permit.

### What If I Need to Reschedule the Exam?

You can change your test date and/or center by contacting Prometric at 1-800-MED-EXAM (1-800-633-3926) or www.prometric.com. Make sure to have your CIN when rescheduling. If you are rescheduling by phone, you must speak with a Prometric representative; leaving a voicemail message will not suffice. To avoid a rescheduling fee, you will need to request a change at least 31 calendar days before your appointment. Please note that your rescheduled test date must fall within your assigned three-month eligibility period.

### When Should I Register for the Exam?

> ▶ Register six months in advance for seating and scheduling preference.

You should plan to register as far in advance as possible ahead of your desired test date (eg, six months), but, depending on your particular test center, new dates and times may open closer to the date. Scheduling early will guarantee that you will get either your test center of choice or one within a 50-mile radius of your first choice. For most US medical students, the desired testing window correlates with the end of the preclerkship curriculum, which is around June for schools on a two-year preclerkship schedule, and around January for schools on an 18-month schedule. Thus US medical students should plan to register before January in anticipation of a June test date, or before August in anticipation of a January test date. The timing of the exam is more flexible for IMGs, as it is related only to when they finish exam preparation. Talk with upperclassmen who have already taken the test so you have real-life experience from students who went through a similar curriculum, then formulate your own strategy.

### Where Can I Take the Exam?

Your testing location is arranged with Prometric when you book your test date (after you receive your scheduling permit). For a list of Prometric locations nearest you, visit www.prometric.com.

### How Long Will I Have to Wait Before I Get My Result?

The USMLE reports results in three to four weeks, unless there are delays in processing. Examinees will be notified via email when their results are available. By following the online instructions, examinees will be able to view, download, and print their exam report online for ~120 days after notification, after which results can only be obtained through requesting an official USMLE transcript. Additional information about results reporting timetables and accessibility is available on the official USMLE website. Between 2021 and 2022, Step 1 pass rates dropped from 95% to 91% across US/Canadian schools and from 77% to 71% across non-US/Canadian schools (see Table 2), following the transition to pass/fail scoring in January 2022.

> ▶ Step 1 pass rates dropped significantly amongst both US/Canadian students and IMGs in 2022.

### What About Time?

Time is of special interest on the CBT exam. Here's a breakdown of the exam schedule:

| | |
|---|---|
| 15 minutes | Tutorial (skip if familiar with test format and features) |
| 7 hours | Seven 60-minute question blocks |
| 45 minutes | Break time (includes time for lunch) |

> ▶ Gain extra break time by skipping the tutorial, or utilize the tutorial time to add personal notes to your scratch paper.

The computer will keep track of how much time has elapsed on the exam. However, the computer will show you only how much time you have remaining in a given block. Therefore, it is up to you to determine if you are pacing yourself properly (at a rate of approximately one question per 90 seconds).

The computer does not warn you if you are spending more than your allotted time for a break. You should therefore budget your time so that you can take a short break when you need one and have time to eat. You must be especially careful not to spend too much time in between blocks (you should keep track of how much time elapses from the time you finish a block of questions to the time you start the next block). After you finish one question block, you'll need to click to proceed to the next block of questions. If you do not click within 30 seconds, you will automatically be entered into a break period.

Break time for the day is 45 minutes, but you are not required to use all of it, nor are you required to use any of it. You can gain extra break time (but not extra time for the question blocks) by skipping the tutorial or by finishing a block ahead of the allotted time. Any time remaining on the clock when you finish a block gets added to your remaining break time. Once a new question block has been started, you may not take a break until you have reached the end of that block. If you do so, this will be recorded as an "unauthorized break" and will be reported on your final exam report.

> ▶ Be careful to watch the clock on your break time.

Finally, be aware that it may take a few minutes of your break time to "check out" of the secure resting room and then "check in" again to resume testing, so plan accordingly. The "check-in" process may include fingerprints, pocket checks, and metal detector scanning. Some students recommend pocketless clothing on exam day to streamline the process.

### If I Freak Out and Leave, What Happens to My Exam?

Your scheduling permit shows a CIN that you will need to enter to start your exam. Entering the CIN is the same as breaking the seal on a test book, and you are considered to have started the exam when you do so. However, no result will be reported if you do not complete the exam. If you leave at any time after starting the test, or do not open every block of your test, your test will not be scored and will be reported as incomplete. Incomplete results count toward the maximum of four attempts for each Step exam. Although a pass or fail result is not posted for incomplete tests, examinees may still be offered an option to request that their scores be calculated and reported if they desire; unanswered questions will be scored as incorrect.

The exam ends when all question blocks have been completed or when their time has expired. As you leave the testing center, you will receive a printed test-completion notice to document your completion of the exam. To receive an official score, you must finish the entire exam.

### What Types of Questions Are Asked?

▶ *Nearly three fourths of Step 1 questions begin with a description of a patient.*

All questions on the exam are **one-best-answer multiple choice items.** Most questions consist of a clinical scenario or a direct question followed by a list of four or more options. You are required to select the single best answer among the options given. There are no "except," "not," or matching questions on the exam. A number of options may be partially correct, in which case you must select the option that best answers the question or completes the statement. Additionally, keep in mind that experimental questions may appear on the exam, which do not affect your exam result.

**TABLE 2. Passing Rates for the 2021-2022 USMLE Step 1.**[2]

| | 2021 | | 2022 | |
|---|---|---|---|---|
| | No. Tested | % Passing | No. Tested | % Passing |
| Allopathic 1st takers | 22,280 | 96% | 22,828 | 93% |
| Repeaters | 798 | 66% | 1,489 | 71% |
| Allopathic total | 23,078 | 95% | 24,317 | 91% |
| Osteopathic 1st takers | 5,309 | 94% | 4,659 | 89% |
| Repeaters | 56 | 75% | 63 | 67% |
| Osteopathic total | 5,365 | 94% | 4,722 | 89% |
| **Total US/Canadian** | **28,443** | **95%** | **29,039** | **91%** |
| IMG 1st takers | 16,952 | 82% | 22,030 | 74% |
| Repeaters | 2,258 | 45% | 2,926 | 45% |
| IMG total | 19,210 | 77% | 24,956 | 71% |
| **Total Step 1 examinees** | **47,653** | **87%** | **53,881** | **82%** |

**How Is the Test Scored?**

The USMLE transitioned to a pass/fail scoring system for Step 1 on January 26, 2022. Examinees now receive an electronic report that will display the outcome of either "Pass" or "Fail." Failing reports include a graphic depiction of the distance between the examinee's score and the minimum passing standard as well as content area feedback. Feedback for the content area shows the examinee's performance relative to examinees with a low pass (lower, same, or higher) and should be used to guide future study plans. Passing exam reports only displays the outcome of "Pass," along with a breakdown of topics covered on that individual examination (which will closely mirror the frequencies listed in Table 1). Note that a number of questions are experimental and are not counted toward or against the examinee's performance.

Examinees who took the test before the transition to pass/fail reporting received an electronic report that includes the examinee's pass/fail status, a three-digit test score, a bar chart comparing the examinee's performance in each content area with their overall Step 1 performance, and a graphic depiction of the examinee's performance by physician task, discipline, and organ system. Changes will not be made to transcripts containing three-digit test scores.

The USMLE does not report the minimum number of correct responses needed to pass, but estimates that it is approximately 60%. The USMLE may update exam result reporting in the future, so please check the USMLE website or www.firstaidteam.com for updates.

> ▶ Depending on the resource used, practice questions may be easier than the actual exam.

**Official NBME/USMLE Resources**

The NBME offers a Comprehensive Basic Science Examination (CBSE) for practice that is a shorter version of the Step 1. The CBSE contains four blocks of 50 questions each and covers material that is typically learned during the basic science years. CBSE scores represent the percent of content mastered and show an estimated probability of passing Step 1. Many schools use this test to gauge whether a student is expected to pass Step 1. If this test is offered by your school, it is usually conducted at the end of regular didactic time before any dedicated Step 1 preparation. If you do not encounter the CBSE before your dedicated study time, you need not worry about taking it. Use the information to help set realistic goals and timetables for your success.

The NBME also offers six forms of Comprehensive Basic Science Self-Assessment (CBSSA). Students who prepared for the exam using this web-based tool reported that they found the format and content highly indicative of questions tested on the actual exam. In addition, the CBSSA is a fair predictor of historical USMLE performance. The test interface, however, does not match the actual USMLE test interface, so practicing with these forms alone is not advised.

The CBSSA exists in two formats: standard-paced and self-paced, both of which consist of four sections of 50 questions each (for a total of 200 multiple choice items). The standard-paced format allows the user up to 75 minutes to complete each section, reflecting time limits similar to the actual exam. By contrast, the self-paced format places a 5-hour time limit on answering all multiple choice questions. Every few years, new forms are released and older ones are retired, reflecting changes in exam content. Therefore, the newer exams tend to be more similar to the actual Step 1, and scores from these exams tend to provide a better estimation of exam day performance.

Keep in mind that this bank of questions is available only on the web. The NBME requires that users start and complete the exam within 90 days of purchase. Once the assessment has begun, users are required to complete the sections within 20 days. Following completion of the questions, the CBSSA provides a performance profile indicating the user's relative strengths and weaknesses, much like the report profile for the USMLE Step 1 exam. In addition to the performance profile, examinees will be informed of the number of questions answered incorrectly. You will have the ability to review the text of all questions with detailed explanations. The NBME charges $60 for each assessment, payable by credit card or money order. For more information regarding the CBSE and the CBSSA, visit the NBME's website at www.nbme.org.

The NBME scoring system is weighted for each assessment exam. While some exams seem more difficult than others, the equated percent correct reported takes into account these inter-test differences. Also, while many students report seeing Step 1 questions "word-for-word" out of the assessments, the NBME makes special note that no live USMLE questions are shown on any NBME assessment.

Lastly, the International Foundations of Medicine (IFOM) offers a Basic Science Examination (BSE) practice exam at participating Prometric test centers for $200. Students may also take the self-assessment test online for $35 through the NBME's website. The IFOM BSE is intended to determine an examinee's relative areas of strength and weakness in general areas of basic science—not to predict performance on the USMLE Step 1 exam— and the content covered by the two examinations is somewhat different. However, because there is substantial overlap in content coverage and many IFOM items were previously used on the USMLE Step 1, it is possible to roughly project IFOM performance onto the historical USMLE Step 1 score scale. More information is available at http://www.nbme.org/ifom/.

## ▶ LEARNING STRATEGIES

Many students feel overwhelmed during the preclinical years and struggle to find an effective learning strategy. Table 3 lists several learning strategies you can try and their estimated effectiveness for Step 1 preparation based on the literature (see References). These are merely suggestions, and it's important to take your learning preferences into account. Your comprehensive learning approach will contain a combination of strategies (eg, elaborative interrogation followed by practice testing, mnemonics review using spaced repetition, etc). Regardless of your choice, the foundation of knowledge you build during your basic science years is the most important resource for success on the USMLE Step 1.

## HIGH EFFICACY

### Practice Testing

Also called "retrieval practice," practice testing has both direct and indirect benefits to the learner.[4] Effortful retrieval of answers does not only identify weak spots—it directly strengthens long-term retention of material.[5] The more effortful the recall, the better the long-term retention. This advantage has been shown to result in higher test scores and GPAs.[6] In fact, research has shown a positive correlation between the number of boards-style practice questions completed and Step 1 performance among medical students.[7]

Practice testing should be done with "interleaving" (mixing of questions from different topics in a single session). Question banks often allow you to intermingle topics. Interleaved practice helps learners develop their ability to

▶ The foundation of knowledge you build during your basic science years is the most important resource for success on the USMLE Step 1.

▶ Research has shown a positive correlation between the number of boards-style practice questions completed and Step 1 performance among medical students.

**TABLE 3. Effective Learning Strategies.**

| Efficacy | Strategy | Example Resources |
|---|---|---|
| *High efficacy* | Practice testing (retrieval practice) | UWorld Qbank<br>NBME Self-Assessments<br>USMLE-Rx QMax<br>Amboss Qbank |
| | Distributed practice | USMLE-Rx Flash Facts<br>Anki<br>Firecracker<br>Memorang<br>Osmosis |
| *Moderate efficacy* | Mnemonics | *Pre-made:*<br>SketchyMedical<br>Picmonic<br>*Self-made:*<br>Mullen Memory |
| | Elaborative interrogation/ self-explanation | |
| | Concept mapping | Coggle<br>FreeMind<br>XMind<br>MindNode |
| *Low efficacy* | Rereading | |
| | Highlighting/underlining | |
| | Summarization | |

focus on the relevant concept when faced with many possibilities. Practicing topics in massed fashion (eg, all cardiology, then all dermatology) may seem intuitive, but there is strong evidence that interleaving correlates with longer-term retention and increased student achievement, especially on tasks that involve problem solving.[5]

In addition to using question banks, you can test yourself by arranging your notes in a question-answer format (eg, via flash cards). Testing these Q&As in random order allows you to reap the benefit of interleaved practice. Bear in mind that the utility of practice testing comes from the practice of information retrieval, so simply reading through Q&As will attenuate this benefit.

### Distributed Practice

Also called "spaced repetition," distributed practice is the opposite of massed practice or "cramming." Learners review material at increasingly spaced out intervals (days to weeks to months). Massed learning may produce more short-term gains and satisfaction, but learners who use distributed practice have better mastery and retention over the long term.[5,9]

Flash cards are a simple way to incorporate both distributed practice and practice testing. Studies have linked spaced repetition learning with flash cards to improved long-term knowledge retention and higher exam scores.[6,8,10] Apps with automated spaced-repetition software (SRS) for flash cards exist for smartphones and tablets, so the cards are accessible anywhere. Proceed with caution: there is an art to making and reviewing cards. The ease of quickly downloading or creating digital cards can lead to flash card overload (it is unsustainable to make 50 flash cards per lecture!). Even at a modest pace, the thousands upon thousands of cards are too overwhelming for Step 1 preparation. Unless you have specific high-yield cards (and have checked the content with high-yield resources), stick to pre-made cards by reputable sources that curate the vast amount of knowledge for you.

If you prefer pen and paper, consider using a planner or spreadsheet to organize your study material over time. Distributed practice allows for some forgetting of information, and the added effort of recall over time strengthens the learning.

### MODERATE EFFICACY

### Mnemonics

A "mnemonic" refers to any device that assists memory, such as acronyms, mental imagery (eg, keywords with or without memory palaces), etc. Keyword mnemonics have been shown to produce superior knowledge retention when compared with rote memorization in many scenarios. However, they are generally more effective when applied to memorization-heavy, keyword-friendly topics and may not be broadly suitable.[5] Keyword mnemonics may not produce long-term retention, so consider combining mnemonics with distributed, retrieval-based practice (eg, via flash cards with SRS).

▶ *Studies have linked spaced repetition learning with flash cards to improved long-term knowledge retention and higher exam scores.*

Self-made mnemonics may have an advantage when material is simple and keyword friendly. If you can create your own mnemonic that accurately represents the material, this will be more memorable. When topics are complex and accurate mnemonics are challenging to create, pre-made mnemonics may be more effective, especially if you are inexperienced at creating mnemonics.[11]

### Elaborative Interrogation/Self-Explanation

Elaborative interrogation ("why" questions) and self-explanation (general questioning) prompt learners to generate explanations for facts. When reading passages of discrete facts, consider using these techniques, which have been shown to be more effective than rereading (eg, improved recall and better problem-solving/diagnostic performance).[5,12,13]

> ▶ Elaborative interrogation and self-explanation prompt learners to generate explanations for facts, which improves recall and problem solving.

### Concept Mapping

Concept mapping is a method for graphically organizing knowledge, with concepts enclosed in boxes and lines drawn between related concepts. Creating or studying concept maps may be more effective than other activities (eg, writing or reading summaries/outlines). However, studies have reached mixed conclusions about its utility, and the small size of this effect raises doubts about its authenticity and pedagogic significance.[14]

## LOW EFFICACY

### Rereading

While the most commonly used method among surveyed students, rereading has not been shown to correlate with grade point average.[9] Due to its popularity, rereading is often a comparator in studies on learning. Other strategies that we have discussed (eg, practice testing) have been shown to be significantly more effective than rereading.

### Highlighting/Underlining

Because this method is passive, it tends to be of minimal value for learning and recall. In fact, lower-performing students are more likely to use these techniques.[9] Students who highlight and underline do not learn how to actively recall learned information and thus find it difficult to apply knowledge to exam questions.

### Summarization

While more useful for improving performance on generative measures (eg, free recall or essays), summarization is less useful for exams that depend on recognition (eg, multiple choice). Findings on the overall efficacy of this method have been mixed.[5]

## ▶ TIMELINE FOR STUDY

### Before Starting

Your preparation for the USMLE Step 1 should begin when you enter medical school. Organize and commit to studying from the beginning so that when the time comes to prepare for the USMLE, you will be ready with a strong foundation.

### Make a Schedule

▶ *Customize your schedule. Tackle your weakest section first.*

After you have defined your goals, map out a study schedule that is consistent with your objectives, your vacation time, the difficulty of your ongoing coursework, and your family and social commitments. Determine whether you want to spread out your study time or concentrate it into 10-hour study days in the final weeks. Then factor in your own history in preparing for standardized examinations (eg, SAT, MCAT). Talk to students at your school who have recently taken Step 1. Ask them for their study schedules, especially those who have study habits and goals similar to yours. Sample schedules can be found at https://firstaidteam.com/schedules/.

Typically, US medical schools allot between four and eight weeks for dedicated Step 1 preparation. The time you dedicate to exam preparation will depend on your confidence in comfortably achieving a passing score as well as your success in preparing yourself during the first two years of medical school. Some students reserve about a week at the end of their study period for final review; others save just a few days. When you have scheduled your exam date, do your best to adhere to it.

Make your schedule realistic, and set achievable goals. Many students make the mistake of studying at a level of detail that requires too much time for a comprehensive review—reading *Gray's Anatomy* in a couple of days is not a realistic goal! Have one catch-up day per week of studying. No matter how well you stick to your schedule, unexpected events happen. But don't let yourself procrastinate because you have catch-up days; stick to your schedule as closely as possible and revise it regularly on the basis of your actual progress. Be careful not to lose focus. Beware of feelings of inadequacy when comparing study schedules and progress with your peers. **Avoid others who stress you out.** Focus on a few top-rated resources that suit your learning style—not on some obscure resource your friends may pass down to you. Accept the fact that you cannot learn it all.

▶ *Avoid burnout. Maintain proper diet, exercise, and sleep habits.*

You will need time for uninterrupted and focused study. Plan your personal affairs to minimize crisis situations near the date of the test. Allot an adequate number of breaks in your study schedule to avoid burnout. Maintain a healthy lifestyle with proper diet, exercise, and sleep.

Another important aspect of your preparation is your studying environment. **Study where you have always been comfortable studying.** Be sure to include everything you need close by (review books, notes, coffee, snacks, etc). If you're the kind of person who cannot study alone, form a study group with other students taking the exam. The main point here is to create a comfortable environment with minimal distractions.

### Year(s) Prior

The knowledge you gained during your first two years of medical school and even during your undergraduate years should provide the groundwork on which to base your test preparation. Student scores on NBME subject tests (commonly known as "shelf exams") have been shown to be highly correlated with subsequent Step 1 performance.[15] Moreover, undergraduate science GPAs as well as MCAT scores are strong predictors of performance on the Step 1 exam.[16]

We also recommend that you buy highly rated review books early in your first year of medical school and use them as you study throughout the two years. When Step 1 comes along, these books will be familiar and personalized to the way in which you learn. It is risky and intimidating to use unfamiliar review books in the final two or three weeks preceding the exam. Some students find it helpful to personalize and annotate *First Aid* throughout the curriculum.

▶ *Buy review resources early (first year) and use while studying for courses.*

### Months Prior

Review test dates and the application procedure. Testing for the USMLE Step 1 is done on a year-round basis. If you have disabilities or special circumstances, contact the NBME as early as possible to discuss test accommodations (see the Section I Supplement at www.firstaidteam.com/bonus).

Use this time to finalize your ideal schedule. Consider upcoming breaks and whether you want to relax or study. Work backward from your test date to make sure you finish at least one question bank. Also add time to redo missed or flagged questions (which may be half the bank). This is the time to build a structured plan with enough flexibility for the realities of life.

▶ *Simulate the USMLE Step 1 under "real" conditions before beginning your studies.*

Begin doing blocks of questions from reputable question banks under "real" conditions. Don't use tutor mode until you're sure you can finish blocks in the allotted time. It is important to continue balancing success in your normal studies with the Step 1 test preparation process.

### Weeks Prior (Dedicated Preparation)

Your dedicated prep time may be one week or two months. You should have a working plan as you go into this period. Finish your schoolwork strong, take a day off, and then get to work. Start by simulating a full-length USMLE Step 1 if you haven't yet done so. Consider doing one NBME CBSSA and the free questions from the NBME website. Alternatively, you could choose 7 blocks of randomized questions from a commercial question bank. Make sure you get feedback on your strengths and weaknesses and adjust your studying accordingly. Many students study from review sources or comprehensive

> ▶ In the final two weeks, focus on review, practice questions, and endurance. Stay confident!

> ▶ One week before the test:
>   ▪ Sleep according to the same schedule you'll use on test day
>   ▪ Review the CBT tutorial one last time
>   ▪ Call Prometric to confirm test date and time

> ▶ No notes, books, calculators, pagers, cell phones, recording devices, or watches of any kind are allowed in the testing area, but they are allowed in lockers and may be accessed during authorized breaks.

programs for part of the day, then do question blocks. Also, keep in mind that reviewing a question block can take upward of two hours. Feedback from CBSSA exams and question banks will help you focus on your weaknesses.

## One Week Prior

Make sure you have your CIN (found on your scheduling permit) as well as other items necessary for the day of the examination, including a current driver's license or another form of photo ID with your signature (make sure the name on your **ID exactly** matches that on your scheduling permit). Confirm the Prometric testing center location and test time. Work out how you will get to the testing center and what parking, traffic, and public transportation problems you might encounter. Exchange cell phone numbers with other students taking the test on the same day in case of emergencies. Check www.prometric.com/closures for test site closures due to unforeseen events. Determine what you will do for lunch. Make sure you have everything you need to ensure that you will be comfortable and alert at the test site. It may be beneficial to adjust your schedule to start waking up at the same time that you will on your test day. And of course, make sure to maintain a healthy lifestyle and get enough sleep.

## One Day Prior

Try your best to relax and rest the night before the test. Double-check your admissions and test-taking materials as well as the comfort measures discussed earlier so that you will not have to deal with such details on the morning of the exam. At this point it will be more effective to review short-term memory material that you're already familiar with than to try to learn new material. The Rapid Review section at the end of this book is high yield for last-minute studying. Remember that regardless of how hard you have studied, you cannot (and need not!) know everything. There will be things on the exam that you have never even seen before, so do not panic. Do not underestimate your abilities.

Many students report difficulty sleeping the night prior to the exam. This is often exacerbated by going to bed much earlier than usual. Do whatever it takes to ensure a good night's sleep (eg, massage, exercise, warm milk, no screens at night). Do not change your daily routine prior to the exam. Exam day is not the day for a caffeine-withdrawal headache.

## Morning of the Exam

On the morning of the Step 1 exam, wake up at your regular time and eat a normal breakfast. If you think it will help you, have a close friend or family member check to make sure you get out of bed. Make sure you have your scheduling permit admission ticket, test-taking materials, and comfort measures as discussed earlier. Wear loose, comfortable clothing. Limiting the number of pockets in your outfit may save time during security screening. Plan for a variable temperature in the testing center. Arrive at the test site 30 minutes before the time designated on the admission ticket; however, do not come too early, as doing so may intensify your anxiety. When you arrive at the test site, the proctor should give you a USMLE information sheet that will explain critical factors such as the proper use of break time. Seating may be assigned, but ask to be reseated if necessary; you need to be seated in an area that will allow you to remain comfortable and to concentrate. Get to know your testing station, especially if you have never been in a Prometric testing center before. Listen to your proctors regarding any changes in instructions or testing procedures that may apply to your test site.

If you are experiencing symptoms of illness on the day of your exam, we strongly recommend you reschedule. If you become ill or show signs of illness (eg, persistent cough) during the exam, the test center may prohibit you from completing the exam due to health and safety risks for test center staff and other examinees.

Finally, remember that it is natural (and even beneficial) to be a little nervous. Focus on being mentally clear and alert. Avoid panic. When you are asked to begin the exam, take a deep breath, focus on the screen, and then begin. Keep an eye on the timer. Take advantage of breaks between blocks to stretch, maybe do some jumping jacks, and relax for a moment with deep breathing or stretching.

> ▶ Arrive at the testing center 30 minutes before your scheduled exam time. If you arrive more than half an hour late, you will not be allowed to take the test.

### After the Test

After you have completed the exam, be sure to have fun and relax regardless of how you may feel. Taking the test is an achievement in itself. Remember, you are much more likely to have passed than not. Enjoy the free time you have before your clerkships. Expect to experience some "reentry" phenomena as you try to regain a real life. Once you have recovered sufficiently from the test (or from partying), we invite you to send us your feedback, corrections, and suggestions for entries, facts, mnemonics, strategies, resource ratings, and the like (see p. xvii, How to Contribute). Sharing your experience will benefit fellow medical students.

## ▶ STUDY MATERIALS

### Quality Considerations

Although an ever-increasing number of review books and software are now available on the market, the quality of such material is highly variable. Some common problems are as follows:

- Certain review books are too detailed to allow for review in a reasonable amount of time or cover subtopics that are not emphasized on the exam.
- Many sample question books were originally written years ago and have not been adequately updated to reflect recent trends.
- Some question banks test to a level of detail that you will not find on the exam.

## Review Books

▶ *If a given review book is not working for you, stop using it no matter how highly rated it may be or how much it costs.*

In selecting review books, be sure to weigh different opinions against each other, read the reviews and ratings in Section IV of this guide, examine the books closely in the bookstore, and choose carefully. You are investing not only money but also your limited study time. Do not worry about finding the "perfect" book, as many subjects simply do not have one, and different students prefer different formats. Supplement your chosen books with personal notes from other sources, including what you learn from question banks.

▶ *Charts and diagrams may be the best approach for physiology and biochemistry, whereas tables and outlines may be preferable for microbiology.*

There are two types of review books: those that are stand-alone titles and those that are part of a series. Books in a series generally have the same style, and you must decide if that style works for you. However, a given style is not optimal for every subject.

You should also find out which books are up to date. Some recent editions reflect major improvements, whereas others contain only cursory changes. Take into consideration how a book reflects the format of the USMLE Step 1.

## Apps

With the explosion of smartphones and tablets, apps are an increasingly popular way to review for the Step 1 exam. The majority of apps are compatible with both iOS and Android. Many popular Step 1 review resources (eg, UWorld, USMLE-Rx) have apps that are compatible with their software. Many popular web references (eg, UpToDate) also now offer app versions. All of these apps offer flexibility, allowing you to study while away from a computer (eg, while traveling).

## Practice Tests

▶ *Most practice exams are shorter and less clinical than the real thing.*

Taking practice tests provides valuable information about potential strengths and weaknesses in your fund of knowledge and test-taking skills. Some students use practice examinations simply as a means of breaking up the monotony of studying and adding variety to their study schedule, whereas other students rely almost solely on practice. You should also subscribe to one or more high-quality question banks.

Additionally, some students preparing for the Step 1 exam have started to incorporate case-based books intended primarily for clinical students on the wards or studying for the Step 2 CK exam. *First Aid Cases for the USMLE Step 1* aims to directly address this need.

▶ *Use practice tests to identify concepts and areas of weakness, not just facts that you missed.*

After taking a practice test, spend time on each question and each answer choice whether you were right or wrong. There are important teaching points in each explanation. Knowing why a wrong answer choice is incorrect is just as important as knowing why the right answer is correct. Do not panic if your practice scores are low as many questions try to trick or distract you to highlight a certain point. Use the questions you missed or were unsure about to develop focused plans during your scheduled catch-up time.

**Textbooks and Course Syllabi**

Limit your use of textbooks and course syllabi for Step 1 review. Many textbooks are too detailed for high-yield review and include material that is generally not tested on the USMLE Step 1 (eg, drug dosages, complex chemical structures). Syllabi, although familiar, are inconsistent across medical schools and frequently reflect the emphasis of individual faculty, which often does not correspond to that of the USMLE Step 1. Syllabi also tend to be less organized than top-rated books and generally contain fewer diagrams and study questions.

**Integration of AI in Medical Education: Transforming USMLE Preparation**

The integration of AI into education signals a paradigm shift in the acquisition and application of medical knowledge. AI's increasing ability to process extensive data sets and adapt to various learning styles makes it an attractive tool in medical training and practice.[17] Studies have demonstrated that AI language models are capable of achieving high accuracy rates when answering USMLE-style questions, underscoring its potential in supporting medical education.[18]

Although undeniably powerful, effectively utilizing AI as a study tool requires both practice and individual trial and error. We suggest the following approaches and prompts that might help learners more effectively harness AI for exam preparation:

*Tailored Mnemonic Creation:* Devise unique mnemonics to aid in memorizing complex medical terms efficiently. AI models can be highly creative in generating new ones, although feedback and iteration will likely be needed to produce mnemonics that are both accurate and memorable.

Example prompt: Create a food-related mnemonic for remembering adverse effects 1, 2, and 3 of Drug A.

*Custom Summarization of Medical Texts:* Efficiently condense extensive medical literature into concise summaries, facilitating efficient and rapid topic reviews.

Example prompt: Summarize this medical school lecture into bullet points. Decrease length by 80%.

*AI-Generated Custom Quizzes:* Create focused practice questions.

Example Prompt: Create three vignette-style multiple choice questions testing presentations of lysosomal storage disorders.

*Clinical Case Simulations:* Utilize AI-powered simulations of realistic clinical scenarios to practice decision-making skills and application of medical knowledge.

Example prompt: Create an exercise to practice analyzing acid-base disorders requiring Winter's formula with step-by-step explanations.

*Personalized Learning Schedules:* Create customized study schedules, adjusting time allocation based on challenging subjects. Modify schedules daily based on progress.

Example prompt: Prepare a schedule to review this book over 4 weeks.

Though both exciting and promising, pitfalls of using AI models for studying include the potential for outdated information or reliance on data that are not validated, resulting in a potential source of misinformation. AI can become unintentionally trained with human biases, and thus produce results that further reinforce or perpetuate potentially harmful biases. When using AI for personal studying, always validate information and maintain a critical eye when creating prompts.

AI is clearly a rapidly evolving study tool, however, how it can be best integrated with proven study methods remains to be seen. For the most recent updates on effectively leveraging AI in medical education, we encourage you to explore our blog at firstaidteam.com and scan a variety of student-centered discussion forums.

## ▶ TEST-TAKING STRATEGIES

▶ *Practice! Develop your test-taking skills and strategies well before the test date.*

Your test performance will be influenced by both your knowledge and your test-taking skills. You can strengthen your performance by considering each of these factors. Test-taking skills and strategies should be developed and perfected well in advance of the test date so that you can concentrate on the test itself. We suggest that you try the following strategies to see if they might work for you.

### Pacing

▶ *Time management is an important skill for exam success.*

You have seven hours to complete up to 280 questions. Note that each one-hour block contains up to 40 questions. This works out to approximately 90 seconds per question. We recommend following the "1 minute rule" to pace yourself. Spend no more than 1 minute on each question. If you are still unsure about the answer after this time, mark the question, make an educated guess, and move on. Following this rule, you should have approximately 20 minutes left after all questions are answered, which you can use to revisit all of your marked questions. Remember that some questions may be experimental and do not count for points (and reassure yourself that these experimental questions are the ones that are stumping you). In the past, pacing errors have been detrimental to the performance of even highly prepared examinees. The bottom line is to keep one eye on the clock at all times!

## Dealing with Each Question

There are several established techniques for efficiently approaching multiple choice questions; find what works for you. One technique begins with identifying each question as easy, workable, or impossible. Your goal should be to answer all easy questions, resolve all workable questions in a reasonable amount of time, and make quick and intelligent guesses on all impossible questions. Most students read the stem, think of the answer, and turn immediately to the choices. A second technique is to first skim the answer choices to get a context, then read the last sentence of the question (the lead-in), and then read through the passage quickly, extracting only information relevant to answering the question. This can be particularly helpful for questions with long clinical vignettes. Try a variety of techniques on practice exams and see what works best for you. If you get overwhelmed, remember that a 30-second time out to refocus may get you back on track.

## Guessing

There is **no penalty** for wrong answers. Thus **no test block should be left with unanswered questions.** If you don't know the answer, first eliminate incorrect choices, then guess among the remaining options. **Note that dozens of questions are unscored experimental questions** meant to obtain statistics for future exams. Therefore, some questions may seem unusual or unreasonably difficult simply because they are part of the development process for future exams.

## Changing Your Answer

The conventional wisdom is not to second-guess your initial answers. However, studies have consistently shown that test takers are more likely to change from a wrong answer to the correct answer than the other way around. Many question banks tell you how many questions you changed from right to wrong, wrong to wrong, and wrong to right. Use this feedback to judge how good a second-guesser you are. If you have extra time, reread the question stem and make sure you didn't misinterpret the question.

> ▶ Go with your first hunch, unless you are certain that you are a good second-guesser.

## ▶ CLINICAL VIGNETTE STRATEGIES

In recent years, the USMLE Step 1 has become increasingly clinically oriented. This change mirrors the trend in medical education toward introducing students to clinical problem solving during the basic science years. The increasing clinical emphasis on Step 1 may be challenging to those students who attend schools with a more traditional curriculum.

> ▶ Be prepared to read fast and think on your feet!

### What Is a Clinical Vignette?

A clinical vignette is a short (usually paragraph-long) description of a patient, including demographics, presenting symptoms, signs, and other information concerning the patient. Sometimes this paragraph is followed by a brief listing of important physical findings and/or laboratory results. The task of assimilating all this information and answering the associated question in the span of one minute can be intimidating. So be prepared to read quickly and think on your feet. Remember that the question is often indirectly asking something you already know.

A pseudovignette is a question that includes a description of a case similar to that of a clinical vignette, but it ends with a declarative recall question; thus the material presented in the pseudovignette is not necessary to answer the question. Question writers strive to avoid pseudovignettes on the USMLE Step 1. Be prepared to tackle each vignette as if the information presented is important to answer the associated question correctly.

### Strategy

Remember that Step 1 vignettes usually describe diseases or disorders in their most classic presentation. So look for cardinal signs (eg, malar rash for lupus or nuchal rigidity for meningitis) in the narrative history. Be aware that the question will contain classic signs and symptoms instead of buzzwords. Sometimes the data from labs and the physical exam will help you confirm or reject possible diagnoses, thereby helping you rule answer choices in or out. In some cases, they will be a dead giveaway for the diagnosis.

Making a diagnosis from the history and data is often not the final answer. Not infrequently, the diagnosis is divulged at the end of the vignette, after you have just struggled through the narrative to come up with a diagnosis of your own. The question might then ask about a related aspect of the diagnosed disease. Consider skimming the answer choices and lead-in before diving into a long stem. However, be careful with skimming the answer choices; going too fast may warp your perception of what the vignette is asking.

> ▶ Practice questions that include case histories or descriptive vignettes are critical for Step 1 preparation.

> ▶ Step 1 vignettes usually describe diseases or disorders in their most classic presentation.

## ▶ IF YOU THINK YOU FAILED

After taking the test, it is normal for many examinees to feel unsure about their performance, despite the majority of them achieving a passing score. Historical pass data are in Table 2. If you remain quite concerned, it may be wise to prepare a course of action should you need to retest. There are several sensible steps you can take to plan for the future in the event that you do not achieve a passing score. First, save and organize all your study materials, including review books, practice tests, and notes. Familiarize yourself with the reapplication procedures for Step 1, including application deadlines and upcoming test dates.

Make sure you know both your school's and the NBME's policies regarding retakes. The total number of attempts an examinee may take per Step examination is four.[18] You may take Step 1 no more than three times within a 12-month period. Your fourth attempt must be at least 12 months after your first attempt at that exam, and at least 6 months after your most recent attempt at that exam.

If you failed, the performance profiles in your score report provide valuable feedback concerning your relative strengths and weaknesses. Study these profiles closely. Set up a study timeline to strengthen gaps in your knowledge as well as to maintain and improve what you already know. Do not neglect high-yield subjects. It is normal to feel somewhat anxious about retaking the test, but if anxiety becomes a problem, seek appropriate counseling.

▶ *If you pass Step 1, you are not allowed to retake the exam.*

## ▶ TESTING AGENCIES

▪ **National Board of Medical Examiners (NBME) / USMLE Secretariat**
Department of Licensing Examination Services
3750 Market Street
Philadelphia, PA 19104-3102
(215) 590-9500 (operator) or
(215) 590-9700 (automated information line)
Email: webmail@nbme.org
www.nbme.org

▪ **Educational Commission for Foreign Medical Graduates (ECFMG)**
3624 Market Street
Philadelphia, PA 19104-2685
(215) 386-5900
Email: info@ecfmg.org
www.ecfmg.org

## ▶ REFERENCES

1. United States Medical Licensing Examination. Available from: https://www.usmle.org/prepare-your-exam/step-1-materials/step-1-content-outline-and-specifications. Accessed January 2024.
2. United States Medical Licensing Examination. Performance Data. Available from: https://www.usmle.org/performance-data. Accessed January 2024.
3. Prober CG, Kolars JC, First LR, et al. A plea to reassess the role of United States Medical Licensing Examination Step 1 scores in residency selection. *Acad Med.* 2016;91(1):12–15.
4. Roediger HL, Butler AC. The critical role of retrieval practice in long-term retention. *Trends Cogn Sci.* 2011;15(1):20–27.
5. Dunlosky J, Rawson KA, Marsh EJ, et al. Improving students' learning with effective learning techniques: promising directions from cognitive and educational psychology. *Psychol Sci Publ Int.* 2013;14(1):4–58.

6. Larsen DP, Butler AC, Lawson AL, et al. The importance of seeing the patient: test-enhanced learning with standardized patients and written tests improves clinical application of knowledge. *Adv Health Sci Educ.* 2013;18(3):409–425.

7. Panus PC, Stewart DW, Hagemeier NE, et al. A subgroup analysis of the impact of self-testing frequency on examination scores in a pathophysiology course. *Am J Pharm Educ.* 2014;78(9):165.

8. Deng F, Gluckstein JA, Larsen DP. Student-directed retrieval practice is a predictor of medical licensing examination performance. *Perspect Med Educ.* 2015;4(6):308–313.

9. McAndrew M, Morrow CS, Atiyeh L, et al. Dental student study strategies: are self-testing and scheduling related to academic performance? *J Dent Educ.* 2016;80(5):542–552.

10. Augustin M. How to learn effectively in medical school: test yourself, learn actively, and repeat in intervals. *Yale J Biol Med.* 2014;87(2):207–212.

11. Bellezza FS. Mnemonic devices: classification, characteristics, and criteria. *Rev Educ Res.* 1981;51(2):247–275.

12. Dyer J-O, Hudon A, Montpetit-Tourangeau K, et al. Example-based learning: comparing the effects of additionally providing three different integrative learning activities on physiotherapy intervention knowledge. *BMC Med Educ.* 2015;15:37.

13. Chamberland M, Mamede S, St-Onge C, et al. Self-explanation in learning clinical reasoning: the added value of examples and prompts. *Med Educ.* 2015;49(2):193–202.

14. Nesbit JC, Adesope OO. Learning with concept and knowledge maps: a meta-analysis. *Rev Educ Res.* 2006;76(3):413–448.

15. Holtman MC, Swanson DB, Ripkey DR, et al. Using basic science subject tests to identify students at risk for failing Step 1. *Acad Med.* 2001;76(10):S48–S51.

16. Basco WT, Way DP, Gilbert GE, et al. Undergraduate institutional MCAT scores as predictors of USMLE Step 1 performance. *Acad Med.* 2002;77(10):S13–S16.

17. Patino GA, Amiel JM, Brown M, et al. The promise and perils of artificial intelligence in health professions education practice and scholarship. *Acad Med.* 2024. doi: 10.1097/ACM.0000000000005636.

18. Kung TH, Cheatham M, Medenilla A, et al. Performance of ChatGPT on USMLE: potential for AI-assisted medical education using large language models. *PLOS Dig Health.* 2023. doi: 10.1371/journal.pdig.0000198.

19. United States Medical Licensing Examination. Number of attempts and time limits. Available from: https://www.usmle.org/bulletin-information/eligibility. Accessed January 2024.

# Special Situations

Please visit **www.firstaidteam.com/bonus/** to view this section.

▶ First Aid for the International Medical Graduate

▶ First Aid for the Osteopathic Medical Student

▶ First Aid for the Podiatric Medical Student

▶ First Aid for the Student Requiring Test Accommodations

▶ NOTES

# SECTION II

# High-Yield
# General Principles

*"I've learned that I still have a lot to learn."*

—Maya Angelou

*"Never regard study as a duty, but as the enviable opportunity to learn."*

—Albert Einstein

*"Live as if you were to die tomorrow. Learn as if you were to live forever."*

—Gandhi

*"Success is the maximum utilization of the ability that you have."*

—Zig Ziglar

*"I didn't want to just know names of things. I remember really wanting to know how it all worked."*

—Elizabeth Blackburn

*"If you do not have time to do it right, how are you going to have time to do it again?"*

—Diana Downs

### ▶ HOW TO USE THE DATABASE

The 2024 edition of *First Aid for the USMLE Step 1* contains a revised and expanded database of basic science material that students, student authors, and faculty authors have identified as high yield for board review. The information is presented in a partially organ-based format. Hence, Section II is devoted to the foundational principles of biochemistry, microbiology, immunology, basic pathology, basic pharmacology, and public health sciences. Section III focuses on organ systems, with subsections covering the embryology, anatomy and histology, physiology, clinical pathology, and clinical pharmacology relevant to each. Each subsection is then divided into smaller topic areas containing related facts. Individual facts are generally presented in a three-column format, with the **Title** of the fact in the first column, the **Description** of the fact in the second column, and the **Mnemonic** or **Special Note** in the third column. Some facts do not have a mnemonic and are presented in a two-column format. Others are presented in list or tabular form in order to emphasize key associations.

The database structure used in Sections II and III is useful for reviewing material already learned. These sections are **not** ideal for learning complex or highly conceptual material for the first time.

The database of high-yield facts is not comprehensive. Use it to complement your core study material and not as your primary study source. The facts and notes have been condensed and edited to emphasize the high-yield material, and as a result, each entry is "incomplete" and arguably "over-simplified." Often, the more you research a topic, the more complex it becomes, with certain topics resisting simplification. Determine your most efficient methods for learning the material, and do not be afraid to abandon a strategy if it is not working for you.

Our database of high-yield facts is updated annually to keep current with new trends in boards emphasis, including clinical relevance. However, we must note that inevitably many other high-yield topics are not yet included in our database.

We actively encourage medical students and faculty to submit high-yield topics, well-written entries, diagrams, clinical images, and useful mnemonics so that we may enhance the database for future students. We also solicit recommendations of alternate tools for study that may be useful in preparing for the examination, such as charts, flash cards, apps, and online resources (see How to Contribute, p. xv).

**Image Acknowledgments**

All images and diagrams marked with ▣ are © USMLE-Rx.com (MedIQ Learning, LLC) and reproduced here by special permission. All images marked with ▣ are © Dr. Richard P. Usatine, author of *The Color Atlas of Family Medicine*, *The Color Atlas of Internal Medicine*, and *The Color Atlas of Pediatrics*, and are reproduced here by special permission (www.usatinemedia.com). Images and diagrams marked with ▣ are adapted or reproduced with permission of other sources as listed on page 755. Images and diagrams with no acknowledgment are part of this book.

**Disclaimer**

The entries in this section reflect student opinions on what is high yield. Because of the diverse sources of material, no attempt has been made to trace or reference the origins of entries individually. We have regarded mnemonics as essentially in the public domain. Errata will gladly be corrected if brought to the attention of the authors, either through our online errata submission form at www.firstaidteam.com or directly by email to firstaid@scholarrx.com.

# Biochemistry

> *"The nitrogen in our DNA, the calcium in our teeth, the iron in our blood, the carbon in our apple pies were made in the interiors of collapsing stars. We are made of starstuff."*
>
> —Carl Sagan

> *"Biochemistry is the study of carbon compounds that crawl."*
>
> —Mike Adams

> *"The power to control our species' genetic future is awesome and terrifying."*
>
> —A Crack in Creation

> *"Nothing in this world is to be feared, it is only to be understood."*
>
> —Marie Curie

This high-yield material includes molecular biology, genetics, cell biology, and principles of metabolism (especially vitamins, cofactors, minerals, and single-enzyme-deficiency diseases). When studying metabolic pathways, emphasize important regulatory steps and enzyme deficiencies that result in disease, as well as reactions targeted by pharmacologic interventions. For example, understanding the defect in Lesch-Nyhan syndrome and its clinical consequences is higher yield than memorizing every intermediate in the purine salvage pathway.

Do not spend time learning details of organic chemistry, mechanisms, or physical chemistry. Detailed chemical structures are infrequently tested; however, many structures have been included here to help students learn reactions and the important enzymes involved. Familiarity with the biochemical techniques that have medical relevance—such as ELISA, immunoelectrophoresis, Southern blotting, and PCR—is useful. Review the related biochemistry when studying pharmacology or genetic diseases as a way to reinforce and integrate the material.

## ▶ BIOCHEMISTRY—MOLECULAR

**Chromatin structure**

DNA exists in the condensed, chromatin form to fit into the nucleus. DNA loops twice around a histone octamer to form a nucleosome ("beads on a string"). H1 binds to the nucleosome and to "linker DNA," thereby stabilizing the chromatin fiber.

DNA has ⊖ charge from phosphate groups. Histones are **large** and have ⊕ charge from lysine and **arginine**.

In mitosis, DNA condenses to form chromosomes. DNA and histone synthesis occurs during S phase.

Mitochondria have their own DNA, which is circular and does not utilize histones.

DNA double-helix

DNA

H1 histone (linker)

Nucleosome (H2A, H2B, H3, H4) ×2

Euchromatin (histone acetylation)

Heterochromatin (histone deacetylation)

Supercoiled structure

Metaphase chromosome ℞

| | | |
|---|---|---|
| **Heterochromatin**  | Condensed, appears darker on EM (labeled H in Ⓐ; Nu, nucleolus). Sterically inaccessible, thus transcriptionally inactive. ↑ methylation, ↓ acetylation. | Heterochromatin = highly condensed (hidden chromatin). Barr bodies (inactive X chromosomes) may be visible on the periphery of nucleus. |
| **Euchromatin** | Less condensed, appears lighter on EM (labeled E in Ⓐ). Transcriptionally active, sterically accessible. | *Eu* = true, "truly transcribed." Euchromatin is expressed. |
| **DNA methylation** | Reversibly changes the expression of a DNA segment without changing its sequence. Involved with aging, carcinogenesis, epigenetics, genomic imprinting, transposable element repression, and X chromosome inactivation (lyonization). | DNA is methylated in imprinting. Methylation within gene promoter (CpG islands) typically represses (silences) gene transcription. CpG methylation makes DNA mute. Dysregulated DNA methylation is implicated in fragile X syndrome. |
| **Histone methylation** | Usually causes reversible transcriptional suppression, but can also cause activation depending on location of methyl groups. | Histone methylation mostly makes DNA mute. Lysine and arginine residues of histones can be methylated. |
| **Histone acetylation** | Removal of histone's ⊕ charge → relaxed DNA coiling → ↑ transcription. | Thyroid hormone synthesis is altered by acetylation of thyroid hormone receptor. Histone acetylation makes DNA active. |
| **Histone deacetylation** | Removal of acetyl groups → tightened DNA coiling → ↓ transcription. | Histone deacetylation may be responsible for altered gene expression in Huntington disease. Histone deacetylation deactivates DNA. |

**Nucleotides**

Nucleoside = base + (deoxy)ribose (sugar).
Nucleotide = base + (deoxy)ribose + phosphate;
  linked by 3'-5' phosphodiester bond.


Purines (A,G)—2 rings.
Pyrimidines (C,U,T)—1 ring.

Deamination reactions:
  Cytosine → uracil
  Adenine → hypoxanthine
  Guanine → xanthine
  5-methylcytosine → thymine

Uracil found in RNA; thymine in DNA.
  Methylation of uracil makes thymine.

5' end of incoming nucleotide bears the
  triphosphate (energy source for the bond).

Pure As Gold.
CUT the pyramid.
Thymine has a methyl.
C-G bond (3 H bonds) stronger than A-T bond
  (2 H bonds). ↑ C-G content → ↑ melting
  temperature of DNA. "C-G bonds are like
  Crazy Glue."

Amino acids necessary for **purine** synthesis (cats
  purr until they **GAG**):
  Glycine
  Aspartate
  Glutamine

Purine (A, G)

Pyrimidine (C, U, T)

**De novo pyrimidine and purine synthesis**

Various immunosuppressive, antineoplastic, and antibiotic drugs function by interfering with nucleotide synthesis:

**Pyrimidine synthesis:**

- Leflunomide: inhibits dihydroorotate dehydrogenase
- 5-fluorouracil (5-FU) and its prodrug capecitabine: form 5-F-dUMP, which inhibits thymidylate synthase (↓ dTMP)

**Purine synthesis:**

- 6-mercaptopurine (6-MP) and its prodrug azathioprine: inhibit de novo purine synthesis (guanine phosphoribosyltransferase); azathioprine is metabolized via purine degradation pathway and can lead to immunosuppression when administered with xanthine oxidase inhibitor
- Mycophenolate and ribavirin: inhibit inosine monophosphate dehydrogenase

**Purine and pyrimidine synthesis:**

- Hydroxyurea: inhibits ribonucleotide reductase
- Methotrexate (MTX), trimethoprim (TMP), and pyrimethamine: inhibit dihydrofolate reductase (↓ deoxythymidine monophosphate [dTMP]) in humans (methotrexate), bacteria (trimethoprim), and protozoa (pyrimethamine)

CPS1 = mitochondria, urea cycle, found in liver
CPS2 = cytwosol, pyrimidine synthesis, found in most cells

## Purine salvage deficiencies

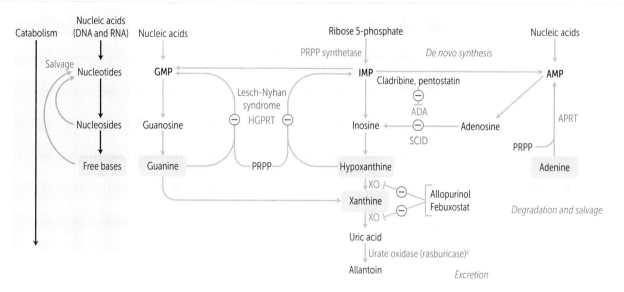

[a]Absent in humans.

ADA, adenosine deaminase; APRT, adenine phosphoribosyltransferase; HGPRT, hypoxanthine guanine phosphoribosyltransferase, XO, xanthine oxidase; SCID, severe combined immune deficiency (autosomal recessive inheritance)

| | | |
|---|---|---|
| **Adenosine deaminase deficiency** | ADA is required for degradation of adenosine and deoxyadenosine. ↓ ADA → ↑ dATP → ↓ ribonucleotide reductase activity → ↓ DNA precursors in cells → ↓ lymphocytes. | One of the major causes of autosomal recessive SCID. |
| **Lesch-Nyhan syndrome** | Defective purine salvage. Absent **HGPRT** → ↓ GMP (from guanine) and ↓ IMP (from hypoxanthine) formation. Compensatory ↑ in purine synthesis (↑ PRPP amidotransferase activity) → excess uric acid production. X-linked recessive. Findings: intellectual disability, self-mutilation, aggression, hyperuricemia (red/orange "sand" [sodium urate crystals] in diaper), gout, dystonia, macrocytosis. | **HGPRT**: Hyperuricemia Gout Pissed off (aggression, self-mutilation) Red/orange crystals in urine Tense muscles (dystonia) Treatment: allopurinol, febuxostat. |

## Genetic code features

| | | |
|---|---|---|
| Unambiguous | Each codon specifies only 1 amino acid. | |
| Degenerate/ redundant | Most amino acids are coded by multiple codons. Wobble hypothesis—first 2 nucleotides of codon are essential for anticodon recognition while the 3rd nucleotide can differ ("wobble"). | Exceptions: methionine (AUG) and tryptophan (UGG) are encoded by only 1 codon. |
| Commaless, nonoverlapping | Read from a fixed starting point as a continuous sequence of bases. | Exceptions: some viruses. |
| Universal | Genetic code is conserved throughout evolution. | Exception in humans: mitochondria. |

| | | |
|---|---|---|
| **DNA replication** | Occurs in 5′ → 3′ direction ("5ynth3sis") in continuous and discontinuous (Okazaki fragment) fashion. Semiconservative. More complex in eukaryotes than in prokaryotes, but shares analogous enzymes. | |
| **Origin of replication** A | Particular consensus sequence in genome where DNA replication begins. May be single (prokaryotes) or multiple (eukaryotes). | AT-rich sequences (eg, TATA box regions) are found in promoters (often upstream) and origins of replication (ori). |
| **Replication fork** B | Y-shaped region along DNA template where leading and lagging strands are synthesized. | |
| **Helicase** C | Unwinds DNA template at replication fork. | Helicase halves DNA. Deficient in **Bloom** syndrome (*BLM* gene mutation). |
| **Single-stranded binding proteins** D | Prevent strands from reannealing or degradation by nucleases. | |
| **DNA topoisomerases** E | Creates a **single-** (topoisomerase I) or **double-** (topoisomerase II) stranded break in the helix to add or remove supercoils (as needed due to underwinding or overwinding of DNA). | In eukaryotes: irinotecan/topotecan inhibit topoisomerase (TOP) I, etoposide/teniposide inhibit TOP II. In prokaryotes: fluoroquinolones inhibit TOP II (DNA gyrase) and TOP IV. |
| **Primase** F | Makes RNA primer for DNA polymerase III to initiate replication. | |
| **DNA polymerase III** G | Prokaryotes only. Elongates leading strand by adding deoxynucleotides to the 3′ end. Elongates lagging strand until it reaches primer of preceding fragment. | DNA polymerase III has 5′ → 3′ synthesis and proofreads with 3′ → 5′ exonuclease. Drugs blocking DNA replication often have a modified 3′ OH, thereby preventing addition of the next nucleotide ("chain termination"). |
| **DNA polymerase I** H | Prokaryotes only. Degrades RNA primer; replaces it with DNA. | Same functions as DNA polymerase III, also excises RNA primer with 5′ → 3′ exonuclease. |
| **DNA ligase** I | Catalyzes the formation of a phosphodiester bond within a strand of double-stranded DNA. | Joins Okazaki fragments. Ligase links DNA. |
| **Telomerase** | Eukaryotes only. A reverse transcriptase (RNA-dependent DNA polymerase) that adds DNA (**TTAGGG**) to 3′ ends of chromosomes to avoid loss of genetic material with every duplication. | Upregulated in progenitor cells and also often in cancer; downregulated in aging and progeria. Telomerase **TAG**s for **G**reatness and **G**lory. |

## DNA repair

### Double strand

| | | |
|---|---|---|
| **Nonhomologous end joining** | Brings together 2 ends of DNA fragments to repair double-stranded breaks. Homology not required. Part of the DNA may be lost or translocated. May be dysfunctional in ataxia telangiectasia. | |
| **Homologous recombination** | Requires 2 homologous DNA duplexes. A strand from damaged dsDNA is repaired using a complementary strand from intact homologous dsDNA as a template. Defective in breast/ovarian cancers with *BRCA1* or *BRCA2* mutations and in Fanconi anemia. Restores duplexes accurately without loss of nucleotides. | |

### Single strand

| | | |
|---|---|---|
| **Nucleotide excision repair** | Specific endonucleases remove the oligonucleotides containing damaged bases; DNA polymerase and ligase fill and reseal the gap, respectively. Repairs bulky helix-distorting lesions (eg, pyrimidine dimers). | Occurs in $G_1$ phase of cell cycle. Defective in xeroderma pigmentosum (inability to repair DNA pyrimidine dimers caused by UV exposure). Presents with dry skin, photosensitivity, skin cancer. |
| **Base excision repair** | Base-specific Glycosylase removes altered base and creates AP site (apurinic/apyrimidinic). One or more nucleotides are removed by AP-Endonuclease, which cleaves 5′ end. AP-Lyase cleaves 3′ end. DNA Polymerase-β fills the gap and DNA ligase seals it. | Occurs throughout cell cycle. Important in repair of spontaneous/toxic deamination. "GEL Please." |
| **Mismatch repair** | Mismatched nucleotides in newly synthesized strand are removed and gap is filled and resealed. | Occurs predominantly in S phase of cell cycle. Defective in Lynch syndrome (hereditary nonpolyposis colorectal cancer [HNPCC]). |

Nucleotide excision repair

Base excision repair

Mismatch repair

A    B    C

| | |
|---|---|
| **Mutations in DNA** | Degree of change: silent ≪ missense < nonsense < frameshift. Single nucleotide substitutions are repaired by DNA polymerase and DNA ligase. Types of single nucleotide (point) mutations:<br> ▪ Transition—purine to purine (eg, A to G) or pyrimidine to pyrimidine (eg, C to T).<br> ▪ Transversion—purine to pyrimidine (eg, A to T) or pyrimidine to purine (eg, C to G). |

### Single nucleotide substitutions

| | |
|---|---|
| **Silent mutation** | Codes for same (synonymous) amino acid; often involves 3rd position of codon (tRNA wobble). |
| **Missense mutation** | Results in changed amino acid (called conservative if new amino acid has similar chemical structure). Examples: sickle cell disease (substitution of glutamic acid with valine). |
| **Nonsense mutation** | Results in early stop codon (UGA, UAA, UAG). Usually generates nonfunctional protein. Stop the nonsense! |

### Other mutations

| | |
|---|---|
| **Frameshift mutation** | Deletion or insertion of any number of nucleotides not divisible by 3 → misreading of all nucleotides downstream. Protein may be shorter or longer, and its function may be disrupted or altered. May occur due to slippage of DNA polymerase during replication at repetitive nucleotide regions. Examples: Duchenne muscular dystrophy, Tay-Sachs disease, cystic fibrosis. |
| **Splice site mutation** | Retained intron in mRNA → protein with impaired or altered function. Examples: rare causes of cancers, dementia, epilepsy, some types of β-thalassemia, Gaucher disease, Marfan syndrome. |

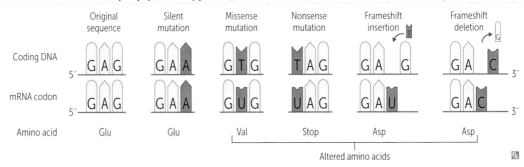

| | **Lac operon** |
|---|---|
| | Classic example of a genetic response to an environmental change. Glucose is the preferred metabolic substrate in *E coli*, but when glucose is absent and lactose is available, the *lac* operon is activated to switch to lactose metabolism. Mechanism of shift:<br> ▪ Low glucose → ↑ adenylate cyclase activity → ↑ generation of cAMP from ATP → activation of catabolite activator protein (CAP) → ↑ transcription.<br> ▪ High lactose → unbinds repressor protein from repressor/operator site → ↑ transcription. |

## Functional organization of a eukaryotic gene

## Regulation of gene expression

| | | |
|---|---|---|
| Promoter | Site where RNA polymerase II and multiple other transcription factors bind to DNA upstream from gene locus (AT-rich upstream sequence with TATA and CAAT boxes, which differ between eukaryotes and prokaryotes). | Promoters increase initiation of transcription. Promoter mutation commonly results in dramatic ↓ in level of gene transcription. |
| Enhancer | DNA locus where regulatory proteins ("**activators**") bind, **increasing** expression of a gene on the same chromosome. | Enhancers and silencers may be located close to, far from, or even within (in an intron) the gene whose expression they regulate. |
| Silencer | DNA locus where regulatory proteins ("**repressors**") bind, **decreasing** expression of a gene on the same chromosome. | |
| Epigenetics | Changes made to gene expression (heritable mitotically/meiotically) without a change in underlying DNA sequence. | Primary mechanisms of epigenetic change include DNA methylation, histone modification, and noncoding RNA. |

**RNA processing (eukaryotes)**

Initial transcript is called heterogeneous nuclear RNA (hnRNA). hnRNA is then modified and becomes mRNA.

The following processes occur in the nucleus:
- Capping of 5′ end (addition of 7-methylguanosine cap; cotranscriptional)
- Polyadenylation of 3′ end (~200 A's → poly-A tail; posttranscriptional)
- Splicing out of introns (posttranscriptional)

Capped, tailed, and spliced transcript is called mRNA.

mRNA is transported out of nucleus to be translated in cytosol.

mRNA quality control occurs at cytoplasmic processing bodies (P-bodies), which contain exonucleases, decapping enzymes, and microRNAs; mRNAs may be degraded or stored in P-bodies for future translation.

Poly-A polymerase does not require a template. AAUAAA = polyadenylation signal. Mutation in polyadenylation signal → early degradation prior to translation.

Kozak sequence—initiation site in most eukaryotic mRNA. Facilitates binding of small subunit of ribosome to mRNA. Mutations in sequence → impairment of initiation of translation → ↓ protein synthesis.

---

**RNA polymerases**

| | | |
|---|---|---|
| **Eukaryotes** | RNA polymerase I makes rRNA, the most common (rampant) type; present only in nucleolus.<br>RNA polymerase II makes mRNA (massive), microRNA (miRNA), and small nuclear RNA (snRNA).<br>RNA polymerase III makes 5S rRNA, tRNA (tiny).<br>No proofreading function, but can initiate chains. RNA polymerase II opens DNA at promoter site. | I, II, and III are numbered in the same order that their products are used in protein synthesis: rRNA, mRNA, then tRNA.<br>α-amanitin, found in *Amanita phalloides* (death cap mushrooms), inhibits RNA polymerase II. Causes dysentery and severe hepatotoxicity if ingested.<br>Dactinomycin inhibits RNA polymerase in both prokaryotes and eukaryotes. |
| **Prokaryotes** | 1 RNA polymerase (multisubunit complex) makes all 3 kinds of RNA. | Rifamycins (rifampin, rifabutin) inhibit DNA-dependent RNA polymerase in prokaryotes. |

**Introns vs exons**

Exons contain the actual genetic information coding for protein or functional RNA.

Introns do not code for protein, but are important in regulation of gene expression.

Different exons are frequently combined by alternative splicing to produce a larger number of unique proteins.

Introns are intervening sequences and stay in the nucleus, whereas exons exit and are expressed.

Alternative splicing—can produce a variety of protein products from a single hnRNA (heterogenous nuclear RNA) sequence (eg, transmembrane vs secreted Ig, tropomyosin variants in muscle, dopamine receptors in the brain, host defense evasion by tumor cells).

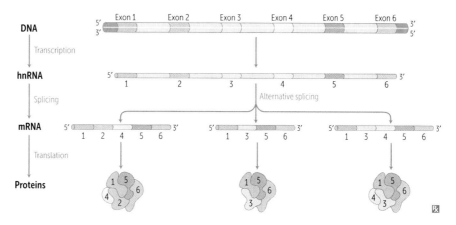

**Splicing of pre-mRNA**

Part of process by which precursor mRNA (pre-mRNA) is transformed into mature mRNA. Introns typically begin with GU and end with AG. Alterations in snRNP assembly can cause clinical disease; eg, in spinal muscular atrophy, snRNP assembly is affected due to ↓ SMN protein → congenital degeneration of anterior horns of spinal cord → symmetric weakness (hypotonia, or "floppy baby syndrome").

snRNPs are snRNA bound to proteins (eg, Smith [Sm]) to form a spliceosome that cleaves pre-mRNA. Anti-U1 snRNP antibodies are associated with SLE, mixed connective tissue disease, other rheumatic diseases.

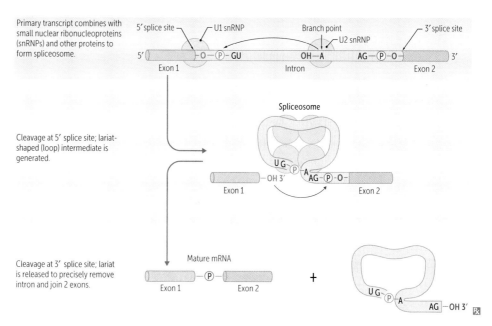

## tRNA

| | |
|---|---|
| **Structure** | 75–90 nucleotides, 2° structure, cloverleaf form, anticodon end is opposite 3′ aminoacyl end. All tRNAs, both eukaryotic and prokaryotic, have CCA at 3′ end along with a high percentage of chemically modified bases. The amino acid is covalently bound to the 3′ end of the tRNA. CCA Can Carry Amino acids.<br>T-arm: contains the TΨC (ribothymidine, pseudouridine, cytidine) sequence necessary for tRNA-ribosome binding. T-arm Tethers tRNA molecule to ribosome.<br>D-arm: contains Dihydrouridine residues necessary for tRNA recognition by the correct aminoacyl-tRNA synthetase. D-arm allows Detection of the tRNA by aminoacyl-tRNA synthetase.<br>Attachment site: 3′-ACC-5′ is the amino acid ACCeptor site. |
| **Charging** | Aminoacyl-tRNA synthetase (uses ATP; 1 unique enzyme per respective amino acid) and binding of charged tRNA to the codon are responsible for the accuracy of amino acid selection. Aminoacyl-tRNA synthetase matches an amino acid to the tRNA by scrutinizing the amino acid before and after it binds to tRNA. If an incorrect amino acid is attached, the bond is hydrolyzed. A mischarged tRNA reads the usual codon but inserts the wrong amino acid. |

## Start and stop codons

| | | |
|---|---|---|
| **mRNA start codon** | AUG. | AUG inAUGurates protein synthesis. |
| Eukaryotes | Codes for methionine, which may be removed before translation is completed. | |
| Prokaryotes | Codes for N-formylmethionine (fMet). | fMet stimulates neutrophil chemotaxis. |
| **mRNA stop codons** | UGA, UAA, UAG.<br>Recognized by release factors. | UGA = U Go Away.<br>UAA = U Are Away.<br>UAG = U Are Gone. |

## Protein synthesis

| | | |
|---|---|---|
| Initiation | 1. Eukaryotic initiation factors (eIFs) identify the 5' cap.<br>2. eIFs help assemble the 40S ribosomal subunit with the initiator tRNA.<br>3. eIFs released when the mRNA and the ribosomal 60S subunit assemble with the complex. Requires GTP. | Eukaryotes: 40S + 60S → 80S (even).<br>Prokaryotes: 30S + 50S → 70S (prime).<br>Synthesis occurs from N-terminus to C-terminus.<br><br>ATP—tRNA **A**ctivation (charging).<br>GTP—tRNA **G**ripping and **G**oing places (translocation). |
| Elongation | ❶ Aminoacyl-tRNA binds to A site (except for initiator methionine, which binds the P site), requires an elongation factor and GTP.<br>❷ rRNA ("ribozyme") catalyzes peptide bond formation, transfers growing polypeptide to amino acid in A site.<br>❸ Ribosome advances 3 nucleotides toward 3' end of mRNA, moving peptidyl tRNA to P site (translocation). | Think of "going **APE**":<br>  **A** site = incoming **A**minoacyl-tRNA.<br>  **P** site = accommodates growing **P**eptide.<br>  **E** site = holds **E**mpty tRNA as it **E**xits.<br><br>Elongation factors are targets of bacterial toxins (eg, *Diphtheria, Pseudomonas*). |
| Termination | Eukaryotic release factors (eRFs) recognize the stop codon and halt translation → completed polypeptide is released from ribosome. Requires GTP. | Shine-Dalgarno sequence—ribosomal binding site in prokaryotic mRNA. Recognized by 16S RNA in ribosomal subunit. Enables protein synthesis initiation by aligning ribosome with start codon so that code is read correctly. |

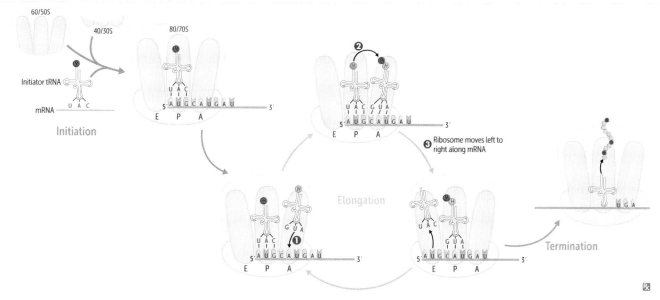

## Posttranslational modifications

| | |
|---|---|
| Trimming | Removal of N- or C-terminal propeptides from zymogen to generate mature protein (eg, trypsinogen to trypsin). |
| Covalent alterations | Phosphorylation, glycosylation, hydroxylation, methylation, acetylation, and ubiquitination. |

## Chaperone protein

Intracellular protein involved in facilitating and maintaining protein folding. In yeast, heat shock proteins (eg, HSP60) are constitutively expressed, but expression may increase with high temperatures, acidic pH, and hypoxia to prevent protein denaturing/misfolding.

▶ BIOCHEMISTRY—CELLULAR

| | |
|---|---|
| **Cell cycle phases** | Checkpoints control transitions between phases of cell cycle. This process is regulated by cyclins, cyclin-dependent kinases (CDKs), and tumor suppressors. M phase (shortest phase of cell cycle) includes mitosis (prophase, prometaphase, metaphase, anaphase, telophase) and cytokinesis (cytoplasm splits in two). $G_1$ is of variable duration. |

REGULATION OF CELL CYCLE

| | |
|---|---|
| **Cyclin-dependent kinases** | Constitutively expressed but inactive when not bound to cyclin. |
| **Cyclin-CDK complexes** | Cyclins are phase-specific regulatory proteins that activate CDKs when stimulated by growth factors. The cyclin-CDK complex can then phosphorylate other proteins (eg, Rb) to coordinate cell cycle progression. This complex must be activated/inactivated at appropriate times for cell cycle to progress. |
| **Tumor suppressors** | p53 → p21 induction → CDK inhibition → Rb hypophosphorylation (activation) → $G_1$-S progression inhibition. Mutations in tumor suppressor genes can result in unrestrained cell division (eg, Li-Fraumeni syndrome). <br> Growth factors (eg, insulin, PDGF, EPO, EGF) bind tyrosine kinase receptors to transition the cell from $G_1$ to S phase. |

CELL TYPES

| | | |
|---|---|---|
| **Permanent** | Remain in $G_0$, regenerate from stem cells. | Neurons, skeletal and cardiac muscle, RBCs. |
| **Stable (quiescent)** | Enter $G_1$ from $G_0$ when stimulated. | Hepatocytes, lymphocytes, PCT, periosteal cells. |
| **Labile** | Never go to $G_0$, divide rapidly with a short $G_1$. Most affected by chemotherapy. | Bone marrow, gut epithelium, skin, hair follicles, germ cells. |

| | | |
|---|---|---|
| **Rough endoplasmic reticulum** | Site of synthesis of secretory (exported) proteins and of N-linked oligosaccharide addition to lysosomal and other proteins.<br>Nissl bodies (RER in neurons)—synthesize peptide neurotransmitters for secretion.<br>Free ribosomes—unattached to any membrane; site of synthesis of cytosolic, peroxisomal, and mitochondrial proteins. | N-linked glycosylation occurs in the eNdoplasmic reticulum.<br>Mucus-secreting goblet cells of small intestine and antibody-secreting plasma cells are rich in RER.<br>Proteins within organelles (eg, ER, Golgi bodies, lysosomes) are formed in RER. |
| **Smooth endoplasmic reticulum** | Site of steroid synthesis and detoxification of drugs and poisons. Lacks surface ribosomes. Location of glucose-6-phosphatase (last step in both glycogenolysis and gluconeogenesis). | Hepatocytes and steroid hormone–producing cells of the adrenal cortex and gonads are rich in SER. |

**Cell trafficking**

Golgi is distribution center for proteins and lipids from ER to vesicles and plasma membrane. Posttranslational events in GOlgi include modifying N-oligosaccharides on asparagine, adding O-oligosaccharides on serine and threonine, and adding mannose-6-phosphate to proteins for lysosomal degradation.

Endosomes are sorting centers for material from outside the cell or from the Golgi, sending it to lysosomes for destruction or back to the membrane/Golgi for further use.

**I-cell disease** (inclusion cell disease/mucolipidosis type II)—inherited lysosomal storage disorder (autosomal recessive); defect in N-acetylglucosaminyl-1-phosphotransferase → failure of the Golgi to phosphorylate mannose residues (↓ mannose-6-phosphate) on glycoproteins → enzymes secreted extracellularly rather than delivered to lysosomes → lysosomes deficient in digestive enzymes → buildup of cellular debris in lysosomes (inclusion bodies). Results in coarse facial features, gingival hyperplasia, corneal clouding, restricted joint movements, claw hand deformities, kyphoscoliosis, and ↑ plasma levels of lysosomal enzymes. Symptoms similar to but more severe than Hurler syndrome. Often fatal in childhood.

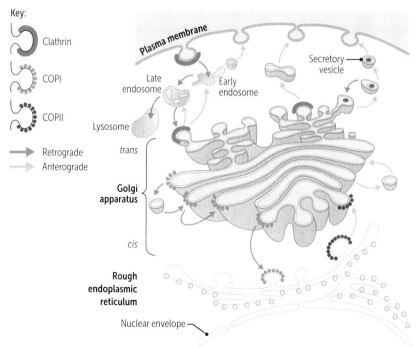

Key:
- Clathrin
- COPI
- COPII
- → Retrograde
- ┈┈▶ Anterograde

Plasma membrane
Secretory vesicle
Late endosome
Early endosome
Lysosome
*trans*
Golgi apparatus
*cis*
Rough endoplasmic reticulum
Nuclear envelope

Signal recognition particle (SRP)—abundant, cytosolic ribonucleoprotein that traffics polypeptide-ribosome complex from the cytosol to the RER. Absent or dysfunctional SRP → accumulation of protein in cytosol.

Vesicular trafficking proteins
- COPI: Golgi → Golgi (retrograde); *cis*-Golgi → ER.
- COPII: ER → *cis*-Golgi (anterograde). "Two (COPII) steps forward (anterograde); one (COPI) step back (retrograde)."
- Clathrin: *trans*-Golgi → lysosomes; plasma membrane → endosomes (receptor-mediated endocytosis [eg, LDL receptor activity]).

**Peroxisome**

Membrane-enclosed organelle involved in:
- β-oxidation of very-long-chain fatty acids (VLCFA) (strictly peroxisomal process)
- α-oxidation of branched-chain fatty acids (strictly peroxisomal process)
- Catabolism of amino acids and ethanol
- Synthesis of bile acids and plasmalogens (important membrane phospholipid, especially in white matter of brain)

Zellweger syndrome—autosomal recessive disorder of peroxisome biogenesis due to mutated *PEX* genes (accumulation of pipecolic acid in peroxisomes). Hypotonia, seizures, jaundice, craniofacial dysmorphia, hepatomegaly, early death.

Refsum disease—autosomal recessive disorder of α-oxidation → buildup of phytanic acid due to inability to degrade it. Vision loss (retinitis pigmentosa), anosmia, hearing loss, ataxia, peripheral neuropathy, ichthyosis, and cardiac conduction defects. Treatment: diet, plasmapheresis.

Adrenoleukodystrophy—X-linked recessive disorder of β-oxidation due to mutation in *ABCD1* gene → VLCFA buildup in **adrenal** glands, white (**leuko**) matter of brain, testes. Progressive disease that can lead to adrenal gland crisis, progressive loss of neurologic function, death.

---

**Proteasome**

Barrel-shaped protein complex that degrades polyubiquitin-tagged proteins. Plays a role in many cellular processes, including immune response (MHC I–mediated). Defects in ubiquitin-proteasome system also implicated in diverse human diseases including neurodegenerative diseases.

---

**Cytoskeletal elements**

A network of protein fibers within the cytoplasm that supports cell structure, cell and organelle movement, and cell division.

| TYPE OF FILAMENT | PREDOMINANT FUNCTION | EXAMPLES |
|---|---|---|
| **Microfilaments** | Muscle contraction, cytokinesis, phagocytosis | Actin, microvilli. |
| **Intermediate filaments** | Maintain cell structure | Vimentin, desmin, cytokeratin, lamins, glial fibrillary acidic protein (GFAP), neurofilaments. |
| **Microtubules** | Movement, cell division | Cilia, flagella, mitotic spindle, axonal trafficking, centrioles. |

---

**Microtubule**

Positive end (+)
Heterodimer
Protofilament
Negative end (−)

Cylindrical outer structure composed of a helical array of polymerized heterodimers of α- and β-tubulin. Each dimer has 2 GTP bound. Incorporated into flagella, cilia, mitotic spindles. Also involved in slow axoplasmic transport in neurons.

Molecular motor proteins—transport cellular cargo toward opposite ends of microtubule.
- Retrograde to microtubule (+ → −)—dynein.
- Anterograde to microtubule (− → +)—kinesin.

*Clostridium tetani* toxin, poliovirus, rabies virus, and herpes simplex virus (HSV) use dynein for retrograde transport to the neuronal cell body. HSV reactivation occurs via anterograde transport from cell body (kinesin mediated).

Slow anterograde transport rate limiting step of peripheral nerve regeneration after injury.

Drugs that act on microtubules (microtubules get constructed very terribly):
- Mebendazole (antihelminthic)
- Griseofulvin (antifungal)
- Colchicine (antigout)
- Vinca alkaloids (anticancer)
- Taxanes (anticancer)

Negative end near nucleus.

Positive end points to periphery.

Ready? Attack!

**Cilia structure**

Motile cilia consist of 9 doublet + 2 singlet arrangement of microtubules (axoneme) .

Basal body (base of cilium below cell membrane) consists of 9 microtubule triplets B with no central microtubules.

Nonmotile (primary) cilia work as chemical signal sensors and have a role in signal transduction and cell growth control. Dysgenesis may lead to polycystic kidney disease, mitral valve prolapse, or retinal degeneration.

Axonemal dynein—ATPase that links peripheral 9 doublets and causes bending of cilium by differential sliding of doublets.

Gap junctions enable coordinated ciliary movement.

**Primary ciliary dyskinesia**

Autosomal recessive. Dynein arm defect → immotile cilia → dysfunctional ciliated epithelia. Most common type is Kartagener syndrome (PCD with situs inversus).

Developmental abnormalities due to impaired migration and orientation (eg, situs inversus A, hearing loss due to dysfunctional eustachian tube cilia); recurrent infections (eg, sinusitis, ear infections, bronchiectasis due to impaired ciliary clearance of debris/pathogens); infertility (↑ risk of ectopic pregnancy due to dysfunctional fallopian tube cilia, immotile spermatozoa).

Lab findings: ↓ nasal nitric oxide (used as screening test).

**Sodium-potassium pump**

Na+/K+-ATPase is located in the plasma membrane with ATP site on cytosolic side. For each ATP consumed, **2 K+** go **in** to the cell (pump dephosphorylated) and **3 Na+** go out of the cell (pump phosphorylated).

2 strikes? **K**, you're still in. 3 strikes? Nah, you're out!

Digoxin directly inhibits Na+/K+-ATPase → indirect inhibition of Na+/Ca2+ exchange → ↑ $[Ca^{2+}]_i$ → ↑ cardiac contractility.

| | | |
|---|---|---|
| **Collagen** | Most abundant protein in the human body. Extensively modified by posttranslational modification. Organizes and strengthens extracellular matrix. Types I to IV are the most common types in humans. | Type I: Skeleton Type II: Cartilage Type III: Arteries Type IV: Basement membrane **SCAB** |
| **Type I** | Most common (90%)—bone (made by osteoblasts), skin, tendon, dentin, fascia, cornea, **late** wound repair. | Type I: bone, tendone. ↓ production in osteogenesis imperfecta type I. |
| **Type II** | Cartilage (including hyaline), vitreous body, nucleus pulposus. | Type II: cartwoII age. |
| **Type III** | Reticulin—skin, **blood vessels**, uterus, fetal tissue, **early** wound repair. | Type III: deficient in **vascular** type of Ehlers-Danlos syndrome (**threE D**). Myofibroblasts are responsible for secretion (proliferative stage) and wound contraction. |
| **Type IV** | Basement membrane/basal lamina (glomerulus, cochlea), lens. | Type IV: under the **floor** (basement membrane). Defective in Alport syndrome; targeted by autoantibodies in Goodpasture syndrome. |

## Collagen synthesis and structure

❶ **Synthesis**—translation of collagen α chains (preprocollagen)—usually Gly-X-Y (X is often proline or lysine and Y is often hydroxyproline or hydroxylysine). Collagen is 1/3 glycine; glycine content of collagen is less variable than that of lysine and proline.

❷ **Hydroxylation**—hydroxylation ("hydroxCylation") of specific proline and lysine residues. Requires vitamin C; deficiency → scurvy.

❸ **Glycosylation**—glycosylation of pro-α-chain hydroxylysine residues and formation of procollagen via hydrogen and disulfide bonds (triple helix of 3 collagen α chains). Problems forming triple helix → osteogenesis imperfecta.

❹ **Exocytosis**—exocytosis of procollagen into extracellular space.

❺ **Proteolytic processing**—cleavage of disulfide-rich terminal regions of procollagen → insoluble tropocollagen.

❻ **Assembly and alignment**—collagen assembles in fibrils and aligns for cross-linking.

❼ **Cross-linking**—reinforcement of staggered tropocollagen molecules by covalent lysine-hydroxylysine cross-linkage (by copper-containing lysyl oxidase) to make collagen fibers. Cross-linking of collagen ↑ with age. Problems with cross-linking → Menkes disease.

**Osteogenesis imperfecta**

Genetic bone disorder (brittle bone disease) caused by a variety of gene defects (most commonly *COL1A1* and *COL1A2*). Most common form is autosomal dominant with ↓ production of otherwise normal type I collagen (altered triple helix formation). Manifestations include:

- Multiple fractures and bone deformities (arrows in A) after minimal trauma (eg, during birth)
- Blue sclerae B due to thin, translucent scleral collagen revealing choroidal veins
- Some forms have tooth abnormalities, including opalescent teeth that wear easily due to lack of dentin (dentinogenesis imperfecta)
- Hearing loss (abnormal ossicles)

May be confused with child abuse.
Treat with bisphosphonates to ↓ fracture risk.
Patients can't **BITE**:
  **B**ones = multiple fractures
  **I** (eye) = blue sclerae
  **T**eeth = dental imperfections
  **E**ar = hearing loss

**Ehlers-Danlos syndrome**

Faulty collagen synthesis causes skin to be hyperextensible and often thin or transparent A, joints to be hypermobile B, and tendency to bleed (easy bruising).

Multiple types. Inheritance and severity vary. Can be autosomal dominant or recessive. May be associated with joint dislocation, berry and aortic aneurysms, organ rupture.

Hypermobility type (joint instability): most common type.

Classical type (joint and skin symptoms): caused by a mutation in type V collagen (eg, *COL5A1*, *COL5A2*).

Vascular type (fragile tissues including vessels [eg, aorta], muscles, and organs that are prone to rupture [eg, gravid uterus]): mutations in type III procollagen (eg, *COL3A1*).

Can be caused by procollagen peptidase deficiency.

**Menkes disease**

X-linked recessive connective tissue disease caused by impaired copper absorption and transport due to defective Menkes protein *ATP7A* (**A**bsent copper), vs *ATP7B* in Wilson disease (copper **B**uildup). Leads to ↓ activity of lysyl oxidase (copper is a necessary cofactor) → defective collagen cross-linking. Results in brittle, "kinky" hair, growth and developmental delay, hypotonia, ↑ risk of cerebral aneurysms.

**Elastin**

Single elastin molecule    **Stretch** ↕ **Relax**    Cross-link

Stretchy protein within skin, lungs, large arteries, elastic ligaments, vocal cords, epiglottis, ligamenta flava (connect vertebrae → relaxed and stretched conformations).

Rich in nonhydroxylated proline, glycine, and lysine residues, vs the hydroxylated residues of collagen.

Tropoelastin with fibrillin scaffolding.

Cross-linking occurs extracellularly via lysyl oxidase and gives elastin its elastic properties.

Broken down by elastase, which is normally inhibited by $\alpha_1$-antitrypsin.

$\alpha_1$-Antitrypsin deficiency results in unopposed elastase activity, which can cause COPD.

**Marfan syndrome**—autosomal dominant (with variable expression) connective tissue disorder affecting skeleton, heart, and eyes. *FBN1* gene mutation on chromosome 15 (fifteen) results in defective fibrillin-1, a glycoprotein that forms a sheath around elastin and sequesters TGF-β. Findings: tall with long extremities; chest wall deformity (pectus carinatum [pigeon chest] or pectus excavatum **A**); hypermobile joints; long, tapering fingers and toes (arachnodactyly); cystic medial necrosis of aorta; aortic root aneurysm rupture or dissection (most common cause of death); mitral valve prolapse; ↑ risk of spontaneous pneumothorax.

**Homocystinuria**—most commonly due to cystathionine synthase deficiency leading to homocysteine buildup. Presentation similar to Marfan syndrome with pectus deformity, tall stature, ↑ arm:height ratio, ↓ upper:lower body segment ratio, arachnodactyly, joint hyperlaxity, skin hyperelasticity, scoliosis, fair complexion (vs Marfan syndrome).

|  | Marfan syndrome | Homocystinuria |
|---|---|---|
| INHERITANCE | Autosomal dominant | Autosomal recessive |
| INTELLECT | Normal | Decreased |
| VASCULAR COMPLICATIONS | Aortic root dilatation | Thrombosis |
| LENS DISLOCATION | Upward/temporal (Marfan fans out) | Downward/nasal |

## ▶ BIOCHEMISTRY—LABORATORY TECHNIQUES

**Polymerase chain reaction**

Molecular biology lab procedure used to amplify a desired fragment of DNA. Useful as a diagnostic tool (eg, neonatal HIV, herpes encephalitis).

❶ **Denaturation**—DNA template, DNA primers, a heat-stable DNA polymerase, and deoxynucleotide triphosphates (dNTPs) are heated to separate the DNA strands.

❷ **Annealing**—sample is cooled. DNA primers anneal to the specific sequence to be amplified on the DNA template.

❸ **Elongation**—temperature is increased. DNA polymerase adds dNTPs to the strand to replicate the sequence after each primer.

Heating and cooling cycles continue until the amount of DNA is sufficient.

**CRISPR/Cas9**

A genome editing tool derived from bacteria. Consists of a guide RNA (gRNA), which is complementary to a target DNA sequence, and an endonuclease (Cas9), which makes a single- or double-strand break at the target site.

Potential applications include removing virulence factors from pathogens, replacing disease-causing alleles of genes with healthy variants (in clinical trials for sickle cell disease), and specifically targeting tumor cells.

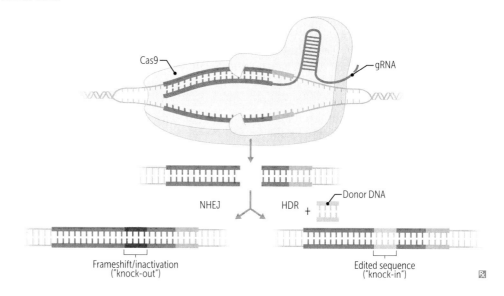

## Blotting procedures

**Southern blot**

1. DNA sample is enzymatically cleaved into smaller pieces, which are separated by gel electrophoresis, and then transferred to a membrane.
2. Membrane is exposed to labeled DNA probe that anneals to its complementary strand.
3. Resulting double-stranded, labeled piece of DNA is visualized when membrane is exposed to film or digital imager.

Useful to identify size of specific sequences (eg, determination of heterozygosity [as seen in image], # of CGG repeats in *FMR1* to diagnose fragile X syndrome)

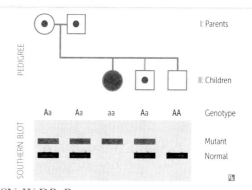

SNoW DRoP:
Southern = DNA
Northern = RNA
Western = Protein

**Northern blot**

Similar to Southern blot, except that an RNA sample is electrophoresed. Useful for studying mRNA levels and size, which are reflective of gene expression. Detects splicing errors.

**Western blot**

Sample protein is separated via gel electrophoresis and transferred to a membrane. Labeled antibody is used to bind relevant protein. This helps identify specific protein and determines quantity.

**Flow cytometry**

Laboratory technique to assess size, granularity, and protein expression (immunophenotype) of individual cells in a sample.

Cells are tagged with antibodies specific to surface or intracellular proteins. Antibodies are then tagged with a unique fluorescent dye. Sample is analyzed one cell at a time by focusing a laser on the cell and measuring light scatter and intensity of fluorescence.

Data are plotted either as histogram (one measure) or scatter plot (any two measures, as shown). In illustration:

- Cells in left lower quadrant ⊖ for both CD8 and CD3.
- Cells in right lower quadrant ⊕ for CD8 and ⊖ for CD3. In this example, right lower quadrant is empty because all CD8-expressing cells also express CD3.
- Cells in left upper quadrant ⊕ for CD3 and ⊖ for CD8.
- Cells in right upper quadrant ⊕ for both CD8 and CD3.

Commonly used in workup of hematologic abnormalities (eg, leukemia, paroxysmal nocturnal hemoglobinuria, fetal RBCs in pregnant person's blood) and immunodeficiencies (eg, CD4+ cell count in HIV).

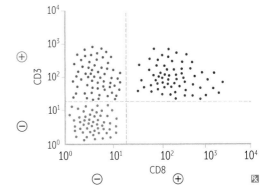

**Microarrays**

Array consisting of thousands of DNA oligonucleotides arranged in a grid on a glass or silicon chip. The DNA or RNA samples being compared are attached to different fluorophores and hybridized to the array. The ratio of fluorescence signal at a particular oligonucleotide reflects the relative amount of the hybridizing nucleic acid in the two samples.

Used to compare the relative transcription of genes in two RNA samples. Can detect single nucleotide polymorphisms (SNPs) and copy number variants (CNVs) for genotyping, clinical genetic testing, forensic analysis, and cancer mutation and genetic linkage analysis when DNA is used.

**Enzyme-linked immunosorbent assay**

Immunologic test used to detect the presence of either a specific antigen (in direct ELISA) or antibody (in indirect ELISA) in a patient's blood sample. Detection involves the use of an antibody linked to an enzyme. Added substrate reacts with the enzyme, producing a detectable signal. Can have high sensitivity and specificity, but is less specific than Western blot. Often used to screen for HIV infection.

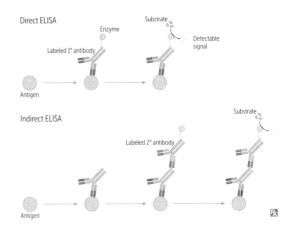

| | | |
|---|---|---|
| **Karyotyping** | Colchicine is added to cultured cells to halt chromosomes in metaphase. Chromosomes are stained, ordered, and numbered according to morphology, size, arm-length ratio, and banding pattern (arrows in  point to extensive abnormalities in a cancer cell).<br><br>Can be performed on a sample of blood, bone marrow, amniotic fluid, or placental tissue.<br><br>Used to diagnose chromosomal imbalances (eg, autosomal trisomies, sex chromosome disorders). | |
| **Fluorescence in situ hybridization** | Fluorescent DNA or RNA probe binds to specific gene or other site of interest on chromosomes.<br><br>Used for specific localization of genes and direct visualization of chromosomal anomalies.<br><br>  ▪ Microdeletion—no fluorescence on a chromosome compared to fluorescence at the same locus on the second copy of that chromosome.<br>  ▪ Translocation— fluorescence signal (from *ABL* gene) that corresponds to one chromosome (chromosome 9) is found in a different chromosome (chromosome 22, next to *BCR* gene).<br>  ▪ Duplication—a second copy of a chromosome, resulting in a trisomy or tetrasomy. | |

der(9)  9   der(22) 22

| | |
|---|---|
| **Molecular cloning** | Production of a recombinant DNA molecule in a bacterial or eukaryotic cell line host. Useful for production of human proteins in bacteria (eg, human growth hormone, insulin). |

| Gene expression modifications | Transgenic strategies in mice involve:<br>• Random insertion of gene into mouse genome<br>• Targeted insertion or deletion of gene through homologous recombination with mouse gene | Knock-out = removing a gene, taking it out.<br>Knock-in = inserting a gene.<br><br>Random insertion—constitutive expression.<br>Targeted insertion—conditional expression. |
|---|---|---|
| RNA interference | Process whereby small non-coding RNA molecules target mRNAs to inhibit gene expression. | |
| MicroRNA | Naturally produced by cell as hairpin structures. Loose nucleotide pairing allows broad targeting of related mRNAs. When miRNA binds to mRNA, it blocks translation of mRNA and sometimes facilitates its degradation. | Abnormal expression of miRNAs contributes to certain malignancies (eg, by silencing an mRNA from a tumor suppressor gene). |
| Small interfering RNA | Usually derived from exogenous dsRNA source (eg, virus). Once inside a cell, siRNA requires complete nucleotide pairing, leading to highly specific mRNA targeting. Results in mRNA cleavage prior to translation. | Can be produced by transcription or chemically synthesized for gene "knockdown" experiments. |

## ▶ BIOCHEMISTRY—GENETICS

### Genetic terms

| TERM | DEFINITION | EXAMPLE |
|---|---|---|
| Codominance | Both alleles contribute to the phenotype of the heterozygote. | Blood groups A, B, AB; $\alpha_1$-antitrypsin deficiency; HLA groups. |
| Variable expressivity | Patients with the same genotype have varying phenotypes. | Two patients with neurofibromatosis type 1 (NF1) may have varying disease severity. |
| Incomplete penetrance | Not all individuals with a pathogenic gene variant show the disease.<br>% penetrance × probability of inheriting genotype = risk of expressing phenotype. | BRCA1 gene mutations do not always result in breast or ovarian cancer. |
| Pleiotropy | One gene contributes to multiple phenotypic effects. | Untreated phenylketonuria (PKU) manifests with light skin, intellectual disability, musty body odor. |
| Anticipation | Increased severity or earlier onset of disease in succeeding generations. | Trinucleotide repeat diseases (eg, Huntington disease). |
| Loss of heterozygosity | If a patient inherits or develops a mutation in a tumor suppressor gene, the wild type allele must be deleted/mutated/eliminated before cancer develops. This is not true of oncogenes. | Retinoblastoma and the "two-hit hypothesis," Lynch syndrome (HNPCC), Li-Fraumeni syndrome. |
| Epistasis | The allele of one gene affects the phenotypic expression of alleles in another gene. | Albinism, alopecia. |
| Aneuploidy | An abnormal number of chromosomes; due to chromosomal nondisjunction during mitosis or meiosis. | Down syndrome (trisomy 21), Turner syndrome (45,XO), oncogenesis. |

## Genetic terms (continued)

| TERM | DEFINITION | EXAMPLE |
|---|---|---|
| Dominant negative mutation | Exerts a dominant effect. A heterozygote produces a nonfunctional altered protein that also prevents the normal gene product from functioning. | A single mutated $p53$ tumor suppressor gene results in a protein that is able to bind DNA and block the wild type p53 from binding to the promoter. |
| Linkage disequilibrium | Tendency for certain alleles to occur in close proximity on the same chromosome more or less often than expected by chance. Measured in a population, not in a family, and often varies in different populations. | $HLA$ gene, $CFTR$ gene. |
| Mosaicism | Presence of genetically distinct cell lines in the same individual.<br>Somatic mosaicism—mutation arises from mitotic errors after fertilization and propagates through multiple tissues or organs.<br>Germline (gonadal) mosaicism—mutation only in egg or sperm cells. If parents and relatives do not have the disease, suspect gonadal (or germline) mosaicism. | McCune-Albright syndrome—due to $G_s$-protein (GNAS) activating mutation. Presents with unilateral café-au-lait spots **A** with ragged edges, polyostotic fibrous dysplasia (bone is replaced by collagen and fibroblasts), and at least one endocrinopathy (eg, precocious puberty). Lethal if mutation occurs before fertilization (affecting all cells), but survivable in patients with mosaicism. |
| Locus heterogeneity | Mutations at different loci result in the same disease. | Albinism, retinitis pigmentosa, familial hypercholesteremia. |
| Allelic heterogeneity | Different mutations in the same locus result in the same disease. | β-thalassemia. |
| Heteroplasmy | Presence of both normal and mutated mtDNA, resulting in variable expression in mitochondrially inherited disease. | mtDNA passed from mother to all children. |
| Uniparental disomy | Offspring receives 2 copies of a chromosome from 1 parent and no copies from the other parent. HeterodIsomy (heterozygous) indicates a meiosis I error. IsodIsomy (homozygous) indicates a meiosis II error or postzygotic chromosomal duplication of one of a pair of chromosomes, and loss of the other of the original pair. | Uniparental is euploid (correct number of chromosomes). Most occurrences of uniparental disomy (UPD) → normal phenotype. Consider isodisomy in an individual manifesting a recessive disorder when only one parent is a carrier. Examples: Prader-Willi and Angelman syndromes. |

## Population genetics

| CONCEPT | DESCRIPTION | EXAMPLE |
|---|---|---|
| Bottleneck effect | Fitness equal across alleles → natural disaster that removes certain alleles by chance → new allelic frequency (by chance, not naturally selected). | The founder effect is a type of bottleneck when cause is due to calamitous population separation. |
| Natural selection | Alleles that increase species fitness are more likely to be passed down to offspring and vice versa. | Human evolution. |
| Genetic drift | Also called allelic drift or Wright effect. A dramatic shift in allelic frequency that occurs by chance (not by natural selection). | Founder effect and bottleneck effect are both examples of genetic drift. |

## Hardy-Weinberg principle

|        | A (p)        | a (q)        |
|--------|--------------|--------------|
| A (p)  | AA ($p^2$)   | Aa (pq)      |
| a (q)  | Aa (pq)      | aa ($q^2$)   |

In a given population where mating is at random, allele and genotype frequencies will be constant. If p and q represent the frequencies of alleles A and a in a population, respectively, then $p + q = 1$, where:

- $p^2$ = frequency of homozygosity for allele A
- $q^2$ = frequency of homozygosity for allele a
- $2pq$ = frequency of heterozygosity (carrier frequency, if an autosomal recessive disease)

Therefore the sum of the frequencies of these genotypes is $p^2 + 2pq + q^2 = 1$.

The frequency of an X-linked recessive disease in males = q and in females = $q^2$.

Hardy-Weinberg law assumptions include:

- No mutation occurring at the locus
- Natural selection is not occurring
- Completely random mating
- No net migration
- Large population

If a population is in Hardy-Weinberg equilibrium, then the values of p and q remain constant from generation to generation. In rare autosomal recessive diseases, $p \approx 1$.

Example: The prevalence of cystic fibrosis (an autosomal recessive disease) in the US is approximately 1/3200, which tells us that $q^2 = 1/3200$, with $q \approx 0.017$ or 1.7% of the population. Since $p + q = 1$, we know that $p = 1 - \sqrt{1/3200} \approx 0.982$, which gives us a heterozygous carrier frequency of $2pq = 0.035$ or 3.5% of the population. Notice that since the disease is relatively rare, we could have approximated $p \approx 1$ and obtained a similar result.

---

## Disorders of imprinting

One gene copy is silenced by methylation, and only the other copy is expressed → parent-of-origin effects. The expressed copy may be mutated, may not be expressed, or may be deleted altogether.

|                        | Prader-Willi syndrome                                                                                 | Angelman syndrome                                                                                                              |
|------------------------|------------------------------------------------------------------------------------------------------|------------------------------------------------------------------------------------------------------------------------------|
| WHICH GENE IS SILENT?  | Maternally derived genes are silenced. Disease occurs when the paternal allele is deleted or mutated  | Paternally derived *UBE3A* is silenced. Disease occurs when the maternal allele is deleted or mutated                         |
| SIGNS AND SYMPTOMS     | Hyperphagia, obesity, intellectual disability, hypogonadism, hypotonia                                | Hand-flapping, Ataxia, severe Intellectual disability, inappropriate Laughter, Seizures. **HAILS** the Angels.                |
| CHROMOSOMES INVOLVED   | Chromosome 15 of paternal origin                                                                     | *UBE3A* on maternal copy of chromosome 15                                                                                     |
| NOTES                  | 25% of cases are due to maternal uniparental disomy                                                   | 5% of cases are due to paternal uniparental disomy                                                                            |
|                        | **POP:** Prader-Willi, Obesity/overeating, Paternal allele deleted                                    | **MAMAS:** Maternal allele deleted, Angelman syndrome, Mood, Ataxia, Seizures                                                 |

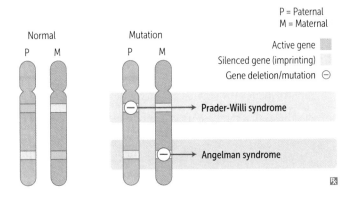

P = Paternal
M = Maternal

Active gene
Silenced gene (imprinting)
Gene deletion/mutation ⊖

## Modes of inheritance

### Autosomal dominant

Often due to defects in structural genes. Many generations, both males and females are affected.

| | A | a |
|---|---|---|
| a | Aa | aa |
| a | Aa | aa |

Often pleiotropic (multiple apparently unrelated effects) and variably expressive (different between individuals). Family history crucial to diagnosis. With one affected (heterozygous) parent, each child has a 50% chance of being affected.

### Autosomal recessive

With 2 carrier (heterozygous) parents, on average: each child has a 25% chance of being affected, 50% chance of being a carrier, and 25% chance of not being affected nor a carrier.

| | A | a |
|---|---|---|
| A | AA | Aa |
| a | Aa | aa |

Often due to enzyme deficiencies. Usually seen in only 1 generation. Commonly more severe than dominant disorders; patients often present in childhood.
↑ risk in consanguineous families.
Unaffected individual with affected sibling has 2/3 probability of being a carrier.

### X-linked recessive

carrier

Sons of heterozygous mothers have a 50% chance of being affected. No male-to-male transmission. Skips generations.

| | X | X | | X | X |
|---|---|---|---|---|---|
| X | XX | XX | X | XX | XX |
| Y | XY | XY | Y | XY | XY |

Commonly more severe in males. Females usually must be homozygous to be affected.

### X-linked dominant

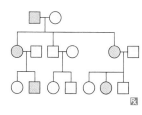

Transmitted through both parents. Children of affected mothers each have a 50% chance of being affected. 100% of daughters and 0% of sons of affected fathers will be affected.

| | X | X | | X | X |
|---|---|---|---|---|---|
| X | XX | XX | X | XX | XX |
| Y | XY | XY | Y | XY | XY |

Examples: fragile X syndrome, Alport syndrome, hypophosphatemic rickets (also called X-linked hypophosphatemia)—phosphate wasting at proximal tubule → ricketslike presentation.

### Mitochondrial inheritance

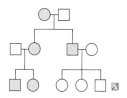

Transmitted only through the mother. All offspring of affected females may show signs of disease.
Variable expression in a population or even within a family due to heteroplasmy.

Caused by mutations in mtDNA.
Examples: mitochondrial myopathies, Leber hereditary optic neuropathy.

☐ = unaffected male;  ▨ = affected male;  ◯ = unaffected female;  ⬤ = affected female.

| | |
|---|---|
| **Autosomal dominant diseases** | Achondroplasia, autosomal dominant polycystic kidney disease, familial adenomatous polyposis, familial hypercholesterolemia, hereditary hemorrhagic telangiectasia (Osler-Weber-Rendu syndrome), hereditary spherocytosis, Huntington disease, Li-Fraumeni syndrome, Marfan syndrome, multiple endocrine neoplasias, myotonic muscular dystrophy, neurofibromatosis type 1 (von Recklinghausen disease), neurofibromatosis type 2, tuberous sclerosis, von Hippel-Lindau disease. |
| **Autosomal recessive diseases** | Mostly consist of enzyme defects. Oculocutaneous albinism, phenylketonuria, cystic fibrosis, sickle cell disease, Wilson disease, sphingolipidoses (except Fabry disease), hemochromatosis, glycogen storage diseases, thalassemia, mucopolysaccharidoses (except Hunter syndrome), Friedreich ataxia, Kartagener syndrome, **ARPKD**. Oh, please! Can students who score high grades tell me features of the kidney disorder **Autosomal Recessive Polycystic Kidney Disease**? |

## Cystic fibrosis

| | |
|---|---|
| GENETICS | Autosomal recessive; defect in CFTR gene on chromosome 7 (deletion; $\Delta$F508). Most common lethal genetic disease in patients with European ancestry. |
| PATHOPHYSIOLOGY | CFTR encodes an ATP-gated $Cl^-$ channel (secretes $Cl^-$ in lungs/GI tract, reabsorbs $Cl^-$ in sweat glands). Phe508 deletion → misfolded protein → improper protein trafficking → protein absent from cell membrane → ↓ $Cl^-$ (and $H_2O$) secretion → compensatory ↑ $Na^+$ reabsorption via epithelial $Na^+$ channels (ENaC) → ↑ $H_2O$ reabsorption → abnormally thick mucus secreted into lungs/GI tract. ↑ $Na^+$ reabsorption → more negative transepithelial potential difference. |
| DIAGNOSIS | ↑ $Cl^-$ concentration in pilocarpine-induced sweat test. Can present with contraction alkalosis and hypokalemia (ECF effects analogous loop diuretic effect) due to ECF $H_2O$/$Na^+$ losses via sweating and concomitant renal $K^+$/$H^+$ wasting. ↑ immunoreactive trypsinogen (newborn screening) due to clogging of pancreatic duct. |
| COMPLICATIONS | Recurrent pulmonary infections (eg, S aureus [infancy and early childhood], P aeruginosa [adulthood], allergic bronchopulmonary aspergillosis [ABPA]), chronic bronchitis and bronchiectasis → reticulonodular pattern on CXR, opacification of sinuses. Nasal polyps, nail clubbing. Pancreatic insufficiency, malabsorption with steatorrhea, and fat-soluble vitamin deficiencies (A, D, E, K) progressing to endocrine dysfunction (CF-related diabetes), biliary cirrhosis, liver disease. Meconium ileus in newborns. Infertility in males (absence of vas deferens, spermatogenesis may be unaffected) and subfertility in females (amenorrhea, abnormally thick cervical mucus). |
| TREATMENT | Multifactorial: chest physiotherapy, aerosolized dornase alfa (DNase), and inhaled hypertonic saline → mucus clearance. Azithromycin prevents acute exacerbations. Ibuprofen for anti-inflammatory effect. Pancreatic enzyme replacement therapy (pancrelipase) for pancreatic insufficiency. CFTR modulators can be used alone or in combination. Efficacy varies by different genetic mutations (pharmacogenomics). Are either potentiators (hold gate of CFTR channel open → $Cl^-$ flows through cell membrane; eg, ivacaftor) or correctors (help CFTR protein to form right 3-D shape → moves to the cell surface; eg, lumacaftor, tezacaftor). |

| | |
|---|---|
| **X-linked recessive diseases** | Bruton agammaglobulinemia, Duchenne and Becker muscular dystrophies, Fabry disease, G6PD deficiency, hemophilia A and B, Hunter syndrome, Lesch-Nyhan syndrome, ocular albinism, ornithine transcarbamylase (OTC) deficiency, Wiskott-Aldrich syndrome. |
| | Females with Turner syndrome (45,XO) are more likely to have an X-linked recessive disorder. |
| | X-inactivation (lyonization)—during development, one of the X chromosomes in each XX cell is randomly deactivated and condensed into a Barr body (methylated heterochromatin). If skewed inactivation occurs, XX individuals may express X-linked recessive diseases (eg, G6PD); penetrance and severity of X-linked dominant diseases in XX individuals may also be impacted. |

## Muscular dystrophies

| | | |
|---|---|---|
| **Duchenne** |  X-linked recessive disorder typically due to **frameshift** deletions or nonsense mutations → truncated or absent dystrophin protein → progressive myofiber damage. Can also result from splicing errors. | Duchenne = deleted dystrophin. Dystrophin gene (*DMD*) is the largest protein-coding human gene → ↑ chance of spontaneous mutation. Dystrophin helps to anchor muscle fibers to the extracellular matrix, primarily in skeletal and cardiac muscles. Loss of dystrophin → myonecrosis. |
| | Weakness begins in pelvic girdle muscles and progresses superiorly. Pseudohypertrophy of calf muscles due to fibrofatty replacement of muscle A. Waddling gait. | ↑ CK and aldolase; genetic testing confirms diagnosis. |
| | Onset before 5 years of age. Dilated cardiomyopathy is common cause of death. |  |
| | **Gowers sign**—patient uses upper extremities to help stand up. Classically seen in Duchenne muscular dystrophy, but also seen in other muscular dystrophies and inflammatory myopathies (eg, polymyositis). | |
| **Becker** | X-linked recessive disorder typically due to **non-frameshift** deletions in dystrophin gene (partially functional instead of truncated). Less severe than Duchenne (Becker is better). Onset in adolescence or early adulthood. | Deletions can cause both Duchenne and Becker muscular dystrophies. ⅔ of cases have large deletions spanning one or more exons. |
| **Myotonic dystrophy** | Autosomal dominant. Onset 20–30 years. CTG trinucleotide repeat expansion in the *DMPK* gene → abnormal expression of myotonin protein kinase → percussion myotonia (eg, difficulty releasing hand from handshake), muscle wasting, cataracts, testicular atrophy, frontal balding, arrhythmia. | Cataracts, Toupee (early balding in males), Gonadal atrophy. Muscle biopsy shows ring fibers and central nuclei. |

| **Mitochondrial diseases** | Rare disorders arising 2° to failure in oxidative phosphorylation. Tissues with ↑ energy requirements are preferentially affected (eg, CNS, skeletal muscle). |
|---|---|
| | **Mitochondrial myopathies**—include **MELAS** (mitochondrial encephalomyopathy with lactic acidosis and strokelike episodes) and **MERRF** (myoclonic epilepsy with ragged red fibers). Light microscopy with stain: ragged red fibers due to compensatory proliferation of mitochondria. Electron microscopy: mitochondrial crystalline inclusions. |
| | **Leber hereditary optic neuropathy**—mutations in complex I of ETC → neuronal death in retina and optic nerve → subacute bilateral vision loss in teens/young adults (males > females). Usually permanent. May be accompanied by neurologic dysfunction (eg, tremors, multiple sclerosis–like illness). |

| **Rett syndrome** | Sporadic disorder caused by de novo mutation of *MECP2* on X chromosome. Seen mostly in females. Embryonically lethal in males. Individuals with **Rett** syndrome experience initial normal development (6–18 months) followed by regression ("**rett**urn") in motor, verbal, and cognitive abilities; ataxia; seizures; scoliosis; and stereotypic hand-wringing. |
|---|---|

| **Fragile X syndrome** | X-linked (atypical) inheritance. Trinucleotide repeats in *FMR1* → hypermethylation of cytosine residues → ↓ expression. Most common inherited cause of intellectual disability (Down syndrome is most common genetic cause, but most cases occur sporadically). | Trinucleotide repeat expansion [$(CGG)_n$] occurs during oogenesis. Premutation (50–200 repeats) → tremor, ataxia, 1° ovarian insufficiency. Full mutation (>200 repeats) → postpubertal macroorchidism (enlarged testes), long face with large jaw, large everted ears, autism, mitral valve prolapse, hypermobile joints. Self-mutilation is common and can be confused with Lesch-Nyhan syndrome. |
|---|---|---|

| **Trinucleotide repeat expansion diseases** | May show genetic anticipation (disease severity ↑ and age of onset ↓ in successive generations). |
|---|---|

| DISEASE | TRINUCLEOTIDE REPEAT | MODE OF INHERITANCE | MNEMONIC |
|---|---|---|---|
| Huntington disease | $(CAG)_n$ | AD | Caudate has ↓ ACh and GABA |
| Myotonic dystrophy | $(CTG)_n$ | AD | Cataracts, Toupee (early balding in males), Gonadal atrophy in males, reduced fertility in females |
| Fragile X syndrome | $(CGG)_n$ | XD | Chin (protruding), Giant Gonads |
| Friedreich ataxia | $(GAA)_n$ | AR | Ataxic GAAit |

| **Autosomal trisomies** | Autosomal trisomies are screened in first and second trimesters with noninvasive prenatal tests. Incidence of trisomies: Down (21) > Edwards (18) > Patau (13). Autosomal monosomies are incompatible with life (high chance of recessive trait expression). |
|---|---|

| **Down syndrome (trisomy 21)**  Single palmar crease ℞ | Findings: intellectual disability, flat facies, prominent epicanthal folds, single palmar crease, incurved 5th finger, gap between 1st 2 toes, duodenal atresia, Hirschsprung disease, congenital heart disease (eg, AVSD), Brushfield spots (whitish spots at the periphery of the iris). Associated with early-onset Alzheimer disease (chromosome 21 codes for amyloid precursor protein), ↑ risk of AML/ALL. 95% of cases due to meiotic nondisjunction, most commonly during meiosis I (↑ with advanced maternal age: from 1:1500 in females < 20 to 1:25 in females > 45). 4% of cases due to unbalanced Robertsonian translocation, most typically between chromosomes 14 and 21. 1% of cases due to postfertilization mitotic error. | Drinking age (21). Most common viable chromosomal disorder and most common cause of genetic intellectual disability. First-trimester ultrasound commonly shows ↑ nuchal translucency and hypoplastic nasal bone. Markers for Down syndrome are **hi** up: ↑ hCG, ↑ inhibin. ↑ risk of umbilical hernia (incomplete closure of umbilical ring). The 5 A's of Down syndrome: <br>▪ Advanced maternal age <br>▪ Atresia (duodenal) <br>▪ Atrioventricular septal defect <br>▪ Alzheimer disease (early onset) <br>▪ AML (<5 years of age)/ALL (>5 years of age) |
|---|---|---|
| **Edwards syndrome (trisomy 18)**  ℞ | Findings: **PRINCE** Edward—**P**rominent occiput, **R**ocker-bottom feet, **I**ntellectual disability, **N**ondisjunction, **C**lenched fists with overlapping fingers, low-set **E**ars, micrognathia (small jaw), congenital heart disease (eg, VSD), omphalocele, myelomeningocele. Death usually occurs by age 1. | Election age (18). 2nd most common autosomal trisomy resulting in live birth (most common is Down syndrome). In Edwards syndrome, every prenatal screening marker decreases. |
| **Patau syndrome (trisomy 13)** Cutis aplasia ℞ | Findings: severe intellectual disability, rocker-bottom feet, microphthalmia, microcephaly, cleft lip/palate, holoprosencephaly, polydactyly, cutis aplasia, congenital heart (pump) disease, polycystic kidney disease, omphalocele. Death usually occurs by age 1. | Puberty at age 13. Defect in fusion of prechordal mesoderm → midline defects. |

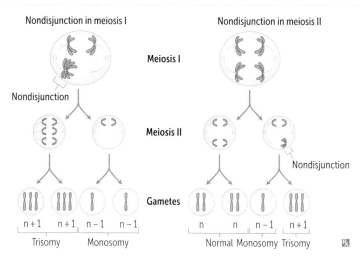

| 1st trimester screening | | |
|---|---|---|
| Trisomy | β-hCG | PAPP-A |
| 21 | ↑ | ↓ |
| 18 | ↓ | ↓ |
| 13 | ↓ | ↓ |

℞

| 2nd trimester (quadruple) screening | | | |
|---|---|---|---|
| Trisomy | hCG | Inhibin A | Estriol | AFP |
| 21 | ↑ | ↑ | ↓ | ↓ |
| 18 | ↓ | — or ↓ | ↓ | ↓ |
| 13 | — | — | — | — |

℞

**Genetic disorders by chromosome**

| CHROMOSOME | SELECTED EXAMPLES |
|---|---|
| 3 | von Hippel-Lindau disease, renal cell carcinoma |
| 4 | ADPKD (*PKD2*), achondroplasia, Huntington disease |
| 5 | Cri-du-chat syndrome, familial adenomatous polyposis |
| 6 | Hemochromatosis (*HFE*) |
| 7 | Williams syndrome, cystic fibrosis |
| 9 | Friedreich ataxia, tuberous sclerosis (*TSC1*) |
| 11 | Wilms tumor, β-globin gene defects (eg, sickle cell disease, β-thalassemia), MEN1 |
| 13 | Patau syndrome, Wilson disease, retinoblastoma (*RB1*), *BRCA2* |
| 15 | Prader-Willi syndrome, Angelman syndrome, Marfan syndrome |
| 16 | ADPKD (*PKD1*), α-globin gene defects (eg, α-thalassemia), tuberous sclerosis (*TSC2*) |
| 17 | Neurofibromatosis type 1, *BRCA1*, *TP53* (Li-Fraumeni syndrome) |
| 18 | Edwards syndrome |
| 21 | Down syndrome |
| 22 | Neurofibromatosis type 2, DiGeorge syndrome (22q11) |
| X | Fragile X syndrome, X-linked agammaglobulinemia, Klinefelter syndrome (XXY) |

**Robertsonian translocation**

Chromosomal translocation that commonly involves chromosome pairs 21, 22, 13, 14, and 15. One of the most common types of translocation. Occurs when the long arms of 2 acrocentric chromosomes (chromosomes with centromeres near their ends) fuse at the centromere and the 2 short arms are lost.

Balanced translocations (no gain or loss of significant genetic material) normally do not cause abnormal phenotype. Unbalanced translocations (missing or extra genes) can result in miscarriage, stillbirth, and chromosomal imbalance (eg, Down syndrome, Patau syndrome).

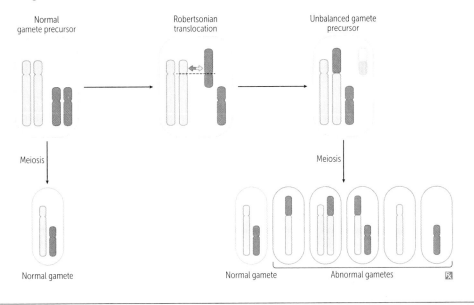

**Cri-du-chat syndrome**

*Cri du chat* = cry of the cat. Congenital deletion on short arm of chromosome 5 (46,XX or XY, 5p–). Findings: microcephaly, moderate to severe intellectual disability, high-pitched **cr**ying, epicanthal folds, cardiac abnormalities (**VSD**). **I cr**y when I am **V**ery **SaD**.

**Williams syndrome**

Congenital microdeletion of long arm of chromosome 7 (deleted region includes elastin gene). Findings: distinctive "elfin" facies, intellectual disability, hypercalcemia, well-developed verbal skills, extreme friendliness with strangers, cardiovascular problems (eg, supravalvular aortic stenosis, pulmonary artery stenosis, renal artery stenosis).

## ▶ BIOCHEMISTRY—NUTRITION

**Essential fatty acids**

Polyunsaturated fatty acids that cannot be synthesized in the body and must be provided in the diet (eg, nuts/seeds, plant oils, seafood). Linoleic acid (omega-6) is metabolized to arachidonic acid, which serves as the precursor to leukotrienes and prostaglandins. Linolenic acid (omega-3) and its metabolites have cardioprotective and antihyperlipidemic effects.

In contrast, consumption of *trans*-unsaturated fatty acids (found in fast food) promotes cardiovascular disease by ↑ LDL and ↓ HDL.

**Vitamins: fat soluble**

A, D, E, K. Absorption dependent on bile emulsification, pancreatic secretions, and intact ileum. Toxicity more common than for water-soluble vitamins because fat-soluble vitamins accumulate in fat.

Malabsorption syndromes with steatorrhea (eg, cystic fibrosis and celiac disease) or mineral oil intake can cause fat-soluble vitamin deficiencies.

**Vitamins: water soluble**

$B_1$ (thiamine: TPP)
$B_2$ (riboflavin: FAD, FMN)
$B_3$ (niacin: $NAD^+$)
$B_5$ (pantothenic acid: CoA)
$B_6$ (pyridoxine: PLP)
$B_7$ (biotin)
$B_9$ (folate)
$B_{12}$ (cobalamin)
C (ascorbic acid)

Wash out easily from body except $B_{12}$ and $B_9$. $B_{12}$ stored in liver for ~ 3–4 years. $B_9$ stored in liver for ~ 3–4 months.
B-complex deficiencies often result in dermatitis, glossitis, and diarrhea.
Can be coenzymes (eg, ascorbic acid) or precursors to coenzymes (eg, FAD, $NAD^+$).

**Dietary supplementation**

| DIET | SUPPLEMENTATION REQUIRED |
| --- | --- |
| Vegetarian/vegan | Vitamin $B_{12}$ <br> Iron <br> Vitamin $B_2$ <br> Frequently, vitamin D (although this is commonly deficient in many diets) |
| High egg white (raw) | Vitamin $B_7$ (avidin in egg whites binds biotin and prevents absorption) |
| Untreated corn | Vitamin $B_3$ (deficiency is common in resource-limited areas) |

## Vitamin A

Includes retinal, retinol, retinoic acid.

| | | |
|---|---|---|
| FUNCTION | Antioxidant; constituent of visual pigments (**retinal**); essential for normal differentiation of epithelial cells into specialized tissue (pancreatic cells, mucus-secreting cells); prevents squamous metaplasia. | **Retinol** is vitamin **A**, so think **retin-A** (used topically for wrinkles and Acne). Found in liver and leafy vegetables. Supplementation in vitamin A-deficient measles patients may improve outcomes. Use oral isotretinoin to treat severe cystic acne. Use *all*-trans retinoic acid to treat acute promyelocytic leukemia. |
| DEFICIENCY | Night blindness (nyctalopia); dry, scaly skin (xerosis cutis); dry eyes (xerophthalmia); conjunctival squamous metaplasia → Bitot spots (keratin debris; foamy appearance on conjunctiva A); corneal degeneration (keratomalacia); immunosuppression. | |
| EXCESS | Acute toxicity—nausea, vomiting, ↑ ICP (eg, vertigo, blurred vision). Chronic toxicity—alopecia, dry skin (eg, scaliness), hepatic toxicity and enlargement, arthralgias, and idiopathic intracranial hypertension. | Teratogenic (interferes with homeobox gene; cleft palate, cardiac abnormalities), therefore a ⊖ pregnancy test and two forms of contraception are required before isotretinoin (vitamin A derivative) is prescribed. Isotretinoin **is teratogenic**. |

## Vitamin B₁

Also called thiamine.

| | |
|---|---|
| FUNCTION | In thiamine pyrophosphate (TPP), a cofactor for several dehydrogenase enzyme reactions (**Be APT**): |
| | ▪ Branched-chain ketoacid dehydrogenase |
| | ▪ α-Ketoglutarate dehydrogenase (TCA cycle) |
| | ▪ Pyruvate dehydrogenase (links glycolysis to TCA cycle) |
| | ▪ Transketolase (HMP shunt) |
| DEFICIENCY | Impaired glucose breakdown → ATP depletion worsened by glucose infusion; highly aerobic tissues (eg, brain, heart) are affected first. In patients with chronic alcohol overuse or malnutrition, give thiamine before dextrose to ↓ risk of precipitating Wernicke encephalopathy. Diagnosis made by ↑ in RBC transketolase activity following vitamin B₁ administration. |

| DISORDER | CHARACTERISTICS | |
|---|---|---|
| **Wernicke encephalopathy** | Acute, reversible, life-threatening neurologic condition. Symptoms: Confusion, Ophthalmoplegia/Nystagmus, Ataxia (**CorONA** beer). | |
| **Korsakoff syndrome** | Amnestic disorder due to chronic alcohol overuse; presents with confabulation, personality changes, memory loss (permanent). | |
| **Wernicke-Korsakoff syndrome** | Damage to medial dorsal nucleus of thalamus, mammillary bodies. Presentation is combination of Wernicke encephalopathy and Korsakoff syndrome. | |
| **Dry beriberi** | Polyneuropathy, symmetric muscle wasting. | Spell beriberi as Ber1Ber1 to remember vitamin B₁. |
| **Wet beriberi** | High-output cardiac failure (due to systemic vasodilation). | |

| **Vitamin B$_2$** | Also called riboflavin. | |
|---|---|---|
| FUNCTION | Component of flavins FAD and FMN, used as cofactors in redox reactions, eg, the succinate dehydrogenase reaction in the TCA cycle. | FAD and FMN are derived from riboFlavin (B$_2$ ≈ 2 ATP). |
| DEFICIENCY | Cheilosis (inflammation of lips, scaling and fissures at the corners of the mouth), "magenta" tongue, corneal vascularization. | The 2 C's of B$_2$. |

| **Vitamin B$_3$** | Also called niacin, nicotinic acid. | |
|---|---|---|
| FUNCTION | Constituent of NAD$^+$, NADP$^+$ (used in redox reactions and as cofactor by dehydrogenases). Derived from tryptophan. Synthesis requires vitamins B$_2$ and B$_6$. Used to treat dyslipidemia (↓ VLDL, ↑ HDL). | NAD derived from Niacin (B$_3$ ≈ 3 ATP). |
| DEFICIENCY | Glossitis. Severe deficiency of B$_3$ leads to pellagra, which can also be caused by Hartnup disease, malignant carcinoid syndrome (↑ tryptophan metabolism → ↑ serotonin synthesis), and isoniazid (↓ vitamin B$_6$). Symptoms of B$_3$ deficiency (pellagra) (the 3 D's): diarrhea, dementia (also hallucinations), dermatitis (C3/C4 dermatome circumferential "broad collar" rash [Casal necklace], hyperpigmentation of sun-exposed limbs ). | **Hartnup disease**—autosomal recessive. Deficiency of neutral amino acid (eg, tryptophan) transporters in proximal renal tubular cells and on enterocytes → neutral aminoaciduria and ↓ absorption from the gut → ↓ tryptophan for conversion to niacin → pellagra-like symptoms. Treat with high-protein diet and nicotinic acid. Pellagra = vitamin B$_3$ levels fell. |
| EXCESS | Facial flushing (induced by prostaglandin, not histamine; can avoid by taking aspirin before niacin), pruritus, hyperglycemia, hyperuricemia. | Podagra = vitamin B$_3$ OD (overdose). |

| **Vitamin B$_5$** | Also called pantothenic acid. B$_5$ is "pento"thenic acid. |
|---|---|
| FUNCTION | Component of coenzyme A (CoA, a cofactor for acyl transfers) and fatty acid synthase. |
| DEFICIENCY | Dermatitis, enteritis, alopecia, adrenal insufficiency may lead to burning sensation of feet ("burning feet syndrome"; distal paresthesias, dysesthesia). |

| **Vitamin B$_6$** | Also called pyridoxine. |
|---|---|
| FUNCTION | Converted to pyridoxal phosphate (PLP), a cofactor used in transamination (eg, ALT and AST), decarboxylation reactions, glycogen phosphorylase. Synthesis of glutathione, cystathionine, heme, niacin, histamine, and neurotransmitters including serotonin, epinephrine, norepinephrine (NE), dopamine, and GABA. |
| DEFICIENCY | Convulsions, hyperirritability, peripheral neuropathy (deficiency inducible by isoniazid and oral contraceptives), sideroblastic anemia (due to impaired hemoglobin synthesis and iron excess). |

| **Vitamin B₇** | Also called biotin. |
| --- | --- |
| FUNCTION | Cofactor for carboxylation enzymes (which add a 1-carbon group):<br>▪ Pyruvate carboxylase (gluconeogenesis): pyruvate (3C) → oxaloacetate (4C)<br>▪ Acetyl-CoA carboxylase (fatty acid synthesis): acetyl-CoA (2C) → malonyl-CoA (3C)<br>▪ Propionyl-CoA carboxylase (fatty acid oxidation and branched-chain amino acid breakdown): propionyl-CoA (3C) → methylmalonyl-CoA (4C) |
| DEFICIENCY | Relatively rare. Dermatitis, enteritis, alopecia. Caused by long-term antibiotic use or excessive ingestion of raw egg whites.<br>"**A**vidin in egg whites avidly binds biotin." |

| **Vitamin B₉** | Also called folate. | |
| --- | --- | --- |
| FUNCTION | Converted to tetrahydrofolic acid (THF), a coenzyme for 1-carbon transfer/methylation reactions.<br>Important for the synthesis of nitrogenous bases in DNA and RNA. | Found in leafy green vegetables. Also produced by gut microbiota. Folate absorbed in jejunum (think foliage in the "jejun"gle).<br>Small reserve pool stored primarily in the liver. |
| DEFICIENCY | Macrocytic, megaloblastic anemia; hypersegmented polymorphonuclear cells (PMNs); glossitis; no neurologic symptoms (as opposed to vitamin B₁₂ deficiency).<br>Labs: ↑ homocysteine, normal methylmalonic acid levels. Seen in chronic alcohol overuse and in pregnancy. | Deficiency can be caused by several drugs (eg, phenytoin, trimethoprim, methotrexate).<br>Supplemental folic acid at least 1 month prior to conception and during pregnancy to ↓ risk of neural tube defects. Give vitamin B₉ for the 9 months of pregnancy, and 1 month prior to conception. |

| **Vitamin B$_{12}$** | Also called cobalamin. | |
|---|---|---|
| FUNCTION | Cofactor for methionine synthase (transfers CH$_3$ groups as methylcobalamin) and methylmalonyl-CoA mutase. Important for DNA synthesis. | Found in animal products. Synthesized only by intestinal microbiota. Site of synthesis in humans is distal to site of absorption; thus B$_{12}$ must be consumed via animal products. |
| DEFICIENCY | Macrocytic, megaloblastic anemia; hypersegmented PMNs; paresthesias and subacute combined degeneration (degeneration of dorsal columns, lateral corticospinal tracts, and spinocerebellar tracts) due to abnormal myelin. Associated with ↑ serum homocysteine and methylmalonic acid levels, along with 2° folate deficiency. Prolonged deficiency → irreversible nerve damage. | Very large reserve pool (several years) stored primarily in the liver. Deficiency caused by malabsorption (eg, sprue, enteritis, *Diphyllobothrium latum*, achlorhydria, bacterial overgrowth, alcohol overuse), lack of intrinsic factor (eg, pernicious anemia, gastric bypass surgery), absence of terminal ileum (surgical resection, eg, for Crohn disease), certain drugs (eg, metformin), or insufficient intake (eg, veganism). B$_9$ (folate) supplementation can mask the hematologic symptoms of B$_{12}$ deficiency, but not the neurologic symptoms. |

| **Vitamin C** | Also called ascorbic acid. | |
|---|---|---|
| FUNCTION | Antioxidant; also facilitates iron absorption by reducing it to Fe$^{2+}$ state. Necessary for hydroxylation of proline and lysine in collagen synthesis. Necessary for dopamine β-hydroxylase (converts dopamine to NE). | Found in fruits and vegetables. Pronounce "**absorbic**" acid. Ancillary treatment for methemoglobinemia by reducing Fe$^{3+}$ to Fe$^{2+}$. |
| DEFICIENCY | Scurvy—swollen gums, easy bruising, petechiae, hemarthrosis, anemia, poor wound healing, perifollicular and subperiosteal hemorrhages, "corkscrew" hair. Weakened immune response. | Deficiency may be precipitated by tea and toast diet. Vitamin C deficiency causes sCurvy due to a Collagen hydroCylation defect. |
| EXCESS | Nausea, vomiting, diarrhea, fatigue, calcium oxalate nephrolithiasis (excess oxalate from vitamin C metabolism). Can ↑ iron toxicity in predisposed individuals by increasing dietary iron absorption (ie, can worsen hemochromatosis or transfusion-related iron overload). | |

| **Vitamin D** | $D_3$ (cholecalciferol) from exposure of skin (stratum basale) to sun, ingestion of fish, milk, plants. $D_2$ (ergocalciferol) from ingestion of plants, fungi, yeasts. Both converted to 25-OH $D_3$ (storage form) in liver and to the active form 1,25-$(OH)_2$ $D_3$ (calcitriol) in kidney. | |
|---|---|---|
| FUNCTION | ↑ intestinal absorption of $Ca^{2+}$ and $PO_4^{3-}$. ↑ bone mineralization at low levels. ↑ bone resorption at higher levels. | |
| REGULATION | ↑ PTH, ↓ $Ca^{2+}$, ↓ $PO_4^{3-}$ → ↑ 1,25-$(OH)_2D_3$ production. 1,25-$(OH)_2D_3$ feedback inhibits its own production. ↑ PTH → ↑ $Ca^{2+}$ reabsorption and ↓ $PO_4^{3-}$ reabsorption in the kidney. | |
| DEFICIENCY | Rickets in children (deformity, such as genu varum "bowlegs" **A**), osteomalacia in adults (bone pain and muscle weakness), hypocalcemic tetany. Caused by malabsorption, ↓ sun exposure, poor diet, chronic kidney disease (CKD), advanced liver disease. Give oral vitamin D to breastfed infants. Darker skin and prematurity predispose to deficiency. | |
| EXCESS | Hypercalcemia, hypercalciuria, loss of appetite, stupor. Seen in granulomatous diseases (↑ activation of vitamin D by epithelioid macrophages). | |

| **Vitamin E** | Includes tocopherol, tocotrienol. | |
|---|---|---|
| FUNCTION | Antioxidant (protects RBCs and neuronal membranes from free radical damage). | |
| DEFICIENCY | Hemolytic anemia, acanthocytosis, muscle weakness, demyelination of posterior columns (↓ proprioception and vibration sensation) and spinocerebellar tract (ataxia). Closely mimics Friedreich ataxia. | Neurologic presentation may appear similar to vitamin $B_{12}$ deficiency, but without megaloblastic anemia, hypersegmented neutrophils, or ↑ serum methylmalonic acid levels. |
| EXCESS | Risk of enterocolitis in enfants (infants) with excess of vitamin E. | High-dose supplementation may alter metabolism of vitamin K–dependent proteins (factors II, VII, IX, X; protein C/S) → enhanced anticoagulant effects of warfarin. |

| **Vitamin K** | Includes phytomenadione, phylloquinone, phytonadione, menaquinone. | |
|---|---|---|
| FUNCTION | Activated by epoxide reductase to the reduced form, which is a cofactor for the γ-carboxylation of glutamic acid residues on various proteins required for blood clotting. Synthesized by intestinal microbiota. | **K** is for **K**oagulation. Necessary for the maturation of clotting factors II, VII, IX, X, and proteins C and S. Warfarin inhibits vitamin K–dependent synthesis of these factors and proteins. |
| DEFICIENCY | Neonatal hemorrhage with ↑ PT and ↑ aPTT but normal bleeding time (neonates have sterile intestines and are unable to synthesize vitamin K). Can also occur after prolonged use of broad-spectrum antibiotics or hepatocellular disease. | Not in breast milk; "breast-fed infants **D**on't **K**now about vitamins **D** and **K**". Neonates are given vitamin K injection at birth to prevent hemorrhagic disease of the newborn. |

| **Zinc** | | |
|---|---|---|
| FUNCTION | Mineral essential for the activity of 100+ enzymes. Important in the formation of zinc fingers (transcription factor motif). | |
| DEFICIENCY  | Delayed wound healing, suppressed immunity, male hypogonadism, ↓ adult hair (axillary, facial, pubic), dysgeusia, anosmia. Associated with acrodermatitis enteropathica A—congenital defect in intestinal zinc absorption manifesting with triad of hair loss, diarrhea, and inflammatory skin rash around body openings (periorificial) and tips of fingers/toes (acral). May predispose to alcoholic cirrhosis. | |

## Protein-energy malnutrition

| Kwashiorkor | Protein malnutrition resulting in skin lesions, edema due to ↓ plasma oncotic pressure (arising from ↓ serum albumin and ↓ antidiuretic hormone), liver malfunction (fatty change due to ↓ apolipoprotein synthesis and deposition). Clinical picture is small child with swollen abdomen A. Kwashiorkor results from protein-deficient **MEALS**: **M**alnutrition **E**dema **A**nemia **L**iver (fatty) **S**kin lesions (eg, hyperkeratosis, dyspigmentation) |  |
|---|---|---|
| Marasmus | Malnutrition not causing edema. Diet is deficient in calories but no nutrients are entirely absent. **M**arasmus results in **m**uscle wasting B. | Linear growth maintained in acute protein-energy malnutrition (vs chronic malnutrition). |

## Ethanol metabolism

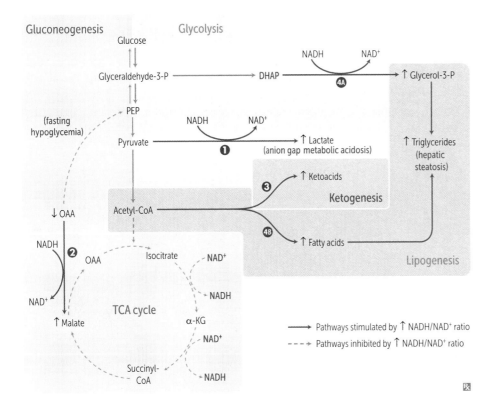

→ Pathways stimulated by ↑ NADH/NAD⁺ ratio
--→ Pathways inhibited by ↑ NADH/NAD⁺ ratio

↑ NADH/NAD⁺ ratio inhibits TCA cycle → ↑ acetyl-CoA used in ketogenesis (→ ketoacidosis), lipogenesis (→ hepatosteatosis).

Females are more susceptible than males to effects of alcohol due to ↓ activity of gastric alcohol dehydrogenase, ↓ body size, ↓ percentage of water in body weight.

NAD⁺ is the limiting reagent.

Alcohol dehydrogenase operates via zero-order kinetics.

Ethanol metabolism ↑ NADH/NAD⁺ ratio in liver, causing:
❶ Lactic acidosis—↑ pyruvate conversion to lactate
❷ Fasting hypoglycemia— ↓ gluconeogenesis due to ↑ conversion of OAA to malate
❸ Ketoacidosis—diversion of acetyl-CoA into ketogenesis rather than TCA cycle
❹ Hepatosteatosis— ↑ conversion of DHAP to glycerol-3-P ❹ⓐ; acetyl-CoA diverges into fatty acid synthesis ❹ⓑ, which combines with glycerol-3-P to synthesize triglycerides

Fomepizole—competitive inhibitor of alcohol dehydrogenase; preferred antidote for overdoses of methanol or ethylene glycol. Alcohol dehydrogenase has higher affinity for ethanol than for methanol or ethylene glycol → ethanol can be used as competitive inhibitor of alcohol dehydrogenase to treat methanol or ethylene glycol poisoning.

Disulfiram—blocks acetaldehyde dehydrogenase → ↑ acetaldehyde → ↑ hangover symptoms → discouraging drinking.

## ▶ BIOCHEMISTRY—METABOLISM

| | |
|---|---|
| **Enzyme terminology** | An enzyme's name often describes its function. For example, glucokinase is an enzyme that catalyzes the phosphorylation of glucose using a molecule of ATP. The following are commonly used enzyme descriptors. |
| Kinase | Catalyzes transfer of a phosphate group from a high-energy molecule (usually ATP) to a substrate (eg, phosphofructokinase). |
| Phosphorylase | Adds inorganic phosphate onto substrate without using ATP (eg, glycogen phosphorylase). |
| Phosphatase | Removes phosphate group from substrate (eg, fructose-1,6-bisphosphatase 1). |
| Dehydrogenase | Catalyzes oxidation-reduction reactions (eg, pyruvate dehydrogenase). |
| Hydroxylase | Adds hydroxyl group (−OH) onto substrate (eg, tyrosine hydroxylase). |
| Carboxylase | Transfers carboxyl groups (−COOH) with the help of biotin (eg, pyruvate carboxylase). |
| Mutase | Relocates a functional group within a molecule (eg, vitamin $B_{12}$–dependent methylmalonyl-CoA mutase). |
| Synthase | Catalyzes synthesis reactions without using ATP as a source of energy |

## Rate-determining enzymes of metabolic processes

| PROCESS | ENZYME | REGULATORS |
|---|---|---|
| Glycolysis | Phosphofructokinase-1 (PFK-1) | AMP ⊕, fructose-2,6-bisphosphate ⊕ ATP ⊖, citrate ⊖ |
| Gluconeogenesis | Fructose-1,6-bisphosphatase 1 | AMP ⊖, fructose-2,6-bisphosphate ⊖ |
| TCA cycle | Isocitrate dehydrogenase | ADP ⊕ ATP ⊖, NADH ⊖ |
| Glycogenesis | Glycogen synthase | Glucose-6-phosphate ⊕, insulin ⊕, cortisol ⊕ Epinephrine ⊖, glucagon ⊖ |
| Glycogenolysis | Glycogen phosphorylase | Epinephrine ⊕, glucagon ⊕, AMP ⊕ Glucose-6-phosphate ⊖, insulin ⊖, ATP ⊖ |
| HMP shunt | Glucose-6-phosphate dehydrogenase (G6PD) | $NADP^+$ ⊕ NADPH ⊖ |
| De novo pyrimidine synthesis | Carbamoyl phosphate synthetase II | ATP ⊕, PRPP ⊕ UTP ⊖ |
| De novo purine synthesis | Glutamine-phosphoribosylpyrophosphate (PRPP) amidotransferase | AMP ⊖, inosine monophosphate (IMP) ⊖, GMP ⊖ |
| Urea cycle | Carbamoyl phosphate synthetase I | N-acetylglutamate ⊕ |
| Fatty acid synthesis | Acetyl-CoA carboxylase (ACC) | Insulin ⊕, citrate ⊕ Glucagon ⊖, palmitoyl-CoA ⊖ |
| Fatty acid oxidation | Carnitine acyltransferase I | Malonyl-CoA ⊖ |
| Ketogenesis | HMG-CoA synthase (HOMG! I'm starving!) | |
| Cholesterol synthesis | HMG-CoA reductase | Insulin ⊕, thyroxine ⊕, estrogen ⊕ Glucagon ⊖, cholesterol ⊖ |

## Metabolic compartmentation

| Mitochondria | Fatty acid oxidation (β-oxidation), acetyl-CoA production, TCA cycle, oxidative phosphorylation, ketogenesis. |
| --- | --- |
| Cytoplasm | Glycolysis, HMP shunt, and synthesis of cholesterol (SER), proteins (ribosomes, RER), fatty acids, and nucleotides. |
| Both | Heme synthesis, urea cycle, gluconeogenesis. Hugs take two (both). |

## Summary of pathways

❶ Galactokinase *(mild galactosemia)*

❷ Galactose-1-phosphate uridyltransferase *(severe galactosemia)*

❸ Hexokinase/glucokinase

❹ Glucose-6-phosphatase *(von Gierke disease)*

❺ Glucose-6-phosphate dehydrogenase

❻ Transketolase

❼ Phosphofructokinase-1

❽ Fructose-1,6-bisphosphatase 1

❾ Fructokinase *(essential fructosuria)*

❿ Aldolase B *(fructose intolerance)*

⓫ Aldolase B *(liver)*, A *(muscle)*

⓬ Triose phosphate isomerase

⓭ Pyruvate kinase

⓮ Pyruvate dehydrogenase

⓯ Pyruvate carboxylase

⓰ PEP carboxykinase

⓱ Citrate synthase

⓲ Isocitrate dehydrogenase

⓳ α-ketoglutarate dehydrogenase

⓴ Carbamoyl phosphate synthetase I

㉑ Ornithine transcarbamylase

㉒ Propionyl-CoA carboxylase

㉓ HMG-CoA reductase

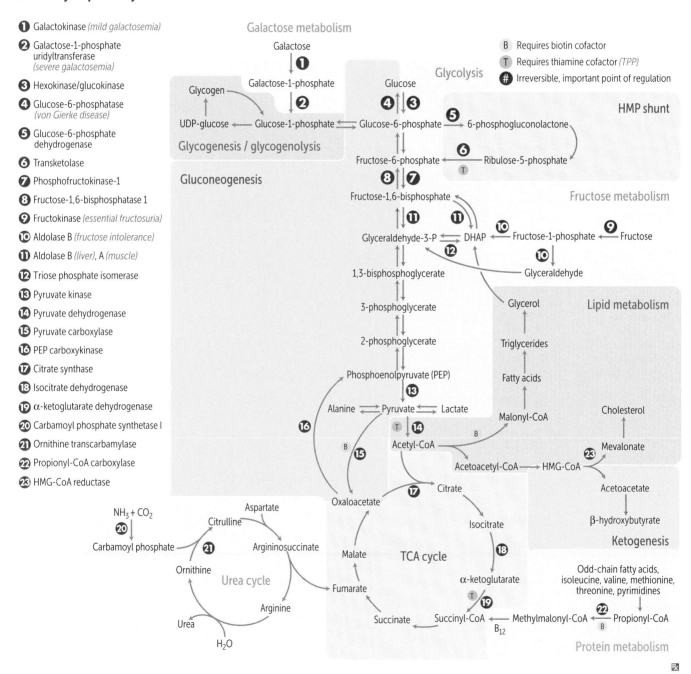

| Activated carriers | CARRIER MOLECULE | CARRIED IN ACTIVATED FORM |
|---|---|---|
| | ATP | Phosphoryl groups |
| | NADH, NADPH, $FADH_2$ | Electrons |
| | CoA, lipoamide | Acyl groups |
| | Biotin | $CO_2$ |
| | Tetrahydrofolates | 1-carbon units |
| | S-adenosylmethionine (SAM) | $CH_3$ groups |
| | TPP | Aldehydes |

**Universal electron acceptors**

Nicotinamides ($NAD^+$, $NADP^+$ from vitamin $B_3$) and flavin nucleotides (FAD from vitamin $B_2$). $NAD^+$ is generally used in **catabolic** processes to carry reducing equivalents away as NADH. NADPH is used in **anabolic** processes (eg, steroid and fatty acid synthesis) as a supply of reducing equivalents.

NADPH is a product of the HMP shunt.
NADPH is used in:
- Anabolic processes
- Respiratory burst
- Cytochrome P-450 system
- Glutathione reductase

**Hexokinase vs glucokinase**

Phosphorylation of glucose to yield glucose-6-phosphate is catalyzed by glucokinase in the liver and hexokinase in other tissues. Hexokinase sequesters glucose in tissues, where it is used even when glucose concentrations are low. At high glucose concentrations, glucokinase helps to store glucose in liver. Glucokinase deficiency (→ ↑↑ glucose needed for activation → impaired insulin release [vs. diabetes mellitus]) is a cause of maturity onset diabetes of the young (MODY) and gestational diabetes.

| | Hexokinase | Glucokinase |
|---|---|---|
| Location | Most tissues, except liver and pancreatic β cells | Liver, β cells of pancreas |
| $K_m$ | Lower (↑ affinity) | Higher (↓ affinity) |
| $V_{max}$ | Lower (↓ capacity) | Higher (↑ capacity) |
| Induced by insulin | No | Yes |
| Feedback inhibition by | Glucose-6-phosphate | Fructose-6-phosphate |

| **Glycolysis regulation, key enzymes** | Net glycolysis (cytoplasm): Glucose + 2 $P_i$ + 2 ADP + 2 $NAD^+$ → 2 pyruvate + 2 ATP + 2 NADH + 2 $H^+$ + 2 $H_2O$. Equation not balanced chemically, and exact balanced equation depends on ionization state of reactants and products. | |

| REQUIRE ATP | Glucose —Hexokinase/glucokinase→ Glucose-6-P | Glucose-6-P ⊖ hexokinase. Fructose-6-P ⊖ glucokinase. |
|---|---|---|
| | Fructose-6-P —Phosphofructokinase-1 (rate-limiting step)→ Fructose-1,6-BP | AMP ⊕, fructose-2,6-bisphosphate ⊕. ATP ⊖, citrate ⊖. |
| PRODUCE ATP | 1,3-BPG ←Phosphoglycerate kinase→ 3-PG | |
| | Phosphoenolpyruvate —Pyruvate kinase→ Pyruvate | Fructose-1,6-bisphosphate ⊕. ATP ⊖, alanine ⊖, glucagon ⊖, epinephrine ⊖. |

| **Regulation by fructose-2,6-bisphosphate** | Fructose bisphosphatase-2 (FBPase-2) and phosphofructokinase-2 (PFK-2) are the same bifunctional enzyme whose function is reversed by phosphorylation by protein kinase A. | |

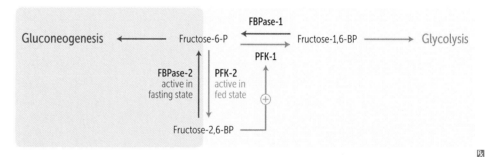

| | Fasting state: ↑ glucagon → ↑ cAMP → ↑ protein kinase A → ↑ FBPase-2, ↓ PFK-2, less glycolysis, more gluconeogenesis. | FaBian the Peasant (**FBP**) has to work hard when starving. |
|---|---|---|
| | Fed state: ↑ insulin → ↓ cAMP → ↓ protein kinase A → ↓ FBPase-2, ↑ PFK-2, more glycolysis, less gluconeogenesis. | Prince FredericK (**PFK**) works only when fed. |

| **Pyruvate dehydrogenase complex** | Mitochondrial enzyme complex linking glycolysis and TCA cycle. Differentially regulated in fed (active)/fasting (inactive) states. Reaction: pyruvate + $NAD^+$ + CoA → acetyl-CoA + $CO_2$ + NADH. Contains 3 enzymes requiring 5 cofactors: 1. Thiamine pyrophosphate ($B_1$) 2. Lipoic acid 3. CoA ($B_5$, pantothenic acid) 4. FAD ($B_2$, riboflavin) 5. $NAD^+$ ($B_3$, niacin) Activated by: ↑ $NAD^+$/NADH ratio, ↑ ADP ↑ $Ca^{2+}$. | The complex is similar to the α-ketoglutarate dehydrogenase complex (same cofactors, similar substrate and action), which converts α-ketoglutarate → succinyl-CoA (TCA cycle). The lovely coenzymes for nerds. Arsenic inhibits lipoic acid. Arsenic poisoning clinical findings: imagine a vampire (pigmentary skin changes, skin cancer), vomiting and having diarrhea, running away from a cutie (QT prolongation) with garlic breath. |

| Pyruvate dehydrogenase complex deficiency | Causes a buildup of pyruvate that gets shunted to lactate (via LDH) and alanine (via ALT). X-linked. |
| --- | --- |
| FINDINGS | Neurologic defects, lactic acidosis, ↑ serum alanine starting in infancy. |
| TREATMENT | ↑ intake of ketogenic nutrients (eg, high fat content or ↑ lysine and leucine), $B_1$ and lipoic acid. |

## Pyruvate metabolism

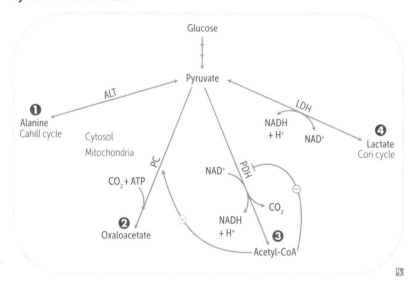

Functions of different pyruvate metabolic pathways (and their associated cofactors):

❶ Alanine aminotransferase ($B_6$): alanine carries amino groups to the liver from muscle

❷ Pyruvate carboxylase ($B_7$): oxaloacetate can replenish TCA cycle or be used in gluconeogenesis

❸ Pyruvate dehydrogenase ($B_1$, $B_2$, $B_3$, $B_5$, lipoic acid): transition from glycolysis to the TCA cycle

❹ Lactic acid dehydrogenase ($B_3$): end of anaerobic glycolysis (major pathway in RBCs, WBCs, kidney medulla, lens, cornea, and Sertoli cells in testes)

## TCA cycle

* Enzymes are irreversible

Also called Krebs cycle. Pyruvate → acetyl-CoA produces 1 NADH, 1 $CO_2$.

The TCA cycle produces 3 NADH, 1 $FADH_2$, 2 $CO_2$, 1 GTP per acetyl-CoA = 10 ATP/acetyl-CoA (2× everything per glucose). TCA cycle reactions occur in the mitochondria.

α-ketoglutarate dehydrogenase complex requires the same cofactors as the pyruvate dehydrogenase complex (vitamins $B_1$, $B_2$, $B_3$, $B_5$, lipoic acid).

Citrate is Krebs' starting substrate for making oxaloacetate.

**Electron transport chain and oxidative phosphorylation**

NADH electrons are transferred to complex I. $FADH_2$ electrons are transferred to complex II (at a lower energy level than NADH).

Oxygen acts as an electron acceptor to provide energy.

The passage of electrons results in the formation of a proton gradient that, coupled to oxidative phosphorylation, drives ATP production. ATP hydrolysis can be coupled to energetically unfavorable reactions.

Uncoupling proteins (found in brown fat, which has more mitochondria than white fat) produce heat by ↑ inner mitochondrial membrane permeability → ↓ proton gradient. ATP synthesis stops, but electron transport continues.

1 NADH → 2.5 ATP; 1 $FADH_2$ → 1.5 ATP

NADH electrons from glycolysis enter mitochondria via the malate-aspartate or glycerol-3-phosphate shuttle.

Aerobic metabolism of one glucose molecule produces 32 net ATP via malate-aspartate shuttle (heart and liver), 30 net ATP via glycerol-3-phosphate shuttle (muscle).

Anaerobic glycolysis produces only 2 net ATP per glucose molecule.

Aspirin overdose can also cause uncoupling of oxidative phosphorylation resulting in hyperthermia.

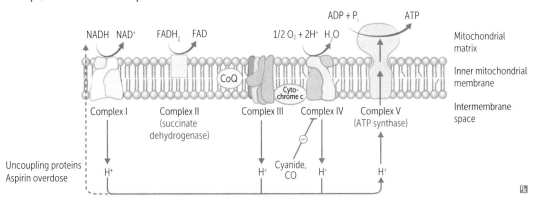

| **Gluconeogenesis, irreversible enzymes** | All enzymes may be subject to activation by glucagon in fasting state. | Pathway produces fresh glucose. |
|---|---|---|
| Pyruvate carboxylase | In mitochondria. Pyruvate → oxaloacetate. | Requires biotin, ATP. Activated by acetyl-CoA. |
| Phosphoenolpyruvate carboxykinase | In cytosol. Oxaloacetate → phosphoenolpyruvate (PEP). | Requires GTP. |
| Fructose-1,6-bisphosphatase 1 | In cytosol. Fructose-1,6-bisphosphate → fructose-6-phosphate. | Citrate ⊕, AMP ⊖, fructose 2,6-bisphosphate ⊖. |
| Glucose-6-phosphatase | In ER. Glucose-6-phosphate → glucose. | |

Occurs primarily in liver; serves to maintain euglycemia during fasting. Enzymes also found in kidney, intestinal epithelium. Deficiency of the key gluconeogenic enzymes causes hypoglycemia. (Muscle cannot participate in gluconeogenesis because it lacks glucose-6-phosphatase).

Odd-chain **fatty acids** yield 1 propionyl-CoA during metabolism, which can enter the TCA cycle (as succinyl-CoA), undergo gluconeogenesis, and serve as a **glucose** source (It's **odd** for **fatty acids** to make **glucose**). Even-chain fatty acids cannot produce new glucose, since they yield only acetyl-CoA equivalents.

| | |
|---|---|
| **Pentose phosphate pathway** | Also called HMP shunt. Provides a source of NADPH from abundantly available glucose-6-P (NADPH is required for reductive reactions, eg, glutathione reduction inside RBCs, fatty acid and cholesterol biosynthesis). Additionally, this pathway yields ribose for nucleotide synthesis. Two distinct phases (oxidative and nonoxidative), both of which occur in the cytoplasm. No ATP is used or produced.<br>Sites: lactating mammary glands, liver, adrenal cortex (sites of fatty acid or steroid synthesis), RBCs. |

REACTIONS

| | |
|---|---|
| Oxidative (irreversible) | |
| Nonoxidative (reversible) | |

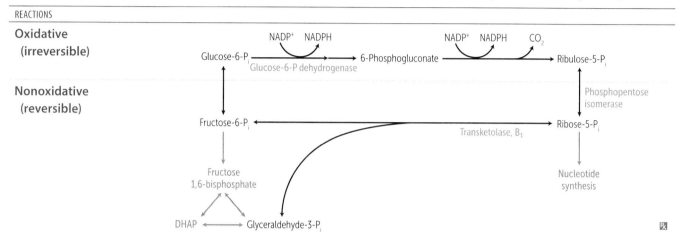

| | |
|---|---|
| **Glucose-6-phosphate dehydrogenase deficiency** | NADPH is necessary to keep glutathione reduced, which in turn detoxifies free radicals and peroxides. ↓ NADPH in RBCs leads to hemolytic anemia due to poor RBC defense against oxidizing agents (eg, fava beans, sulfonamides, nitrofurantoin, primaquine). Infection (most common cause) can also precipitate hemolysis; inflammatory response produces free radicals that diffuse into RBCs, causing oxidative damage. | X-linked recessive disorder; most common human enzyme deficiency; more prevalent among descendants of populations in malaria-endemic regions (eg, sub-Saharan Africa, Southeast Asia).<br>Heinz bodies—denatured globin chains precipitate within RBCs due to oxidative stress.<br>Bite cells—result from the phagocytic removal of Heinz bodies by splenic macrophages. Think, "Bite into some Heinz ketchup." |

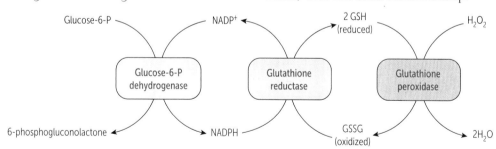

## Disorders of fructose metabolism

|  | Essential fructosuria | Hereditary fructose intolerance |
|---|---|---|
| ENZYME DEFICIENCY | Fructokinase (autosomal recessive) | Aldolase B (autosomal recessive) |
| PATHOPHYSIOLOGY | Fructose is not trapped into cells. Hexokinase becomes 1° pathway for converting fructose to fructose-6-phosphate. | Fructose-1-phosphate accumulates → ↓ available phosphate → inhibition of glycogenolysis and gluconeogenesis. |
| PRESENTATION (SIGNS/SYMPTOMS) | Asymptomatic, benign. Fructose appears in blood and urine (fructokinase deficiency is kinder). | Hypoglycemia, jaundice, cirrhosis, vomiting. Symptoms only present following consumption of fruit, juice, or honey. |
| ADDITIONAL REMARKS | Urine dipstick will be ⊖ (tests for glucose only); reducing sugar can be detected in the urine (nonspecific test for inborn errors of carbohydrate metabolism). | |
| TREATMENT | – | ↓ intake of fructose, sucrose (glucose + fructose), and sorbitol (metabolized to fructose). |

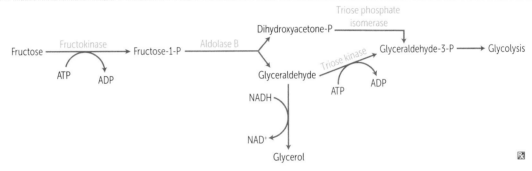

## Disorders of galactose metabolism

|  | Galactokinase deficiency | Classic galactosemia |
|---|---|---|
| ENZYME DEFICIENCY | Galactokinase (autosomal recessive). | Galactose-1-phosphate uridyltransferase (autosomal recessive). |
| PATHOPHYSIOLOGY | Galactitol accumulates if diet has galactose. | Damage caused by accumulation of toxic substances (eg, galactitol). |
| PRESENTATION (SIGNS/SYMPTOMS) | Relatively mild/benign condition (galactokinase deficiency is kinder). Galactose appears in blood (galactosemia) and urine (galactosuria); infantile cataracts. May present as failure to track objects or develop social smile. | Symptoms start when infant is fed formula or breast milk → failure to thrive, jaundice, hepatomegaly, infantile cataracts (galacitol deposition in eye lens), intellectual disability. Can predispose neonates to *E coli* sepsis. |
| TREATMENT | – | Exclude galactose and lactose (galactose + glucose) from diet. |

Galactose → (Galactokinase, ATP → ADP) → Galactose-1-P → (Uridylyltransferase) → Glucose-1-P

Galactose → (Aldose reductase) → Galactitol

Galactose-1-P → UDP-Glu / UDP-Gal (4-Epimerase) → Glucose-1-P → Glycolysis/glycogenesis

**Sorbitol**

An alternative method of trapping glucose in the cell is to convert it to its alcohol counterpart, sorbitol, via aldose reductase. Some tissues then convert sorbitol to fructose using sorbitol dehydrogenase; tissues with an insufficient amount/activity of this enzyme are at risk of intracellular sorbitol accumulation, causing osmotic damage (eg, cataracts, retinopathy, and peripheral neuropathy seen with chronic hyperglycemia in diabetes).

High blood levels of galactose also result in conversion to the osmotically active galactitol via aldose reductase.

Liver, ovaries, and seminal vesicles have both enzymes (they lose sorbitol).

Lens has primarily Aldose reductase. Retina, Kidneys, and Schwann cells have only aldose reductase (LARKS).

---

**Lactase deficiency**

Insufficient lactase enzyme → dietary lactose intolerance. Lactase functions on the intestinal brush border to digest lactose (in milk and milk products) into glucose and galactose.

Primary: age-dependent decline after childhood (absence of lactase-persistent allele), common in people of Asian, African, or Native American descent.

Secondary: loss of intestinal brush border due to gastroenteritis (eg, rotavirus), autoimmune disease.

Congenital lactase deficiency: rare, due to defective gene.

Stool demonstrates ↓ pH and breath shows ↑ hydrogen content with lactose hydrogen breath test ($H^+$ is produced when colonic bacteria ferment undigested lactose). Intestinal biopsy reveals normal mucosa in patients with hereditary lactose intolerance.

FINDINGS

Bloating, cramps, flatulence (all due to fermentation of lactose by colonic bacteria → gas), and osmotic diarrhea (undigested lactose).

TREATMENT

Avoid dairy products or add lactase pills to diet; lactose-free milk.

---

**Amino acids**

Only L-amino acids are found in proteins.

**Essential**

PVT TIM HaLL: Phenylalanine, Valine, Tryptophan, Threonine, Isoleucine, Methionine, Histidine, Leucine, Lysine.

Glucogenic: Methionine, histidine, valine. We met his valentine, who is so sweet (glucogenic).

Glucogenic/ketogenic: Isoleucine, phenylalanine, threonine, tryptophan.

Ketogenic: leucine, lysine. The only purely ketogenic amino acids.

**Acidic**

Aspartic acid, glutamic acid.
Negatively charged at body pH.

**Basic**

Histidine, lysine, arginine.
Arginine is most basic. Histidine has no charge at body pH.
Arginine and histidine are required during periods of growth.
Arginine and lysine are ↑ in histones which bind negatively charged DNA.
His lys (lies) are basic.

## Urea cycle

Amino acid catabolism generates common metabolites (eg, pyruvate, acetyl-CoA), which serve as metabolic fuels. Excess nitrogen is converted to urea and excreted by the kidneys.

Ordinarily, Careless Crappers Are Also Frivolous About Urination.

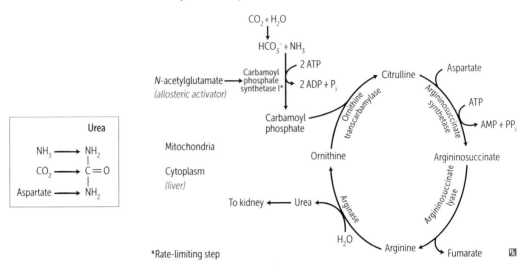

Urea

$$NH_3 \longrightarrow NH_2$$
$$CO_2 \longrightarrow C=O$$
$$Aspartate \longrightarrow NH_2$$

Mitochondria

Cytoplasm
(liver)

*Rate-limiting step

## Transport of ammonia by alanine

## Hyperammonemia

Asterixis

Can be acquired (eg, liver disease) or hereditary (eg, urea cycle enzyme deficiencies).
Presents with flapping tremor (asterixis), slurring of speech, somnolence, vomiting, cerebral edema, blurring of vision.
↑ $NH_3$ changes relative amounts of α-ketoglutarate, glutamate, GABA, and glutamine. CNS toxicity mainly involves:
  ▪ ↑ GABAergic tone (↑ GABA)
  ▪ TCA cycle inhibition (↓ α-ketoglutarate)
  ▪ Cerebral edema (glutamine induced osmotic shifts)

Treatment: limit protein in diet.
May be given to ↓ ammonia levels:
  ▪ Lactulose to acidify GI tract and trap $NH_4^+$ for excretion.
  ▪ Antibiotics (eg, rifaximin) to ↓ ammoniagenic bacteria.
  ▪ Benzoate, phenylacetate, or phenylbutyrate react with glycine or glutamine, forming products that are excreted renally.

**Ornithine transcarbamylase deficiency**

Most common urea cycle disorder. X-linked recessive (vs other urea cycle enzyme deficiencies, which are autosomal recessive). Interferes with the body's ability to eliminate ammonia. Often evident in the first few days of life, but may present later. Excess carbamoyl phosphate is converted to orotic acid (part of the pyrimidine synthesis pathway; vs. carbamoyl phosphate synthetase I deficiency).

Findings: ↑ orotic acid in blood and urine, ↓ BUN, symptoms of hyperammonemia. No megaloblastic anemia (vs orotic aciduria).

**Amino acid derivatives**

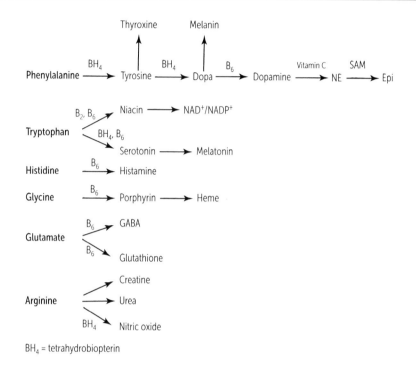

BH₄ = tetrahydrobiopterin

**Catecholamine synthesis/tyrosine catabolism**

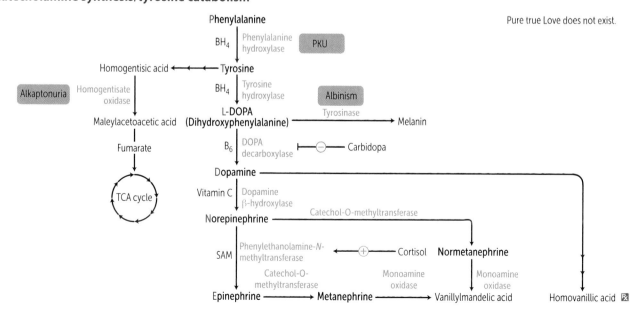

Pure true Love does not exist.

**Phenylketonuria**

Caused by ↓ phenylalanine hydroxylase (PAH). Tyrosine becomes essential. ↑ phenylalanine → ↑ phenyl ketones in urine.

Tetrahydrobiopterin ($BH_4$) deficiency—$BH_4$ essential cofactor for PAH. $BH_4$ deficiency → ↑ phenylalanine. Varying degrees of clinical severity. Untreated patients typically die in infancy.

Phenylalanine embryopathy—↑ phenylalanine levels in pregnant patients with untreated PKU can cause fetal growth restriction, microcephaly, intellectual disability, congenital heart defects. Can be prevented with dietary measures.

Autosomal recessive.

Screening occurs 2–3 days after birth (normal at birth because of maternal enzyme during fetal life).

Findings: intellectual disability, microcephaly, seizures, hypopigmented skin, eczema, musty body odor. Findings are rare due to neonatal screening.

Treatment: ↓ phenylalanine and ↑ tyrosine in diet (eg, soy products, chicken, fish, milk), tetrahydrobiopterin supplementation.

Phenyl ketones—phenylacetate, phenyllactate, and phenylpyruvate.

Disorder of aromatic amino acid metabolism → musty body odor.

Patients with PKU must avoid the artificial sweetener aspartame, which contains phenylalanine.

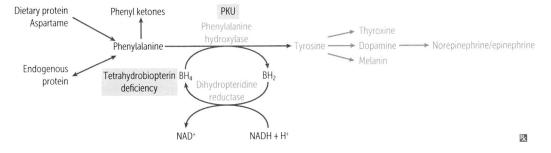

**Maple syrup urine disease**

Blocked degradation of branched amino acids (isoleucine, leucine, valine) due to ↓ branched-chain α-ketoacid dehydrogenase ($B_1$). Causes ↑ α-ketoacids in the blood, especially those of leucine.

Treatment: restriction of isoleucine, leucine, valine in diet, and thiamine supplementation.

Autosomal recessive.

Presentation: vomiting, poor feeding, urine smells like maple syrup/burnt sugar. Causes progressive neurological decline.

I love Vermont maple syrup from maple trees (with $B_1$ranches).

**Alkaptonuria**

Congenital deficiency of homogentisate oxidase in the degradative pathway of tyrosine to fumarate → pigment-forming homogentisic acid builds up in tissue. Autosomal recessive. Usually benign.

Findings: bluish-black connective tissue, ear cartilage, and sclerae (ochronosis ); urine turns black on prolonged exposure to air. May have debilitating arthralgias (homogentisic acid toxic to cartilage).

**Homocystinuria**

Causes (all autosomal recessive):
- Cystathionine synthase deficiency (treatment: ↓ methionine, ↑ cysteine, ↑ $B_6$, $B_{12}$, and folate in diet)
- ↓ affinity of cystathionine synthase for pyridoxal phosphate (treatment: ↑↑ $B_6$ and ↑ cysteine in diet)
- Methionine synthase (homocysteine methyltransferase) deficiency (treatment: ↑ methionine in diet)
- Methylenetetrahydrofolate reductase (MTHFR) deficiency (treatment: ↑ folate in diet)

All forms result in excess homocysteine. HOMOCYstinuria: ↑↑ Homocysteine in urine, Osteoporosis, Marfanoid habitus, Ocular changes (downward and inward lens subluxation), Cardiovascular effects (thrombosis and atherosclerosis → stroke and MI), kYphosis, intellectual disability, hypopigmented skin. In homocystinuria, lens subluxes "down and in" (vs Marfan, "up and fans out").

**Cystinuria**

Hereditary defect of renal PCT and intestinal amino acid transporter that prevents reabsorption of Cystine, Ornithine, Lysine, and Arginine (COLA).

Cystine is made of 2 cysteines connected by a disulfide bond.

Excess cystine in the urine can lead to recurrent precipitation of hexagonal cystine stones.

Treatment: urinary alkalinization (eg, potassium citrate, acetazolamide) and chelating agents (eg, penicillamine) ↑ solubility of cystine stones; good hydration; diet low in methionine.

Autosomal recessive. Common (1:7000).

Cystinuria detected with urinary sodium-cyanide nitroprusside test and proton nuclear magnetic resonance spectroscopy of urine.

**Organic acidemias**

Most commonly present in infancy with poor feeding, vomiting, hypotonia, high anion gap metabolic acidosis, hepatomegaly, seizures. Organic acid accumulation:
- Inhibits gluconeogenesis → ↓ fasting blood glucose levels, ↑ ketoacidosis → high anion gap metabolic acidosis
- Inhibits urea cycle → hyperammonemia

**Propionic acidemia**

Deficiency of propionyl-CoA carboxylase → ↑ propionyl-CoA, ↓ methylmalonic acid.

Treatment: low-protein diet limited in substances that metabolize into propionyl-CoA: Valine, Odd-chain fatty acids, Methionine, Isoleucine, Threonine (VOMIT).

**Methylmalonic acidemia**

Deficiency of methylmalonyl-CoA mutase or vitamin $B_{12}$.

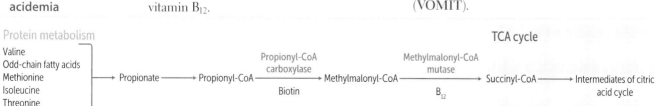

## Glycogen regulation by insulin and glucagon/epinephrine

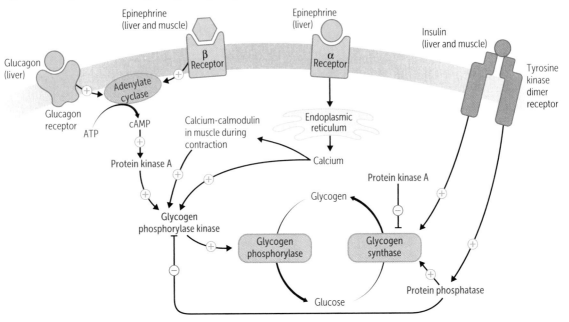

| Glycogen | Branches have α-(1,6) bonds; linear linkages have α-(1,4) bonds. |
|---|---|
| **Skeletal muscle** | Glycogen undergoes glycogenolysis → glucose-1-phosphate → glucose-6-phosphate, which is rapidly metabolized during exercise. |
| **Hepatocytes** | Glycogen is stored and undergoes glycogenolysis to maintain blood sugar at appropriate levels. Glycogen phosphorylase ❺ liberates glucose-1-phosphate residues off branched glycogen until 4 glucose units remain on a branch. Then 4-α-D-glucanotransferase (debranching enzyme ❻) moves 3 of the 4 glucose units from the branch to the linear linkage. Then α-1,6-glucosidase (debranching enzyme ❼) cleaves off the last residue, liberating a free glucose.<br>Limit dextrin—2–4 residues remaining on a branch after glycogen phosphorylase has shortened it. |

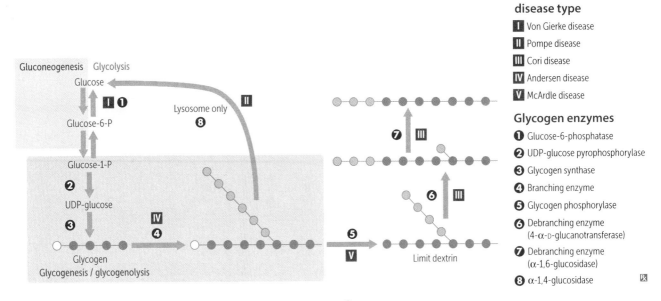

**Glycogen storage disease type**

**I** Von Gierke disease
**II** Pompe disease
**III** Cori disease
**IV** Andersen disease
**V** McArdle disease

**Glycogen enzymes**

❶ Glucose-6-phosphatase
❷ UDP-glucose pyrophosphorylase
❸ Glycogen synthase
❹ Branching enzyme
❺ Glycogen phosphorylase
❻ Debranching enzyme (4-α-D-glucanotransferase)
❼ Debranching enzyme (α-1,6-glucosidase)
❽ α-1,4-glucosidase

Note: A small amount of glycogen is degraded in lysosomes by ❽ α-1,4-glucosidase (acid maltase).

**Glycogen storage diseases**

At least 15 types have been identified, all resulting in abnormal glycogen metabolism and an accumulation of glycogen within cells. Periodic acid–Schiff stain identifies glycogen and is useful in identifying these diseases.

Vice president can't accept money. Types I-V are autosomal recessive. Andersen: Branching. Cori: Debranching. (ABCD)

| DISEASE | FINDINGS | DEFICIENT ENZYME | COMMENTS |
|---|---|---|---|
| **Von Gierke disease (type I)** | Severe fasting hypoglycemia, ↑↑ Glycogen in liver and kidneys, ↑ blood lactate, ↑ triglycerides, ↑ uric acid (Gout), and hepatomegaly, renomegaly. Liver does not regulate blood glucose. | Glucose-6-phosphatase. | Treatment: frequent oral glucose/cornstarch; avoidance of fructose and galactose. Impaired gluconeogenesis and glycogenolysis. |
| **Pompe disease (type II)** | Cardiomyopathy, hypotonia, exercise intolerance, enlarged tongue, and systemic findings lead to early death. | Lysosomal acid $\alpha$-1,4-glucosidase (acid maltase). | Pompe trashes the pump (1st and 4th letter; heart, liver, and muscle). |
| **Cori disease (type III)** | Similar to von Gierke disease, but milder symptoms and normal blood lactate levels. Can lead to cardiomyopathy. Limit dextrin–like structures accumulate in cytosol; can lead to hepatomegaly, cirrhosis, and hepatic adenomas. | Debranching enzymes ($\alpha$-1,6-glucosidase and 4-$\alpha$-D-glucanotransferase). | Gluconeogenesis is intact. |
| **Andersen disease (type IV)** | Most commonly presents with hepatosplenomegaly and failure to thrive in early infancy. Other findings include infantile cirrhosis, muscular weakness, hypotonia, cardiomyopathy early childhood death. | Branching enzyme. Neuromuscular form can present at any age. | Hypoglycemia occurs late in the disease. |
| **McArdle disease (type V)** | ↑ glycogen in muscle, but muscle cannot break it down → painful muscle cramps, myoglobinuria (red urine) with strenuous exercise, and arrhythmia from electrolyte abnormalities. Second-wind phenomenon noted during exercise due to ↑ muscular blood flow. | Skeletal muscle glycogen phosphorylase (myophosphorylase). Characterized by a flat venous lactate curve with normal rise in ammonia levels during exercise. | Blood glucose levels typically unaffected. McArdle = muscle. |

**Lysosomal storage diseases**

Lysosomal enzyme deficiency → accumulation of abnormal metabolic products. ↑ incidence of Tay-Sachs, Niemann-Pick, and some forms of Gaucher disease in Ashkenazi Jews.

| DISEASE | FINDINGS | DEFICIENT ENZYME | ACCUMULATED SUBSTRATE | INHERITANCE |
|---|---|---|---|---|
| **Sphingolipidoses** | | | | |
| **Tay-Sachs disease** | Progressive neurodegeneration, developmental delay, hyperreflexia, hyperacusis, "cherry-red" spot on macula A (lipid accumulation in ganglion cell layer), lysosomes with onion skin, no hepatosplenomegaly (vs Niemann-Pick). | ❶ Hexosaminidase A ("TAy-Sax"). | $GM_2$ ganglioside. | AR |
| **Fabry disease** | Early: triad of episodic peripheral neuropathy, angiokeratomas B, hypohidrosis. Late: progressive renal failure, cardiovascular disease. | ❷ α-galactosidase A; treat with recombinant α-galactosidase. | Ceramide trihexoside (globotriaosylce-ramide). | XR |
| **Metachromatic leukodystrophy** | Central and peripheral demyelination with ataxia, dementia. | ❸ Arylsulfatase A. | Cerebroside sulfate. | AR |
| **Krabbe disease** | Peripheral neuropathy, destruction of oligodendrocytes, developmental delay, CN II atrophy, globoid cells. | ❹ Galactocerebrosi-dase (galactosylce-ramidase). | Galactocerebroside, psychosine. | AR |
| **Gaucher disease** | Most common. Hepatosplenomegaly, pancytopenia, osteoporosis, avascular necrosis of femur, bone crises, Gaucher cells (lipid-laden macrophages resembling crumpled tissue paper C). | ❺ Glucocerebrosidase (β-glucosidase); treat with recombinant glucocerebrosidase. | Glucocerebroside. | AR |
| **Niemann-Pick disease** | Progressive neurodegeneration, hepatosplenomegaly, foam cells (lipid-laden macrophages) D, "cherry-red" spot on macula A. | ❻ Sphingomyelinase. | Sphingomyelin. | AR |
| **Mucopolysaccharidoses** | | | | |
| **Hurler syndrome** | Developmental delay, hirsutism, skeletal anomalies, airway obstruction, clouded cornea, hepatosplenomegaly. | α-L-iduronidase. | Heparan sulfate, dermatan sulfate. | AR |
| **Hunter syndrome** | Mild Hurler + aggressive behavior, no corneal clouding. | Iduronate-2 (two)-sulfatase. | | XR |

Hunters see clearly (no corneal clouding) and aggressively aim for the X (X-linked recessive).

## Fatty acid metabolism

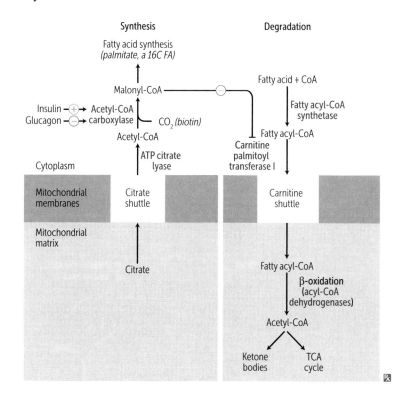

Fatty acid synthesis requires transport of citrate from mitochondria to cytosol. Predominantly occurs in liver, lactating mammary glands, and adipose tissue.

Long-chain fatty acid (LCFA) degradation requires carnitine-dependent transport into the mitochondrial matrix.

"Sytrate" = synthesis.

Carnitine = carnage of fatty acids.

**Systemic 1° carnitine deficiency**—no cellular uptake of carnitine → no transport of LCFAs into mitochondria → toxic accumulation of LCFAs in the cytosol. Causes weakness, hypotonia, hypoketotic hypoglycemia, dilated cardiomyopathy.

**Medium-chain acyl-CoA dehydrogenase deficiency**—↓ ability to break down fatty acids into acetyl-CoA → accumulation of fatty acyl carnitines and dicarboxylic acids in the blood with hypoketotic hypoglycemia. Causes vomiting, lethargy, seizures, coma, liver dysfunction, hyperammonemia. Can lead to sudden death in infants or children. Treat by avoiding fasting.

## Ketone bodies

In the liver, fatty acids and amino acids are metabolized to acetoacetate and β-hydroxybutyrate (to be used in muscle and brain).

In prolonged starvation and diabetic ketoacidosis, oxaloacetate is depleted for gluconeogenesis. With chronic alcohol overuse, high NADH state leads to accumulation of oxaloacetate (downregulated TCA cycle), shunting it to malate.

Ketone bodies: acetone (ketone), acetoacetate (ketoacid), β-hydroxybutyrate (ketoacid).

Breath smells like acetone (fruity odor).

Urine test for ketones can detect acetoacetate, but not β-hydroxybutyrate.

RBCs cannot utilize ketone bodies; they strictly use glucose. Liver cells lack β ketoacyl-CoA transferase → cannot use ketone bodies as fuel.

HMG-CoA lyase for ketone body production.

HMG-CoA reductase for cholesterol synthesis.

| | Hyperammonemia | Hypoketosis | Ketosis |
|---|---|---|---|
| KETONE LEVELS | Normal | ↓ | ↑ |
| GLUCOSE LEVELS | Normal | ↓ | ↓ |
| DEFICIENCY | OTC (urea cycle) | MCAD deficiency | Methylmalonic acidemia, propionic acidemia |

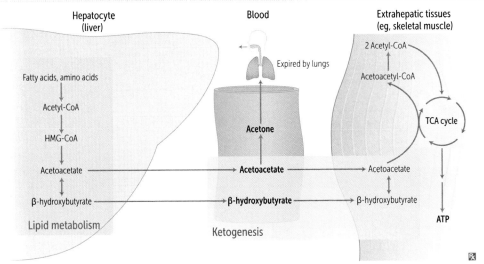

## Fasted vs fed state

## Metabolic fuel use

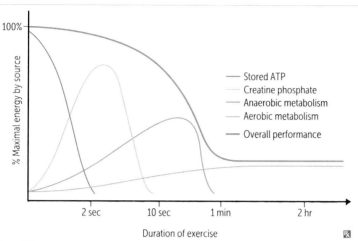

1g carb/protein = 4 kcal
1g alcohol = 7 kcal
1g fatty acid = 9 kcal
(# letters = # kcal)

| Fasting and starvation | Priorities are to supply sufficient glucose to the brain and RBCs and to preserve protein. | |
|---|---|---|
| Fed state (after a meal) | Glycolysis and aerobic respiration. | Insulin stimulates triglycerides (lipids) and glycogen (carbohydrate) storage plus protein synthesis. |
| Fasting (between meals) | Hepatic glycogenolysis (major); hepatic gluconeogenesis, adipose release of FFA (minor). | Glucagon and epinephrine stimulate use of fuel reserves. |
| Starvation days 1–3 | Blood glucose levels maintained by:<br>▪ Hepatic glycogenolysis<br>▪ Adipose release of FFA<br>▪ Muscle and liver, which shift fuel use from glucose to FFA<br>▪ Hepatic gluconeogenesis from peripheral tissue lactate and alanine, and from adipose tissue glycerol and propionyl-CoA (from odd-chain FFA—the only triacylglycerol component that contributes to gluconeogenesis) | Glycogen reserves depleted after day 1. RBCs lack mitochondria and therefore cannot use ketone bodies. |
| Starvation after day 3 | Adipose stores (ketone bodies become the main source of energy for the brain). After these are depleted, vital protein degradation accelerates, leading to organ failure and death. Amount of excess stores determines survival time. | |

# Lipid transport

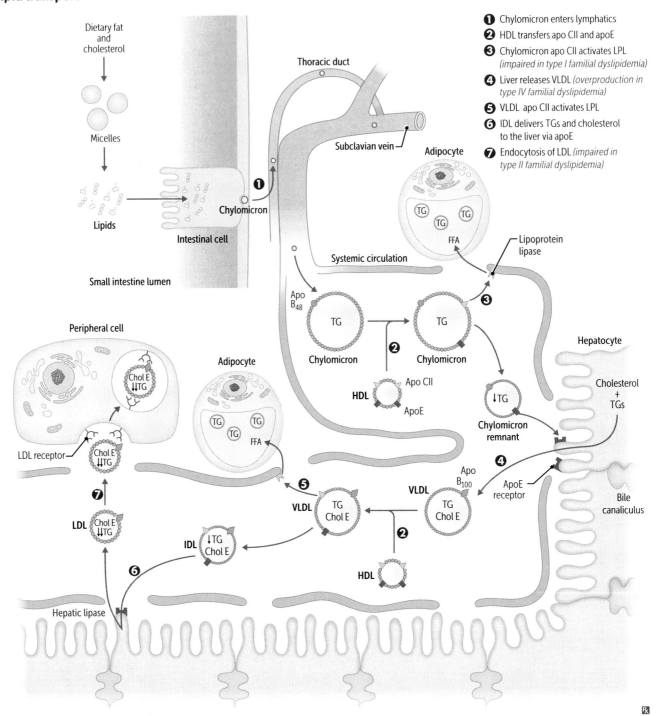

Dietary fat
and
cholesterol

Micelles

Lipids

Small intestine lumen

Intestinal cell

Thoracic duct

Subclavian vein

Chylomicron

❶

Systemic circulation

Adipocyte

TG   TG

TG

FFA

Lipoprotein
lipase

Apo
B₄₈

TG

Chylomicron

❷

TG

Chylomicron

❸

Hepatocyte

HDL

Apo CII

ApoE

↓TG

Chylomicron
remnant

Cholesterol
+
TGs

❹

Apo
B₁₀₀

VLDL

TG
Chol E

ApoE
receptor

Bile
canaliculus

Peripheral cell

Chol E
↓↓TG

Adipocyte

TG   TG

TG  FFA

LDL receptor

Chol E
↓↓TG

❼

❺

VLDL

TG
Chol E

VLDL

❷

HDL

LDL

Chol E
↓↓TG

IDL

↓TG
Chol E

❻

Hepatic lipase

❶ Chylomicron enters lymphatics
❷ HDL transfers apo CII and apoE
❸ Chylomicron apo CII activates LPL
   (impaired in type I familial dyslipidemia)
❹ Liver releases VLDL (overproduction in
   type IV familial dyslipidemia)
❺ VLDL apo CII activates LPL
❻ IDL delivers TGs and cholesterol
   to the liver via apoE
❼ Endocytosis of LDL (impaired in
   type II familial dyslipidemia)

℞

## Key enzymes in lipid transport

| | |
|---|---|
| Cholesteryl ester transfer protein | Mediates transfer of cholesteryl esters to other lipoprotein particles. |
| Hepatic lipase | Degrades TGs remaining in IDL and chylomicron remnants. |
| Hormone-sensitive lipase | Degrades TGs stored in adipocytes. Promotes gluconeogenesis by releasing glycerol. |
| Lecithin-cholesterol acyltransferase | Catalyzes esterification of $\frac{2}{3}$ of plasma cholesterol (ie, required for HDL maturation). |
| Lipoprotein lipase | Degrades TGs in circulating chylomicrons and VLDL. |
| Pancreatic lipase | Degrades dietary TGs in small intestine. |
| PCSK9 | Degrades LDL receptor → ↑ serum LDL. Inhibition → ↑ LDL receptor recycling → ↓ serum LDL. |

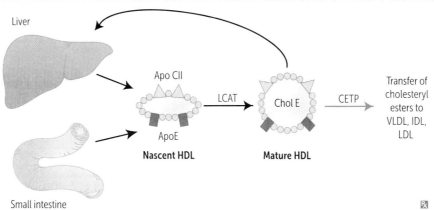

## Major apolipoproteins

| APOLIPOPROTEIN | FUNCTION | CHYLOMICRON | CHYLOMICRON REMNANT | VLDL | IDL | LDL | HDL |
|---|---|---|---|---|---|---|---|
| E | Mediates remnant uptake (everything except LDL) | ✓ | ✓ | ✓ | ✓ | | ✓ |
| AI | Found only on alpha-lipoproteins (HDL), activates LCAT | | | | | | ✓ |
| CII | Lipoprotein lipase cofactor that catalyzes cleavage | ✓ | | ✓ | ✓ | | ✓ |
| $B_{48}$ | Mediates chylomicron secretion into lymphatics. Only on particles originating from the intestines | ✓ | ✓ | | | | |
| $B_{100}$ | Binds LDL receptor. Only on particles originating from the liver (I hope I live to Be 100) | | | ✓ | ✓ | ✓ | |

| | |
|---|---|
| **Lipoprotein functions** | Lipoproteins are composed of varying proportions of proteins, cholesterol, TGs, and phospholipids. LDL and HDL carry the most cholesterol.<br>Cholesterol is needed to maintain cell membrane integrity and synthesize bile acids, steroids, and vitamin D. |
| **Chylomicron** | Delivers dietary TGs to peripheral tissues. Delivers cholesterol to liver in the form of chylomicron remnants, which are mostly depleted of their TGs. Secreted by intestinal epithelial cells. |
| **VLDL** | Delivers hepatic TGs to peripheral tissue. Secreted by liver. |
| **IDL** | Delivers TGs and cholesterol to liver. Formed from degradation of VLDL. |
| **LDL** | Delivers hepatic cholesterol to peripheral tissues. Formed by hepatic lipase modification of IDL in the liver and peripheral tissue. Taken up by target cells via receptor-mediated endocytosis. LDL is Lethal. |
| **HDL** | Mediates reverse cholesterol transport from peripheral tissues to liver. Acts as a repository for apoC and apoE (which are needed for chylomicron and VLDL metabolism). Secreted from both liver and intestine. Alcohol ↑ synthesis. HDL is Healthy. |

| | |
|---|---|
| **Abetalipoproteinemia**<br> | Autosomal recessive. Mutation in gene that encodes microsomal transfer protein ($MTP$). Chylomicrons, VLDL, LDL absent. Deficiency in apo $B_{48}$– and apo $B_{100}$–containing lipoproteins. Affected infants present with severe fat malabsorption, steatorrhea, failure to thrive. Later manifestations include retinitis pigmentosa, spinocerebellar degeneration due to vitamin E deficiency, progressive ataxia, acanthocytosis. Intestinal biopsy shows lipid-laden enterocytes (arrow in A).<br>Treatment: restriction of long-chain fatty acids, large doses of oral vitamin E. |

### Familial dyslipidemias

| TYPE | INHERITANCE | PATHOGENESIS | ↑ BLOOD LEVEL | CLINICAL |
|---|---|---|---|---|
| I—Hyper-chylomicronemia | AR | Lipoprotein lipase or apo CII deficiency | Chylomicrons, TG, cholesterol | Pancreatitis, hepatosplenomegaly, and eruptive/pruritic xanthomas (no ↑ risk for atherosclerosis). Creamy layer in supernatant. |
| II—Hyper-cholesterolemia | AD | Absent or defective LDL receptors, or defective apo $B_{100}$ | IIa: LDL, cholesterol<br>IIb: LDL, cholesterol, VLDL | Heterozygotes (1:500) have cholesterol ≈ 300 mg/dL; homozygotes (very rare) have cholesterol ≥ 700 mg/dL. Accelerated atherosclerosis (may have MI before age 20), tendon (Achilles) xanthomas, and corneal arcus. |
| III—Dysbeta-lipoproteinemia | AR | ApoE (defective in type thrEE) | Chylomicrons, VLDL, TG | Premature atherosclerosis, tuberoeruptive and palmar xanthomas. |
| IV—Hyper-triglyceridemia | AD | Hepatic overproduction of VLDL | VLDL, TG | Hypertriglyceridemia (> 1000 mg/dL) can cause acute pancreatitis. Related to insulin resistance. |

# Immunology

*"I hate to disappoint you, but my rubber lips are immune to your charms."*
—*Batman & Robin*

*"Imagine the action of a vaccine not just in terms of how it affects a single body, but also in terms of how it affects the collective body of a community."*
—Eula Biss

*"Some people are immune to good advice."*
—Saul Goodman, *Breaking Bad*

Learning the components of the immune system and their roles in host defense at the cellular level is essential for both the understanding of disease pathophysiology and clinical practice. Know the immune mechanisms of responses to vaccines. Both congenital and acquired immunodeficiencies are very testable. Cell surface markers are high yield for understanding immune cell interactions and for laboratory diagnosis. Know the roles and functions of major cytokines and chemokines.

### ▶ IMMUNOLOGY—LYMPHOID STRUCTURES

| | |
|---|---|
| **Immune system organs** | 1° organs:<br>■ Bone marrow—immune cell production, B cell maturation<br>■ Thymus—T cell maturation<br>2° organs:<br>■ Spleen, lymph nodes, tonsils, adenoids, appendix, Peyer patches<br>■ Allow immune cells to interact with antigen |
| **Lymph node** | A 2° lymphoid organ that has many afferents, 1 or more efferents. Encapsulated, with trabeculae 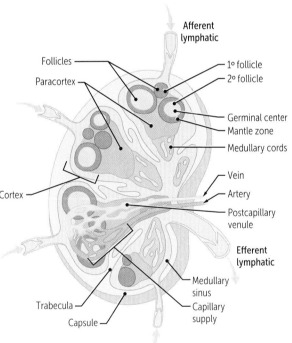.<br>Functions are nonspecific filtration by macrophages, circulation of B and T cells, and immune response activation. |
| **Follicle** | Located in outer cortex; site of B-cell localization and proliferation. 1° follicles are dense and quiescent. 2° follicles have pale central germinal centers and are active. |
| **Medulla** | Consists of medullary cords (closely packed lymphocytes and plasma cells) and medullary sinuses (contain reticular cells and macrophages). Medullary sinuses communicate with efferent lymphatics. |
| **Paracortex** | Contains T cells. Region of cortex between follicles and medulla. Contains high endothelial venules through which T and B cells enter from blood. Underdeveloped in patients with DiGeorge syndrome.<br>Paracortex enlarges in an extreme cellular immune response (eg, EBV and other viral infections → paracortical hyperplasia → lymphadenopathy). |

## Lymphatic drainage associations

| Lymph node cluster | Area of body drained | Associated pathology |
|---|---|---|
| Submandibular, submental | Oral cavity, anterior tongue, lower lip | Malignancy of and metastasis to the oral cavity |
| Deep cervical | Head, neck, oropharynx | Upper respiratory tract infection Infectious mononucleosis Kawasaki disease Malignancy of head, neck, oropharynx |
| Supraclavicular | Right: right hemithorax Left (Virchow node): left hemithorax, abdomen, pelvis | Malignancies of thorax, abdomen, pelvis |
| Mediastinal | Trachea, esophagus | Pulmonary TB (unilateral hilar) Sarcoidosis (bilateral hilar) Lung cancer Granulomatous disease |
| Hilar | Lungs | |
| Axillary | Upper limb, breast, skin above umbilicus | Mastitis Metastasis (especially breast cancer) |
| Epitrochlear | Hand, forearm | Secondary syphilis |
| Celiac | Liver, stomach, spleen, pancreas, upper duodenum | Mesenteric lymphadenitis Inflammatory bowel disease Celiac disease |
| Superior mesenteric | Lower duodenum, jejunum, ileum, colon to splenic flexure | |
| Inferior mesenteric | Colon from splenic flexure to upper rectum | |
| Periumbilical (Sister Mary Joseph node) | Abdomen, pelvis | Gastric cancer |
| Para-aortic | Pair of testes, ovaries, kidneys, fallopian tubes, fundus of uterus | Metastasis |
| External iliac | Body of uterus, cervix, superior bladder | Sexually transmitted infections Medial foot/leg cellulitis (superficial inguinal) |
| Internal iliac | Cervix, proximal vagina, corpus cavernosum, prostate, inferior bladder, lower rectum to anal canal (above pectinate line) | |
| Superficial inguinal | Distal vagina, vulva, scrotum, urethra, anal canal (below pectinate line), skin below umbilicus (except popliteal area) | |
| Popliteal ("pop-lateral") | Dorsolateral foot, posterior calf | Lateral foot/leg cellulitis |

○ Palpable lymph node
◎ Nonpalpable lymph node

▮ Right lymphatic duct drains right side of body above diaphragm into junction of the right subclavian and internal jugular vein

▯ Thoracic duct drains below the diaphragm and left thorax and upper limb into junction of left subclavian and internal jugular veins (rupture of thoracic duct can cause chylothorax)  ℞

## Spleen

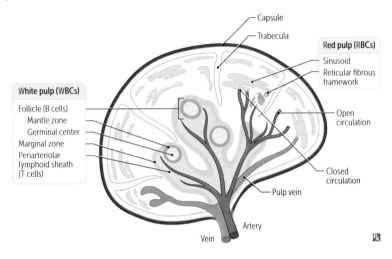

White pulp (WBCs)
- Follicle (B cells)
  - Mantle zone
  - Germinal center
- Marginal zone
- Periarteriolar lymphoid sheath (T cells)

Capsule
Trabecula

Red pulp (RBCs)
- Sinusoid
- Reticular fibrous framework

Open circulation
Closed circulation
Pulp vein
Artery
Vein

Located in LUQ of abdomen, anterolateral to left kidney, protected by 9th-11th ribs. Splenic dysfunction (eg, postsplenectomy, sickle cell disease autosplenectomy) → ↓ IgM → ↓ complement activation → ↓ C3b opsonization → ↑ susceptibility to encapsulated organisms.

Postsplenectomy findings:
- Howell-Jolly bodies (nuclear remnants)
- Target cells
- Thrombocytosis (loss of sequestration and removal)
- Lymphocytosis (loss of sequestration)

Vaccinate patients undergoing splenectomy or with splenic dysfunction against encapsulated organisms (pneumococci, Hib, meningococci).

| | |
|---|---|
| **Periarteriolar lymphatic sheath** | Contains T cells. Located within white pulp. |
| **Follicle** | Contains B cells. Located within white pulp. |
| **Marginal zone** | Contains macrophages and specialized B cells. Site where antigen-presenting cells (APCs) capture blood-borne antigens for recognition by lymphocytes. Located between red pulp and white pulp. |

## Thymus

Located in the anterosuperior mediastinum. Site of T-cell differentiation and maturation. Encapsulated. Thymus epithelium is derived from third pharyngeal pouch (endoderm), whereas thymic lymphocytes are of mesodermal origin. Cortex is dense with immature T cells; medulla is pale with mature T cells and Hassall corpuscles containing epithelial reticular cells.

Normal neonatal thymus "sail-shaped" on CXR (arrows in A), involutes by age 3 years.

T cells = Thymus
B cells = Bone marrow
Absent thymic shadow or hypoplastic thymus seen in some immunodeficiencies (eg, SCID, DiGeorge syndrome).

**Thymoma**—neoplasm of thymus. Associated with myasthenia gravis, superior vena cava syndrome, pure red cell aplasia, Good syndrome.

## ▶ IMMUNOLOGY—CELLULAR COMPONENTS

### Innate vs adaptive immunity

| | Innate immunity | Adaptive immunity |
|---|---|---|
| COMPONENTS | Neutrophils, macrophages, monocytes, dendritic cells, natural killer (NK) cells (lymphoid origin), complement, physical epithelial barriers, secreted enzymes | T cells, B cells, circulating antibodies |
| MECHANISM | Germline encoded | Variation through V(D)J recombination during lymphocyte development |
| RESPONSE TO PATHOGENS | Nonspecific<br>Occurs rapidly (minutes to hours)<br>No memory response | Highly specific, refined over time<br>Develops over long periods; memory response is faster and more robust |
| SECRETED PROTEINS | Lysozyme, complement, C-reactive protein (CRP), defensins, cytokines | Immunoglobulins, cytokines |
| KEY FEATURES IN PATHOGEN RECOGNITION | Toll-like receptors (TLRs): pattern recognition receptors that recognize pathogen-associated molecular patterns (PAMPs) and lead to activation of NF-κB. Examples of PAMPs: LPS (gram ⊖ bacteria), flagellin (bacteria), nucleic acids (viruses) | Memory cells: activated B and T cells; subsequent exposure to a previously encountered antigen → stronger, quicker immune response<br>Adaptive immune responses decrease with age (immunosenescence) |

**Immune privilege**    Organs (eg, eye, brain, placenta, testes) and tissues where chemical or physical mechanisms limit immune responses to foreign antigens to avoid damage that would occur from inflammatory sequelae. Allograft rejection at these sites is less likely.

**Major histocompatibility complex I and II**

MHC encoded by HLA genes. Present antigen fragments to T cells and bind T-cell receptors (TCRs).

| | MHC I | MHC II |
|---|---|---|
| LOCI | HLA-A, HLA-B, HLA-C<br>MHC I loci have 1 letter | HLA-DP, HLA-DQ, HLA-DR<br>MHC II loci have 2 letters |
| BINDING | TCR and CD8 (CD8 × MHC 1 = 8) | TCR and CD4 (CD4 × MHC 2 = 8) |
| STRUCTURE | 1 long chain, 1 short chain | 2 equal-length chains (2 $\alpha$, 2 $\beta$) |
| EXPRESSION | All nucleated cells, APCs, platelets (except RBCs) | APCs |
| FUNCTION | Present endogenous antigens (eg, viral or cytosolic proteins) to CD8+ cytotoxic T cells | Present exogenous antigens (eg, bacterial proteins) to CD4+ helper T cells |
| ANTIGEN LOADING | Antigen peptides loaded onto MHC I in RER after delivery via TAP (transporter associated with antigen processing) | Antigen loaded following release of invariant chain in an acidified endosome |
| ASSOCIATED PROTEINS | $\beta_2$-microglobulin | Invariant chain |
| STRUCTURE | | |

**HLA subtypes associated with diseases**

| HLA SUBTYPE | DISEASE | MNEMONIC |
|---|---|---|
| B27 | Psoriatic arthritis, Ankylosing spondylitis, IBD-associated arthritis, Reactive arthritis | PAIR |
| B57 | Abacavir hypersensitivity | |
| DQ2/DQ8 | Celiac disease | I ate (8) too (2) much gluten at Dairy Queen |
| DR3 | DM type 1, SLE, Graves disease, Hashimoto thyroiditis, Addison disease | DM type 1: HLA-3 and -4 (1 + 3 = 4)<br>SL3 (SLE) |
| DR4 | Rheumatoid arthritis, DM type 1, Addison disease | There are 4 walls in 1 "rheum" (room) |

| **Functions of natural killer cells** | Lymphocyte member of innate immune system. |
|---|---|
| | Use perforin and granzymes to induce apoptosis of virally infected cells and tumor cells. |
| | Activity enhanced by IL-2, IL-12, IFN-$\alpha$, and IFN-$\beta$. |
| | Induced to kill when exposed to a nonspecific activation signal on target cell and/or to an absence of an inhibitory signal such as MHC I on target cell surface. |
| | Also kills via antibody-dependent cell-mediated cytotoxicity (CD16 binds Fc region of bound IgG, activating the NK cell). |

### Major functions of B and T cells

| B cells | Humoral immunity. |
|---|---|
| | Recognize and present antigen—undergo somatic hypermutation to optimize antigen specificity. |
| | Produce antibody—differentiate into plasma cells to secrete specific immunoglobulins. |
| | Maintain immunologic memory—memory B cells persist and accelerate future response to antigen. |
| T cells | Cell-mediated immunity. |
| | CD4+ T cells help B cells make antibodies and produce cytokines to recruit phagocytes and activate other leukocytes. |
| | CD8+ T cells directly kill virus-infected and tumor cells via perforin and granzymes (similar to NK cells). |
| | Type IV hypersensitivity reaction. |
| | Acute and chronic cellular organ rejection. |

## Differentiation of T cells

| Positive selection | Thymic cortex. Keeps T cells that recognize self-peptides to allow for cooperation in immune responses. Double positive thymocytes expressing TCRs that recognize self-peptide MHC complexes receive a survival signal. |
| --- | --- |
| Negative selection | Thymic medulla. Removes T cells that bind too strongly to self-peptides. Thymocytes expressing TCRs with high affinity for self antigens undergo apoptosis or become regulatory T cells. The autoimmune regulator (**AIRE**) protein drives negative selection, and deficiency leads to autoimmune polyendocrine syndrome (**C**hronic mucocutaneous candidiasis, **H**ypoparathyroidism, **A**drenal insufficiency, **R**ecurrent *Candida* infections). "Without **AIRE**, your body will **CHAR**". |

| Macrophage-lymphocyte interaction | Th1 cells secrete IFN-γ, which enhances the ability of monocytes and macrophages to kill microbes they ingest. This function is also enhanced by interaction of T cell CD40L with CD40 on macrophages. Macrophages also activate lymphocytes via antigen presentation. |
| --- | --- |
| Cytotoxic T cells | Kill virus-infected, neoplastic, and donor graft cells by inducing apoptosis. Release cytotoxic granules containing preformed proteins (eg, perforin, granzyme B). Cytotoxic T cells have CD8, which binds to MHC I on virus-infected cells. |
| Regulatory T cells | Help maintain specific immune tolerance by suppressing CD4+ and CD8+ T-cell effector functions. Identified by expression of CD3, CD4, CD25, and FOXP3. Activated regulatory T cells (Tregs) produce anti-inflammatory cytokines (eg, IL-10, TGF-β). **IPEX (Immune dysregulation, Polyendocrinopathy, Enteropathy, X-linked) syndrome**— genetic deficiency of FOXP3 → autoimmunity. Characterized by enteropathy, endocrinopathy, nail dystrophy, dermatitis, and/or other autoimmune dermatologic conditions. Associated with diabetes in male infants. |

| **T- and B-cell activation** | APCs: B cells, dendritic cells, Langerhans cells, macrophages. Two signals are required for T-cell activation, B-cell activation, and class switching. |
|---|---|

| **T-cell activation** | ❶ APC ingests and processes antigen, then migrates to the draining lymph node. <br> ❷ T-cell activation (signal 1): exogenous antigen is presented on MHC II and recognized by TCR on Th (CD4+) cell. Endogenous or cross-presented antigen is presented on MHC I to Tc (CD8+) cell. <br> ❸ Proliferation and survival (signal 2): costimulatory signal via interaction of B7 protein (CD80/86) on dendritic cell and CD28 on naïve T cell. <br> ❹ Activated Th cell produces cytokines. Tc cell able to recognize and kill virus-infected cell. |  |

| **B-cell activation and class switching** | ❶ Th-cell activation as above. <br> ❷ B-cell receptor–mediated endocytosis. <br> ❸ Exogenous antigen is presented on MHC II and recognized by TCR on Th cell. <br> ❹ CD40 receptor on B cell binds CD40 ligand (CD40L) on Th cell. <br> ❺ Th cells secrete cytokines that determine Ig class switching of B cells. <br> ❻ B cells are activated and produce IgM. They undergo class switching and affinity maturation. | 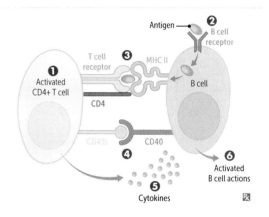 |

▶ **IMMUNOLOGY—IMMUNE RESPONSES**

**Antibody structure and function**

Fab fragment consisting of light (L) and heavy (H) chains recognizes antigens. Fc region of IgM and IgG fixes complement. Heavy chain contributes to Fc and Fab regions. Light chain contributes only to Fab region.

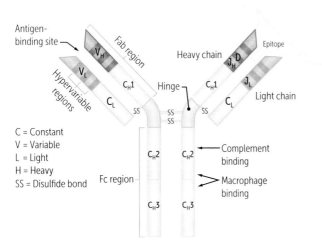

C = Constant
V = Variable
L = Light
H = Heavy
SS = Disulfide bond

Fab:
- Fragment, antigen binding
- Determines idiotype: unique antigen-binding pocket; only 1 antigenic specificity expressed per B cell

Fc (5 C's):
- Constant
- Carboxy terminal
- Complement binding
- Carbohydrate side chains
- Confers (determines) isotype (IgM, IgD, etc)

**Generation of antibody diversity** (antigen independent)
1. Random recombination of VJ (light-chain) or V(D)J (heavy-chain) genes by RAG1 and RAG2
2. Random addition of nucleotides to DNA during recombination by terminal deoxynucleotidyl transferase (TdT)
3. Random combination of heavy chains with light chains

**Generation of antibody specificity** (antigen dependent)
4. Somatic hypermutation and affinity maturation (variable region)
5. Isotype switching (constant region)

**Neutralization**

Antibody prevents bacterial adherence

**Opsonization**

Antibody promotes phagocytosis

**Complement activation**

Membrane attack complex (MAC)

C3b

Antibody activates complement, enhancing opsonization and lysis

| | |
|---|---|
| **Immunoglobulin isotypes** | All isotypes can exist as monomers. Mature, naïve B cells prior to activation express IgM and IgD on their surfaces. They may differentiate in germinal centers of lymph nodes by isotype switching (gene rearrangement; induced by cytokines and CD40L) into plasma cells that secrete IgA, IgG, or IgE. "For B cells, IgMom and IgDad mature to plasma cells as they AGE. Affinity refers to the individual antibody-antigen interaction, while avidity describes the cumulative binding strength of all antibody-antigen interactions in a multivalent molecule. |
| **IgG** | Main antibody in 2° response to an antigen. Most abundant isotype in serum. Fixes complement, opsonizes bacteria, neutralizes bacterial toxins and viruses. Only isotype that crosses the placenta (provides infants with passive immunity that starts to wane after birth). "IgG Greets the Growing fetus." Associated with warm autoimmune hemolytic anemia ("warm weather is Good!"). |
| **IgA** | Prevents attachment of bacteria and viruses to mucous membranes; does not fix complement. Monomer (in circulation) or dimer (with J chain when secreted). Crosses epithelial cells by transcytosis. Produced in GI tract (eg, by Peyer patches) and protects against gut infections (eg, *Giardia*). Most produced antibody overall, but has lower serum concentrations. Released into secretions (tears, saliva, mucus) and breast milk. Picks up secretory component from epithelial cells, which protects the Fc portion from luminal proteases. |
| **IgM** | First antibody to be produced during an immune response. Fixes complement. Antigen receptor on the surface of B cells. Monomer on B cell, pentamer with J chain when secreted. Pentamer enables avid binding to antigen while humoral response evolves. Associated with cold autoimmune hemolytic anemia. |
| **IgD** | Expressed on the surface of mature, naïve B cells. Normally, low levels are detectable in serum. |
| **IgE** | Binds mast cells and basophils; cross-links when exposed to allergen, mediating immediate (type I) hypersensitivity through release of inflammatory mediators such as histamine. Contributes to immunity to parasites by activating Eosinophils. |

## Antigen type and memory

| | |
|---|---|
| **Thymus-independent antigens** | Antigens lacking a peptide component (eg, lipopolysaccharides from gram ⊖ bacteria); cannot be presented by MHC to T cells. Weakly immunogenic; vaccines often require boosters and adjuvants (eg, capsular polysaccharide subunit of *Streptococcus pneumoniae* PPSV23 vaccine). |
| **Thymus-dependent antigens** | Antigens containing a protein component (eg, diphtheria toxoid). Class switching and immunologic memory occur as a result of direct contact of B cells with Th cells. |

| | | |
|---|---|---|
| **Complement** | System of hepatically synthesized plasma proteins that play a role in innate immunity and inflammation. Membrane attack complex (MAC) defends against gram ⊖ bacteria. The $CH_{50}$ test is used to screen for activation of the classical complement pathway. | |
| ACTIVATION PATHWAYS | Classic—IgG or IgM mediated. Alternative—microbe surface molecules. Lectin—mannose or other sugars on microbe surface. | General Motors makes classic cars. |
| FUNCTIONS | C3b—opsonization. C3a, C4a, C5a—anaphylaxis. C5a—neutrophil chemotaxis. C5b-9 (MAC)—cytolysis. | C3b binds to lipopolysaccharides on bacteria. MAC complex is important for neutralizing *Neisseria* species. Deficiency results in recurrent infection. Get "Neis" (nice) Big MACs from 5-9 pm. |
| | **Opsonins**—C3b and IgG are the two 1° opsonins in bacterial defense; enhance phagocytosis. C3b also helps clear immune complexes. | *Opsonin* (Greek) = to prepare for eating. |
| | **Inhibitors**—decay-accelerating factor (DAF, also called CD55) and C1 esterase inhibitor help prevent complement activation on self cells (eg, RBCs). | |

## Complement disorders

### Complement protein deficiencies

| | |
|---|---|
| Early complement deficiencies (C1–C4) | ↑ risk of severe, recurrent pyogenic sinus and respiratory tract infections. C3b used in clearance of antigen-antibody complexes → ↑ risk of SLE (think SLEarly). |
| Terminal complement deficiencies (C5–C9) | ↑ susceptibility to recurrent *Neisseria* bacteremia. |

### Complement regulatory protein deficiencies

| | |
|---|---|
| C1 esterase inhibitor deficiency | Causes hereditary angioedema due to unregulated activation of kallikrein → ↑ bradykinin. Characterized by ↓ C4 levels. ACE inhibitors are contraindicated (also ↑ bradykinin). |
| Paroxysmal nocturnal hemoglobinuria  | A defect in the *PIGA* gene prevents the formation of glycosylphosphatidylinositol (GPI) anchors for complement inhibitors, such as decay-accelerating factor (DAF/CD55) and membrane inhibitor of reactive lysis (MIRL/CD59). Causes complement-mediated intravascular hemolysis → ↓ haptoglobin, dark urine A. <br> Can cause atypical venous thrombosis (eg, Budd-Chiari syndrome; portal vein, cerebral, or dermal thrombosis). |

| **Important cytokines** | Acute (IL-1, IL-6, TNF-α), then recruit (IL-8, IL-12). | |
|---|---|---|
| **Secreted by macrophages** | | |
| Interleukin-1 | Causes fever, acute inflammation. Activates endothelium to express adhesion molecules. Induces chemokine secretion to recruit WBCs. Also called osteoclast-activating factor. | "Hot T-bone stEAK": IL-1: fever (hot). IL-2: stimulates T cells. IL-3: stimulates bone marrow. IL-4: stimulates IgE production. IL-5: stimulates IgA production. IL-6: stimulates aKute-phase protein production. |
| Interleukin-6 | Causes fever and stimulates production of acute-phase proteins. | |
| Tumor necrosis factor-α | Activates endothelium. Causes WBC recruitment, vascular leak. | Causes cachexia in malignancy. Maintains granulomas in TB. IL-1, IL-6, TNF-α can mediate fever and sepsis. |
| Interleukin-8 | Major chemotactic factor for neutrophils. | "Clean up on aisle 8." Neutrophils are recruited by IL-8 to clear infections. |
| Interleukin-12 | Induces differentiation of T cells into Th1 cells. Activates NK cells. | Facilitates granuloma formation in TB. |
| **Secreted by T cells** | | |
| Interleukin-2 | Stimulates growth of helper, cytotoxic, and regulatory T cells, and NK cells. | |
| Interleukin-3 | Supports growth and differentiation of bone marrow stem cells. Functions like GM-CSF. | Stimulates proliferation of eosinophils, basophils, neutrophils, monocytes. |
| **From Th1 cells** | | |
| Interferon-γ | Secreted by NK cells and T cells in response to antigen or IL-12 from macrophages; stimulates macrophages to kill phagocytosed pathogens. Inhibits differentiation of Th2 cells. Induces IgG isotype switching in B cells. | Increases MHC expression and antigen presentation by all cells. Activates macrophages to induce granuloma formation. |
| **From Th2 cells** | | |
| Interleukin-4 | Induces differentiation of T cells into Th (helper) 2 cells. Promotes growth of B cells. Enhances class switching to IgE and IgG. | Ain't too proud 2 BEG 4 help. |
| Interleukin-5 | Promotes growth and differentiation of B cells. Enhances class switching to IgA. Stimulates growth and differentiation of Eosinophils. | I have 5 BAEs. |
| Interleukin-10 | Attenuates inflammatory response. Decreases expression of MHC class II and Th1 cytokines. Inhibits activated macrophages and dendritic cells. Also secreted by regulatory T cells. | TGF-β and IL-10 both attenuate the immune response. |
| Interleukin-13 | Promotes IgE production by B cells. Induces alternative macrophage activation. | Interleukin thirtEEn promotes IgE. |

**Respiratory burst**

Also called oxidative burst. Involves the activation of the phagocyte NADPH oxidase complex (eg, in neutrophils, monocytes), which utilizes $O_2$ as a substrate. Plays an important role in the immune response → rapid release of reactive oxygen species (ROS). NADPH plays a role in both the creation and neutralization of ROS. Myeloperoxidase contains a blue-green, heme-containing pigment that gives sputum its color. **NO Safe Microbe** (**N**ADPH **O**xidase → **S**uperoxide dismutase → **M**yeloperoxidase).

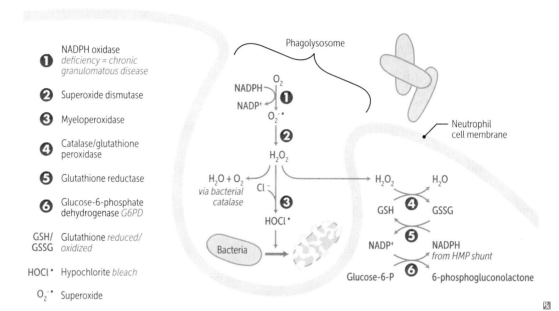

Phagocytes of patients with CGD can utilize $H_2O_2$ generated by invading organisms and convert it to ROS. Patients are at ↑ risk for infection by catalase ⊕ species (eg, S *aureus*, *Aspergillus*) capable of neutralizing their own $H_2O_2$, leaving phagocytes without ROS for fighting infections.

Pyocyanin of *P aeruginosa* generates ROS to kill competing pathogens. Oxidative burst leads to release of lysosomal enzymes.

---

**Interferons**

IFN-α, IFN-β, IFN-γ.

MECHANISM

A part of innate host defense, **interferons interfere** with both RNA and DNA viruses. Cells infected with a virus synthesize these glycoproteins, which act on local cells, priming them for viral defense by downregulating protein synthesis to resist potential viral replication and by upregulating MHC expression to facilitate recognition of infected cells. Also play a major role in activating antitumor immunity.

CLINICAL USE

Chronic HBV, Kaposi sarcoma, hairy cell leukemia, condyloma acuminatum, renal cell carcinoma, malignant melanoma, multiple sclerosis, chronic granulomatous disease.

ADVERSE EFFECTS

Flulike symptoms, depression, neutropenia, myopathy, interferon-induced autoimmunity.

## Cell surface proteins

| | |
|---|---|
| T cells | TCR (binds antigen-MHC complex), CD3 (associated with TCR for signal transduction), CD28 (binds B7 on APC) |
| Helper T cells | CD4, CD40L, CXCR4/CCR5 (coreceptors for HIV) |
| Cytotoxic T cells | CD8 |
| Regulatory T cells | CD4, CD25 |
| B cells | Ig (binds antigen), CD19, CD20, CD21 (receptor for Epstein-**Barr** virus), CD40, MHC II, B7 (CD80/86) — Must be **21** to drink at a **Barr** |
| NK cells | CD16 (binds Fc of IgG), CD56 (suggestive marker for NK cells) |
| Macrophages | CD14 (receptor for PAMPs [eg, LPS]), CD40, CCR5, MHC II, B7, Fc and C3b receptors (enhanced phagocytosis) |
| Hematopoietic stem cells | CD34 |

**Anergy**    State during which a cell cannot become activated by exposure to its antigen. T and B cells become anergic when exposed to their antigen without costimulatory signal (signal 2). Another mechanism of self-tolerance.

## Passive vs active immunity

| | Passive | Active |
|---|---|---|
| MEANS OF ACQUISITION | Receiving preformed antibodies | Exposure to exogenous antigens |
| ONSET | Rapid | Slow |
| DURATION | Short span of antibodies (half-life = 3 weeks) | Long-lasting protection (memory) |
| EXAMPLES | IgA in breast milk, maternal IgG crossing placenta, antitoxin, humanized monoclonal antibody | Natural infection, vaccines, toxoid |
| NOTES | IVIG and other immune globulin preparations can be administered to provide temporary but specific passive immunity to a target pathogen. | Combined passive and active immunizations can be given for hepatitis B or rabies exposure |

## Vaccination

Induces an active immune response (humoral and/or cellular) to specific pathogens.

| VACCINE TYPE | DESCRIPTION | PROS/CONS | EXAMPLES |
|---|---|---|---|
| **Live attenuated vaccine** | Microorganism rendered nonpathogenic but retains capacity for transient growth within inoculated host. MMR and varicella vaccines can be given to people living with HIV without evidence of immunity if CD4+ cell count ≥ 200 cells/mm$^3$. | Pros: induces cellular and humoral responses. Induces strong, often lifelong immunity. Cons: may revert to virulent form. Contraindicated in pregnancy and patients with immunodeficiency. | Adenovirus (nonattenuated, given to military recruits), typhoid (Ty21a, oral), polio (Sabin), varicella (chickenpox), smallpox, BCG, yellow fever, influenza (intranasal), **MMR**, rotavirus. "Attention teachers! Please vaccinate small, Beautiful young infants with **MMR** routinely!" |
| **Killed or inactivated vaccine** | Pathogen is inactivated by heat or chemicals. Maintaining epitope structure on surface antigens is important for immune response. Mainly induces a humoral response. | Pros: safer than live vaccines. Cons: weaker cell-mediated immune response; mainly induces a humoral response. Booster shots usually needed. | Hepatitis A, Typhoid (Vi polysaccharide, intramuscular), Rabies, Influenza (intramuscular), Polio (SalK). A **TRIP** could Kill you. |
| **Subunit, recombinant, polysaccharide, and conjugate** | All use specific antigens that best stimulate the immune system. | Pros: targets specific epitopes of antigen; lower chance of adverse reactions. Cons: expensive; weaker immune response. | HBV (antigen = HBsAg), HPV, acellular pertussis (aP), *Neisseria meningitidis* (various strains), *Streptococcus pneumoniae* (PPSV23 polysaccharide primarily T-cell–independent response; PCV13, PCV15, and PCV20 polysaccharide produces T-cell–dependent response), *Haemophilus influenzae* type b, herpes zoster. |
| **Toxoid** | Denatured bacterial toxin with an intact receptor binding site. Stimulates immune system to make antibodies without potential for causing disease. | Pros: protects against the bacterial toxins. Cons: antitoxin levels decrease with time, thus booster shots may be needed. | *Clostridium tetani*, *Corynebacterium diphtheriae*. |
| **mRNA** | A lipid nanoparticle delivers mRNA, causing cells to synthesize foreign protein (eg, spike protein of SARS-CoV-2). | Pros: high efficacy; induces cellular and humoral immunity. Safe in pregnancy. Cons: local and transient systemic (fatigue, headache, myalgia) reactions are common. Rare myocarditis, pericarditis particularly in young males. | SARS-CoV-2 |

| **Hypersensitivity types** | Four types: Anaphylactic and atopic (type I), antibody-mediated (type II), immune complex (type III), cell-mediated (type IV). Types I, II, and III are all antibody-mediated. | |
|---|---|---|
| **Type I hypersensitivity**<br><br>Allergen — Allergen-specific IgE<br>Fc receptor for IgE<br>Degranulation ℞ | Anaphylactic and atopic—two phases:<br>▪ Immediate (minutes): antigen crosslinks preformed IgE on presensitized mast cells → immediate degranulation → release of histamine (a vasoactive amine), tryptase (marker of mast cell activation), and leukotrienes.<br>▪ Late (hours): chemokines (attract inflammatory cells, eg, eosinophils) and other mediators from mast cells → inflammation and tissue damage. | First (type) and Fast (anaphylaxis).<br>Test: skin test or blood test (ELISA) for allergen-specific IgE.<br>Example:<br>▪ Anaphylaxis (eg, food, drug, or bee sting allergies)<br>▪ Allergic asthma |
| **Type II hypersensitivity**<br>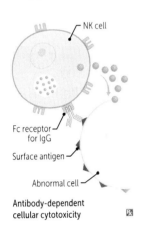<br>NK cell<br>Fc receptor for IgG<br>Surface antigen<br>Abnormal cell<br>Antibody-dependent cellular cytotoxicity ℞ | Antibodies bind to cell-surface antigens or extracellular matrix → cellular destruction, inflammation, and cellular dysfunction.<br><br>Cellular destruction—cell is opsonized (coated) by antibodies, leading to either:<br>▪ Phagocytosis and/or activation of complement system.<br>▪ NK cell killing (antibody-dependent cellular cytotoxicity).<br>Inflammation—binding of antibodies to cell surfaces → activation of complement system and Fc receptor-mediated inflammation.<br><br>Cellular dysfunction—antibodies bind to cell-surface receptors → abnormal blockade or activation of downstream process. | Direct Coombs test—detects antibodies attached directly to the RBC surface.<br>Indirect Coombs test—detects presence of unbound antibodies in the serum.<br><br>Examples:<br>▪ Autoimmune hemolytic anemia (including drug-induced form)<br>▪ Immune thrombocytopenia<br>▪ Transfusion reactions<br>▪ Hemolytic disease of the newborn<br>Examples:<br>▪ Goodpasture syndrome<br>▪ Rheumatic fever<br>▪ Hyperacute transplant rejection<br>Examples:<br>▪ Myasthenia gravis<br>▪ Graves disease<br>▪ Pemphigus vulgaris |

## Hypersensitivity types *(continued)*

### Type III hypersensitivity

Neutrophils

Enzymes from neutrophils damage endothelial cells

Immune complex—antigen-antibody (mostly IgG) complexes activate complement, which attracts neutrophils; neutrophils release lysosomal enzymes.
Can be associated with vasculitis and systemic manifestations.

**Serum sickness**—the prototypic immune complex disease. Antibodies to foreign proteins are produced and 1–2 weeks later, antibody-antigen complexes form and deposit in tissues → complement activation → inflammation and tissue damage (↓ serum C3, C4).

**Arthus reaction**—a local subacute immune complex-mediated hypersensitivity reaction. Intradermal injection of antigen into a presensitized (has circulating IgG) individual leads to immune complex formation in the skin (eg, enhanced local reaction to a booster vaccination). Characterized by edema, fibrinoid necrosis, activation of complement.

In type III reaction, imagine an immune complex as 3 things stuck together: antigen-antibody-complement.
Examples:
- SLE
- Rheumatoid arthritis
- Reactive arthritis
- Polyarteritis nodosa
- Poststreptococcal glomerulonephritis
- IgA vasculitis

Fever, urticaria, arthralgia, proteinuria, lymphadenopathy occur 1–2 weeks after antigen exposure. Serum sickness–like reactions are associated with some drugs (may act as haptens, eg, penicillin, monoclonal antibodies) and infections (eg, hepatitis B).

### Type IV hypersensitivity

Antigen-presenting cell

Antigen

Sensitized Th1 cell

Cytokines

Activated macrophage

Delayed-type hypersensitivity

Two mechanisms, each involving T cells:
1. Direct cell cytotoxicity: CD8+ cytotoxic T cells kill targeted cells.
2. Inflammatory reaction: effector CD4+ T cells recognize antigen and release inflammation-inducing cytokines (shown in illustration).

Response does not involve antibodies (vs types I, II, and III).
Examples:
- Contact dermatitis (eg, poison ivy, nickel allergy)
- Drug reaction with eosinophilia and systemic symptoms (DRESS)
- Graft-versus-host disease

Tests: PPD for TB infection; patch test for contact dermatitis; *Candida* skin test for T cell immune function.
4T's: T cells, Transplant rejections, TB skin tests, Touching (contact dermatitis).

Fourth (type) and last (delayed).

## Immunologic blood transfusion reactions

| TYPE | PATHOGENESIS | TIMING | CLINICAL PRESENTATION | DONOR BLOOD | HOST BLOOD |
|---|---|---|---|---|---|
| **Allergic/ anaphylactic reaction** | Type I hypersensitivity reaction against plasma proteins in transfused blood<br>IgA-deficient individuals should receive blood products without IgA | Within minutes to 2–3 hr (due to release of preformed inflammatory mediators in degranulating mast cells) | Allergies: urticaria, pruritus<br>Anaphylaxis: wheezing, hypotension, respiratory arrest, shock | Donor plasma proteins, including IgA | IgE (anti-IgA)<br><br>Host mast cell |
| **Acute hemolytic transfusion reaction** | Type II hypersensitivity reaction<br>Typically causes intravascular hemolysis (ABO blood group incompatibility) | During transfusion or within 24 hr (due to preformed antibodies) | Fever, hypotension, tachypnea, tachycardia, flank pain, hemoglobinuria (intravascular), jaundice (extravascular) | Donor RBC with A and/ or B group antigens | Host anti-A, anti-B IgG, IgM |
| **Febrile nonhemolytic transfusion reaction** | Cytokines created by donor WBCs accumulate during storage of blood products<br>Reactions prevented by leukoreduction of blood products | Within 1–6 hr (due to preformed cytokines) | Fever, headaches, chills, flushing<br>More common in children | Donor WBC releases preformed cytokines | |
| **Transfusion-related acute lung injury** | Two-hit mechanism:<br>▫ Neutrophils are sequestered and primed in pulmonary vasculature due to recipient risk factors<br>▫ Neutrophils are activated by a product (eg, antileukocyte antibodies) in the transfused blood and release inflammatory mediators → ↑ capillary permeability → pulmonary edema | Within minutes to 6 hr | Respiratory distress, noncardiogenic pulmonary edema | Donor antileukocyte antibody | Host neutrophils |
| **Delayed hemolytic transfusion reaction** | Anamnestic response to a foreign antigen on donor RBCs (Rh [D] or other minor blood group antigens) previously encountered by recipient<br>Typically causes extravascular hemolysis | Onset over 24 hr<br>Usually presents within 1–2 wk (due to slow destruction by reticuloendothelial system) | Generally self limited and clinically silent<br>Mild fever, hyperbilirubinemia | | |

**Autoantibodies**

| AUTOANTIBODY | ASSOCIATED DISORDER |
| --- | --- |
| Anti-postsynaptic ACh receptor | Myasthenia gravis |
| Anti-presynaptic voltage-gated $Ca^{2+}$ channel | Lambert-Eaton myasthenic syndrome |
| Anti-$\beta_2$ glycoprotein I | Antiphospholipid syndrome |
| Antinuclear (ANA) | Nonspecific screening antibody, often associated with SLE |
| Anticardiolipin, lupus anticoagulant | SLE, antiphospholipid syndrome |
| Anti-dsDNA, anti-Smith | SLE |
| Antihistone | Drug-induced lupus |
| Anti-U1 RNP (ribonucleoprotein) | Mixed connective tissue disease |
| Rheumatoid factor (IgM antibody against IgG Fc region), anti-cyclic citrullinated peptide (anti-CCP, more specific) | Rheumatoid arthritis |
| Anti-Ro/SSA, anti-La/SSB | Sjögren syndrome |
| Anti-Scl-70 (anti-DNA topoisomerase I) | Scleroderma (diffuse) |
| Anticentromere | Limited scleroderma (CREST syndrome) |
| Antisynthetase (eg, anti-Jo-1), anti-SRP, anti-helicase (anti-Mi-2) | Polymyositis, dermatomyositis |
| Antimitochondrial | 1° biliary cholangitis |
| Anti-smooth muscle, anti-liver/kidney microsomal-1 | Autoimmune hepatitis |
| Myeloperoxidase-antineutrophil cytoplasmic antibody (MPO-ANCA)/perinuclear ANCA (p-ANCA) | Microscopic polyangiitis, eosinophilic granulomatosis with polyangiitis, ulcerative colitis, 1° sclerosing cholangitis |
| PR3-ANCA/cytoplasmic ANCA (c-ANCA) | Granulomatosis with polyangiitis |
| Anti-phospholipase $A_2$ receptor | 1° membranous nephropathy |
| Anti-hemidesmosome | Bullous pemphigoid |
| Anti-desmoglein (anti-desmosome) | Pemphigus vulgaris |
| Antithyroglobulin, antithyroid peroxidase (antimicrosomal) | Hashimoto thyroiditis |
| Anti-TSH receptor | Graves disease |
| IgA anti-endomysial, IgA anti-tissue transglutaminase, IgA and IgG deamidated gliadin peptide | Celiac disease |
| Anti-glutamic acid decarboxylase, islet cell cytoplasmic antibodies | Type 1 diabetes mellitus |
| Antiparietal cell, anti-intrinsic factor | Pernicious anemia |
| Anti-glomerular basement membrane | Goodpasture syndrome |

## Immunodeficiencies

| DISEASE | DEFECT | PRESENTATION | FINDINGS |
|---|---|---|---|
| **B-cell disorders** | | | |
| **X-linked (Bruton) agammaglobulinemia** | Defect in *BTK*, a tyrosine kinase gene → no B-cell maturation; X-linked recessive (↑ in Boys) | Recurrent bacterial and enteroviral infections after 6 months (↓ maternal IgG) | Absent B cells in peripheral blood, ↓ Ig of all classes. Absent/scanty lymph nodes and tonsils (1° follicles and germinal centers absent) → live vaccines contraindicated |
| **Selective IgA deficiency** | Cause unknown Most common 1° immunodeficiency | Majority Asymptomatic Can see Airway and GI infections, Autoimmune disease, Atopy, Anaphylaxis to IgA in blood products | ↓ IgA with normal IgG, IgM levels ↑ susceptibility to giardiasis Can cause false-negative celiac disease test and false-positive serum pregnancy test |
| **Common variable immunodeficiency** | Defect in B-cell differentiation. Cause unknown in most cases | May present in childhood but usually diagnosed after puberty ↑ risk of autoimmune disease, bronchiectasis, lymphoma, sinopulmonary infections | ↓ plasma cells, ↓ immunoglobulins |
| **T-cell disorders** | | | |
| **Thymic aplasia** | 22q11 microdeletion; failure to develop 3rd and 4th pharyngeal pouches → absent thymus and parathyroids DiGeorge syndrome—thymic, parathyroid, cardiac defects Velocardiofacial syndrome—palate, facial, cardiac defects | CATCH-22: Cardiac defects (conotruncal abnormalities [eg, tetralogy of Fallot, truncus arteriosus]), Abnormal facies, Thymic hypoplasia → T-cell deficiency (recurrent viral/fungal infections), Cleft palate, Hypocalcemia 2° to parathyroid aplasia → tetany | ↓ T cells, ↓ PTH, ↓ $Ca^{2+}$ Thymic shadow absent on CXR |
| **IL-12 receptor deficiency** | ↓ Th1 response; autosomal recessive | Disseminated mycobacterial and fungal infections; may present after administration of BCG vaccine | ↓ IFN-γ Most common cause of Mendelian susceptibility to mycobacterial diseases (MSMD) |
| **Autosomal dominant hyper-IgE syndrome (Job syndrome)** | Deficiency of Th17 cells due to *STAT3* mutation → impaired recruitment of neutrophils to sites of infection | Cold (noninflamed) staphylococcal Abscesses, retained Baby teeth, Coarse facies, Dermatologic problems (eczema), ↑ IgE, bone Fractures from minor trauma | ↑ IgE ↑ eosinophils Learn the ABCDEF's to get a Job STAT! |
| **Chronic mucocutaneous candidiasis** | T-cell dysfunction Impaired cell-mediated immunity against *Candida* sp Classic form caused by defects in *AIRE* | Persistent noninvasive *Candida albicans* infections of skin and mucous membranes | Absent in vitro T-cell proliferation in response to *Candida* antigens Absent cutaneous reaction to *Candida* antigens |

## Immunodeficiencies *(continued)*

| DISEASE | DEFECT | PRESENTATION | FINDINGS |
|---|---|---|---|
| **B- and T-cell disorders** | | | |
| **Severe combined immunodeficiency** | Several types including defective IL-2R gamma chain (most common, X-linked recessive); adenosine deaminase deficiency (autosomal recessive); *RAG* mutation → VDJ recombination defect | Failure to thrive, chronic diarrhea, thrush<br>Recurrent viral, bacterial, fungal, and protozoal infections | ↓ T-cell receptor excision circles (TRECs)<br>Part of newborn screening for SCID<br>Absence of thymic shadow (CXR), germinal centers (lymph node biopsy), and T cells (flow cytometry) |
| **Ataxia-telangiectasia**<br> | Defects in *ATM* gene → failure to detect DNA damage → failure to halt progression of cell cycle → mutations accumulate; autosomal recessive | Triad: cerebellar defects (Ataxia), spider Angiomas (telangiectasia A), IgA deficiency<br>↑↑ sensitivity to radiation (limit x-ray exposure) | ↑ AFP<br>↓ IgA, IgG, and IgE<br>Lymphopenia, cerebellar atrophy<br>↑ risk of lymphoma and leukemia |
| **Hyper-IgM syndrome** | Most commonly due to defective CD40L on Th cells → class switching defect; X-linked recessive | Severe pyogenic infections early in life; opportunistic infection with *Pneumocystis*, *Cryptosporidium*, CMV | Normal or ↑ IgM<br>↓↓ IgG, IgA, IgE<br>Failure to make germinal centers |
| **Wiskott-Aldrich syndrome** | Mutation in *WAS* gene; leukocytes and platelets unable to reorganize actin cytoskeleton → defective antigen presentation; X-linked recessive | WATER: Wiskott-Aldrich: Thrombocytopenia, Eczema, Recurrent (pyogenic) infections<br>↑ risk of autoimmune disease and malignancy | ↓ to normal IgG, IgM<br>↑ IgE, IgA<br>Fewer and smaller platelets |
| **Phagocyte dysfunction** | | | |
| **Leukocyte adhesion deficiency (type 1)** | Autosomal recessive defect in LFA-1 integrin (CD18) protein on phagocytes leads to impaired migration and chemotaxis by C5a, IL-8, and leukotriene B4 | Late separation (>30 days) of umbilical cord, absent pus, dysfunctional neutrophils → recurrent skin and mucosal bacterial infections | ↑ neutrophils in blood<br>Absence of neutrophils at infection sites → impaired wound healing |
| **Chédiak-Higashi syndrome**<br> | Defect in lysosomal trafficking regulator gene (*LYST*)<br>Microtubule dysfunction in phagosome-lysosome fusion; autosomal recessive | PLAIN: Progressive neurodegeneration, Lymphohistiocytosis, Albinism (partial), recurrent pyogenic Infections, peripheral Neuropathy | Giant granules (B, arrows) in granulocytes and platelets<br>Pancytopenia<br>Mild coagulation defects |
| **Chronic granulomatous disease** | Defect of NADPH oxidase → ↓ reactive oxygen species (eg, superoxide) and ↓ respiratory burst in neutrophils; X-linked form most common | ↑ susceptibility to catalase ⊕ organisms<br>Recurrent infections and granulomas | Abnormal dihydrorhodamine (flow cytometry) test (↓ green fluorescence)<br>Nitroblue tetrazolium dye reduction test (obsolete) fails to turn blue |

## Infections in immunodeficiency

| PATHOGEN | ↓ T CELLS | ↓ B CELLS | ↓ GRANULOCYTES | ↓ COMPLEMENT |
|---|---|---|---|---|
| **Bacteria** | Sepsis | Encapsulated (Please **SHINE** my SK**i**S): *Pseudomonas aeruginosa*, *Streptococcus pneumoniae*, *Haemophilus Influenzae* type b, *Neisseria meningitidis*, *Escherichia coli*, *Salmonella*, *Klebsiella pneumoniae*, group B *Streptococcus* | Some Bacteria Produce No Serious granules: *Staphylococcus*, *Burkholderia cepacia*, *Pseudomonas aeruginosa*, *Nocardia*, *Serratia* | Encapsulated species with early complement deficiencies *Neisseria* with late complement (C5–C9) deficiencies |
| **Viruses** | CMV, EBV, JC virus, VZV, chronic infection with respiratory/GI viruses | Enteroviral encephalitis, poliovirus (live vaccine contraindicated) | N/A | N/A |
| **Fungi/parasites** | *Candida* (local), PCP, *Cryptococcus* | GI giardiasis (no IgA) | *Candida* (systemic), *Aspergillus*, *Mucor* | N/A |

Note: B-cell deficiencies tend to produce recurrent bacterial infections, whereas T-cell deficiencies produce more fungal and viral infections.

## Transplant rejection

| TYPE OF REJECTION | ONSET | PATHOGENESIS | FEATURES |
|---|---|---|---|
| Hyperacute | Within minutes | Pre-existing recipient antibodies react to donor antigen (type II hypersensitivity reaction), activate complement | Widespread thrombosis of graft vessels (arrows within glomerulus **A**) → ischemia and fibrinoid necrosis<br>Graft must be removed |
| Acute | Weeks to months | Cellular: CD8+ T cells and/or CD4+ T cells activated against donor MHCs (type IV hypersensitivity reaction)<br>Humoral: similar to hyperacute, except antibodies develop after transplant (associated with C4d deposition) | Vasculitis of graft vessels with dense interstitial lymphocytic infiltrate **B**<br>Prevent/reverse with immunosuppressants |
| Chronic | Months to years | CD4+ T cells respond to recipient APCs presenting donor peptides, including allogeneic MHC<br>Both cellular and humoral components (type II and IV hypersensitivity reactions) | Dominated by arteriosclerosis **C**<br>Recipient T cells react and secrete cytokines → proliferation of vascular smooth muscle, parenchymal atrophy, interstitial fibrosis<br>Organ-specific examples:<br>▪ Chronic allograft nephropathy<br>▪ Bronchiolitis obliterans<br>▪ Accelerated atherosclerosis (heart)<br>▪ Vanishing bile duct syndrome |
| Graft-versus-host disease | Varies | Grafted immunocompetent T cells proliferate in the immunocompromised host and reject host cells with "foreign" proteins → severe organ dysfunction<br>HLA mismatches (most importantly HLA-A, -B, and -DR antigens) ↑ the risk for GVHD<br>Type IV hypersensitivity reaction | Maculopapular rash, jaundice, diarrhea, hepatosplenomegaly<br>Usually in bone marrow and liver transplants (rich in lymphocytes)<br>Potentially beneficial in bone marrow transplant for leukemia (graft-versus-tumor effect)<br>For patients who are immunocompromised, irradiate blood products prior to transfusion to prevent GVHD |

▶ **IMMUNOLOGY—IMMUNOSUPPRESSANTS**

**Immunosuppressants**    Agents that block lymphocyte activation and proliferation. Reduce acute transplant rejection by suppressing cellular immunity (used as prophylaxis). Frequently combined to achieve greater efficacy with ↓ toxicity. Chronic suppression ↑ risk of infection and malignancy.

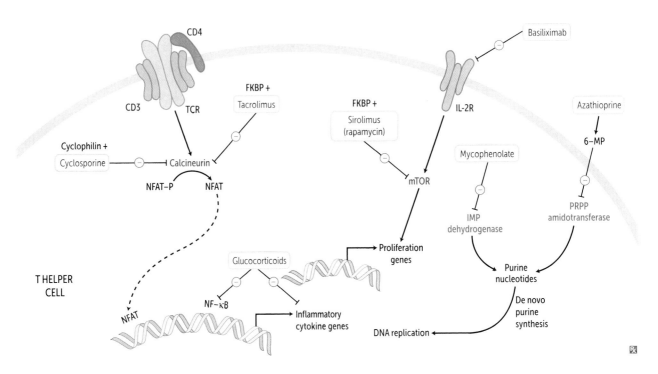

| DRUG | MECHANISM | INDICATIONS | TOXICITY | NOTES |
|---|---|---|---|---|
| **Cyclosporine** | Calcineurin inhibitor; binds cyclophilin. Blocks T-cell activation by **preventing IL-2 transcription** | Psoriasis, rheumatoid arthritis | **Nephrotoxicity,** hypertension, hyperlipidemia, neurotoxicity, gingival hyperplasia, hirsutism | Both calcineurin inhibitors are highly nephrotoxic, especially in higher doses or in patients with ↓ renal function |
| **Tacrolimus (FK506)** | Calcineurin inhibitor; binds FK506 binding protein (FKBP). Blocks T-cell activation by **preventing IL-2 transcription** | Immunosuppression after solid organ transplant | Similar to cyclosporine, ↑ risk of diabetes and neurotoxicity; no gingival hyperplasia or hirsutism | |
| **Sirolimus (Rapamycin)** | mTOR inhibitor; binds FKBP. Blocks T-cell activation and B-cell differentiation by **preventing response to IL-2** | Kidney transplant rejection prophylaxis specifically. Sir Basil's kidney transplant | "Pansirtopenia" (pancytopenia), insulin resistance, hyperlipidemia; **not nephrotoxic** | Kidney "sir-vives." Synergistic with cyclosporine. Also used in drug-eluting stents |
| **Basiliximab** | Monoclonal antibody; blocks IL-2R | | Edema, hypertension, tremor | |

## Immunosuppressants (continued)

| DRUG | MECHANISM | INDICATIONS | TOXICITY | NOTES |
|---|---|---|---|---|
| Azathioprine | Antimetabolite precursor of 6-mercaptopurine Inhibits lymphocyte proliferation by blocking nucleotide synthesis | Rheumatoid arthritis, Crohn disease, glomerulonephritis, other autoimmune conditions | Pancytopenia | 6-MP degraded by xanthine oxidase; toxicity ↑ by allopurinol Pronounce "azathio-purine" |
| Mycophenolate mofetil | Reversibly inhibits IMP dehydrogenase, preventing purine synthesis of B and T cells | Glucocorticoid-sparing agent in rheumatic disease | GI upset, pancytopenia, hypertension Less nephrotoxic and neurotoxic | Associated with invasive CMV infection |
| Glucocorticoids | Inhibit NF-κB Suppress both B- and T-cell function by ↓ transcription of many cytokines Induce T cell apoptosis | Many autoimmune and inflammatory disorders, adrenal insufficiency, asthma, CLL, non-Hodgkin lymphoma | Cushing syndrome, osteoporosis, hyperglycemia, diabetes, amenorrhea, adrenocortical atrophy, peptic ulcers, psychosis, cataracts, avascular necrosis (femoral head) | Demargination of WBCs causes artificial leukocytosis Adrenal insufficiency may develop if drug is stopped abruptly after chronic use |

## Recombinant cytokines and clinical uses

| CYTOKINE | AGENT | CLINICAL USES |
|---|---|---|
| **Bone marrow stimulation** | | |
| Erythropoietin | Epoetin alfa (EPO analog) | Anemias (especially in renal failure) Associated with ↑ risk of hypertension, thromboembolic events |
| Colony stimulating factors | Filgrastim (G-CSF), sargramostim (GM-CSF) | Leukopenia; recovery of granulocyte and monocyte counts |
| Thrombopoietin | Romiplostim (TPO analog), eltrombopag (think "elthrombopag." TPO receptor agonist) | Autoimmune thrombocytopenia Platelet stimulator |
| **Immunotherapy** | | |
| Interleukin-2 | Aldesleukin | Renal cell carcinoma, metastatic melanoma |
| Interferons | IFN-α | Chronic hepatitis C (not preferred) and B, renal cell carcinoma |
| | IFN-β | Multiple sclerosis |
| | IFN-γ | Chronic granulomatous disease |

▶ NOTES

# Microbiology

*"Within one linear centimeter of your lower colon there lives and works more bacteria (about 100 billion) than all humans who have ever been born. Yet many people continue to assert that it is we who are in charge of the world."*

—Neil deGrasse Tyson

*"What lies behind us and what lies ahead of us are tiny matters compared to what lies within us."*

—Henry S. Haskins

*"Wise and humane management of the patient is the best safeguard against infection."*

—Florence Nightingale

*"I sing and play the guitar, and I'm a walking, talking bacterial infection."*

—Kurt Cobain

Microbiology questions on the Step 1 exam often require two (or more) steps: Given a certain clinical presentation, you will first need to identify the most likely causative organism, and you will then need to provide an answer regarding some features of that organism or relevant antimicrobial agents. For example, a description of a child with fever and a petechial rash will be followed by a question that reads, "From what site does the responsible organism usually enter the blood?"

This section therefore presents organisms in two major ways: in individual microbial "profiles" and in the context of the systems they infect and the clinical presentations they produce. You should become familiar with both formats. When reviewing the systems approach, remind yourself of the features of each microbe by returning to the individual profiles. Also be sure to memorize the laboratory characteristics that allow you to identify microbes.

## ▶ MICROBIOLOGY—BASIC BACTERIOLOGY

### Bacterial structures

| STRUCTURE | CHEMICAL COMPOSITION | FUNCTION |
|---|---|---|
| **Appendages** | | |
| **Flagellum** | Proteins | Motility |
| **Pilus/fimbria** | Glycoprotein | Mediate adherence of bacteria to cell surface; sex pilus forms during conjugation |
| **Specialized structures** | | |
| **Spore** | Keratinlike coat, dipicolinic acid, peptidoglycan, DNA | Survival: resist dehydration, heat, chemicals |
| **Cell envelope** | | |
| **Capsule** | Discrete layer usually made of polysaccharides (and rarely proteins) | Protects against phagocytosis |
| **Slime (S) layer** | Loose network of polysaccharides | Mediates adherence to surfaces, plays a role in biofilm formation (eg, indwelling catheters) |
| **Outer membrane** | Outer leaflet: contains endotoxin (LPS/LOS) Embedded proteins: porins and other outer membrane proteins (OMPs) Inner leaflet: phospholipids | Gram ⊖ only Endotoxin: lipid A induces TNF and IL-1; antigenic O polysaccharide component Most OMPs are antigenic Porins: transport across outer membrane |
| **Periplasm** | Space between cytoplasmic membrane and outer membrane in gram ⊖ bacteria (peptidoglycan in middle) | Accumulates components exiting gram ⊖ cells, including hydrolytic enzymes (eg, β-lactamases) |
| **Cell wall** | Peptidoglycan is a sugar backbone with peptide side chains cross-linked by transpeptidase | Netlike structure gives rigid support, protects against osmotic pressure damage |
| **Cytoplasmic membrane** | Phospholipid bilayer sac with embedded proteins (eg, penicillin-binding proteins [PBPs]) and other enzymes Lipoteichoic acids (gram positive) only extend from membrane to exterior | Site of oxidative and transport enzymes; PBPs involved in cell wall synthesis Lipoteichoic acids induce TNF-α and IL-1 |

### Cell envelope

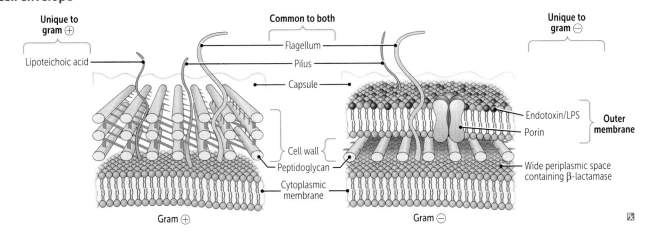

## Stains

| | | |
|---|---|---|
| **Gram stain** | First-line lab test in bacterial identification. Bacteria with thick peptidoglycan layer retain crystal violet dye (gram ⊕); bacteria with thin peptidoglycan layer turn red or pink (gram ⊖) with counterstain. | |
| | These bugs do not Gram stain well (These Little Microbes May Unfortunately Lack Real Color But Are Everywhere): | |
| | Treponema, *Leptospira* | Too thin to be visualized |
| | Mycobacteria | Cell wall has high lipid content |
| | *Mycoplasma, Ureaplasma* | No cell wall |
| | *Legionella, Rickettsia, Chlamydia, Bartonella, Anaplasma, Ehrlichia* | Primarily intracellular; also, *Chlamydia* lack classic peptidoglycan because of ↓ muramic acid |
| **Giemsa stain** | *H pylori, Chlamydia, Borrelia, Rickettsia, Trypanosomes* , *Plasmodium* | Help! Certain Bugs Really Try my Patience |
| **Periodic acid–Schiff stain** | Stains glycogen, mucopolysaccharides; used to diagnose Whipple disease (*Tropheryma whipplei* ) | |
| **Ziehl-Neelsen stain (carbol fuchsin)** | Acid-fast bacteria (eg, *Mycobacteria* , *Nocardia*; stains mycolic acid in cell wall); protozoa (eg, *Cryptosporidium* oocysts) | Auramine-rhodamine stain is more often used for screening (inexpensive, more sensitive) |
| **India ink stain** | *Cryptococcus neoformans* ; mucicarmine can also be used to stain thick polysaccharide capsule red | |
| **Silver stain** | *Helicobacter pylori, Legionella, Bartonella henselae*, and fungi (eg, *Coccidioides* ▣, *Pneumocystis jirovecii, Aspergillus fumigatus*) | HeLiCoPters Are silver |
| **Fluorescent antibody stain** | Used to identify many bacteria, viruses, *Pneumocystis jirovecii, Giardia*, and *Cryptosporidium* | Example is FTA-ABS for syphilis |

## Special culture requirements

| BUG | MEDIA USED FOR ISOLATION | MEDIA CONTENTS/OTHER |
|---|---|---|
| *H influenzae* | Chocolate agar | Factors V (NAD⁺) and X (hematin) |
| *N gonorrhoeae, N meningitidis* | Thayer-Martin agar | Selectively favors growth of *Neisseria* by inhibiting growth of gram ⊕ organisms with vancomycin, gram ⊖ organisms except *Neisseria* with trimethoprim and colistin, and fungi with nystatin <br> Very typically cultures *Neisseria* |
| *B pertussis* | Bordet-Gengou agar (**Bordet** for *Bordetella*) <br> Regan-Lowe medium | Potato extract <br> Charcoal, blood, and antibiotic |
| *C diphtheriae* | Tellurite agar, Löffler medium | |
| *M tuberculosis* | Löwenstein-Jensen medium, Middlebrook medium, rapid automated broth cultures | |
| *M pneumoniae* | Eaton agar | Requires cholesterol |
| Lactose-fermenting enterics | MacConkey agar | Fermentation produces acid, causing colonies to turn pink |
| *E coli* | Eosin–methylene blue (EMB) agar | Colonies with green metallic sheen |
| *Brucella, Francisella, Legionella, Pasteurella* | Charcoal yeast extract agar buffered with cysteine and iron | The **Ella** siblings, **Bruce**, **Francis**, a **legion**naire, and a **pasteur** (pastor), built the **Sistine** (cysteine) chapel out of **charcoal** and **iron** |
| Fungi | Sabouraud agar | "**Sab**'s a fun guy!" |

| **Anaerobes** | Examples include *Clostridium, Bacteroides, Fusobacterium,* and *Actinomyces israelii.* They lack catalase and/or superoxide dismutase and are thus susceptible to oxidative damage. Generally foul smelling (short-chain fatty acids), are difficult to culture, and produce gas in tissue ($CO_2$ and $H_2$). | Anaerobes Can't Breathe Fresh Air. Anaerobes are normal microbiota in GI tract, typically pathogenic elsewhere (eg, causes aspiration pneumonia). Amin$O_2$glycosides are ineffective against anaerobes because these antibiotics require $O_2$ to enter into bacterial cell. |
|---|---|---|
| **Facultative anaerobes** | May use $O_2$ as a terminal electron acceptor to generate ATP, but can also use fermentation and other $O_2$-independent pathways. | Streptococci, staphylococci, and enteric gram ⊖ bacteria. |

**Intracellular bacteria**

| **Obligate intracellular** | *Rickettsia, Chlamydia, Coxiella* Rely on host ATP | Stay inside (cells) when it is Really Chilly and Cold |
|---|---|---|
| **Facultative intracellular** | *Salmonella, Neisseria, Brucella, Mycobacterium, Listeria, Francisella, Legionella, Yersinia pestis* | Some Nasty Bugs May Live FacultativeLY |

| **Encapsulated bacteria**<br> | Examples are *Pseudomonas aeruginosa, Streptococcus pneumoniae* Ⓐ, *Haemophilus influenzae* type b, *Neisseria meningitidis, Escherichia coli, Salmonella, Klebsiella pneumoniae,* and group B Strep. Their capsules serve as an antiphagocytic virulence factor.<br>Capsular polysaccharide +/– protein conjugate can serve as an antigen in vaccines. A polysaccharide antigen alone cannot be presented to T cells; immunogenicity can be enhanced by conjugating capsule antigens to a carrier protein. | Please SHiNE my SKiS.<br>Are opsonized, and then cleared by spleen. Asplenics (No Spleen Here) have ↓ opsonizing ability and thus ↑ risk for severe infections; need vaccines to protect against:<br>▪ *N meningitidis*<br>▪ *S pneumoniae*<br>▪ *H influenzae* |
|---|---|---|

| **Urease-positive organisms** | *Proteus, Cryptococcus, H pylori, Ureaplasma, Nocardia, Klebsiella, S epidermidis, S saprophyticus.* Urease hydrolyzes urea to release ammonia and $CO_2 \rightarrow$ ↑ pH. Predisposes to struvite (magnesium ammonium phosphate) stones, particularly *Proteus.* | Pee CHUNKSS. |
|---|---|---|

**Catalase-positive organisms**

Catalase degrades $H_2O_2$ into $H_2O$ and bubbles of $O_2$  before it can be converted to microbicidal products by the enzyme myeloperoxidase. People with chronic granulomatous disease (NADPH oxidase deficiency) have recurrent infections with certain catalase $\oplus$ organisms.

Catalase $\oplus$ organisms include *Candida, Pseudomonas, Nocardia, Bordetella pertussis, Burkholderia cepacia, Helicobacter pylori, Aspergillus, Staphylococci, Serratia, Listeria, E coli.* Catalase Positive: Notoriously Big Bubbling **HASSLE**.

---

**Pigment-producing bacteria**

| | |
|---|---|
| *Actinomyces israelii*—yellow "sulfur" granules, which are composed of filaments of bacteria | Israel has yellow sand |
| *S aureus*—**gold**en yellow pigment | *Aureus* (Latin) = **gold** |
| *P aeruginosa*—blue-**green** pigment (pyocyanin and pyoverdin) | A**erug**ula is **green** |
| *Serratia marcescens*—**red** pigment | Think **red Sriracha** hot sauce |

---

**In vivo biofilm-producing bacteria**

| | |
|---|---|
| *S epidermidis* | Catheter and prosthetic device infections |
| Viridans streptococci (*S mutans, S sanguinis*) | Dental plaques, infective endocarditis |
| *P aeruginosa* | Respiratory tree colonization in patients with cystic fibrosis, ventilator-associated pneumonia Contact lens–associated keratitis |
| Nontypeable (unencapsulated) *H influenzae* | Otitis media |

| | | |
|---|---|---|
| **Spore-forming bacteria** | Some gram ⊕ bacteria can form spores when nutrients are limited. Spores lack metabolic activity and are highly resistant to heat and chemicals. Core contains dipicolinic acid (responsible for heat resistance). Must autoclave to kill spores (as is done to surgical equipment) by steaming at 121°C for 15 minutes. Hydrogen peroxide and iodine-based agents are also sporicidal. | Examples: *B anthracis* (anthrax), *B cereus* (food poisoning), *C botulinum* (botulism), *C difficile* (pseudomembranous colitis), *C perfringens* (gas gangrene), *C tetani* (tetanus). Autoclave to kill Bacillus and Clostridium (ABC). |

| | |
|---|---|
| **Bacterial virulence factors** | These promote evasion of host immune response. |
| Capsular polysaccharide | Highly charged, hydrophilic structure. Acts as barrier to phagocytosis and complement-mediated lysis. Major determinant of virulence. |
| Protein A | Binds Fc region of IgG. Prevents opsonization and phagocytosis. Expressed by *S aureus.* |
| IgA protease | Enzyme that cleaves IgA, allowing bacteria to adhere to and colonize mucous membranes. Secreted by *S pneumoniae*, *H influenzae* type b, and *Neisseria* (SHiN). |
| M protein | Helps prevent phagocytosis. Expressed by group A streptococci. Sequence homology with human cardiac myosin (molecular mimicry); possibly underlies the autoimmune response seen in acute rheumatic fever. |

| | |
|---|---|
| **Bacterial genetics** | Horizontal gene transfer is the main mechanism for transfer of antibiotic resistance among bacteria. |

### Transformation

Competent bacteria can bind and import short pieces of environmental naked bacterial chromosomal DNA (from bacterial cell lysis). The transfer and expression of newly transferred genes is called transformation. A feature of many bacteria, especially *S pneumoniae*, *H influenzae* type b, and *Neisseria* (**SHiN**).

Adding deoxyribonuclease degrades naked DNA, preventing transformation.

Naked DNA → Recipient cell → Transformed cell

Degraded uncombined DNA, Recipient DNA, Donor DNA

### Conjugation

#### F⁺ × F⁻

F⁺ plasmid contains genes required for sex pilus and conjugation. Bacteria without this plasmid are termed F⁻. Sex pilus on F⁺ bacterium contacts F⁻ bacterium. A single strand of plasmid DNA is transferred across the conjugal bridge ("mating bridge"). No transfer of chromosomal DNA.

F⁺ plasmid contains genes for sex pilus and conjugation. Sex pilus forming congugal bridge "mating bridge". Single strand of plasmid DNA transferred. No transfer of chromosomal DNA.

F⁺ cell F⁻ cell | F⁺ cell F⁻ cell | F⁺ cell F⁻ cell | F⁺ cell F⁺ cell

#### Hfr × F⁻

F⁺ plasmid can become incorporated into bacterial chromosomal DNA, termed high-frequency recombination (Hfr) cell. Transfer of leading part of plasmid and a few flanking chromosomal genes. High-frequency recombination may integrate some of those bacterial genes. Recipient cell remains F⁻ but now may have new bacterial genes.

High-frequency recombination (Hfr) cell contains F⁺ plasmid incorporated into bacterial DNA. Leading portion of plasmid transfers along with flanking bacterial chromosome.

Plasmid

F⁺ cell F⁻ cell | Hfr cell F⁻ cell | Hfr cell F⁻ cell | Hfr cell Recombinant F⁻ cell

F⁻ cell bacterial DNA + F⁺ cell bacterial DNA + plasmid copy

### Transduction

#### Generalized

A "packaging" error. Lytic phage infects bacterium, leading to cleavage of bacterial DNA. Parts of bacterial chromosomal DNA may become packaged in phage capsid. Phage infects another bacterium, transferring these genes.

Lytic phage, Bacteria, Cleavage of bacterial DNA, Bacterial DNA packaged in phage capsids

Release of new phage from lysed cell, Infects other bacteria, Genes transferred to new bacteria

#### Specialized

An "excision" event. Lysogenic phage infects bacterium; viral DNA incorporates into bacterial chromosome. When phage DNA is excised, flanking bacterial genes may be excised with it. DNA is packaged into phage capsid and can infect another bacterium.

Genes for the following 5 bacterial toxins are encoded in a lysogenic phage (**ABCD'S**): Group A strep erythrogenic toxin, Botulinum toxin, Cholera toxin, Diphtheria toxin, Shiga toxin.

Lysogenic phage, Viral DNA, Bacteria, Viral DNA incorporates in bacterial DNA, Phage particles carry bacterial DNA

Release of new phage from lysed cell, Infects other bacteria, Genes different from donor and recipient

## Bacterial genetics (continued)

| | |
|---|---|
| Transposition | A "jumping" process involving a transposon (specialized segment of DNA), which can copy and excise itself and then insert into the same DNA molecule or an unrelated DNA (eg, plasmid or chromosome). Critical in creating plasmids with multiple drug resistance and transfer across species lines (eg, Tn*1546* with *vanA* from *Enterococcus* to *S aureus*). |

## Main features of exotoxins and endotoxins

| | Exotoxins | Endotoxins |
|---|---|---|
| SOURCE | Certain species of gram ⊕ and gram ⊖ bacteria | Outer cell membrane of most gram ⊖ bacteria |
| SECRETED FROM CELL | Yes | No |
| CHEMISTRY | Polypeptide | Lipid A component of LPS (structural part of bacteria; released when lysed) |
| LOCATION OF GENES | Plasmid or bacteriophage | Bacterial chromosome |
| TOXICITY | High (fatal dose on the order of 1 μg) | Low (fatal dose on the order of hundreds of micrograms) |
| CLINICAL EFFECTS | Various effects (see following pages) | Fever, shock (hypotension), DIC |
| MODE OF ACTION | Various modes (see following pages) | Induces TNF, IL-1, and IL-6 |
| ANTIGENICITY | Induces high-titer antibodies called antitoxins | Poorly antigenic |
| VACCINES | Toxoids used as vaccines | No toxoids formed and no vaccine available |
| HEAT STABILITY | Destroyed rapidly at 60°C (except staphylococcal enterotoxin and *E coli* heat-stable toxin, and *B cereus* emetic toxin) | Stable at 100°C for 1 hr |
| TYPICAL DISEASES | Tetanus, botulism, diphtheria, cholera | Meningococcemia; sepsis by gram ⊖ rods |

## Bacteria with exotoxins

| BACTERIA | TOXIN | MECHANISM | MANIFESTATION |
|---|---|---|---|
| **Inhibit protein synthesis** | | | |
| *Corynebacterium diphtheriae* | Diphtheria toxin[a] | Inactivate elongation factor (EF-2) through ADP-ribosylation | Pharyngitis with pseudomembranes in throat and severe lymphadenopathy (bull neck), myocarditis |
| *Pseudomonas aeruginosa* | Exotoxin A[a] | | Host cell death |
| *Shigella* spp  <br>**Enterohemorrhagic *E coli*** | Shiga toxin[a] | Inactivate 60S ribosome by removing adenine from rRNA | Damages GI mucosa → dysentery  <br>Toxin-mediated injury and cytokine release → hemolytic-uremic syndrome (HUS; prototypically in EHEC serotype O157:H7)  <br>Unlike *Shigella*, EHEC does not invade host cells |
| **Increase fluid secretion** | | | |
| **Enterotoxigenic *E coli*** | Heat-labile toxin (LT)[a] | Overactivates adenylate cyclase ($\uparrow$ cAMP) → $\uparrow$ Cl⁻ secretion in gut and $H_2O$ efflux | Watery diarrhea: "labile in the Air (Adenylate cyclase), stable on the Ground (Guanylate cyclase)"  <br>Bacteria that $\uparrow$ cAMP include cholera, anthracis, pertussis, *E coli* |
| | Heat-stable toxin (ST) | Overactivates guanylate cyclase ($\uparrow$ cGMP) → $\downarrow$ resorption of NaCl and $H_2O$ in gut | |
| *Bacillus anthracis* | Anthrax toxin[a] | Mimics adenylate cyclase ($\uparrow$ cAMP) | Likely responsible for characteristic edematous borders of black eschar in cutaneous anthrax |
| *Vibrio cholerae* | Cholera toxin[a] | Overactivates adenylate cyclase ($\uparrow$ cAMP) by permanently activating $G_s$ | Voluminous "rice-water" diarrhea |
| **Inhibit phagocytic ability** | | | |
| *Bordetella pertussis* | Pertussis toxin[a] | Activates adenylate cyclase ($\uparrow$ cAMP) by inactivating inhibitory subunit ($G_i$). | Whooping cough—child coughs on expiration and "whoops" on inspiration; can cause "100-day cough" in adults; associated with posttussive emesis |
| **Inhibit release of neurotransmitter** | | | |
| *Clostridium tetani* | Tetanospasmin[a] | Both are proteases that cleave SNARE (soluble NSF attachment protein receptor), a set of proteins required for neurotransmitter release via vesicular fusion | Toxin prevents release of **inhibitory** (GABA and glycine) neurotransmitters from Renshaw cells in spinal cord → spastic paralysis, risus sardonicus, trismus (lockjaw), opisthotonos |
| *Clostridium botulinum* | Botulinum toxin[a] | | Infant botulism—caused by ingestion of spores (eg, from soil, raw honey). Toxin produced in vivo  <br>Foodborne botulism—caused by ingestion of preformed toxin (eg, from canned foods) |

[a]An AB toxin (also called two-component toxin [or three for anthrax]) with B enabling Binding and triggering uptake (endocytosis) of the Active A component. The A components are usually ADP ribosyltransferases; others have enzymatic activities as listed in chart.

**Bacteria with exotoxins** *(continued)*

| BACTERIA | TOXIN | MECHANISM | MANIFESTATION |
|---|---|---|---|
| **Lyse cell membranes** | | | |
| *Clostridium perfringens* | Alpha toxin | Phospholipase (lecithinase) that degrades tissue and cell membranes | Degradation of phospholipids → myonecrosis ("gas gangrene") and hemolysis ("double zone" of hemolysis on blood agar) |
| *Streptococcus pyogenes* | Streptolysin O | Protein that degrades cell membrane | Lyses RBCs; contributes to β-hemolysis; host antibodies against toxin (ASO) used to diagnose rheumatic fever (do not confuse with immune complexes of poststreptococcal glomerulonephritis) |
| **Superantigens causing shock** | | | |
| *Staphylococcus aureus* | Toxic shock syndrome toxin (TSST-1) | Cross-links β region of TCR to MHC class II on APCs outside of the antigen binding site → overwhelming release of IL-1, IL-2, IFN-γ, and TNF-α → shock | Toxic shock syndrome: fever, rash, shock; other toxins cause scalded skin syndrome (exfoliative toxin) and food poisoning (heat-stable enterotoxin) |
| *Streptococcus pyogenes* | Erythrogenic exotoxin A | | Toxic shock–like syndrome: fever, rash, shock; scarlet fever |

| **Endotoxin** | LPS found in outer membrane of gram ⊖ bacteria (both cocci and rods). Composed of O-antigen + core polysaccharide + lipid A (the toxic component). *Neisseria* have lipooligosaccharide.<br>Released upon cell lysis or by living cells by blebs detaching from outer surface membrane (vs exotoxin, which is actively secreted).<br>Three main effects: macrophage activation (TLR4/CD14), complement activation, and tissue factor activation. | ENDOTOXINS:<br>Edema<br>Nitric oxide<br>DIC/Death<br>Outer membrane<br>TNF-α<br>O-antigen + core polysaccharide + lipid A<br>eXtremely heat stable<br>IL-1 and IL-6<br>Neutrophil chemotaxis<br>Shock |
|---|---|---|

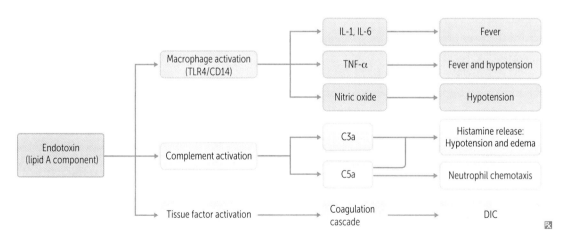

▶ MICROBIOLOGY—CLINICAL BACTERIOLOGY

### Gram-positive lab algorithm

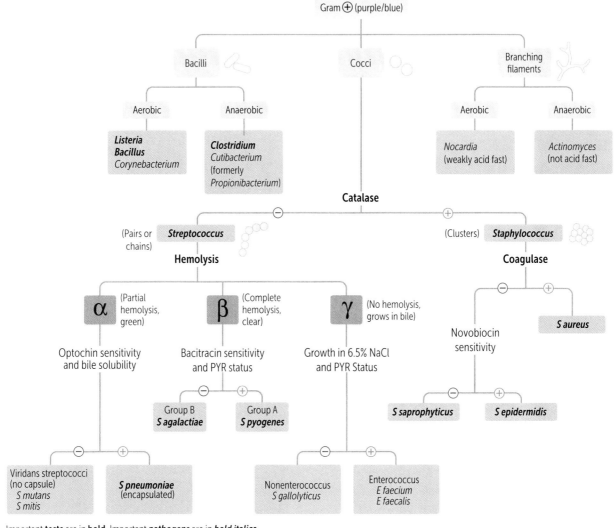

Important **tests** are in **bold.** Important *pathogens* are in ***bold italics.***
Note: Enterococcus is either α- or γ-hemolytic.
*PYR,* Pyrrolidonyl aminopeptidase.

## Hemolytic bacteria

| | | |
|---|---|---|
| α-hemolytic bacteria | Partial oxidation of hemoglobin → greenish or brownish color without clearing around growth on blood agar A. Include *Streptococcus pneumoniae* and viridans streptococci. |  |
| β-hemolytic bacteria | Complete lysis of RBCs → pale/clear area surrounding colony on blood agar A. Include *Staphylococcus aureus, Streptococcus pyogenes* (group A strep), *Streptococcus agalactiae* (group B strep), *Listeria monocytogenes*. | |

### *Staphylococcus aureus*

Gram ⊕, β-hemolytic, catalase ⊕, coagulase ⊕ cocci in clusters A. Protein A (virulence factor) binds Fc-IgG, inhibiting complement activation and phagocytosis. Commonly colonizes the skin, nares, ears, axilla, and groin.

Causes:

- Inflammatory disease—skin infections, organ abscesses, pneumonia (often after influenza virus infection), infective endocarditis, septic arthritis, and osteomyelitis.
- Toxin-mediated disease—toxic shock syndrome (TSST-1), scalded skin syndrome (exfoliative toxin), rapid-onset food poisoning (enterotoxins).

MRSA (methicillin-resistant *S aureus*)—important cause of serious healthcare-associated and community-acquired infections. Resistance due to altered penicillin-binding proteins (conferred by *mecA* gene). Some strains release Panton-Valentine leukocidin (PVL), which kills leukocytes and causes tissue necrosis.

TSST-1 is a superantigen that binds to MHC II and T-cell receptor, resulting in polyclonal T-cell activation and cytokine release.

Staphylococcal toxic shock syndrome (TSS)—fever, vomiting, diarrhea, rash, desquamation, shock, end-organ failure. TSS results in ↑ AST, ↑ ALT, ↑ bilirubin. Associated with prolonged use of vaginal tampons or nasal packing.

Compare with *Streptococcus pyogenes* TSS (a toxic shock–like syndrome associated with painful skin infection).

*S aureus* food poisoning due to ingestion of preformed toxin → short incubation period (2–6 hr) followed by nonbloody diarrhea and emesis. Enterotoxin is heat stable → not destroyed by cooking.

*S aureus* makes coagulase and toxins. Forms fibrin clot around itself → abscess.

### *Staphylococcus epidermidis*

Gram ⊕, catalase ⊕, coagulase ⊖, urease ⊕ cocci in clusters. Novobiocin sensitive. Does not ferment mannitol (vs *S aureus*).

Normal microbiota of skin; contaminates blood cultures.

Infects prosthetic devices (eg, hip implant, heart valve) and IV catheters by producing adherent biofilms.

### *Staphylococcus saprophyticus*

Gram ⊕, catalase ⊕, coagulase ⊖, urease ⊕ cocci in clusters. Novobiocin resistant.

Normal microbiota of female genital tract and perineum.

Second most common cause of uncomplicated UTI in young females (most common is *E coli*).

| | | |
|---|---|---|
| ***Streptococcus pneumoniae***<br> | Gram ⊕, α-hemolytic, lancet-shaped diplococci A.<br>Encapsulated. IgA protease. Optochin sensitive and bile soluble.<br>Most commonly causes MOPS:<br>▪ Meningitis<br>▪ Otitis media (in children)<br>▪ Pneumonia<br>▪ Sinusitis | Pneumococcal pneumonia is associated with "rusty" sputum.<br>Patients with anatomic or functional hyposplenia or asplenia are predisposed to infection.<br>No virulence without capsule.<br>Pneumococcal vaccines are available in both conjugate (PCV13, PCV15, PCV20) and polysaccharide (PPSV23) formulations. |
| **Viridans group streptococci** | Gram ⊕, α-hemolytic cocci. Optochin resistant and bile insoluble. Normal microbiota of the oropharynx.<br>*Streptococcus mutans* and *S mitis* cause dental caries.<br>*S sanguinis* makes dextrans that bind to fibrin-platelet aggregates on damaged heart valves, causing infective endocarditis. | Viridans group strep live in the mouth, because they are not afraid of-the-chin (op-to-chin resistant).<br>*Sanguinis* = blood. Think, "there is lots of blood in the heart" (infective endocarditis). |
| ***Streptococcus pyogenes* (group A streptococci)**<br> | Gram ⊕ cocci in chains A. Group A strep cause:<br>▪ Pyogenic—pharyngitis, cellulitis, impetigo ("honey-crusted" lesions), erysipelas<br>▪ Toxigenic—scarlet fever, toxic shock–like syndrome, necrotizing fasciitis<br>▪ Immunologic—rheumatic fever, glomerulonephritis<br>Bacitracin sensitive, β-hemolytic, pyrrolidonyl arylamidase (PYR) ⊕. Hyaluronic acid capsule and M protein inhibit phagocytosis. Antibodies to M protein enhance host defenses. Structurally similar to host proteins (ie, myosin); can lead to autoimmunity (ie, carditis seen in acute rheumatic fever).<br>Diagnose strep pharyngitis via throat swab, which can be tested with an antigen detection assay (rapid, in-office results) or cultured on blood agar (results in 48 hours). | "Ph"yogenes pharyngitis can result in rheumatic "phever" and glomerulonephritis.<br>Strains causing impetigo can induce glomerulonephritis.<br>Key virulence factors include DNase, erythrogenic exotoxin, streptokinase, streptolysin O. ASO titer or anti-DNase B antibodies indicate recent *S pyogenes* infection.<br>Scarlet fever—fine, blanching, generalized sandpaperlike rash sparing palms and soles, strawberry tongue, and circumoral pallor in the setting of group A streptococcal pharyngitis (erythrogenic toxin ⊕). |

| | | |
|---|---|---|
| ***Streptococcus agalactiae* (group B streptococci)** | Gram ⊕ cocci, bacitracin resistant, β-hemolytic, colonizes vagina; causes pneumonia, meningitis, and sepsis, mainly in babies. Polysaccharide capsule confers virulence. Produces CAMP factor, which enlarges the area of hemolysis formed by *S aureus*. (Note: CAMP stands for the authors of the test, not cyclic AMP.) Hippurate test ⊕. PYR ⊖. Screen pregnant patients at 35–37 weeks of gestation with rectal and vaginal swabs. Patients with ⊕ culture receive intrapartum penicillin/ampicillin prophylaxis. | Group B for Babies! |
| **Streptococcus gallolyticus** | Formerly *S bovis*. Gram ⊕ cocci, colonizes the gut. Can cause bacteremia and infective endocarditis. Patients with *S gallolyticus* endocarditis have ↑ incidence of colon cancer. | Bovis in the blood = cancer in the colon. |
| **Enterococci** | Gram ⊕ cocci. Enterococci (*E faecalis* and *E faecium*) are normal colonic microbiota that are penicillin G resistant and cause UTI, biliary tract infections, and infective endocarditis (following GI/GU procedures). Catalase ⊖, PYR ⊕, typically nonhemolytic. VRE (vancomycin-resistant enterococci) are an important cause of healthcare-associated infection. | Enterococci are more resilient than streptococci, can grow in 6.5% NaCl and bile (lab test). *Entero* = intestine, *faecalis* = feces, *strepto* = twisted (chains), *coccus* = berry. |
| ***Bacillus anthracis***  | Gram ⊕, spore-forming rod that produces anthrax toxin, exotoxins consisting of protective antigen, lethal factor (inhibits MAP kinase → macrophage apoptosis), and edema factor (acts as adenylyl cyclase → ↑ intracellular cAMP, upsetting homeostasis → edema, necrosis). Has a polypeptide capsule (poly D-glutamate). Colonies show a halo of projections, sometimes called "medusa head" appearance. **Cutaneous anthrax**—painless papule surrounded by vesicles → ulcer with black eschar **A** (painless, necrotic) → uncommonly progresses to bacteremia and death. **Pulmonary anthrax**—inhalation of spores, most commonly from contaminated animals or animal products, although also a potential bioweapon → flulike symptoms that rapidly progress to fever, pulmonary hemorrhage, mediastinitis (CXR may show widened mediastinum), and shock. Also called woolsorter's disease. Prophylaxis with ciprofloxacin or doxycycline when exposed. Both cutaneous and pulmonary anthrax may be complicated by hemorrhagic meningitis. | |

| | |
|---|---|
| ***Bacillus cereus*** | Gram ⊕ rod. Causes food poisoning. Spores survive cooking rice (reheated rice syndrome). Keeping rice warm results in germination of spores and enterotoxin formation. Emetic type causes nausea and vomiting within 1–5 hours. Caused by cereulide, a preformed toxin. Diarrheal type causes watery, nonbloody diarrhea and GI pain within 8–18 hours. Management: supportive care (antibiotics are ineffective against toxins). | |

***Clostridioides difficile***

Produces toxins A and B, which damage enterocytes. Both toxins lead to watery diarrhea → pseudomembranous colitis A. Often 2° to antibiotic use, especially clindamycin, ampicillin, cephalosporins, fluoroquinolones; associated with PPIs.
Fulminant infection: toxic megacolon, ileus, shock.

*Difficile* causes diarrhea.
Diagnosed by PCR or antigen detection of one or both toxins in stool.
Treatment: oral vancomycin or fidaxomicin. For recurrent cases, consider repeating prior regimen or fecal microbiota transplant.

***Clostridia***

Gram ⊕, spore-forming, obligate anaerobic rods. Tetanus toxin and botulinum toxin are proteases that cleave SNARE proteins involved in neurotransmission.

***Clostridium tetani***

Pathogen is noninvasive and remains localized to wound site. Produces tetanospasmin, an exotoxin causing tetanus. Tetanospasmin spreads by retrograde axonal transport to CNS and blocks release of GABA and glycine from Renshaw cells in spinal cord.
Causes spastic paralysis, trismus (lockjaw), risus sardonicus (raised eyebrows and open grin), opisthotonos (spasms of spinal extensors).

Tetanus is tetanic paralysis.
Prevent with tetanus vaccine. Treat with antitoxin +/– vaccine booster, antibiotics, diazepam (for muscle spasms), and wound debridement.

***Clostridium botulinum***

Produces a heat-labile toxin that damages SNARE proteins, thus preventing ACh release at the neuromuscular junction, causing botulism. In babies, ingestion of spores (eg, in honey) leads to disease (floppy baby syndrome). In adults, disease is caused by ingestion of preformed toxin (eg, in canned food).
Symptoms of botulism (the 5 D's): diplopia, dysarthria, dysphagia, dyspnea, descending flaccid paralysis. Does not present with sensory deficits.

*Botulinum* is from bad bottles of food, juice, and honey.
Treatment: human botulinum immunoglobulin.
Local botulinum toxin A (Botox) injections used to treat focal dystonia, hyperhidrosis, muscle spasms, and cosmetic reduction of facial wrinkles.

***Clostridium perfringens***

Produces α-toxin (lecithinase, a phospholipase) that can cause myonecrosis (gas gangrene A; presents as soft tissue crepitus) and hemolysis.
If heavily spore-contaminated food is cooked but left standing too long at < 60°C, spore germinate → vegetative bacteria ingested → enterotoxin → late-onset (10–12 hours) food poisoning symptoms, resolution in 24 hours.

*Perfringens* perforates a gangrenous leg.
Spontaneous gas gangrene (via hematogenous seeding; associated with colonic malignancy) is most commonly caused by *Clostridium septicum*.

| | | |
|---|---|---|
| **Corynebacterium diphtheriae** | Gram ⊕ rods occurring in angular arrangements; transmitted via respiratory droplets. Causes diphtheria via exotoxin encoded by β-prophage. Potent exotoxin inhibits protein synthesis via ADP-ribosylation of EF-2, leading to possible necrosis in pharynx, cardiac, and CNS tissue. | *Coryne* = club shaped (metachromatic granules on Löffler media). |

Gram ⊕ rods occurring in angular arrangements; transmitted via respiratory droplets. Causes diphtheria via exotoxin encoded by β-prophage. Potent exotoxin inhibits protein synthesis via ADP-ribosylation of EF-2, leading to possible necrosis in pharynx, cardiac, and CNS tissue.

Symptoms include pseudomembranous pharyngitis (grayish-white membrane ) with lymphadenopathy ("bull's neck" appearance). Toxin dissemination may cause myocarditis, arrhythmias, neuropathies.

Lab diagnosis based on gram ⊕ rods with metachromatic (blue and red) granules and ⊕ Elek test for toxin.

Toxoid vaccine prevents diphtheria.

*Coryne* = club shaped (metachromatic granules on Löffler media).
Black colonies on cystine-tellurite agar.
ABCDEFG:
- ADP-ribosylation
- β-prophage
- *Corynebacterium*
- *Diphtheriae*
- Elongation Factor 2
- Granules

Treatment: diphtheria antitoxin +/− erythromycin or penicillin.

---

**Listeria monocytogenes**

Gram ⊕, facultative intracellular rod; acquired by ingestion of unpasteurized dairy products and cold deli meats, transplacental transmission, and by vaginal transmission during birth. Grows well at refrigeration temperatures ("cold enrichment").

Forms "rocket tails" (red in ) via actin polymerization that allow intracellular movement and cell-to-cell spread across cell membranes, thereby avoiding antibody. Listeriolysin generates pores in phagosomes, allowing its escape into cytoplasm. Characteristic tumbling motility in broth.

Can cause amnionitis, sepsis, and spontaneous abortion in pregnant patients; granulomatosis infantiseptica; meningitis in immunocompromised patients, neonates, and older adults; mild, self-limited gastroenteritis in healthy individuals.

Treatment: ampicillin.

---

**Nocardia vs Actinomyces**

Both are gram ⊕ and form long, branching filaments resembling fungi.

| Nocardia | Actinomyces |
|---|---|
| Aerobe, catalase ⊕ | Anaerobe, catalase ⊖ |
| Acid fast (weak)  | Not acid fast  |
| Found in soil | Normal oral, reproductive, and GI microbiota |
| Causes pulmonary infections in immunocompromised (can mimic TB but with ⊖ PPD); cutaneous infections after trauma in immunocompetent; can spread to CNS → cerebral abscess | Causes oral/facial abscesses that drain through sinus tracts; often associated with dental caries/extraction and other maxillofacial trauma; forms yellow "sulfur granules"; can also cause PID with IUDs |
| Treat with sulfonamides (TMP-SMX) | Treat with penicillin |

Treatment is a **SNAP**: Sulfonamides—*Nocardia*; *Actinomyces*—Penicillin

## Mycobacteria

Acid-fast rods (pink rods, arrows in **A**). Grows slowly in culture.

*Mycobacterium tuberculosis* (TB, often resistant to multiple drugs).

*M avium–intracellulare* (causes disseminated, non-TB disease in AIDS; often resistant to multiple drugs).

*M scrofulaceum* (cervical lymphadenitis in children).

*M marinum* (skin infection in aquarium handlers).

TB symptoms include fever, night sweats, weight loss, cough (nonproductive or productive), hemoptysis.

Cord factor creates a "serpentine cord" appearance in virulent *M tuberculosis* strains; activates macrophages (promoting granuloma formation) and induces release of TNF-α. Sulfatides (surface glycolipids) inhibit phagolysosomal fusion.

## Tuberculosis

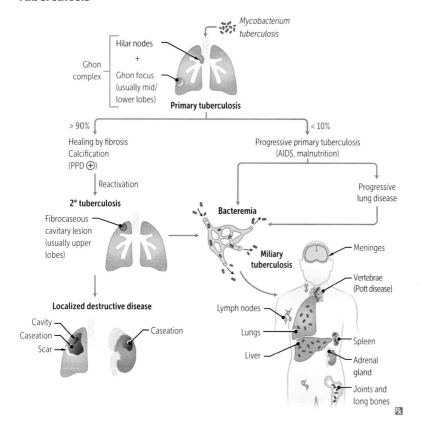

PPD ⊕ if current or past infection.

PPD ⊖ if no infection and in immunocompromised patients (especially with low CD4+ cell count).

Interferon-γ release assay (IGRA) has fewer false positives from BCG vaccination.

Caseating granulomas with central necrosis and Langhans giant cell (single example in **A**) are characteristic of 2° tuberculosis. Do not confuse Langhans giant cell (fused macrophages) with Langerhans cell (dermal APC).

TB reactivation risk highest in immunocompromised individuals (eg, HIV, organ transplant recipients, TNF-α inhibitor use). Reactivation has a predilection for the apices of the lung (due to the bacteria being highly aerobic).

### Leprosy

Also called Hansen disease. Caused by *Mycobacterium leprae*, an acid-fast bacillus that likes cool temperatures (infects skin and superficial nerves—"glove and stocking" loss of sensation) and cannot be grown in vitro. Diagnosed via skin biopsy or tissue PCR. Reservoir in United States: armadillos.

Leprosy has 2 forms (many cases fall temporarily between two extremes):

- Lepromatous—presents diffusely over the skin, with leonine (lionlike) facies **A**, and is communicable (high bacterial load); characterized by low cell-mediated immunity with a largely Th2 response. Lepromatous form can be lethal.
- Tuberculoid—limited to a few hypoesthetic, hairless skin plaques **B**; characterized by high cell-mediated immunity with a largely Th1 response and low bacterial load.

Treatment: dapsone and rifampin for tuberculoid form; clofazimine is added for lepromatous form.

### Gram-negative lab algorithm

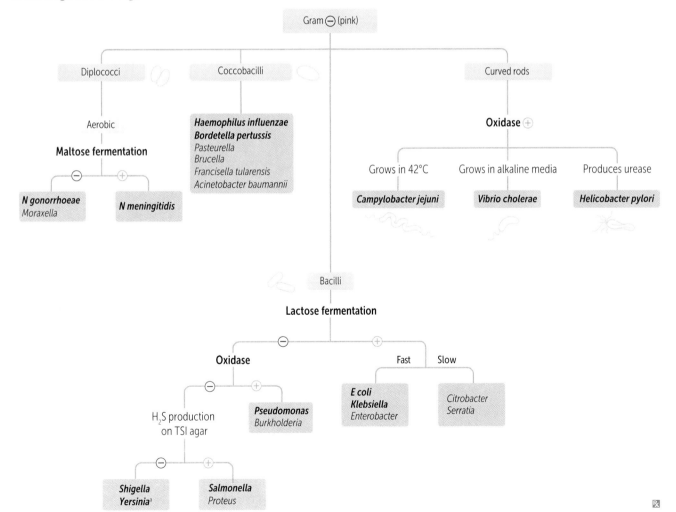

Important **tests** are in **bold**. Important **pathogens** are in ***bold italics***.
[a]Pleomorphic rod/coccobacillus

## Neisseria

Gram ⊖ diplococci. Metabolize glucose and produce IgA proteases. Contain lipooligosaccharides (LOS) with strong endotoxin activity.

N gonorrhoeae is often intracellular (within neutrophils)  **A**.

Acid production: meningococci—maltose and glucose; gonococci—glucose.

| Gonococci | Meningococci |
| --- | --- |
| No polysaccharide capsule | Polysaccharide capsule |
| No maltose acid detection | Maltose acid detection |
| No vaccine due to antigenic variation of pilus proteins | Vaccine (type B vaccine available for at-risk individuals) |
| Sexually or perinatally transmitted | Transmitted via respiratory and oral secretions. More common among individuals in close quarters (eg, army barracks, college dorms) |
| Causes gonorrhea, septic arthritis, neonatal conjunctivitis (2–5 days after birth), pelvic inflammatory disease (PID), and Fitz-Hugh–Curtis syndrome | Causes meningococcemia with petechial hemorrhages and gangrene of toes **B**, meningitis, Waterhouse-Friderichsen syndrome (acute hemorrhagic adrenal insufficiency) |
| Diagnosed with NAAT | Diagnosed via culture-based tests or PCR |
| Condoms ↓ sexual transmission, erythromycin eye ointment prevents neonatal blindness | Rifampin, ciprofloxacin, or ceftriaxone prophylaxis in close contacts |
| Treatment: single dose IM ceftriaxone; if chlamydial coinfection not excluded by molecular testing, add doxycycline | Treatment: ceftriaxone or penicillin G |

## Haemophilus influenzae

Small gram ⊖ (coccobacillary) rod. Transmitted through respiratory droplets. Nontypeable (unencapsulated) strains are the most common cause of mucosal infections (otitis media, conjunctivitis, bronchitis) as well as invasive infections since the vaccine for capsular type b was introduced. Produces IgA protease.

Culture on chocolate agar, which contains factors V (NAD⁺) and X (hematin) for growth; can also be grown with S aureus, which provides factor V via RBC hemolysis.

*Haemophilus* causes epiglottitis (endoscopic appearance can be "cherry red" in children; "thumb sign" on lateral neck x-ray **A**), meningitis, otitis media, and pneumonia.

Vaccine contains type b capsular polysaccharide (polyribosylribitol phosphate) conjugated to diphtheria toxoid or other protein. Given between 2 and 18 months of age.

Does not cause the flu (influenza virus does).

Treatment: amoxicillin +/− clavulanate for mucosal infections; ceftriaxone for meningitis; rifampin prophylaxis for close contacts.

## Burkholderia cepacia complex

Aerobic, catalase ⊕, gram ⊖ rod. Causes pneumonia in patients with underlying lung disease, such as cystic fibrosis. Often multidrug resistant. Infection is a relative contraindication to undergoing lung transplant due to its association with poor outcomes.

**Bordetella pertussis**

Gram ⊖, aerobic coccobacillus. Virulence factors include pertussis toxin (disables G$_i$), adenylate cyclase toxin (↑ cAMP), and tracheal cytotoxin. Three clinical stages:

- Catarrhal—low-grade fevers, coryza.
- Paroxysmal—paroxysms of intense cough followed by inspiratory "whoop" ("whooping cough"), posttussive vomiting.
- Convalescent—gradual recovery of chronic cough.

Prevented by Tdap, DTaP vaccines.
Produces lymphocytosis (unlike most acute bacterial infections).
Treatment: macrolides; if allergic use TMP-SMX.

**Brucella**

Gram ⊖, aerobic coccobacillus. Transmitted via ingestion of contaminated animal products (eg, unpasteurized milk). Survives in macrophages in the reticuloendothelial system. Can form non-caseating granulomas. Typically presents with undulant fever, night sweats, and arthralgia.
Treatment: doxycycline + rifampin or streptomycin.

**Legionella pneumophila**

Gram ⊖ rod. Gram stains poorly—use **silver** stain. Grow on **charcoal** yeast extract medium with **iron** and **cysteine**. Detected by presence of antigen in urine. Labs may show hyponatremia and elevated transaminases.

Aerosol transmission from environmental water source (eg, air conditioning systems, hot water tanks). Outbreaks associated with cruise ships, nursing homes. No person-to-person transmission.

Treatment: macrolide or quinolone.

Think of a French **legionnaire** (soldier) with his **silver** helmet, sitting around a campfire (**charcoal**) with his **iron** dagger—he is missing his **sister** (cysteine).

Legionnaires' disease—severe pneumonia (often unilateral and lobar A), fever, GI and CNS symptoms. Risk factors include older age, tobacco smoking, chronic lung disease.

Pontiac fever—mild flulike symptoms.

**Pseudomonas aeruginosa**

*Aeruginosa*—aerobic; motile, catalase ⊕, gram ⊖ rod. Non-lactose fermenting. Oxidase ⊕. Frequently found in water. Increased virulence in acidic environments. Has a grapelike odor.
**PSEUDOMONAS** is associated with: Pneumonia, Sepsis, Ecthyma gangrenosum, UTIs, Diabetes, Osteomyelitis, Mucoid polysaccharide capsule, Otitis externa (swimmer's ear), Nosocomial (healthcare-associated) infections (eg, catheters, equipment), Addiction (injection drug use), Skin infections (eg, hot tub folliculitis, wound infection in burn victims).
Mucoid polysaccharide capsule may contribute to chronic pneumonia in patients with cystic fibrosis due to biofilm formation.
Produces **PEEP**: Phospholipase C (degrades cell membranes); Endotoxin (fever, shock); Exotoxin A (inactivates EF-2); green Pigment A.

Corneal ulcers/keratitis in contact lens wearers/ minor eye trauma.

Ecthyma gangrenosum—rapidly progressive, necrotic cutaneous lesion B caused by *Pseudomonas* bacteremia. Typically seen in immunocompromised patients.

Treatments:

- Antipseudomonal penicillins in combination with β-lactamase inhibitor (eg, piperacillin-tazobactam)
- 3rd- and 4th-generation cephalosporins (eg, ceftazidime, cefepime)
- Monobactams
- Fluoroquinolones
- Carbapenems

Despite antipseudomonal activity, aminoglycoside monotherapy is avoided due to poor performance in acidic environments.

**Salmonella vs Shigella** — Both *Salmonella* and *Shigella* are gram ⊖ rods, non-lactose fermenters, oxidase ⊖, and can invade the GI tract via M cells of Peyer patches.

| | *Salmonella typhi* (ty-Vi) | *Salmonella* spp. except *S typhi* | *Shigella* |
|---|---|---|---|
| RESERVOIRS | Humans only | Humans and animals | Humans only |
| SPREAD | Hematogenous spread | Hematogenous spread | Cell to cell; no hematogenous spread |
| H₂S PRODUCTION | Yes | Yes | No |
| FLAGELLA | Yes (salmon swim) | Yes (salmon swim) | No |
| VIRULENCE FACTORS | Endotoxin; **Vi** capsule (pronounce "tyVi") | Endotoxin | Endotoxin; Shiga toxin (enterotoxin) |
| INFECTIOUS DOSE (ID₅₀) | High—large inoculum required; acid-labile (inactivated by gastric acids) | High | Low—very small inoculum required; acid stable (resistant to gastric acids) |
| EFFECT OF ANTIBIOTICS ON FECAL EXCRETION | Prolongs duration | Prolongs duration | Shortens duration (shortens *Shigella*) |
| IMMUNE RESPONSE | Primarily monocytes | PMNs in disseminated disease | Primarily PMN infiltration |
| GI MANIFESTATIONS | Constipation, followed by diarrhea | Diarrhea (possibly bloody) | Crampy abdominal pain → tenesmus, bloody mucoid stools (bacillary dysentery) |
| VACCINE | Oral vaccine contains live attenuated *S typhi* IM vaccine contains Vi capsular polysaccharide | No vaccine | No vaccine |
| UNIQUE PROPERTIES | Causes typhoid fever (salmon-colored truncal macular rash, abdominal pain, fever [pulse-temperature dissociation]; later GI ulceration and hemorrhage); treat with ceftriaxone or fluoroquinolone Carrier state with gallbladder colonization | Poultry, eggs, pets, and turtles are common sources Treatment is supportive; antibiotics are not indicated in immunocompetent individuals | 4 F's: fingers, flies, food, feces In order of decreasing severity (less toxin produced): S *dysenteriae*, S *flexneri*, S *boydii*, S *sonnei* Invasion of M cells is key to pathogenicity; infectious dose is low |

**Yersinia enterocolitica** — Gram ⊖ pleomorphic rod/coccobacillus with bipolar staining. Usually transmitted from pet feces (eg, cats, dogs), contaminated milk, or pork. Can cause acute bloody diarrhea, pseudoappendicitis (right lower abdominal pain due to mesenteric adenitis and/or terminal ileitis), reactive arthritis in adults.

**Lactose-fermenting enteric bacteria** — Fermentation of lactose → pink colonies on MacConkey agar. Examples include *Citrobacter, E coli, Enterobacter, Klebsiella, Serratia*.

McCowkey **CEEKS** milk.
EMB agar—lactose fermenters grow as purple/black colonies. *E coli* grows colonies with a green sheen.

| *Escherichia coli* | Gram ⊖, indole ⊕ rod. *E coli* virulence factors: fimbriae (ie, P pili)—cystitis and pyelonephritis; K capsule—pneumonia, neonatal meningitis; LPS endotoxin—septic shock. | |
|---|---|---|
| STRAIN | TOXIN AND MECHANISM | PRESENTATION |
| Enteroinvasive *E coli* | Microbe invades intestinal mucosa and causes necrosis and inflammation. | EIEC is Invasive; dysentery. Clinical manifestations similar to *Shigella*. |
| Enterotoxigenic *E coli* | Produces heat-labile and heat-stable enteroToxins. No inflammation or invasion. | ETEC; Traveler's diarrhea (watery). |
| Enteropathogenic *E coli* | No toxin produced. Adheres to apical surface, flattens villi, prevents absorption. | Diarrhea, usually in children (think EPEC and Pediatrics). |
| Enterohemorrhagic *E coli* | O157:H7 is most common serotype in US. Often transmitted via undercooked meat, raw leafy vegetables. Shiga toxin causes hemolytic-uremic syndrome—triad of anemia, thrombocytopenia, and acute kidney injury due to microthrombi forming on damaged endothelium → mechanical hemolysis (with schistocytes on peripheral blood smear), platelet consumption → thrombocytopenia, and ↓ renal blood flow. | Dysentery (toxin alone causes necrosis and inflammation). Does not ferment sorbitol (vs other *E coli*). EHEC associated with hemorrhage, hamburgers, hemolytic-uremic syndrome. |

| *Klebsiella* | Gram ⊖ rod; intestinal microbiota that causes lobar pneumonia; more common in patients with heavy alcohol use or with impaired host defenses. Very mucoid colonies  caused by abundant polysaccharide capsules. Dark red "currant jelly" sputum (blood/mucus). Also cause of healthcare-associated UTIs. Associated with evolution of multidrug resistance (MDR). | ABCDE's of Klebsiella: Aspiration pneumonia aBscess in lungs and liver "Currant jelly" sputum Diabetes mellitus EtOH overuse |
|---|---|---|

| *Campylobacter jejuni* | Gram ⊖, comma or S shaped (with polar flagella) , oxidase ⊕, grows at 42°C ("*Campylobacter* likes the hot campfire"). Major cause of bloody diarrhea, especially in children. Fecal-oral transmission through person-to-person contact or via ingestion of undercooked contaminated poultry or meat, unpasteurized milk. Contact with infected animals (dogs, cats, pigs) is also a risk factor. Common antecedent to Guillain-Barré syndrome and reactive arthritis. |
|---|---|

| *Proteus mirabilis* | Gram ⊖, urease ⊕, facultative anaerobe, long flagellae with "swarming" motility. Common cause of UTIs. Urease (virulence factor) hydrolyzes urea to carbon dioxide and ammonia → net increase in pH → promotes formation of struvite stones. Significant blockage of renal calyces results in branched stones called staghorn calculi. |
|---|---|

### Vibrio cholerae

Gram ⊖, flagellated, comma shaped , oxidase ⊕, grows in alkaline media. Endemic to developing countries. Produces profuse rice-water diarrhea via enterotoxin that permanently activates $G_s$, ↑ cAMP. Sensitive to stomach acid (acid labile); requires large inoculum (high $ID_{50}$) unless host has ↓ gastric acidity. Transmitted via ingestion of contaminated water or uncooked food (eg, raw shellfish). Treat promptly with oral rehydration solution.

*Vibrio vulnificus*—gram ⊖ bacillus, usually found in marine environments. Causes severe wound infections or septicemia due to exposure to contaminated sea water. Presents as cellulitis that can progress to necrotizing fasciitis in high-risk patients, especially those with high serum iron (eg, cirrhosis, hemochromatosis). Serious wound infection requires surgical debridement.

### Helicobacter pylori

Curved, flagellated (motile), gram ⊖ rod  that is **triple** ⊕: catalase ⊕, oxidase ⊕, and urease ⊕ (can use urea breath test or fecal antigen test for diagnosis). Urease produces ammonia, creating an alkaline environment, which helps *H pylori* survive in acidic mucosa. Colonizes mainly antrum of stomach; causes gastritis and peptic ulcers (especially duodenal). Risk factor for peptic ulcer disease, gastric adenocarcinoma, and MALT lymphoma.

Most common initial treatment is **triple** therapy: amoxicillin (metronidazole if penicillin allergy) + clarithromycin + proton pump inhibitor; antibiotics cure *Pylori*. Bismuth-based quadruple therapy if concerned about macrolide resistance.

### Spirochetes

Spiral-shaped bacteria  with axial filaments. Includes *Leptospira*, *Treponema*, and *Borrelia*. Only *Borrelia* can be visualized using aniline dyes (Wright or Giemsa stain) in light microscopy due to size. *Treponema* is visualized by dark-field microscopy or direct fluorescent antibody (DFA) microscopy.

Little Twirling Bacteria.

Jarisch-Herxheimer reaction—flulike symptoms (fever, chills, headache, myalgia) after antibiotics are started due to host response to sudden release of bacterial antigens. Usually occurs during treatment of spirochetal infections.

### Lyme disease

Caused by *Borrelia burgdorferi*, which is transmitted by the *Ixodes* deer tick  (also vector for *Anaplasma* spp. and protozoa *Babesia*). Natural reservoir is the mouse; deer are essential to tick life cycle but do not harbor *Borrelia*.

Common in northeastern United States.

Stage 1—early localized: erythema migrans (typical "bulls-eye" configuration B is pathognomonic but not always present), flulike symptoms.

Stage 2—early disseminated: secondary lesions, carditis, AV block, facial nerve (Bell) palsy, migratory myalgias/transient arthritis.

Stage 3—late disseminated: encephalopathy, chronic arthritis, peripheral neuropathy.

A Key Lyme pie to the FACE:
   Facial nerve palsy (typically bilateral)
   Arthritis
   Cardiac block
   Erythema migrans
Treatment: doxycycline (1st line); amoxicillin (pregnant patients, children < 8 years old); ceftriaxone if IV therapy required

| | |
|---|---|
| ***Leptospira interrogans*** | Spirochete with hook-shaped ends found in water contaminated with animal urine. |
| | **Leptospirosis**—flulike symptoms, myalgias (classically of calves), jaundice, photophobia with conjunctival suffusion (erythema without exudate). Prevalent among surfers and in tropics (eg, Hawaii). |
| | **Weil disease** (icterohemorrhagic leptospirosis)—severe form with jaundice and azotemia from liver and kidney dysfunction, fever, hemorrhage, and anemia. |

| | |
|---|---|
| **Syphilis** | Caused by spirochete *Treponema pallidum*. Treatment: penicillin G. |
| Primary syphilis | Localized disease presenting with **painless** chancre. Use fluorescent or dark-field microscopy to visualize treponemes in fluid from chancre A. VDRL ⊕ in ~ 80% of patients. |
| Secondary syphilis | Disseminated disease with constitutional symptoms, maculopapular rash B (including palms C and soles), condylomata lata D (smooth, painless, wartlike white lesions on genitals), lymphadenopathy, patchy hair loss; also confirmable with dark-field microscopy. Serologic testing: VDRL/RPR (nonspecific), confirm diagnosis with specific test (eg, FTA-ABS). Secondary syphilis = systemic. Latent syphilis (⊕ serology without symptoms) may follow. |
| Tertiary syphilis | Gummas E (chronic granulomas), aortitis (vasa vasorum destruction), neurosyphilis (tabes dorsalis, "general paresis"), Argyll Robertson pupil (constricts with accommodation but is not reactive to light). Signs: broad-based ataxia, ⊕ Romberg, Charcot joint, stroke without hypertension. |
| Congenital syphilis | Presents with facial abnormalities such as rhagades (linear scars at angle of mouth, black arrow in F), snuffles (nasal discharge, red arrow in F), saddle nose, notched (Hutchinson) teeth G, mulberry molars, and short maxilla; saber shins; CN VIII deafness. To prevent, treat patient early in pregnancy, as placental transmission typically occurs after first trimester. |

| | | |
|---|---|---|
| **Diagnosing syphilis** | VDRL and RPR detects nonspecific antibody that reacts with beef cardiolipin. Quantitative, inexpensive, and widely available test for syphilis (sensitive but not specific). Nontreponemal tests (VDRL, RPR) and direct testing revert to negative after treatment. Antibodies detected by treponemal tests (FTA-ABS, TP-PA) will remain positive. | False-Positive results on VDRL with: Pregnancy Viral infection (eg, EBV, hepatitis) Drugs (eg, chlorpromazine, procainamide) Rheumatic fever (rare) Lupus (anticardiolipin antibody) and Leprosy |

| | | |
|---|---|---|
| **Chlamydiae**  | Chlamydiae cannot make their own ATP. They are obligate intracellular organisms that cause mucosal infections. 2 forms: <ul><li>Elementary body (small, dense) is "enfectious" and enters cell via endocytosis; transforms into reticulate body.</li><li>Reticulate body replicates in cell by fission; reorganizes into elementary bodies.</li></ul> *Chlamydia trachomatis* causes neonatal and follicular adult conjunctivitis **A**, nongonococcal urethritis, PID, and reactive arthritis. *Chlamydophila pneumoniae* and *Chlamydophila psittaci* cause atypical pneumonia; transmitted by aerosol. | Chlamydial cell wall lacks classic peptidoglycan (due to reduced muramic acid), rendering β-lactam antibiotics ineffective. *Chlamys* = cloak (intracellular). *C psittaci*—has an avian reservoir (parrots), causes atypical pneumonia. Lab diagnosis: PCR, NAAT. Cytoplasmic inclusions (reticulate bodies) seen on Giemsa or fluorescent antibody–stained smear. Treatment: doxycycline, azithromycin (for pregnant patients). Add ceftriaxone if concurrent gonorrhea testing is positive. |

### *Chlamydia trachomatis* serotypes

| | | |
|---|---|---|
| **Types A, B, and C** | Chronic infection, cause blindness due to follicular conjunctivitis in resource-limited areas. | ABC = Africa, Blindness, Chronic infection. |
| **Types D–K** | Urethritis/PID, ectopic pregnancy, neonatal pneumonia (staccato cough) with eosinophilia, neonatal conjunctivitis (1–2 weeks after birth). | D–K = everything else. Neonatal disease can be acquired during vaginal birth if pregnant patient is infected. |
| **Types L1, L2, and L3** | Lymphogranuloma venereum—small, painless ulcers on genitals → swollen, painful inguinal lymph nodes that ulcerate (buboes). Treat with doxycycline. | |

**Gardnerella vaginalis**

A pleomorphic, gram-variable rod involved in bacterial vaginosis. Presents as a gray vaginal discharge with a fishy smell; nonpainful (vs vaginitis). Associated with sexual activity, but not sexually transmitted. Bacterial vaginosis is also characterized by overgrowth of certain anaerobic bacteria in vagina (due to ↓ lactobacilli). Clue cells (vaginal epithelial cells covered with *Gardnerella*) have stippled appearance along outer margin (arrow in A).

Amine whiff test—mixing discharge with 10% KOH enhances fishy odor.
Vaginal pH >4.5 during infection.
Treatment: metronidazole or clindamycin.

| **Zoonotic bacteria** | Zoonosis—infectious disease transmitted between animals and humans. | |
| --- | --- | --- |
| SPECIES | DISEASE | TRANSMISSION AND SOURCE |
| *Anaplasma* spp | Anaplasmosis | *Ixodes* ticks (live on deer and mice) |
| *Bartonella* spp | Cat scratch disease, bacillary angiomatosis | Cat scratch |
| *Borrelia burgdorferi* | Lyme disease | *Ixodes* ticks (live on deer and mice) |
| *Borrelia recurrentis* | Relapsing fever | Louse (recurrent due to variable surface antigens) |
| *Brucella* spp | Brucellosis/undulant fever | Unpasteurized dairy; inhalation of or contact with infected animal tissue or fluids |
| *Campylobacter* | Bloody diarrhea | Feces from infected pets/animals; contaminated meats/foods/hands |
| *Chlamydophila psittaci* | Psittacosis | Parrots, other birds |
| *Coxiella burnetii* | Q fever | Aerosols of cattle/sheep amniotic fluid |
| *Ehrlichia chaffeensis* | Ehrlichiosis | *Amblyomma* (Lone Star tick) |
| *Francisella tularensis* | Tularemia | Ticks, rabbits, deer flies |
| *Leptospira* spp | Leptospirosis | Animal urine in water; recreational water use |
| *Mycobacterium leprae* | Leprosy | Humans with lepromatous leprosy; armadillo (rare) |
| *Pasteurella multocida* | Cellulitis, osteomyelitis | Animal bite, cats, dogs |
| *Rickettsia prowazekii* | Epidemic typhus | Human to human via human body louse |
| *Rickettsia rickettsii* | Rocky Mountain spotted fever | *Dermacentor* (dog tick) |
| *Rickettsia typhi* | Endemic typhus | Fleas |
| *Salmonella* spp (except *S typhi*) | Diarrhea (which may be bloody), vomiting, fever, abdominal cramps | Reptiles and poultry |
| *Yersinia pestis* | Plague | Fleas (rats and prairie dogs are reservoirs) |

## Rickettsial diseases and vector-borne illnesses

Treatment: doxycycline.

### RASH COMMON

| | | |
|---|---|---|
| **Rocky Mountain spotted fever** | *Rickettsia rickettsii*, vector is tick. Despite its name, disease occurs primarily in the South Atlantic states, especially North Carolina. Rash typically starts at wrists  and ankles and then spreads to trunk, palms, and soles. | Classic triad—headache, fever, rash (vasculitis). Palms and soles rash is seen in Coxsackievirus A infection (hand, foot, and mouth disease), Rocky Mountain spotted fever, and 2° Syphilis (you drive **CARS** using your palms and soles). |
| **Typhus** | Endemic (fleas)—*R typhi*. Epidemic (human body louse)—*R prowazekii*. Rash starts centrally and spreads out, sparing palms and soles. | *Rickettsii* on the wrists, typhus on the trunk. |

### RASH RARE

| | | |
|---|---|---|
| **Ehrlichiosis** | *Ehrlichia*, vector is tick. Monocytes with morulae **B** (mulberrylike inclusions) in cytoplasm. | **MEGA:** Monocytes = Ehrlichiosis Granulocytes = Anaplasmosis |
| **Anaplasmosis** | *Anaplasma*, vector is tick. Granulocytes with morulae **C** in cytoplasm. | |
| **Q fever** | *Coxiella burnetii*, no arthropod vector. Bacterium inhaled as aerosols from cattle/sheep amniotic fluid. Presents with headache, cough, flulike symptoms, pneumonia, possibly in combination with hepatitis. Common cause of culture ⊖ endocarditis. | Q fever is caused by a Quite Complicated bug because it has no rash or vector and its causative organism can survive outside in its endospore form. Not in the *Rickettsia* genus, but closely related. |

| | |
|---|---|
| ***Mycoplasma pneumoniae***  | Classic cause of atypical "walking pneumonia" (insidious onset, headache, nonproductive cough, patchy or diffuse interstitial infiltrate, macular rash). Occurs frequently in those <30 years old; outbreaks in military recruits, prisons, colleges. Treatment: macrolides, doxycycline, or fluoroquinolone (penicillin ineffective since *Mycoplasma* has no cell wall). | Not seen on Gram stain. Pleomorphic **A**. Bacterial membrane contains sterols for stability. Grown on Eaton agar. CXR appears more severe than patient presentation. High titer of cold agglutinins (IgM), which can agglutinate RBCs. *Mycoplasma* gets cold without a coat (no cell wall). |

## ▶ MICROBIOLOGY—MYCOLOGY

**Systemic mycoses**

All of the following can cause pneumonia and can disseminate.

All are caused by dimorphic fungi: cold (20°C) = **mold**; heat (37°C) = **yeast**. Only exception is *Coccidioides*, which is a spherule (not yeast) in tissue.

Systemic mycoses can form granulomas (like TB); cannot be transmitted person-to-person (unlike TB).

Treatment: fluconazole or itraconazole for **local** infection; amphotericin B for **systemic** infection.

| DISEASE | ENDEMIC LOCATION | PATHOLOGIC FEATURES | UNIQUE SIGNS/SYMPTOMS | NOTES |
|---|---|---|---|---|
| **Histoplasmosis** | Mississippi and Ohio River Valleys | Macrophage filled with *Histoplasma* (smaller than RBC) A Tuberculate macroconidia on culture | Palatal/tongue ulcers, splenomegaly, pancytopenia, erythema nodosum | Histo hides (within macrophages) Associated with bird or bat droppings (eg, caves) Diagnosis via urine/ serum antigen |
| **Blastomycosis** B | Eastern and Central US, Great Lakes | Broad-based budding of *Blastomyces* (same size as RBC) B | Inflammatory lung disease Disseminates to bone/ skin (verrucous lesions C, may mimic SCC). | Blasto buds broadly |
| **Coccidioidomycosis** D | Southwestern US, California | Spherule filled with endospores of *Coccidioides* (much larger than RBC) D | Disseminates to bone/ skin Erythema nodosum (desert bumps) or multiforme Arthralgias (desert rheumatism) Can cause meningitis | Associated with dust exposure in endemic areas (eg, archeological excavations, earthquakes) |
| **Para-coccidioidomycosis** E | Latin America | Budding yeast of *Paracoccidioides* with "captain's wheel" formation (much larger than RBC) E | Similar to blastomycosis, males > females | Paracoccidio parasails with the captain's wheel all the way to Latin America |

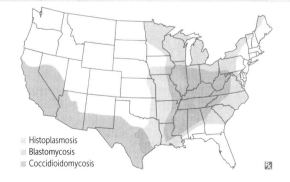

Histoplasmosis
Blastomycosis
Coccidioidomycosis

## Opportunistic fungal infections

| | |
|---|---|
| *Candida albicans* | *alba* = white. Dimorphic; forms pseudohyphae and budding yeasts at 20°C **A**, germ tubes at 37°C **B**.<br><br>Systemic or superficial fungal infection. Causes oral **C** and esophageal thrush in immunocompromised (neonates, steroids, diabetes, AIDS), vulvovaginitis (diabetes, use of antibiotics), diaper rash, infective endocarditis (people who inject drugs), disseminated candidiasis (especially in neutropenic patients as host defense relies on phagocytes), chronic mucocutaneous candidiasis.<br><br>Treatment: oral fluconazole/topical azoles for vaginal; nystatin, azoles, or, rarely, echinocandins for oral; fluconazole, echinocandins, or amphotericin B for esophageal or systemic disease. |
| *Aspergillus fumigatus* | Acute angle (45°) **D** branching of septate hyphae.<br>Causes invasive aspergillosis in immunocompromised patients, especially those with neutrophil dysfunction (eg, chronic granulomatous disease) because *Aspergillus* is catalase ⊕.<br>Can cause aspergillomas **E** in pre-existing lung cavities, especially after TB infection.<br>Some species of Aspergillus produce aflatoxins (induce TP53 mutations leading to hepatocellular carcinoma).<br>Treatment: voriconazole or echinocandins (2nd-line).<br><br>Allergic bronchopulmonary aspergillosis (ABPA)—hypersensitivity response to *Aspergillus* growing in lung mucus. Associated with asthma and cystic fibrosis; may cause bronchiectasis and eosinophilia. |
| *Cryptococcus neoformans* | 5–10 μm with narrow budding. Heavily encapsulated yeast. Not dimorphic. ⊕ PAS staining.<br>Found in soil, pigeon droppings. Acquired through inhalation with hematogenous dissemination to meninges. Highlighted with India ink (clear halo **F**) and mucicarmine (red inner capsule **G**). Latex agglutination test detects polysaccharide capsular antigen and is more sensitive and specific.<br>Causes cryptococcosis, which can manifest with meningitis, pneumonia, and/or encephalitis ("soap bubble" lesions in brain), primarily in immunocompromised.<br>Treatment: amphotericin B + flucytosine followed by fluconazole for cryptococcal meningitis. |
| *Mucor* and *Rhizopus* spp | Irregular, broad, nonseptate hyphae branching at wide angles **H**.<br>Causes mucormycosis, mostly in patients with DKA and/or neutropenia (eg, leukemia). Inhalation of spores → fungi proliferate in blood vessel walls, penetrate cribriform plate, and enter brain. Rhinocerebral, frontal lobe abscess; cavernous sinus thrombosis. Headache, facial pain, black necrotic eschar on face **I**; may have cranial nerve involvement.<br>Treatment: surgical debridement, amphotericin B or isavuconazole. |

**Pneumocystis jirovecii**

Causes *Pneumocystis* pneumonia (PCP), a diffuse interstitial pneumonia **A**. Yeastlike fungus (originally classified as protozoan). Most infections are asymptomatic. Immunosuppression (eg, AIDS) predisposes to disease. Diffuse, bilateral ground-glass opacities on chest imaging, with pneumatoceles **B**. Diagnosed by bronchoalveolar lavage or lung biopsy. Disc-shaped yeast seen on methenamine silver stain of lung tissue **C** or with fluorescent antibody.

Treatment/prophylaxis: TMP-SMX, pentamidine, dapsone (prophylaxis as single agent, or treatment in combination with TMP), atovaquone. Start prophylaxis when CD4+ cell count drops to < 200 cells/mm$^3$ in people living with HIV.

**Sporothrix schenckii**

Causes sporotrichosis. Dimorphic fungus. Exists as a **cigar**-shaped yeast at 37 °C in the human body and as hyphae with spores in soil (conidia). Lives on vegetation. When spores are traumatically introduced into the skin, typically by a thorn ("**rose gardener**'s disease"), causes local pustule or ulcer with nodules along draining lymphatics (ascending lymphangitis **A**). Disseminated disease possible in immunocompromised host.

Treatment: itraconazole or **pot**assium iodide (only for cutaneous/lymphocutaneous).

Think of a **rose gardener** who smokes a **cigar** and **pot**.

## ▶ MICROBIOLOGY—PARASITOLOGY

### Protozoa—gastrointestinal infections

| ORGANISM | DISEASE | TRANSMISSION | DIAGNOSIS | TREATMENT |
|---|---|---|---|---|
| *Giardia lamblia* | **Giardiasis**—bloating, flatulence, foul-smelling, nonbloody, fatty diarrhea (often seen in campers/hikers)—think fat-rich Ghirardelli chocolates for **fatty** stools of *Giardia* | Cysts in water | Multinucleated trophozoites **A** or cysts **B** in stool, antigen detection, PCR | Tinidazole, nitazoxanide, or metronidazole |
| *Entamoeba histolytica* | **Amebiasis**—bloody diarrhea (dysentery), liver abscess ("anchovy paste" exudate), RUQ pain; histology of colon biopsy shows flask-shaped ulcers **C** | Cysts in water | Serology, antigen testing, PCR, and/ or trophozoites (with engulfed RBCs **D** in the cytoplasm) or cysts with up to 4 nuclei in stool **E**; *Entamoeba* Eats Erythrocytes | Metronidazole; paromomycin for asymptomatic cyst passers |
| *Cryptosporidium* | Severe diarrhea in AIDS Mild disease (watery diarrhea) in immunocompetent hosts | Oocysts in water | Oocysts on acid-fast stain **F**, antigen detection, PCR | Prevention (eg, filtering); nitazoxanide (severe disease and/or immuno-compromised) |

## Protozoa—CNS infections

| ORGANISM | DISEASE | TRANSMISSION | DIAGNOSIS | TREATMENT |
|---|---|---|---|---|
| *Toxoplasma gondii* | Immunocompetent: mononucleosis-like symptoms, ⊖ heterophile antibody test<br>Reactivation in AIDS → brain abscesses usually seen as multiple ring-enhancing lesions on MRI A<br>Congenital toxoplasmosis: classic triad of chorioretinitis, hydrocephalus, and intracranial calcifications | Cysts in meat (most common); oocysts in cat feces; crosses placenta (pregnant patients should avoid cats) | Serology, biopsy (tachyzoite) B; PCR of amniotic fluid for possible intrauterine disease | Sulfadiazine + pyrimethamine Prophylaxis with TMP-SMX when CD4+ cell count < 100 cells/mm³ |
| *Naegleria fowleri* | Rapidly fatal meningoencephalitis | Swimming in warm freshwater; enters CNS through olfactory nerve via cribriform plate | Amoebas in CSF C | Amphotericin B has been effective for a few survivors |
| *Trypanosoma brucei* | **African sleeping sickness**— enlarged lymph nodes, recurring fever (due to antigenic variation), somnolence, coma | Tsetse fly, a painful bite | Trypomastigote in blood smear D | Suramin for blood-borne disease or melarsoprol for CNS penetration ("I sure am mellow when I'm sleeping") |

**Protozoa—hematologic infections**

| ORGANISM | DISEASE | TRANSMISSION | DIAGNOSIS | TREATMENT |
|---|---|---|---|---|
| *Plasmodium* | Malaria—cyclic fevers, headache, anemia, splenomegaly; hypoglycemia in severe disease | *Anopheles* mosquito | Peripheral blood smear (also allows for identification of species) | If sensitive, chloroquine; if resistant, mefloquine, doxycycline or atovaquone/proguanil If life threatening, use intravenous quinine or artesunate (test for G6PD deficiency) |
| *P malariae* | 72-hr fever cycle (quartan) | | Trophozoite ring within RBC | |
| *P vivax/ovale* | 48-hr fever cycle (tertian); dormant form (hypnozoite) in liver | | Trophozoites and Schüffner stippling (small red granules) within RBC cytoplasm A | Add primaquine to target hypnozoites |
| *P falciparum* | Severe, irregular fever pattern; parasitized RBCs may occlude capillaries in brain (cerebral malaria), kidneys, lungs | | Trophozoite ring (headphone shaped) within RBC B; crescent-shaped gametocytes C | |
| *Babesia* | Babesiosis—fever and hemolytic anemia; predominantly in northeastern and north central United States; asplenia ↑ risk of severe disease due to inability to clear infected RBCs | *Ixodes* tick (also vector for *Borrelia burgdorferi* and *Anaplasma* spp) | Ring form D1, "Maltese cross" D2; PCR | Atovaquone + azithromycin |

## Protozoa—others

| ORGANISM | DISEASE | TRANSMISSION | DIAGNOSIS | TREATMENT |
|---|---|---|---|---|
| **Visceral infections** | | | | |
| *Trypanosoma cruzi* | **Chagas disease**—dilated cardiomyopathy with apical atrophy, **mega**colon, **mega**esophagus; (*T cruzi* causes **big** problems); predominantly in South America. Unilateral periorbital swelling (Romaña sign) characteristic of acute stage | Triatomine insect (kissing bug) bites and defecates around the mouth or eyes → fecal transmission into bite site or mucosa | Trypomastigote in blood smear A | Benznidazole or nifurtimox |
| *Leishmania* spp | Visceral leishmaniasis (kala-azar)—spiking fevers, hepatosplenomegaly, pancytopenia. Cutaneous leishmaniasis—skin ulcers B | Sandfly | Macrophages containing amastigotes C | Amphotericin B, sodium stibogluconate |
| **Sexually transmitted infections** | | | | |
| *Trichomonas vaginalis* | Vaginitis—foul-smelling, greenish discharge; itching and burning; do not confuse with *Gardnerella vaginalis*, a gram-variable bacterium associated with bacterial vaginosis | Sexual (cannot exist outside human because it cannot form cysts) | Trophozoites (motile) D on wet mount; punctate cervical hemorrhages ("strawberry cervix") | Metronidazole for patient and partner(s) (prophylaxis; check for STI) |

| **Nematode routes of infection** | Ingested—*Enterobius, Ascaris, Toxocara, Trichinella, Trichuris* | You'll get sick if you **EATTT** these! |
|---|---|---|
| | Cutaneous—*Strongyloides, Ancylostoma, Necator* | These get into your feet from the **SAN**d |
| | Bites—*Loa loa, Onchocerca volvulus, Wuchereria bancrofti* | Lay **LOW** to avoid getting bitten |

## Nematodes (roundworms)

| ORGANISM | DISEASE | TRANSMISSION | TREATMENT |
|---|---|---|---|
| **Intestinal** | | | |
| *Enterobius vermicularis* (pinworm) | Causes anal pruritus, worse at night (eggs A visualized via tape test). Most common in children aged 5–10. | Fecal-oral. | Bendazoles, pyrantel pamoate. |
| *Ascaris lumbricoides* (giant roundworm) | May cause obstruction at ileocecal valve, biliary obstruction, intestinal perforation, migrates from nose/mouth. Migration of larvae to alveoli → Löeffler syndrome (pulmonary eosinophilia). | Fecal-oral; knobby-coated, oval eggs seen in feces under microscope B. | Bendazoles. |
| *Strongyloides stercoralis* (threadworm) | GI (eg, duodenitis), pulmonary (eg, dry cough, hemoptysis), and cutaneous (eg, pruritus) symptoms. Hyperinfection syndrome can be caused by accelerated autoinfection in the immunocompromised. | Larvae in soil penetrate skin; rhabditiform larvae seen in feces under microscope. | Ivermectin or bendazoles. |
| *Ancylostoma* spp, *Necator americanus* (hookworms) | Cause microcytic anemia by sucking blood from intestinal wall. Cutaneous larva migrans—pruritic, serpiginous rash C. | Larvae penetrate skin from walking barefoot on contaminated beach/soil. | Bendazoles or pyrantel pamoate. |
| *Trichinella spiralis* | Larvae enter bloodstream, encyst in striated muscle D → myositis. Trichinosis—fever, vomiting, nausea, periorbital edema, myalgia. | Undercooked meat (especially pork); fecal-oral (less likely). | Bendazoles. |
| *Trichuris trichiura* (whipworm) | Often asymptomatic; loose stools, anemia, rectal prolapse in children. | Fecal-oral. | Bendazoles. |
| **Tissue** | | | |
| *Toxocara canis* | Visceral larva migrans—migration into blood → inflammation of liver, eyes (visual impairment), CNS (seizures, coma), heart (myocarditis). Patients often asymptomatic. | Fecal-oral. | Bendazoles. |
| *Onchocerca volvulus* | Black skin nodules, river blindness ("**black** sight"). | Female **black** fly. | Ivermectin (**iver**mectin for **river** blindness). |
| *Loa loa* | Swelling in skin, worm in conjunctiva. | Deer fly, horse fly, mango fly. | Diethylcarbamazine. |
| *Wuchereria bancrofti*, *Brugia malayi* | Lymphatic filariasis (elephantiasis)— worms invade lymph nodes → inflammation → lymphedema E; symptom onset after 9 mo–1 yr. | Female mosquito. | Diethylcarbamazine. |

## Cestodes (tapeworms)

| ORGANISM | DISEASE | TRANSMISSION | TREATMENT |
|---|---|---|---|
| *Taenia solium* A | Intestinal tapeworm | Ingestion of larvae encysted in undercooked pork | Praziquantel |
| | Cysticercosis, neurocysticercosis (cystic CNS lesions, seizures) B | Ingestion of eggs in food contaminated with human feces | Praziquantel; albendazole for neurocysticercosis |
| *Diphyllobothrium latum* | Vitamin $B_{12}$ deficiency (tapeworm competes for $B_{12}$ in intestine) → megaloblastic anemia | Ingestion of larvae in raw freshwater fish | Praziquantel, niclosamide |
| *Echinococcus granulosus* C | Hydatid cysts D ("eggshell calcification") most commonly in liver E and lungs; cyst rupture can cause anaphylaxis | Ingestion of eggs in food contaminated with dog feces Sheep are an intermediate host | Albendazole; surgery for complicated cysts |

## Trematodes (flukes)

| ORGANISM | DISEASE | TRANSMISSION | TREATMENT |
|---|---|---|---|
| *Schistosoma* | Liver and spleen enlargement (A shows *S mansoni* egg with lateral spine), fibrosis, inflammation, portal hypertension; *S mansoni* and *S japonicum* can both also cause intestinal schistosomiasis, presenting with diarrhea, abdominal pain, iron deficiency anemia Chronic infection with *S haematobium* (egg with terminal spine B) can lead to squamous cell carcinoma of the bladder (painless hematuria) and pulmonary hypertension | Snails are intermediate host; cercariae penetrate skin of humans in contact with contaminated fresh water (eg, swimming or bathing) | Praziquantel |
| *Clonorchis sinensis* | Biliary tract inflammation → pigmented gallstones Associated with cholangiocarcinoma | Undercooked fish | Praziquantel |

### Ectoparasites

| | | |
|---|---|---|
| *Sarcoptes scabiei*  | Mites burrow into stratum corneum and cause scabies—pruritus (worse at night) and serpiginous burrows (lines) often between fingers and toes Ⓐ. | Common in children, crowded populations (jails, nursing homes); transmission through skin-to-skin contact (most common) or via fomites. Treatment: permethrin cream, oral ivermectin, washing/drying all clothing/bedding, treat close contacts. |
| *Pediculus humanus* and *Phthirus pubis*  | Blood-sucking lice that cause intense pruritus with associated excoriations, commonly on scalp and neck (head lice), waistband and axilla (body lice), or pubic and perianal regions (pubic lice). | Body lice can transmit *Rickettsia prowazekii* (epidemic typhus), *Borrelia recurrentis* (relapsing fever), *Bartonella quintana* (trench fever). Treatment: pyrethroids, malathion, or ivermectin lotion, and nit Ⓑ combing. Children with head lice can be treated at home without interrupting school attendance. |
| *Cimex lectularius* and *Cimex hemipterus* | Bed bugs. Blood-feeding insects that infest dwellings. Painless bites result in a range of skin reactions, typically pruritic, erythematous papules with central hemorrhagic punctum. A clustered or linear pattern of bites seen upon awakening is suggestive. Diagnosis is confirmed by direct identification of bed bugs in patient's dwelling. | Bed bugs can spread among rooms; cohabitants may exhibit similar symptoms. Infestations can also spread via travelers from infested hotels and the use of unwashed, used bedding. Treatment: bites self resolve within 1 week. Eradication of the infestation is critical. |

### Parasite hints

| ASSOCIATIONS | ORGANISM |
|---|---|
| Biliary tract disease, cholangiocarcinoma | *Clonorchis sinensis* |
| Brain cysts, seizures | *Taenia solium* (neurocysticercosis) |
| Hematuria, squamous cell bladder cancer | *Schistosoma haematobium* |
| Liver (hydatid) cysts, exposure to infected dogs | *Echinococcus granulosus* |
| Iron deficiency anemia | *Ancylostoma, Necator* |
| Myalgias, periorbital edema | *Trichinella spiralis* |
| Nocturnal perianal pruritus | *Enterobius* |
| Portal hypertension | *Schistosoma mansoni, Schistosoma japonicum* |
| Vitamin $B_{12}$ deficiency | *Diphyllobothrium latum* |

## ▶ MICROBIOLOGY—VIROLOGY

### Viral structure—general features

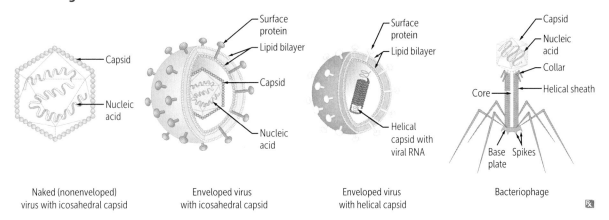

Naked (nonenveloped) virus with icosahedral capsid

Enveloped virus with icosahedral capsid

Enveloped virus with helical capsid

Bacteriophage

### Viral genetics

| | | |
|---|---|---|
| **Recombination** | Exchange of genes between 2 chromosomes by crossing over within regions of significant base sequence homology. | |
| **Reassortment** | When viruses with segmented genomes (eg, influenza virus) exchange genetic material. For example, the 2009 novel H1N1 influenza A pandemic emerged via complex viral reassortment of genes from human, swine, and avian viruses. Has potential to cause antigenic shift. Reassortment of genome segments. | |
| **Complementation** | When 1 of 2 viruses that infect the cell has a mutation that results in a nonfunctional protein, the nonmutated virus "complements" the mutated one by making a functional protein that serves both viruses. For example, hepatitis D virus requires the presence of replicating hepatitis B virus to supply HBsAg, the envelope protein for HDV. | Functional   Nonfunctional   Functional |
| **Phenotypic mixing** | Occurs with simultaneous infection of a cell with 2 viruses. For progeny 1, genome of virus A can be partially or completely coated (forming pseudovirion) with the surface proteins of virus B. Type B protein coat determines the tropism (infectivity) of the hybrid virus. Progeny from subsequent infection of a cell by progeny 1 will have a type A coat that is encoded by its type A genetic material. | Virus A   Virus B   Progeny 1   Progeny 2 |

| **Viral genomes** | Naked nucleic acids of most dsDNA viruses (except poxviruses and HBV) and ⊕ strand ssRNA viruses are infectious. Naked nucleic acids of ⊖ strand ssRNA and dsRNA viruses are not infectious because they lack the required polymerases to replicate. Virions of ⊖ strand ssRNA viruses carry RNA-dependent RNA polymerases to transcribe ⊖ strand to ⊕. | |
|---|---|---|

| | CHARACTERISTICS | MNEMONIC |
|---|---|---|
| **DNA viruses** | All have dsDNA genomes (like our cells) except Parvoviridae (ssDNA).<br>All are linear except papilloma-, polyoma-, and hepadnaviruses (circular). | Part of a virus |
| **RNA viruses** | All have ssRNA genomes except Reoviridae (dsRNA).<br>⊕ stranded (≈ mRNA): retro-, toga-, flavi-, corona-, hepe-, calici-, and picornaviruses.<br>⊖ stranded: arena-, bunya-, paramyxo-, orthomyxo-, filo-, and rhabdoviruses.<br>Segmented: Bunya-, Orthomyxo-, Arena-, and Reoviruses. | Repeato-virus<br><br>While at a retro toga party, I drank flavored Corona and ate hippie California pickles. Always bring polymerase or fail replication.<br><br>BOAR |
| **Viral envelopes** | Generally, enveloped viruses acquire their envelopes from plasma membrane when they exit from cell. Exceptions include herpesviruses, which acquire envelopes from nuclear membrane. | Enveloped DNA viruses (herpesvirus, hepadnavirus, poxvirus) have helpful protection. |

## DNA viruses

All are icosahedral and replicate in the nucleus (except poxvirus). "Pox is out of the box (nucleus)."

| VIRAL FAMILY | ENVELOPE | DNA STRUCTURE | MEDICAL IMPORTANCE |
|---|---|---|---|
| Herpesviruses | Yes | DS and linear | See Herpesviruses entry |
| Poxvirus | Yes | DS and linear (largest DNA virus) | Smallpox eradicated world wide by use of the live-attenuated vaccine<br>Cowpox ("milkmaid blisters")<br>**Molluscum contagiosum**—flesh-colored papule with central umbilication; keratinocytes contain molluscum bodies **A** |
| Hepadnavirus | Yes | Partially DS and circular | HBV:<br>▪ Acute or chronic hepatitis<br>▪ Not a retrovirus but has reverse transcriptase |
| Adenovirus | No | DS and linear | Febrile pharyngitis **B**—sore throat<br>Acute hemorrhagic cystitis<br>Pneumonia<br>Conjunctivitis—"pink eye"<br>Gastroenteritis<br>Myocarditis |
| Papillomavirus | No | DS and circular | HPV—warts, cancer (cervical, anal, penile, or oropharyngeal); serotypes 1, 2, 6, 11 associated with warts; serotypes 16, 18 associated with cancer |
| Polyomavirus | No | DS and circular | JC virus—progressive multifocal leukoencephalopathy (PML) in immunocompromised patients (eg, HIV)<br>BK virus—transplant patients, commonly targets kidney<br>JC: **J**unky **C**erebrum; **BK**: **B**ad **K**idney |
| Parvovirus | No | SS and linear (smallest DNA virus; *parvus* = small) | B19 virus—aplastic crises in sickle cell disease, "slapped cheek" rash in children (erythema infectiosum, or fifth disease); infects RBC precursors and endothelial cells → RBC destruction → hydrops fetalis and death in fetus, pure RBC aplasia and rheumatoid arthritis–like symptoms in adults |

**Herpesviruses**  Enveloped, DS, and linear viruses. Recent data suggest both HSV-1 and HSV-2 can affect both genital and extragenital areas.

| VIRUS | ROUTE OF TRANSMISSION | CLINICAL SIGNIFICANCE | NOTES |
|---|---|---|---|
| **Herpes simplex virus-1** | Respiratory secretions, saliva | Gingivostomatitis, keratoconjunctivitis **A**, herpes labialis (cold sores) **B**, herpetic whitlow on finger, temporal lobe encephalitis, esophagitis, erythema multiforme. Responsible for a growing percentage of herpes genitalis. | Most commonly latent in trigeminal ganglia  <br> Most common cause of sporadic encephalitis, can present as altered mental status, seizures, and/or aphasia |
| **Herpes simplex virus-2** | Sexual contact, perinatal | Herpes genitalis, neonatal herpes **C** | Most commonly latent in sacral ganglia  <br> Viral meningitis more common with HSV-2 than with HSV-1 |
| **Varicella-zoster virus (HHV-3)** | Respiratory secretions, contact with fluid from vesicles | Varicella-zoster (chickenpox **D**, shingles **E**), encephalitis, pneumonia  <br> Most common complication of shingles is post-herpetic neuralgia | Latent in dorsal root or trigeminal ganglia; CN $V_1$ branch involvement can cause herpes zoster ophthalmicus |
| **Epstein-Barr virus (HHV-4)** | Respiratory secretions, saliva; also called "kissing disease," (common in teens, young adults) | **Mononucleosis**—fever, hepatosplenomegaly **F**, pharyngitis, and lymphadenopathy (especially posterior cervical nodes); avoid contact sports until resolution due to risk of splenic rupture  <br> Associated with lymphomas (eg, endemic Burkitt lymphoma), nasopharyngeal carcinoma (especially Asian adults), lymphoproliferative disease in transplant patients | Infects B cells through CD21, "Must be 21 to drink Beer in a Barr"  <br> Atypical lymphocytes on peripheral blood smear **G**—not infected B cells but reactive cytotoxic T cells  <br> ⊕ Monospot test—heterophile antibodies detected by agglutination of sheep or horse RBCs  <br> Use of amoxicillin (eg, for presumed strep pharyngitis) can cause maculopapular rash |
| **Cytomegalo-virus (HHV-5)** | Congenital, transfusion, sexual contact, saliva, urine, transplant | Mononucleosis (⊖ Monospot) in immunocompetent patients; infection in immunocompromised, especially pneumonia in transplant patients; esophagitis; colitis; AIDS retinitis ("sightomegalovirus"): hemorrhage, cotton-wool exudates, vision loss  <br> Congenital CMV | Infected cells have characteristic "owl eye" intranuclear inclusions **H**  <br> Latent in mononuclear cells |
| **Human herpes-viruses 6 and 7** | Saliva | Roseola infantum (exanthem subitum): high fevers for several days that can cause seizures, followed by diffuse macular rash (starts on trunk then spreads to extremities) **I**; usually seen in children < 2 years old | Roseola: fever first, Rosy (rash) later  <br> Self-limited illness  <br> HHV-7—less common cause of roseola |
| **Human herpesvirus 8** | Sexual contact | Kaposi sarcoma (neoplasm of endothelial cells). Seen in HIV/AIDS and transplant patients. Dark/violaceous plaques or nodules **J** representing vascular proliferations | Can also affect GI tract and lungs |

## Herpesviruses *(continued)*

| | |
|---|---|
| **HSV identification**  | PCR of skin lesions is test of choice. |
| | CSF PCR for herpes encephalitis. |
| | Tzanck test (outdated)—a smear of an opened skin vesicle to detect multinucleated giant cells **A** commonly seen in HSV-1, HSV-2, and VZV infection. |
| | Intranuclear eosinophilic Cowdry A inclusions also seen with HSV-1, HSV-2, VZV. |

## Receptors used by viruses

| VIRUS | RECEPTOR(S) |
|---|---|
| CMV | Integrins (heparan sulfate) |
| EBV | CD21 |
| HIV | CD4, CXCR4, CCR5 |
| Parvovirus B19 | P antigen on RBCs |
| Rabies | Nicotinic AChR |
| Rhinovirus | ICAM-1 (**I CAM**e to see the rhino) |
| SARS-CoV-2 | ACE2 |

## RNA viruses

All replicate in the cytoplasm (except retrovirus and influenza virus). "**Retro flu** is outta **cyt** (sight)."

| VIRAL FAMILY | ENVELOPE | RNA STRUCTURE | MEDICAL IMPORTANCE |
|---|---|---|---|
| **Reoviruses** | No | DS linear Multisegmented | Rotavirus—important cause of diarrhea in young children; may be fatal. |
| **Picornaviruses** | No | SS ⊕ linear | Poliovirus—polio-Salk/Sabin vaccines—IPV/OPV<br>Echovirus—aseptic meningitis<br>Rhinovirus—"common cold"<br>Coxsackievirus—aseptic meningitis; herpangina (mouth blisters, fever); hand, foot, and mouth disease; myocarditis; pericarditis<br>HAV—acute viral hepatitis         **PERCH** |
| **Hepevirus** | No | SS ⊕ linear | HEV |
| **Caliciviruses** | No | SS ⊕ linear | Norovirus—viral gastroenteritis |
| **Flaviviruses** | Yes | SS ⊕ linear | HCV<br>Yellow fever[a]<br>Dengue[a]<br>West Nile virus[a]—meningoencephalitis, acute asymmetric flaccid paralysis<br>Zika virus[a] |
| **Togaviruses** | Yes | SS ⊕ linear | **Toga CREW**—**C**hikungunya virus[a] (co-infection with dengue virus can occur), **R**ubella (formerly a togavirus), **E**astern and **W**estern equine encephalitis[a] |
| **Matonavirus** | Yes | SS ⊕ linear | Rubella |
| **Retroviruses** | Yes | SS ⊕ linear | Have reverse transcriptase<br>HTLV—T-cell leukemia<br>HIV—AIDS |
| **Coronaviruses** | Yes | SS ⊕ linear | "Common cold," SARS, COVID-19, MERS |
| **Orthomyxoviruses** | Yes | SS ⊖ linear Multisegmented | Influenza virus |
| **Paramyxoviruses** | Yes | SS ⊖ linear | PaRaMyxovirus:<br>    Parainfluenza—croup<br>    RSV—bronchiolitis in babies<br>    Measles, Mumps |
| **Pneumoviruses** | Yes | SS ⊖ linear | RSV—bronchiolitis in babies |
| **Rhabdoviruses** | Yes | SS ⊖ linear | Rabies |
| **Filoviruses** | Yes | SS ⊖ linear | Ebola/Marburg hemorrhagic fever—often fatal. |
| **Arenaviruses** | Yes | SS ⊕ and ⊖ circular Multisegmented | LCMV—lymphocytic choriomeningitis virus<br>Lassa fever encephalitis—spread by rodents |
| **Bunyaviruses** | Yes | SS ⊖ circular Multisegmented | California encephalitis[a]<br>Sandfly/Rift Valley fevers[a]<br>Crimean-Congo hemorrhagic fever[a]<br>Hantavirus—hemorrhagic fever, pneumonia |
| **Delta virus** | Yes | SS ⊖ circular | HDV is "Defective"; requires presence of HBV to replicate |

SS, single-stranded; DS, double-stranded; ⊕, positive sense; ⊖, negative sense; [a]= **ar**bovirus, **ar**thropod borne (mosquitoes, ticks).

| **Picornavirus** | Includes Poliovirus, Echovirus, Rhinovirus, Coxsackievirus, and HAV. RNA is translated into 1 large polypeptide that is cleaved by virus-encoded proteases into functional viral proteins. Poliovirus, echovirus, and coxsackievirus are enteroviruses and can cause aseptic (viral) meningitis. | PicoRNAvirus = small **RNA** virus. **PERCH** on a "peak" (pico). |
|---|---|---|
| **Rhinovirus** | A picornavirus. Nonenveloped RNA virus. Cause of common cold; > 100 serologic types. Acid labile—destroyed by stomach acid; therefore, does not infect the GI tract (unlike the other picornaviruses). | **Rhino** has a runny nose. |
| **Rotavirus**  | Segmented dsRNA virus (a reovirus) . Most important global cause of infantile gastroenteritis. Major cause of acute diarrhea in the United States during winter, especially in day care centers, kindergartens. Villous destruction with atrophy leads to ↓ absorption of $Na^+$ and loss of $K^+$. | Rotavirus = right out the anus. CDC recommends routine vaccination of all infants except those with a history of intussusception (rare adverse effect of rotavirus vaccination) or SCID. |

**Influenza viruses**

Orthomyxoviruses. Enveloped, ⊖ ssRNA viruses with segmented genome. Contain hemagglutinin (binds sialic acid and promotes viral entry) and neuraminidase (promotes progeny virion release) antigens. Patients at risk for fatal bacterial superinfection, most commonly *S aureus*, *S pneumoniae*, and *H influenzae*. Treatment: supportive +/– neuraminidase inhibitor (eg, oseltamivir, zanamivir).

Hemagglutinin: lets the virus in
Neuraminidaways: sends the virus away
Reformulated vaccine ("the flu shot") contains viral strains most likely to appear during the flu season, due to the virus' rapid genetic change.
Killed viral vaccine is most frequently used.
Live attenuated vaccine contains temperature-sensitive mutant that replicates in the nose but not in the lung; administered intranasally.
Sudden shift is more deadly than gradual drift.

**Genetic/antigenic shift**

Infection of 1 cell by 2 different segmented viruses (eg, swine influenza and human influenza viruses) → RNA segment reassortment → dramatically different virus (genetic shift) → major global outbreaks (pandemics).

**Genetic/antigenic drift**

Random mutation in hemagglutinin (HA) or neuraminidase (NA) genes → minor changes in HA or NA protein (drift) occur frequently → local seasonal outbreaks (epidemics).

**Rubella virus**

A matonavirus. Causes rubella, formerly called German (3-day) measles. Fever, postauricular and other lymphadenopathy, arthralgias, and fine, maculopapular rash that starts on face and spreads centrifugally to involve trunk and extremities Ⓐ.
Causes mild disease in children but serious congenital disease (a TORCH infection). Congenital rubella findings include classic triad of sensorineural deafness, cataracts, and patent ductus arteriosus. "Blueberry muffin" appearance may be seen due to dermal extramedullary hematopoiesis.

**Paramyxoviruses**

Paramyxoviruses cause disease in children. They include those that cause parainfluenza (croup), mumps, measles, RSV, and human metapneumovirus. All subtypes can cause respiratory tract infection (bronchiolitis, pneumonia) in infants. All contain surface F (fusion) protein, which causes respiratory epithelial cells to fuse and form multinucleated cells. Palivizumab (monoclonal antibody against F protein) prevents pneumonia caused by RSV infection in premature infants.
Palivizumab for paramyxovirus (RSV) prophylaxis in preemies.

**Acute laryngotracheobronchitis**

Also called croup. Caused by parainfluenza viruses. Virus membrane contains hemagglutinin (binds sialic acid and promotes viral entry) and neuraminidase (promotes progeny virion release) antigens. Results in a "seal-like" barking cough and inspiratory stridor. Narrowing of upper trachea and subglottis leads to characteristic steeple sign on x-ray .

**Measles (rubeola) virus**

Usual presentation involves prodromal fever with cough, coryza, and conjunctivitis, then eventually Koplik spots (bright red spots with blue-white center on buccal mucosa ), followed 1–2 days later by a maculopapular rash that starts at the head/neck and spreads downward.

Lymphadenitis with Warthin-Finkeldey giant cells (fused lymphocytes) in a background of paracortical hyperplasia. Possible sequelae:
- Subacute sclerosing panencephalitis (SSPE): personality changes, dementia, autonomic dysfunction, death (occurs years later)
- Encephalitis (1:1000): symptoms appear within few days of rash
- Giant cell pneumonia (rare except in immunosuppressed)

4 C's of measles:
  Cough
  Coryza
  Conjunctivitis
  "C"oplik spots
Vitamin A supplementation can reduce morbidity and mortality from measles, particularly in malnourished children.
Pneumonia is the most common cause of measles-associated death in children.

**Mumps virus**

Uncommon due to effectiveness of MMR vaccine.
Symptoms: Parotitis , Orchitis (inflammation of testes), aseptic Meningitis, and Pancreatitis. Can cause sterility (especially after puberty).

Mumps makes your parotid glands and testes as big as POM-Poms.

## Arboviruses transmitted by *Aedes* mosquitoes

|  | Chikungunya virus | Dengue virus |
|---|---|---|
| VIRUS TYPE | Alphavirus/togavirus | Flavivirus |
| SYMPTOMS | High fever, maculopapular rash, headache, lymphadenopathy, and inflammatory polyarthritis<br>Arthralgias are more commonly reported (vs dengue); joint swelling is highly specific for Chikungunya.<br>Thrombocytopenia, leukopenia, and hemorrhagic manifestations are less common. | Dengue fever: fever, rash, headache, myalgias, arthralgias, retro-orbital pain, neutropenia.<br>Dengue hemorrhagic fever: dengue fever + bleeding and plasma leakage due to severe thrombocytopenia and RBC perturbations. Most common if infected with a different serotype after initial infection due to antibody-dependent enhancement of disease.<br>May progress to dengue shock syndrome: plasma leakage → circulatory collapse. |
| DIAGNOSIS | RT-PCR, serology | |
| TREATMENT | Supportive.<br>Steroids or DMARDs for chronic arthritis. | Supportive. Intravascular volume repletion or blood transfusion if severe shock. |
| PREVENTION | Minimize mosquito exposure.<br>No vaccine currently available. | Live, recombinant vaccine available. Derived from the yellow fever virus backbone with insertion of genes for the envelope and pre-membrane proteins of dengue virus. |

## Yellow fever virus

A flavivirus (also an arbovirus) transmitted by *Aedes* mosquito bites. Virus has monkey or human reservoir. *Flavi* = yellow, jaundice.

Symptoms: high fever, black vomitus, jaundice, hemorrhage, backache. May see Councilman bodies (eosinophilic apoptotic globules) on liver biopsy.

Live, attenuated vaccine recommended for travelers to endemic countries.

## Zika virus

A flavivirus most commonly transmitted by *Aedes* mosquito bites.

Causes conjunctivitis, low-grade pyrexia, and itchy rash in 20% of cases. Outbreaks more common in tropical and subtropical climates. May be complicated by Guillain-Barré syndrome. Supportive care, no definitive treatment.

Diagnose with RT-PCR or serology.

Sexual and vertical transmission occurs.

In pregnancy, can lead to miscarriage or congenital Zika syndrome: brain imaging shows ventriculomegaly, subcortical calcifications. Clinical features in the affected newborn include

- Microcephaly
- Ocular anomalies
- Motor abnormalities (spasticity, seizures)

## Rabies virus

Bullet-shaped virus . Negri bodies (cytoplasmic inclusions ) commonly found in Purkinje cells of cerebellum and in hippocampal neurons. Rabies has long incubation period (weeks to months) before symptom onset. Postexposure prophylaxis is wound cleaning plus immunization with killed vaccine and rabies immunoglobulin. Example of passive-active immunity.

Travels to the CNS by migrating in a retrograde fashion (via dynein motors) up nerve axons after binding to ACh receptors.

Progression of disease: fever, malaise → agitation, photophobia, hydrophobia, hypersalivation → paralysis, coma → death.

Infection more commonly from bat, raccoon, and skunk bites than from dog bites in the United States; aerosol transmission (eg, bat caves) also possible.

## Ebola virus

A filovirus . Following an incubation period of up to 21 days, presents with abrupt onset of flulike symptoms, diarrhea/vomiting, high fever, myalgia. Can progress to DIC, diffuse hemorrhage, shock.

Diagnosed with RT-PCR within 48 hr of symptom onset. High mortality rate.

Transmission requires direct contact with bodily fluids, fomites (including dead bodies), infected bats or primates (apes/monkeys); high incidence of healthcare-associated infection.

Supportive care, no definitive treatment. Vaccination of contacts, strict isolation of infected individuals, and barrier practices for healthcare workers are key to preventing transmission.

**Severe acute respiratory syndrome coronavirus 2**

SARS-CoV-2 is a novel ⊕ ssRNA coronavirus and the cause of the COVID-19 pandemic. Predominant presenting symptoms differ by variant and vary from asymptomatic to critical:
- Common: fever, myalgia, headache, nasal congestion, sneezing, cough, sore throat, GI symptoms (eg, nausea, diarrhea).
- More specific: anosmia (loss of smell), dysgeusia (altered taste).

Complications include pneumonia, acute respiratory distress syndrome, hypercoagulability (→ thromboembolic complications including DVT, PE, stroke), myocardial injury, neurologic sequelae, shock, organ failure, death.

Strongest risk factors for severe illness or death include advanced age and pre-existing medical comorbidities (eg, obesity, hypertension).

Diagnosed by NAAT (most commonly RT-PCR). Tests detecting viral antigen are rapid and more accessible, but typically less sensitive than NAATs; negative results may warrant additional testing if there is a high suspicion of disease.

Spreads through respiratory particles. Host cell entry occurs by attachment of viral spike protein to ACE2 receptor on cell membranes. Anti-spike protein antibodies confer immunity.

Vaccination (primary series and booster) induces humoral and cellular immunity, which decreases risk of contracting or transmitting the virus and confers high rates of protection against severe disease and death.

Nirmatrelvir-ritonavir recommended for mild-to-moderate disease in patients at increased risk for severe disease.

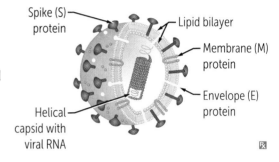

Spike (S) protein — Lipid bilayer — Membrane (M) protein — Envelope (E) protein — Helical capsid with viral RNA

**Hepatitis viruses**

Signs and symptoms of all hepatitis viruses: episodes of fever, jaundice, ↑ ALT and AST. Naked viruses (HAV and HEV) lack an envelope and are not destroyed by the gut: the **vowels** hit your **bowels**.

HBV DNA polymerase has DNA- and RNA-dependent activities. Upon entry into nucleus, the polymerase completes the partial dsDNA. Host RNA polymerase transcribes mRNA from viral DNA to make viral proteins. The DNA polymerase then reverse transcribes viral RNA to DNA, which is the genome of the progeny virus.

HCV lacks 3′-5′ exonuclease activity → no proofreading ability → antigenic variation of HCV envelope proteins. Host antibody production lags behind production of new mutant strains of HCV.

| Virus | HAV | HBV | HCV | HDV | HEV |
|---|---|---|---|---|---|
| FAMILY | RNA picornavirus | DNA hepadnavirus | RNA flavivirus | RNA deltavirus | RNA hepevirus |
| TRANSMISSION | Fecal-oral (shellfish, travelers, day care) | Parenteral (**Blood**), sexual (**Bedroom**), perinatal (**Birthing**) | Primarily blood (injection drug use, posttransfusion) | Parenteral, sexual, perinatal | Fecal-oral, especially waterborne |
| INCUBATION | Short (weeks) | Long (months) | Long | Superinfection (HDV after HBV) = short Coinfection (HDV with HBV) = long | Short |
| CLINICAL COURSE | Acute and self limiting (adults), Asymptomatic (children) | Initially like serum sickness (fever, arthralgias, rash); may progress to carcinoma | May progress to Cirrhosis or Carcinoma | Similar to HBV | Fulminant hepatitis in Expectant (pregnant) patients |
| PROGNOSIS | Good | Adults → mostly full resolution; neonates → worse prognosis | Majority develop stable, Chronic hepatitis C | Superinfection → worse prognosis | High mortality in pregnant patients |
| HCC RISK | No | Yes | Yes | Yes | No |
| LIVER BIOPSY | Hepatocyte swelling, monocyte infiltration, Councilman bodies | Granular eosinophilic "ground glass" appearance due to accumulation of surface antigen within infected hepatocytes; cytotoxic T cells mediate damage | Lymphoid aggregates with focal areas of macrovesicular steatosis | Similar to HBV | Patchy necrosis |
| NOTES | Absent (no) carrier state | Carrier state common | Carrier state very common | Defective virus, Depends on HBV HBsAg coat for entry into hepatocytes | Enteric, Epidemic (eg, in parts of Asia, Africa, Middle East), no carrier state |

## Extrahepatic manifestations of hepatitis B and C

| | Hepatitis B | Hepatitis C |
|---|---|---|
| HEMATOLOGIC | Aplastic anemia | Essential mixed cryoglobulinemia, ↑ risk B-cell NHL, ITP, autoimmune hemolytic anemia |
| RENAL | Membranous GN > membranoproliferative GN | Membranoproliferative GN > membranous GN |
| VASCULAR | Polyarteritis nodosa | Leukocytoclastic vasculitis |
| DERMATOLOGIC | | Sporadic porphyria cutanea tarda, lichen planus |
| ENDOCRINE | | ↑ risk of diabetes mellitus, autoimmune hypothyroidism |

## Hepatitis serologic markers

| | |
|---|---|
| **Anti-HAV (IgM)** | IgM antibody to HAV; best test to detect acute hepatitis A. |
| **Anti-HAV (IgG)** | IgG antibody indicates prior HAV infection and/or prior vaccination; protects against reinfection. |
| **HBsAg** | Antigen found on surface of HBV; indicates hepatitis B infection. |
| **Anti-HBs** | Antibody to HBsAg; indicates immunity to hepatitis B due to vaccination or recovery from infection. |
| **HBcAg** | Antigen associated with core of HBV. |
| **Anti-HBc** | Antibody to HBcAg; IgM = acute/recent infection; IgG = prior exposure or chronic infection. IgM anti-HBc may be the sole ⊕ marker of infection during window period. |
| **HBeAg** | Secreted by infected hepatocyte into circulation. Not part of mature HBV virion. Indicates active viral replication and therefore high transmissibility and poorer prognosis. |
| **Anti-HBe** | Antibody to HBeAg; indicates low transmissibility. |

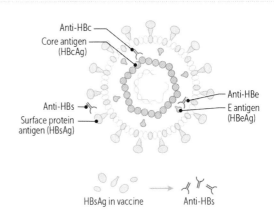

| | HBsAg | Anti-HBs | Anti-HBc | HBeAg | Anti-HBe |
|---|---|---|---|---|---|
| Incubation | + | | | | |
| Acute infection | + | | + (IgM) | + | |
| Window | | | + (IgM) | | + |
| Recovery | | + | + (IgM) | | + |
| Chronic infection (high infectivity) | + | | + (IgG) | + | |
| Chronic infection (low infectivity) | + | | + (IgG) | | + |
| Immunized | | + | | | |

## HIV

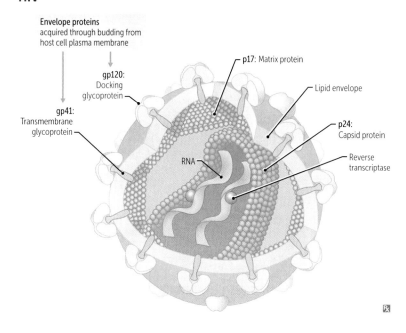

Envelope proteins
acquired through budding from
host cell plasma membrane

gp120:
Docking
glycoprotein

gp41:
Transmembrane
glycoprotein

p17: Matrix protein

Lipid envelope

p24:
Capsid protein

RNA

Reverse
transcriptase

Diploid genome (2 molecules of RNA).
The 3 structural genes (protein coded for):
- *Env* (gp120 and gp41)—formed from cleavage of gp160 to form envelope glycoproteins.
    - gp120—attachment to host CD4+ T cell.
    - gp41 (forty-one)—fusion and entry.
- *gag* (p24 and p17)—capsid and matrix proteins, respectively.
- *pol*—Reverse transcriptase, Integrase, Protease; RIP "Pol" (Paul)

Reverse transcriptase synthesizes dsDNA from genomic RNA; dsDNA integrates into host genome.

Virus binds CD4 as well as a coreceptor, either CCR5 on macrophages (early infection) or CXCR4 on T cells (late infection).

Homozygous CCR5 mutation = immunity.

Heterozygous CCR5 mutation = slower course.

## HIV diagnosis

HIV-1/2 antibodies and p24 antigen combination immunoassay

⊕　⊖

Negative for HIV-1 and HIV-2
antibodies and p24 Ag

HIV-1/HIV-2 antibody
differentiation immunoassay

HIV-1 ⊕
HIV-2 ⊖
HIV-1 infection

HIV-1 ⊖
HIV-2 ⊕
HIV-2 infection

HIV-1 ⊕
HIV-2 ⊕
HIV-1 and HIV-2
infection

HIV-1 ⊖ or indeterminate
HIV-2 ⊖

HIV-1 NAT

HIV-1 NAT ⊕
Acute HIV-1 infection

HIV-1 NAT ⊖
Negative for HIV-1

⊕ Indicates reactive test results
⊖ Indicates nonreactive test results
NAT: nucleic acid test
　Diagnostic tests
　True positive tests
　True negative tests

HIV-1/2 Ag/Ab immunoassays detect viral p24 antigen capsid protein and IgG and/or IgM to HIV-1/2.
- Use for diagnosis. Very high sensitivity/specificity, but may miss early HIV disease if tested within first 2 weeks of infection.
- A positive screening test is followed by a confirmatory HIV-1/2 differentiation immunoassay.

HIV RNA tests detect elevated HIV RNA and can be qualitative or quantitative.
- NAAT is qualitative, and is a sensitive method to detect HIV viremia in antibody-negative patients.
- Viral load tests (RT-PCR) are quantitative and determine amount of viral RNA in the plasma. Use to monitor response to treatment and transmissibility.

Western blot tests are no longer recommended by the CDC for confirmatory testing.

HIV-1/2 Ag/Ab testing is not recommended in babies with suspected HIV due to maternally transferred antibody. Use HIV viral load instead.

AIDS diagnosis: ≤ 200 CD4+ cells/mm$^3$ (normal: 500–1500 cells/mm$^3$) or HIV ⊕ with AIDS-defining condition (eg, *Pneumocystis pneumonia*).

**Common diseases of HIV-positive adults**

↓ CD4+ cell count → reactivation of past infections (eg, TB, HSV, shingles), dissemination of bacterial infections and fungal infections (eg, coccidioidomycosis), and non-Hodgkin lymphomas.

| PATHOGEN | PRESENTATION | FINDINGS |
| --- | --- | --- |
| **CD4+ cell count < 500/mm$^3$** | | |
| *Candida albicans* | Oral thrush | Scrapable white plaque, pseudohyphae on microscopy |
| EBV | Oral hairy leukoplakia | Unscrapable white plaque on lateral tongue |
| HHV-8 | Kaposi sarcoma, localized cutaneous disease | Perivascular spindle cells invading and forming vascular tumors on histology |
| HPV | Squamous cell carcinoma at site(s) of sexual contact (most commonly anus, cervix, oropharynx) | |
| *Mycobacterium tuberculosis* | Increased risk of reactivation of latent TB infection | |
| **CD4+ cell count < 200/mm$^3$** | | |
| *Histoplasma capsulatum* | Fever, weight loss, fatigue, cough, dyspnea, nausea, vomiting, diarrhea | Oval yeast cells within macrophages |
| HIV | Dementia, HIV-associated nephropathy | Cerebral atrophy on neuroimaging |
| JC virus (reactivation) | Progressive multifocal leukoencephalopathy | Nonenhancing areas of demyelination on MRI |
| HHV-8 | Kaposi sarcoma, disseminated disease (pulmonary, GI, lymphatic) | |
| *Pneumocystis jirovecii* | *Pneumocystis* pneumonia | "Ground-glass" opacities on chest imaging |
| **CD4+ cell count < 100/mm$^3$** | | |
| *Bartonella* spp | Bacillary angiomatosis | Multiple red to purple papules or nodules Biopsy with neutrophilic inflammation |
| *Candida albicans* | Esophagitis | White plaques on endoscopy; yeast and pseudohyphae on biopsy |
| CMV | Colitis, Retinitis, Esophagitis, Encephalitis, Pneumonitis (**CREEP**) | Linear ulcers on endoscopy, cotton-wool spots on fundoscopy Biopsy reveals cells with intranuclear (owl eye) inclusion bodies |
| *Cryptococcus neoformans* | Meningitis | Encapsulated yeast on India ink stain or capsular antigen ⊕ |
| *Cryptosporidium* spp | Chronic, watery diarrhea | Acid-fast oocysts in stool |
| EBV | B-cell lymphoma (eg, non-Hodgkin lymphoma, CNS lymphoma) | CNS lymphoma—ring enhancing, may be solitary (vs *Toxoplasma*) |
| *Mycobacterium avium–intracellulare, Mycobacterium avium* complex | Nonspecific systemic symptoms (fever, night sweats, weight loss, diarrhea) or superficial lymphadenitis | Most common if CD4+ cell count < 50/mm$^3$ |
| *Toxoplasma gondii* | Brain abscesses | Multiple ring-enhancing lesions on MRI |

**Prions**

Prion diseases are caused by the conversion of a normal (predominantly α-helical) protein termed prion protein ($PrP^c$) to a β-pleated form ($PrP^{sc}$), which is transmissible via CNS-related tissue (iatrogenic CJD) or food contaminated by BSE-infected animal products (variant CJD). $PrP^{sc}$ resists protease degradation and facilitates the conversion of still more $PrP^c$ to $PrP^{sc}$. Resistant to standard sterilizing procedures, including standard autoclaving. Accumulation of $PrP^{sc}$ results in spongiform encephalopathy and dementia, ataxia, startle myoclonus, and death.

**Creutzfeldt-Jakob disease**—rapidly progressive dementia, typically sporadic (some familial forms).

**Bovine spongiform encephalopathy**—also called "mad cow disease."

**Kuru**—acquired prion disease noted in tribal populations practicing human cannibalism.

## ▶ MICROBIOLOGY—SYSTEMS

**Normal microbiota: dominant**

Neonates delivered by C-section have microbiota enriched in skin commensals.

| LOCATION | MICROORGANISM |
| --- | --- |
| Skin | *S epidermidis* |
| Nose | *S epidermidis*; colonized by *S aureus* |
| Oropharynx | Viridans group streptococci |
| Dental plaque | *S mutans* |
| Colon | *B fragilis* > *E coli* |
| Vagina | *Lactobacillus*; colonized by *E coli* and group B strep |

**Bugs causing food-borne illness**

*S aureus* and *B cereus* food poisoning starts quickly and ends quickly (exotoxin-mediated).

| MICROORGANISM | SOURCE OF INFECTION |
| --- | --- |
| *B cereus* | Reheated rice. "Food poisoning from reheated rice? **Be serious!**" (*B cereus*) |
| *C botulinum* | Improperly canned foods (toxins), raw honey (spores) |
| *C perfringens* | Reheated meat |
| *E coli* O157:H7 | Undercooked meat |
| *L monocytogenes* | Deli meats, soft cheeses |
| *Salmonella* | Poultry, meat, and eggs |
| *S aureus* | Meats, mayonnaise, custard; preformed toxin |
| *V parahaemolyticus* and *V vulnificus*[a] | Raw/undercooked seafood |

[a]*V vulnificus* predominantly causes wound infections from contact with contaminated water or shellfish.

## Bugs causing diarrhea

### Bloody diarrhea

| | |
|---|---|
| *Campylobacter* | Comma- or S-shaped organisms; growth at 42°C |
| *E histolytica* | Protozoan; amebic dysentery; liver abscess |
| Enterohemorrhagic *E coli* | O157:H7; can cause HUS; makes Shiga toxin |
| Enteroinvasive *E coli* | Invades colonic mucosa |
| *Salmonella* (non-typhoidal) | Lactose ⊖; flagellar motility; has animal reservoir, especially poultry and eggs |
| *Shigella* | Lactose ⊖; very low $ID_{50}$; produces Shiga toxin; human reservoir only; bacillary dysentery |
| *Y enterocolitica* | Day care outbreaks; pseudoappendicitis |

### Watery diarrhea

| | |
|---|---|
| *C difficile* | Pseudomembranous colitis; associated with antibiotics and PPIs; occasionally bloody diarrhea |
| *C perfringens* | Also causes gas gangrene |
| Enterotoxigenic *E coli* | Travelers' diarrhea; produces heat-labile (LT) and heat-stable (ST) toxins |
| Protozoa | *Giardia*, *Cryptosporidium* |
| *V cholerae* | Comma-shaped organisms; rice-water diarrhea; often from infected seafood |
| Viruses | Norovirus (most common cause in developed countries), rotavirus (↓ incidence in developed countries due to vaccination), enteric adenovirus |

## Common causes of pneumonia

| NEONATES (< 4 WK) | CHILDREN (4 WK–18 YR) | ADULTS (18–40 YR) | ADULTS (40–65 YR) | ADULTS (65 YR +) |
|---|---|---|---|---|
| Group B streptococci *E coli* | Viruses (**RSV**) *Mycoplasma* *C trachomatis* (infants–3 yr) *C pneumoniae* (school-aged children) *S pneumoniae* Runts May Cough Chunky Sputum | *Mycoplasma* *C pneumoniae* *S pneumoniae* Viruses (eg, influenza) | *S pneumoniae* *H influenzae* Anaerobes Viruses *Mycoplasma* | *S pneumoniae* Influenza virus Anaerobes *H influenzae* Gram ⊖ rods |

### Special groups

| | |
|---|---|
| Alcohol overuse | *Klebsiella*, anaerobes usually due to aspiration (eg, *Peptostreptococcus, Fusobacterium, Prevotella, Bacteroides*) |
| Injection drug use | *S pneumoniae, S aureus* |
| Aspiration | Anaerobes |
| Atypical | *Mycoplasma, Chlamydophila, Legionella,* viruses (RSV, CMV, influenza, adenovirus) |
| Cystic fibrosis | *Pseudomonas, S aureus, S pneumoniae, Burkholderia cepacia* |
| Immunocompromised | *S aureus*, enteric gram ⊖ rods, fungi, viruses, *P jirovecii* (with HIV) |
| Healthcare-associated | *S aureus, Pseudomonas,* other enteric gram ⊖ rods |
| Postviral | *S pneumoniae, S aureus, H influenzae* |
| COPD | *S pneumoniae, H influenzae, M catarrhalis, Pseudomonas* |

## Common causes of meningitis

| NEWBORN (0–6 MO) | CHILDREN (6 MO–6 YR) | 6–60 YR | 60 YR + |
| --- | --- | --- | --- |
| Group B *Streptococcus* | *S pneumoniae* | *S pneumoniae* | *S pneumoniae* |
| *E coli* | *N meningitidis* | *N meningitidis* | *N meningitidis* |
| *Listeria* | *H influenzae* type b | Enteroviruses | *H influenzae* type b |
| | Group B *Streptococcus* | HSV | Group B *Streptococcus* |
| | Enteroviruses | | *Listeria* |

Give ceftriaxone and vancomycin empirically (add ampicillin if *Listeria* is suspected; add acyclovir if viral encephalitis is suspected).

Viral causes of meningitis: enteroviruses (especially coxsackievirus), HSV-2 (HSV-1 = encephalitis), HIV, West Nile virus (also causes encephalitis), VZV.

In HIV: *Cryptococcus* spp.

Note: Incidence of Group B streptococcal meningitis in neonates has ↓ greatly due to screening and antibiotic prophylaxis in pregnancy. Incidence of *H influenzae* meningitis has ↓ greatly due to conjugate *H influenzae* vaccinations. Today, cases are usually seen in unimmunized children.

## Cerebrospinal fluid findings in meningitis

| | OPENING PRESSURE | CELL TYPE | PROTEIN | GLUCOSE |
| --- | --- | --- | --- | --- |
| **Bacterial** | ↑ | ↑ PMNs | ↑ | ↓ |
| **Fungal/TB** | ↑ | ↑ lymphocytes | ↑ | ↓ |
| **Viral** | Normal/↑ | ↑ lymphocytes | Normal/↑ | Normal |

| | |
| --- | --- |
| **Infections causing brain abscess** | Most commonly viridans streptococci and *Staphylococcus aureus*. If dental infection or extraction precedes abscess, oral anaerobes commonly involved. Multiple abscesses are usually from bacteremia; single lesions from contiguous sites: otitis media and mastoiditis → temporal lobe and cerebellum; sinusitis or dental infection → frontal lobe. *Toxoplasma* reactivation in AIDS. |

## Osteomyelitis

| RISK FACTOR | ASSOCIATED INFECTION |
| --- | --- |
| Assume if no other information is available | *S aureus* (most common overall) |
| Sexually active | *Neisseria gonorrhoeae* (rare), septic arthritis more common |
| Sickle cell disease | *Salmonella, S aureus* |
| Prosthetic joint replacement | *S aureus, S epidermidis* |
| Vertebral involvement | *S aureus, M tuberculosis* (Pott disease) |
| Cat and dog bites | *Pasteurella multocida* |
| Injection drug use | *S aureus*; also *Pseudomonas, Candida* |

Elevated ESR and CRP sensitive but not specific.

Radiographs are insensitive early but can be useful in chronic osteomyelitis (A, left). MRI is best for detecting acute infection and detailing anatomic involvement (A, right). Biopsy or aspiration with culture necessary to identify organism.

## Red rashes of childhood

| AGENT | ASSOCIATED SYNDROME/DISEASE | CLINICAL PRESENTATION |
|---|---|---|
| Coxsackievirus type A | Hand-foot-mouth disease | Oval-shaped vesicles on palms and soles ; vesicles and ulcers in oral mucosa (herpangina) |
| Human herpesvirus 6 | Roseola (exanthem subitum) | Asymptomatic rose-colored macules appear on body after several days of high fever; can present with febrile seizures; usually affects infants |
| Measles virus | Measles (rubeola) | Confluent rash beginning at head and moving down ; preceded by cough, coryza, conjunctivitis, and blue-white (Koplik) spots on buccal mucosa |
| Parvovirus B19 | Erythema infectiosum (fifth disease) | "Slapped cheek" rash on face  |
| Rubella virus | Rubella | Pink macules and papules begin at head and move down, remain discrete → fine desquamating truncal rash; postauricular lymphadenopathy |
| *Streptococcus pyogenes* | Scarlet fever | Sore throat, Circumoral pallor, group A strep, Rash (sandpaperlike , from neck to trunk and extremities), Lymphadenopathy, Erythrogenic toxin, strawberry Tongue (**SCARLET**) |
| Varicella-zoster virus | Chickenpox | Vesicular rash begins on trunk , spreads to face and extremities with lesions of different stages |

| Urinary tract infections | Cystitis presents with dysuria, frequency, urgency, suprapubic pain, and WBCs (but not WBC casts) in urine. Primarily caused by ascension of microbes from urethra to bladder. Ascension to kidney results in pyelonephritis, which presents with fever, chills, flank pain, costovertebral angle tenderness, hematuria, and WBC casts.<br>Ten times more common in females (shorter urethras colonized by fecal microbiota).<br>Risk factors: obstruction (eg, kidney stones, enlarged prostate), kidney surgery, catheterization, congenital GU malformation (eg, vesicoureteral reflux), diabetes, pregnancy. | |
|---|---|---|

| SPECIES | FEATURES | COMMENTS |
|---|---|---|
| *Escherichia coli* | Leading cause of UTI. Colonies show strong pink lactose-fermentation on MacConkey agar. | Diagnostic markers:<br>⊕ Leukocyte esterase = evidence of WBC activity.<br>⊕ Nitrite test = reduction of urinary nitrates by gram ⊖ bacterial species (eg, *E coli*). |
| *Staphylococcus saprophyticus* | 2nd leading cause of UTI, particularly in young, sexually active females. | |
| *Klebsiella pneumoniae* | 3rd leading cause of UTI. Large mucoid capsule and viscous colonies. | |
| *Serratia marcescens* | Some strains produce a red pigment; often healthcare-associated and drug resistant. | |
| *Enterococcus* | Often healthcare-associated and drug resistant. | |
| *Proteus mirabilis* | Motility causes "swarming" on agar; associated with struvite stones. Produces urease. | |
| *Pseudomonas aeruginosa* | Blue-green pigment and fruity odor; usually healthcare-associated and drug resistant. | |

## Common vaginal infections

| | Bacterial vaginosis | *Trichomonas* vaginitis | *Candida* vulvovaginitis |
|---|---|---|---|
| SIGNS AND SYMPTOMS | No inflammation<br>Thin, white discharge A with fishy odor | Inflammation B ("strawberry cervix")<br>Frothy, yellow-green, foul-smelling discharge | Inflammation<br>Thick, white, "cottage cheese" discharge D |
| LAB FINDINGS | Clue cells (bacteria-coated epithelial cells)<br>pH > 4.5<br>⊕ KOH whiff test | Motile pear-shaped trichomonads C<br>pH > 4.5 | Pseudohyphae<br>pH normal (4.0–4.5) |
| TREATMENT | Metronidazole or clindamycin | Metronidazole<br>Treat sexual partner(s) | Azoles |

## Sexually transmitted infections

| DISEASE | CLINICAL FEATURES | PATHOGEN |
|---------|-------------------|----------|
| AIDS | Opportunistic infections, Kaposi sarcoma, lymphoma | HIV |
| Chancroid | Painful genital ulcer(s) with exudate, inguinal adenopathy A | *Haemophilus ducreyi* (it's so painful, you "do cry") |
| Chlamydia | Urethritis, cervicitis, epididymitis, conjunctivitis, reactive arthritis, PID | *Chlamydia trachomatis* (D–K) |
| Condylomata acuminata | Genital warts B, koilocytes | HPV-6 and -11 |
| Herpes genitalis | Painful penile, vulvar, or cervical vesicles and ulcers C with bilateral tender inguinal lymphadenopathy; can cause systemic symptoms such as fever, headache, myalgia | HSV-2, less commonly HSV-1 |
| Gonorrhea | Urethritis, cervicitis, PID, prostatitis, epididymitis, arthritis, creamy purulent discharge | *Neisseria gonorrhoeae* |
| Granuloma inguinale (Donovanosis) | Painless, beefy red ulcer that bleeds readily on contact D  Uncommon in US | *Klebsiella* (*Calymmatobacterium*) *granulomatis*; cytoplasmic Donovan bodies (bipolar staining) seen on microscopy |
| Hepatitis B | Jaundice | HBV |
| Lymphogranuloma venereum | Infection of lymphatics; painless genital ulcers, painful lymphadenopathy (ie, buboes E) | *C trachomatis* (L1–L3) |
| Primary syphilis | Painless chancre F, regional lymphadenopathy | *Treponema pallidum* |
| Secondary syphilis | Fever, diffuse lymphadenopathy, generalized rash, condylomata lata | |
| Tertiary syphilis | Gummas, tabes dorsalis, general paresis, aortitis, Argyll Robertson pupil | |
| Trichomoniasis | Vaginitis, strawberry cervix, motile in wet prep | *Trichomonas vaginalis* |

**TORCH infections**  Microbes that may pass from mother to fetus. Transmission is transplacental in most cases, or via vaginal delivery (especially HSV-2). Nonspecific signs common to many ToRCHHeS infections include hepatosplenomegaly, jaundice, thrombocytopenia, and growth restriction.

Other important infectious agents include *Streptococcus agalactiae* (group B streptococci), *E coli*, and *Listeria monocytogenes*—all causes of meningitis in neonates. Parvovirus B19 causes hydrops fetalis.

| AGENT | MATERNAL ACQUISITION | MATERNAL MANIFESTATIONS | NEONATAL MANIFESTATIONS |
|---|---|---|---|
| *Toxoplasma gondii* | Cat feces or ingestion of undercooked meat | Usually asymptomatic; lymphadenopathy (rarely) | Classic triad: chorioretinitis, hydrocephalus, and intracranial calcifications, +/– "blueberry muffin" rash  |
| Rubella | Respiratory droplets | Rash, lymphadenopathy, polyarthritis, polyarthralgia | Classic triad: abnormalities of eye (cataracts ) and ear (deafness) and congenital heart disease (PDA); +/– "blueberry muffin" rash. "I (eye) ♥ ruby (rubella) earrings" |
| Cytomegalovirus | Sexual contact, organ transplants | Usually asymptomatic; mononucleosis-like illness | Hearing loss, seizures, petechial rash, "blueberry muffin" rash, chorioretinitis, periventricular calcifications  CMV = Chorioretinitis, Microcephaly, periVentricular calcifications |
| HIV | Sexual contact, needlestick | Variable presentation depending on CD4+ cell count | Recurrent infections, chronic diarrhea |
| Herpes simplex virus-2 | Skin or mucous membrane contact | Usually asymptomatic; herpetic (vesicular) lesions | Meningoencephalitis, herpetic (vesicular) lesions |
| Syphilis | Sexual contact | Chancre (1°) and disseminated rash (2°) are the two stages likely to result in fetal infection | Often results in stillbirth, hydrops fetalis; if child survives, presents with facial abnormalities (eg, notched teeth, saddle nose, rhinitis, short maxilla), saber shins, CN VIII deafness |

## Pelvic inflammatory disease

Ascending infection causing inflammation of the female gynecologic tract. PID may include salpingitis, endometritis, hydrosalpinx, and tubo-ovarian abscess.

Signs include cervical motion tenderness, adnexal tenderness, purulent cervical discharge **A**.

Top bugs—*Chlamydia trachomatis* (subacute, often undiagnosed), *Neisseria gonorrhoeae* (acute).

*C trachomatis*—most common bacterial STI in the United States.

Salpingitis is a risk factor for ectopic pregnancy, infertility, chronic pelvic pain, and adhesions. Can lead to perihepatitis (**Fitz-Hugh–Curtis syndrome**)—infection and inflammation of liver capsule and "violin string" adhesions of peritoneum to liver **B**.

## Healthcare-associated infections

*E coli* (UTI) and *S aureus* (wound infection) are the two most common causes.

| RISK FACTOR | PATHOGEN | UNIQUE SIGNS/SYMPTOMS |
| --- | --- | --- |
| Antibiotic use, PPIs | *Clostridioides difficile* | Watery diarrhea, leukocytosis |
| Aspiration (2° to altered mental status, old age) | Polymicrobial, gram ⊖ bacteria, often anaerobes | Right lower lobe infiltrate or right upper/middle lobe (patient recumbent); purulent malodorous sputum |
| Decubitus ulcers, surgical wounds, drains | *S aureus* (including MRSA), gram ⊖ anaerobes (*Bacteroides, Prevotella, Fusobacterium*) | Erythema, tenderness, induration, drainage from surgical wound sites |
| Intravascular catheters | *S aureus* (including MRSA), *S epidermidis* (long term) | Erythema, induration, tenderness, drainage from access sites |
| Mechanical ventilation, endotracheal intubation | Late onset: *P aeruginosa, Klebsiella, Acinetobacter, S aureus* | New infiltrate on CXR, ↑ sputum production; sweet odor (*Pseudomonas*) |
| Exposure to blood products, shared medical equipment, needlesticks | HBV, HCV | |
| Urinary catheterization | *Proteus* spp, *E coli, Klebsiella* (PEcK) | Dysuria, leukocytosis, flank pain or costovertebral angle tenderness |
| Water aerosols | *Legionella* | Signs of pneumonia, GI symptoms (diarrhea, nausea, vomiting), neurologic abnormalities |

**Bugs affecting unvaccinated children**

| CLINICAL PRESENTATION | FINDINGS/LABS | PATHOGEN |
|---|---|---|
| **Dermatologic** | | |
| **Rash** | Beginning at head and moving down with postauricular, posterior cervical, and suboccipital lymphadenopathy | Rubella virus |
| | Beginning at head and moving down; preceded by cough, coryza, conjunctivitis, and Koplik spots | Measles virus |
| **Neurologic** | | |
| **Meningitis** | Microbe colonizes nasopharynx | *H influenzae* type b |
| | Can also lead to myalgia and paralysis | Poliovirus |
| **Tetanus** | Muscle spasms and spastic paralysis (eg, lockjaw, opisthotonus) | *Clostridium tetani* |
| **Respiratory** | | |
| **Epiglottitis** | Fever with dysphagia, drooling, inspiratory stridor, and difficulty breathing due to edema | *H influenzae* type b (also capable of causing epiglottitis in fully immunized children) |
| **Pertussis** | Low-grade fevers, coryza → whooping cough, posttussive vomiting → gradual recovery | *Bordetella pertussis* |
| **Pharyngitis** | Grayish pseudomembranes (may obstruct airways) | *Corynebacterium diphtheriae* |

## ▶ MICROBIOLOGY—ANTIMICROBIALS

### Antimicrobial therapy

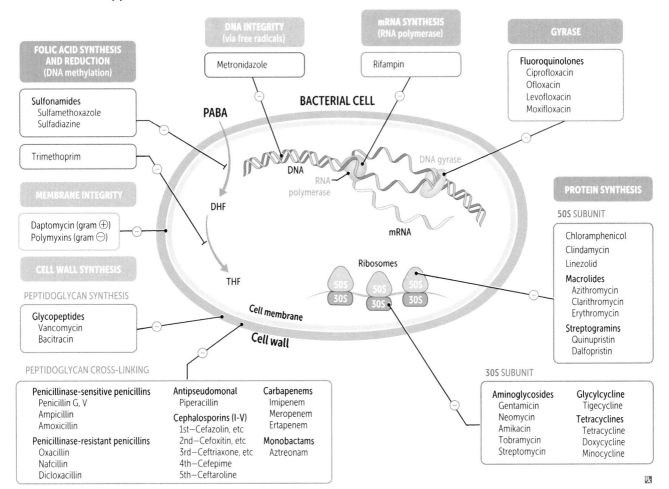

| **Penicillin G, V** | Penicillin G (IV and IM form), penicillin V (oral). Prototype β-lactam antibiotics. |
|---|---|
| MECHANISM | D-Ala-D-Ala structural analog. Bind penicillin-binding proteins (transpeptidases). Block transpeptidase cross-linking of peptidoglycan in cell wall. Activate autolytic enzymes. |
| CLINICAL USE | Mostly used for gram ⊕ organisms (*S pneumoniae, S pyogenes, Actinomyces*). Also used for gram ⊖ cocci (mainly *N meningitidis*) and spirochetes (mainly *T pallidum*). Bactericidal for gram ⊕ cocci, gram ⊕ rods, gram ⊖ cocci, and spirochetes. β-lactamase sensitive. |
| ADVERSE EFFECTS | Hypersensitivity reactions, direct Coombs ⊕ hemolytic anemia, drug-induced interstitial nephritis. |
| RESISTANCE | β-lactamase cleaves the β-lactam ring. Mutations in PBPs. |

| **Penicillinase-sensitive penicillins** | Amoxicillin, ampicillin; aminopenicillins. | |
| --- | --- | --- |
| MECHANISM | Same as penicillin. Wider spectrum; penicillinase sensitive. Also combine with clavulanic acid to protect against destruction by β-lactamase. | Aminopenicillins are amped-up penicillin. Amoxicillin has greater oral bioavailability than ampicillin. |
| CLINICAL USE | Extended-spectrum penicillin—*H influenzae*, *H pylori*, *E coli*, Enterococci, *Listeria monocytogenes*, *Proteus mirabilis*, *Salmonella*, *Shigella*. | Coverage: ampicillin/amoxicillin **HHEELPSS** kill enterococci. |
| ADVERSE EFFECTS | Hypersensitivity reactions, rash, pseudomembranous colitis. | |
| MECHANISM OF RESISTANCE | Penicillinase (a type of β-lactamase) cleaves β-lactam ring. | |

| **Penicillinase-resistant penicillins** | Dicloxacillin, nafcillin, oxacillin. | |
| --- | --- | --- |
| MECHANISM | Same as penicillin. Narrow spectrum; penicillinase resistant because bulky R group blocks access of β-lactamase to β-lactam ring. | |
| CLINICAL USE | *S aureus* (except MRSA). | "Use **naf** (nafcillin) for staph." |
| ADVERSE EFFECTS | Hypersensitivity reactions, interstitial nephritis. | |
| MECHANISM OF RESISTANCE | MRSA has altered penicillin-binding protein target site. | |

| **Piperacillin** | Antipseudomonal penicillin. |
| --- | --- |
| MECHANISM | Same as penicillin. Extended spectrum. Penicillinase sensitive; use with β-lactamase inhibitors. |
| CLINICAL USE | *Pseudomonas* spp., gram ⊖ rods, anaerobes. |
| ADVERSE EFFECTS | Hypersensitivity reactions. |

## Cephalosporins

| | | |
|---|---|---|
| MECHANISM | β-lactam drugs that inhibit cell wall synthesis but are less susceptible to penicillinases. Bactericidal. | Organisms typically not covered by 1st–4th generation cephalosporins are LAME: *Listeria*, Atypicals (*Chlamydia*, *Mycoplasma*), MRSA, and Enterococci. |
| CLINICAL USE | 1st generation (cefazolin, cephalexin)—gram ⊕ cocci, *Proteus mirabilis*, *E coli*, *Klebsiella pneumoniae*. Cefazolin used prior to surgery to prevent *S aureus* wound infections. | 1st generation—⊕ PEcK. |
| | 2nd generation (cefaclor, cefoxitin, cefuroxime, cefotetan)—gram ⊕ cocci, *H influenzae*, *Enterobacter aerogenes*, *Neisseria* spp., *Serratia marcescens*, *Proteus mirabilis*, *E coli*, *Klebsiella pneumoniae*. | 2nd graders wear fake fox fur to tea parties. 2nd generation—⊕ HENS PEcK. |
| | 3rd generation (ceftriaxone, cefpodoxime, ceftazidime, cefixime)—serious gram ⊖ infections resistant to other β-lactams. | Can cross blood-brain barrier. Ceftriaxone—meningitis, gonorrhea, disseminated Lyme disease. Ceftazidime for pseudomonaz. |
| | 4th generation (cefepime)—gram ⊖ organisms, with ↑ activity against *Pseudomonas* and gram ⊕ organisms. | |
| | 5th generation (ceftaroline)—broad gram ⊕ and gram ⊖ organism coverage; unlike 1st–4th generation cephalosporins, ceftaroline covers MRSA, and *Enterococcus faecalis*—does not cover *Pseudomonas*. | |
| ADVERSE EFFECTS | Hypersensitivity reactions, autoimmune hemolytic anemia, disulfiram-like reaction, vitamin K deficiency. Low rate of cross-reactivity even in penicillin-allergic patients. ↑ nephrotoxicity of aminoglycosides. | |
| MECHANISM OF RESISTANCE | Inactivated by cephalosporinases (a type of β-lactamase). Structural change in penicillin-binding proteins (transpeptidases). | |

| | | |
|---|---|---|
| **β-lactamase inhibitors** | Include Clavulanic acid, Avibactam, Sulbactam, Tazobactam. Often added to penicillin antibiotics to protect the antibiotic from destruction by β-lactamase. | CAST (eg, amoxicillin-clavulanate, ceftazidime-avibactam, ampicillin-sulbactam, piperacillin-tazobactam). |

## Carbapenems

Imipenem, meropenem, ertapenem.

| | | |
|---|---|---|
| MECHANISM | Imipenem is a broad-spectrum, β-lactamase–resistant carbapenem. Binds penicillin-binding proteins → inhibition of cell wall synthesis → cell death. Always administered with cilastatin (inhibitor of renal dehydropeptidase I) to ↓ inactivation of drug in renal tubules. | With imipenem, "the kill is **lastin'** with cilastatin."<br>Unlike other carbapenems, ertapenem is not active against *Pseudomonas*. |
| CLINICAL USE | Gram ⊕ cocci, gram ⊖ rods, and anaerobes. Wide spectrum and significant adverse effects limit use to life-threatening infections or after other drugs have failed. Meropenem has a ↓ risk of seizures and is stable to dehydropeptidase I. | |
| ADVERSE EFFECTS | GI distress, rash, and CNS toxicity (seizures) at high plasma levels. | |
| MECHANISM OF RESISTANCE | Inactivated by carbapenemases produced by, eg, *K pneumoniae*, *E coli*, *E aerogenes*. | |

## Aztreonam

| | |
|---|---|
| MECHANISM | Less susceptible to β-lactamases. Prevents peptidoglycan cross-linking by binding to penicillin-binding protein 3. Synergistic with aminoglycosides. No cross-allergenicity with penicillins. |
| CLINICAL USE | Gram ⊖ rods only—no activity against gram ⊕ rods or anaerobes. For penicillin-allergic patients and those with renal insufficiency who cannot tolerate aminoglycosides. |
| ADVERSE EFFECTS | Usually nontoxic; occasional GI upset. |

## Vancomycin

| | |
|---|---|
| MECHANISM | Inhibits cell wall peptidoglycan formation by binding D-Ala-D-Ala portion of cell wall precursors. Bactericidal against most bacteria (bacteriostatic against *C difficile*). Not susceptible to β-lactamases. |
| CLINICAL USE | Gram ⊕ bugs only—for serious, multidrug-resistant organisms, including MRSA, *S epidermidis*, sensitive *Enterococcus* species, and *Clostridium difficile* (oral route). |
| ADVERSE EFFECTS | Well tolerated in general but **not** trouble free: nephrotoxicity, ototoxicity, thrombophlebitis, diffuse flushing (vancomycin infusion reaction 🅰—idiopathic reaction largely preventable by pretreatment with antihistamines and slower infusion rate), DRESS syndrome. |
| MECHANISM OF RESISTANCE | Occurs in bacteria (eg, *Enterococcus*) via amino acid modification of D-Ala-D-Ala to D-Ala-D-Lac. "If you **Lack** a D-Ala (dollar), you can't ride the van (vancomycin)." |

| | |
|---|---|
| **Protein synthesis inhibitors** | Specifically target smaller bacterial ribosome (70S, made of 30S and 50S subunits), leaving human ribosome (80S) unaffected.<br>All are bacteriostatic, except aminoglycosides (bactericidal) and linezolid (variable). |
| **30S inhibitors** | Aminoglycosides<br>Tetracyclines      "Buy at 30, ccel (sell) at 50." |
| **50S inhibitors** | Chloramphenicol, Clindamycin<br>Erythromycin (macrolides)<br>Linezolid |

| | |
|---|---|
| **Aminoglycosides** | Gentamicin, Neomycin, Amikacin, Tobramycin, Streptomycin.<br>"Mean" (aminoglycoside) **GNATS** cannot kill anaerobes. |
| MECHANISM | Bactericidal; irreversible inhibition of initiation complex through binding of the 30S subunit. Can cause misreading of mRNA. Also block translocation. Require $O_2$ for uptake; therefore ineffective against anaerobes. |
| CLINICAL USE | Severe gram ⊖ rod infections. Synergistic with β-lactam antibiotics.<br>Neomycin for bowel surgery. |
| ADVERSE EFFECTS | Nephrotoxicity, neuromuscular blockade (absolute contraindication with myasthenia gravis), ototoxicity (especially with loop diuretics), teratogenicity. |
| MECHANISM OF RESISTANCE | Bacterial transferase enzymes inactivate the drug by acetylation, phosphorylation, or adenylation. |

## Tetracyclines

Tetracycline, doxycycline, minocycline.

| | |
|---|---|
| MECHANISM | Bacteriostatic; bind to 30S and prevent attachment of aminoacyl-tRNA. Limited CNS penetration. Doxycycline is fecally eliminated and can be used in patients with renal failure. Do not take tetracyclines with milk ($Ca^{2+}$), antacids (eg, $Ca^{2+}$ or $Mg^{2+}$), or iron-containing preparations because divalent cations inhibit drugs' absorption in the gut. |
| CLINICAL USE | *Borrelia burgdorferi*, M *pneumoniae*. Drugs' ability to accumulate intracellularly makes them very effective against *Rickettsia* and *Chlamydia*. Also used to treat acne. Doxycycline effective against community-acquired MRSA. |
| ADVERSE EFFECTS | GI distress, discoloration of teeth and inhibition of bone growth in children, photosensitivity. "Teratocylines" are **terato**genic; generally avoided in pregnancy and in children (except doxycycline). |
| MECHANISM OF RESISTANCE | ↓ uptake or ↑ efflux out of bacterial cells by plasmid-encoded transport pumps. |

## Tigecycline

| | |
|---|---|
| MECHANISM | Tetracycline derivative. Binds to 30S, inhibiting protein synthesis. Generally bacteriostatic. |
| CLINICAL USE | Broad-spectrum anaerobic, gram ⊖, and gram ⊕ coverage. Multidrug-resistant organisms (eg, MRSA, VRE). |
| ADVERSE EFFECTS | Nausea, vomiting. |

## Chloramphenicol

| | |
|---|---|
| MECHANISM | Blocks peptidyltransferase at 50S ribosomal subunit. Bacteriostatic. |
| CLINICAL USE | Meningitis (*Haemophilus influenzae*, *Neisseria meningitidis*, *Streptococcus pneumoniae*) and rickettsial diseases (eg, Rocky Mountain spotted fever [*Rickettsia rickettsii*]). Limited use due to toxicity but often still used in developing countries because of low cost. |
| ADVERSE EFFECTS | Anemia (dose dependent), aplastic anemia (dose independent), gray baby syndrome (in premature infants because they lack liver UDP-glucuronosyltransferase). |
| MECHANISM OF RESISTANCE | Plasmid-encoded acetyltransferase inactivates the drug. |

## Clindamycin

| | |
|---|---|
| MECHANISM | Blocks peptide transfer (translocation) at 50S ribosomal subunit. Bacteriostatic. |
| CLINICAL USE | Anaerobic infections (eg, *Bacteroides* spp., *Clostridium perfringens*) in aspiration pneumonia, lung abscesses, and oral infections. Also effective against invasive group A streptococcal infection. Treats anaerobic infections above the diaphragm vs metronidazole (anaerobic infections below diaphragm). |
| ADVERSE EFFECTS | Pseudomembranous colitis (C *difficile* overgrowth), fever, diarrhea. |

## Linezolid

| | |
|---|---|
| MECHANISM | Inhibits protein synthesis by binding to the 23S rRNA of the 50S ribosomal subunit and preventing formation of the initiation complex. |
| CLINICAL USE | Gram ⊕ species including MRSA and VRE. |
| ADVERSE EFFECTS | Myelosuppression (especially thrombocytopenia), peripheral neuropathy, serotonin syndrome (due to partial MAO inhibition). |
| MECHANISM OF RESISTANCE | Point mutation of ribosomal RNA. |

## Macrolides

| | Azithromycin, clarithromycin, erythromycin. |
|---|---|
| MECHANISM | Inhibit protein synthesis by blocking **trans**location ("macro**slides**"); bind to the 50S ribosomal subunit. Bacteriostatic. |
| CLINICAL USE | Atypical pneumonias (*Mycoplasma*, *Chlamydia*, *Legionella*), STIs (*Chlamydia*), gram ⊕ cocci (streptococcal infections in patients allergic to penicillin), and *B pertussis*. |
| ADVERSE EFFECTS | **MACRO**: Gastrointestinal **M**otility issues, **A**rrhythmia caused by prolonged QT interval, acute **C**holestatic hepatitis, **R**ash, e**O**sinophilia. Increases serum concentration of theophylline, oral anticoagulants. Clarithromycin and erythromycin inhibit cytochrome P-450. |
| MECHANISM OF RESISTANCE | Methylation of 23S rRNA-binding site prevents binding of drug. |

## Polymyxins

| | Colistin (polymyxin E), polymyxin B. |
|---|---|
| MECHANISM | Cation polypeptides that bind to phospholipids on cell membrane of gram ⊖ bacteria. Disrupt cell membrane integrity → leakage of cellular components → cell death. |
| CLINICAL USE | Salvage therapy for multidrug-resistant gram ⊖ bacteria (eg, *P aeruginosa*, *E coli*, *K pneumoniae*). Polymyxin B is a component of a triple antibiotic ointment used for superficial skin infections. |
| ADVERSE EFFECTS | Nephrotoxicity, neurotoxicity (eg, slurred speech, weakness, paresthesias), respiratory failure. |

| **Sulfonamides** | Sulfamethoxazole (SMX), sulfisoxazole, sulfadiazine. |
|---|---|
| MECHANISM | Inhibit dihydropteroate synthase, thus inhibiting folate synthesis. Bacteriostatic (bactericidal when combined with trimethoprim). |
| CLINICAL USE | Gram ⊕, gram ⊖, *Nocardia*. TMP-SMX for simple UTI. |
| ADVERSE EFFECTS | Stevens-Johnson syndrome, urticaria, liver damage, folate deficiency, optic neuritis, nephrotoxicity, agranulocytosis, hemolysis if G6PD deficient, kernicterus in infants. |
| MECHANISM OF RESISTANCE | Altered enzyme (bacterial dihydropteroate synthase), ↓ uptake, or ↑ PABA synthesis. |

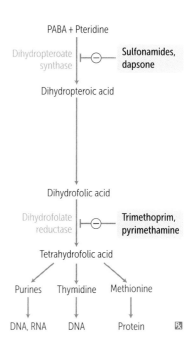

| **Dapsone** | |
|---|---|
| MECHANISM | Similar to sulfonamides, but structurally distinct agent. |
| CLINICAL USE | Leprosy (lepromatous and tuberculoid), *Pneumocystis jirovecii* prophylaxis, or treatment when used in combination with TMP. |
| ADVERSE EFFECTS | Hemolysis if G6PD deficient, methemoglobinemia, agranulocytosis. |

| **Trimethoprim** | |
|---|---|
| MECHANISM | Inhibits bacterial dihydrofolate reductase. Bacteriostatic. |
| CLINICAL USE | Used in combination with sulfonamides (trimethoprim-sulfamethoxazole [TMP-SMX]), causing sequential block of folate synthesis. Combination used for UTIs, *Shigella*, *Salmonella*, *Pneumocystis jirovecii* pneumonia treatment and prophylaxis, toxoplasmosis prophylaxis. |
| ADVERSE EFFECTS | Hyperkalemia (at high doses; similar mechanism as potassium-sparing diuretics), megaloblastic anemia, leukopenia, granulocytopenia, which may be avoided with coadministration of leucovorin (folinic acid). TMP Treats Marrow Poorly. |

| **Fluoroquinolones** | Ciprofloxacin, ofloxacin; respiratory fluoroquinolones: levofloxacin, moxifloxacin. | |
| --- | --- | --- |
| MECHANISM | Inhibit prokaryotic enzymes topoisomerase II (DNA gyrase) and topoisomerase IV. Bactericidal. Concurrent ingestion of divalent cations (eg, dairy, antacids) markedly decreases oral absorption. | |
| CLINICAL USE | Gram ⊖ rods of urinary and GI tracts (including *Pseudomonas*), some gram ⊕ organisms, otitis externa, community-acquired pneumonia. | |
| ADVERSE EFFECTS | GI upset, superinfections, skin rashes, headache, dizziness. Less commonly, can cause leg cramps and myalgias. Contraindicated during pregnancy or breastfeeding and in children < 18 years old due to possible damage to cartilage. Some may prolong QT interval. | May cause tendonitis or tendon rupture in people > 60 years old and in patients taking prednisone. Ciprofloxacin inhibits cytochrome P-450. Fluoroquinolones hurt attachments to your bones. |
| MECHANISM OF RESISTANCE | Chromosome-encoded mutation in DNA gyrase, plasmid-mediated resistance, efflux pumps. | |

| **Daptomycin** | | |
| --- | --- | --- |
| MECHANISM | Lipopeptide that disrupts cell membranes of gram ⊕ cocci by creating transmembrane channels. | |
| CLINICAL USE | *S aureus* skin infections (especially MRSA), bacteremia, infective endocarditis, VRE. | Not used for pneumonia (avidly binds to and is inactivated by surfactant). "Dapto-myo-skin" is used for skin infections but can cause myopathy. |
| ADVERSE EFFECTS | Myopathy, rhabdomyolysis. | |

| **Metronidazole** | | |
| --- | --- | --- |
| MECHANISM | Forms toxic free radical metabolites in the bacterial cell that damage DNA. Bactericidal, antiprotozoal. | |
| CLINICAL USE | Treats *Giardia*, *Entamoeba*, *Trichomonas*, *Gardnerella vaginalis*, Anaerobes (*Bacteroides*, *C difficile*). Can be used in place of amoxicillin in *H pylori* "triple therapy" in case of penicillin allergy. | GET GAP on the Metro with metronidazole! Treats anaerobic infection **below** the diaphragm vs clindamycin (anaerobic infections **above** diaphragm). |
| ADVERSE EFFECTS | Disulfiram-like reaction (severe flushing, tachycardia, hypotension) with alcohol; headache, metallic taste. | |

## Antituberculous drugs

| DRUG | MECHANISM | ADVERSE EFFECTS | NOTES |
|---|---|---|---|
| **Rifamycins**<br>Rifampin, rifabutin, rifapentine | Inhibit DNA-dependent RNA polymerase → ↓ mRNA synthesis<br>Rifamycin resistance arises due to mutations in gene encoding RNA polymerase | Minor hepatotoxicity, drug interactions (CYP450 induction), red-orange discoloration of body fluids (nonhazardous adverse effect) | Rifabutin favored over rifampin in patients with HIV infection due to less CYP450 induction<br>Monotherapy rapidly leads to resistance |
| **Isoniazid** | Inhibits mycolic acid synthesis → ↓ cell wall synthesis<br>Bacterial catalase-peroxidase (encoded by *kat*G) is needed to convert INH to active form<br>INH resistance arises due to mutations in *kat*G | Vitamin $B_6$ deficiency (peripheral neuropathy, sideroblastic anemia), hepatotoxicity, drug interactions (CYP450 inhibition), drug-induced lupus<br>INH overdose can lead to seizures (often refractory to benzodiazepines) | Administer with pyridoxine (vitamin $B_6$)<br>INH Injures Neurons and Hepatocytes (↑ risk of hepatotoxicity with ↑ age and alcohol overuse)<br>Different INH half-lives in fast vs slow acetylators |
| **Pyrazinamide** | Mechanism uncertain | Hepatotoxicity, hyperuricemia | Works best at acidic pH (eg, in host phagolysosomes) |
| **Ethambutol** | Inhibits arabinosyltransferase → ↓ arabinogalactan synthesis → ↓ cell wall synthesis | Optic neuropathy (red-green color blindness or ↓ visual acuity, typically reversible) | Pronounce "eyethambutol" |

## Antimycobacterial therapy

| BACTERIUM | PROPHYLAXIS | TREATMENT |
| --- | --- | --- |
| *M tuberculosis* | Rifamycin-based regimen for 3–4 months | Rifampin, Isoniazid, Pyrazinamide, Ethambutol (**RIPE** for treatment) |
| *M avium–intracellulare* | Azithromycin, rifabutin | Azithromycin or clarithromycin + ethambutol Can add rifabutin or ciprofloxacin |
| *M leprae* | N/A | Long-term treatment with dapsone and rifampin for tuberculoid form Add clofazimine for lepromatous form |

## Antimicrobial prophylaxis

| CLINICAL SCENARIO | MEDICATION |
| --- | --- |
| Exposure to meningococcal infection | Ceftriaxone, ciprofloxacin, or rifampin |
| High risk for infective endocarditis and undergoing surgical or dental procedures | Amoxicillin |
| History of recurrent UTIs | TMP-SMX |
| Malaria prophylaxis for travelers | Atovaquone-proguanil, mefloquine, doxycycline, primaquine, or chloroquine (for areas with sensitive species) |
| Pregnant patients carrying group B strep | Intrapartum penicillin G or ampicillin |
| Prevention of gonococcal conjunctivitis in newborn | Erythromycin ointment on eyes |
| Prevention of postsurgical infection due to *S aureus* | Cefazolin; vancomycin if ⊕ for MRSA |
| Prophylaxis of strep pharyngitis in child with prior rheumatic fever | Benzathine penicillin G or oral penicillin V |

## Prophylaxis in HIV infection/AIDS

| CELL COUNT | PROPHYLAXIS | INFECTION |
| --- | --- | --- |
| CD4+ < 200 cells/mm$^3$ | TMP-SMX | *Pneumocystis* pneumonia |
| CD4+ < 100 cells/mm$^3$ | TMP-SMX | *Pneumocystis* pneumonia and toxoplasmosis |

## Antifungal therapy

## Amphotericin B

| | | |
|---|---|---|
| MECHANISM | Binds ergosterol (unique to fungi); forms membrane pores that allow leakage of electrolytes. | Amphotericin "tears" holes in the fungal membrane by forming pores. |
| CLINICAL USE | Serious, systemic mycoses. *Cryptococcus* (amphotericin B +/– flucytosine for cryptococcal meningitis), *Blastomyces, Coccidioides, Histoplasma, Candida, Mucor.* Intrathecally for coccidioidal meningitis. | Supplement $K^+$ and $Mg^{2+}$ because of altered renal tubule permeability. |
| ADVERSE EFFECTS | Fever/chills ("shake and bake"), hypotension, nephrotoxicity, arrhythmias, anemia, IV phlebitis ("**amphoterrible**"). | Hydration ↓ nephrotoxicity. Liposomal amphotericin ↓ toxicity. |

## Nystatin

| | |
|---|---|
| MECHANISM | Same as amphotericin B. Topical use only as too toxic for systemic use. |
| CLINICAL USE | "Swish and swallow" for oral candidiasis (thrush); topical for diaper rash or vaginal candidiasis. |

## Flucytosine

| | |
|---|---|
| MECHANISM | Inhibits DNA and RNA biosynthesis by conversion to 5-fluorouracil by cytosine deaminase. |
| CLINICAL USE | Systemic fungal infections (especially meningitis caused by *Cryptococcus*) in combination with amphotericin B. |
| ADVERSE EFFECTS | Myelosuppression. |

| **Azoles** | Clotrimazole, fluconazole, isavuconazole, itraconazole, ketoconazole, miconazole, voriconazole. |
|---|---|
| MECHANISM | Inhibit fungal sterol (ergosterol) synthesis by inhibiting the cytochrome P-450 enzyme that converts lanosterol to ergosterol. |
| CLINICAL USE | Local and less serious systemic mycoses. Fluconazole for chronic suppression of cryptococcal meningitis in people living with HIV and candidal infections of all types. Itraconazole may be used for *Blastomyces, Coccidioides, Histoplasma, Sporothrix schenckii*. Clotrimazole and miconazole for topical fungal infections. Voriconazole for *Aspergillus* and some *Candida*. Isavuconazole for serious *Aspergillus* and *Mucor* infections. |
| ADVERSE EFFECTS | Testosterone synthesis inhibition (gynecomastia, especially with ketoconazole), liver dysfunction (inhibits cytochrome P-450), QT interval prolongation. |

| **Terbinafine** | |
|---|---|
| MECHANISM | Inhibits the fungal enzyme squalene epoxidase. |
| CLINICAL USE | Dermatophytoses (especially onychomycosis—fungal infection of finger or toe nails). |
| ADVERSE EFFECTS | GI upset, headaches, hepatotoxicity, taste disturbance. |

| **Echinocandins** | Anidulafungin, caspofungin, micafungin. |
|---|---|
| MECHANISM | Inhibit cell wall synthesis by inhibiting synthesis of β-glucan. |
| CLINICAL USE | Invasive aspergillosis, *Candida*. |
| ADVERSE EFFECTS | GI upset, flushing (by histamine release). |

| **Griseofulvin** | |
|---|---|
| MECHANISM | Interferes with microtubule function; disrupts mitosis. Deposits in keratin-containing tissues (eg, nails). |
| CLINICAL USE | Oral treatment of superficial infections; inhibits growth of dermatophytes (tinea, ringworm). |
| ADVERSE EFFECTS | Teratogenic, carcinogenic, confusion, headaches, disulfiram-like reaction, ↑ cytochrome P-450 and warfarin metabolism. |

| **Antiprotozoal therapy** | Pyrimethamine-sulfadiazine (toxoplasmosis), suramin and melarsoprol (*Trypanosoma brucei*), nifurtimox (*T cruzi*), sodium stibogluconate (leishmaniasis). |
|---|---|

| **Anti-mite/louse therapy** | Permethrin, malathion (acetylcholinesterase inhibitor), topical or oral ivermectin. Used to treat scabies (*Sarcoptes scabiei*) and lice (*Pediculus* and *Pthirus*). |
|---|---|

| **Chloroquine** | |
|---|---|
| MECHANISM | Blocks detoxification of heme into hemozoin. Heme accumulates and is toxic to plasmodia. |
| CLINICAL USE | Treatment of plasmodial species other than *P falciparum* (due to drug resistance from membrane pump that ↓ intracellular concentration of drug). |
| ADVERSE EFFECTS | Retinopathy (dependent on cumulative dose); pruritus (especially in dark-skinned individuals). |

| **Antihelminthic therapy** | Pyrantel pamoate, ivermectin, mebendazole (treats "bendy worms" by disrupting microtubules and cellular motility), praziquantel ($\uparrow$ Ca$^{2+}$ permeability, $\uparrow$ vacuolization), diethylcarbamazine. |
|---|---|

### Oseltamivir, zanamivir

| MECHANISM | Inhibit influenza neuraminidase $\rightarrow$ $\downarrow$ release of progeny virus. |
|---|---|
| CLINICAL USE | Treatment and prevention of influenza A and B. Beginning therapy within 48 hours of symptom onset may shorten duration of illness. |

### Baloxavir

| MECHANISM | Inhibits the "cap snatching" (transfer of the 5′ cap from cell mRNA onto viral mRNA) endonuclease activity of the influenza virus RNA polymerase $\rightarrow$ $\downarrow$ viral replication. |
|---|---|
| CLINICAL USE | Treatment within 48 hours of symptom onset shortens duration of illness. |

### Remdesivir

| MECHANISM | Prodrug of an ATP analog. The active metabolite inhibits viral RNA-dependent RNA polymerase and evades proofreading by viral exoribonuclease (ExoN) $\rightarrow$ $\downarrow$ viral RNA production. |
|---|---|
| CLINICAL USE | Recently approved for treatment of COVID-19 requiring hospitalization. |

### Acyclovir, famciclovir, valacyclovir

| MECHANISM | Guanosine analogs. Monophosphorylated by HSV/VZV thymidine kinase and not phosphorylated in uninfected cells $\rightarrow$ few adverse effects. Triphosphate formed by cellular enzymes. Preferentially inhibit viral DNA polymerase by chain termination. |
|---|---|
| CLINICAL USE | No activity against CMV because CMV lacks the thymidine kinase necessary to activate guanosine analogs. Used for HSV-induced mucocutaneous and genital lesions as well as for encephalitis. Prophylaxis in patients who are immunocompromised. Also used as prophylaxis for immunocompetent patients with severe or recurrent infection. No effect on latent forms of HSV and VZV. Valacyclovir, a prodrug of acyclovir, has better oral bioavailability. For herpes zoster, use famciclovir. |
| ADVERSE EFFECTS | Obstructive crystalline nephropathy and acute kidney injury if not adequately hydrated. |
| MECHANISM OF RESISTANCE | Mutated viral thymidine kinase. |

### Ganciclovir

| MECHANISM | Guanosine analog. 5′-monophosphate formed by a CMV viral kinase. Triphosphate formed by cellular kinases. Preferentially inhibits viral DNA polymerase. |
|---|---|
| CLINICAL USE | CMV, especially in patients who are immunocompromised. Valganciclovir, a prodrug of ganciclovir, has better oral bioavailability. |
| ADVERSE EFFECTS | Myelosuppression (leukopenia, neutropenia, thrombocytopenia), renal toxicity. More toxic to host enzymes than acyclovir. |
| MECHANISM OF RESISTANCE | Mutated viral kinase. |

## Foscarnet

| | |
|---|---|
| MECHANISM | Viral DNA/RNA polymerase inhibitor and HIV reverse transcriptase inhibitor. Binds to pyrophosphate-binding site of enzyme. Does not require any kinase activation. Foscarnet = pyrofosphate analog. |
| CLINICAL USE | CMV retinitis in immunocompromised patients when ganciclovir fails; acyclovir-resistant HSV. |
| ADVERSE EFFECTS | Nephrotoxicity, multiple electrolyte abnormalities can lead to seizures. |
| MECHANISM OF RESISTANCE | Mutated DNA polymerase. |

## Cidofovir

| | |
|---|---|
| MECHANISM | Preferentially inhibits viral DNA polymerase. Does not require phosphorylation by viral kinase. |
| CLINICAL USE | CMV retinitis in immunocompromised patients. Long half-life. |
| ADVERSE EFFECTS | Nephrotoxicity (coadminister cidofovir with probenecid and IV saline to ↓ toxicity). |
| MECHANISM OF RESISTANCE | Mutations in the viral DNA polymerase gene. |

## HIV therapy

Antiretroviral therapy (ART): often initiated at the time of HIV diagnosis.

Strongest indication for use with patients presenting with AIDS-defining illness, low CD4+ cell counts (< 500 cells/mm$^3$), or high viral load. Regimen consists of 3 drugs to prevent resistance: 2 NRTIs and preferably an integrase inhibitor.

Most ARTs are active against both HIV-1 and HIV-2 (exceptions: NNRTIs and enfuvirtide not effective against HIV-2).

Tenofovir + emtricitabine can be administered as pre-exposure prophylaxis.

| DRUG | MECHANISM | ADVERSE EFFECTS |
|---|---|---|
| **NRTIs** | | |
| Abacavir (ABC) Emtricitabine (FTC) Lamivudine (3TC) Tenofovir (TDF) Zidovudine (ZDV, formerly AZT) | Competitively inhibit nucleotide binding to reverse transcriptase and terminate the DNA chain (lack a 3′ OH group). Tenofovir is a nucleoTide; the others are nucleosides. All need to be phosphorylated to be active. ZDV can be used for general prophylaxis and during pregnancy to ↓ risk of fetal transmission. Have you dined (**vudine**) with my **nuclear** (**nucleosides**) family? | Myelosuppression (can be reversed with granulocyte colony-stimulating factor [G-CSF] and erythropoietin), nephrotoxicity. Abacavir contraindicated if patient has HLA-B*5701 mutation due to ↑ risk of hypersensitivity. |
| **NNRTIs** | | |
| Doravirine Efavirenz Rilpivirine | Bind to reverse transcriptase at site different from NRTIs. Do not require phosphorylation to be active or compete with nucleotides. | Rash and hepatotoxicity are common to all NNRTIs. Vivid dreams and CNS symptoms are common with efavirenz. |
| **Integrase strand transfer inhibitors** | | |
| Bictegravir Dolutegravir | Also called integrase inhibitors. Inhibit HIV genome integration into host cell chromosome by reversibly inhibiting HIV integrase. | ↑ creatine kinase, weight gain. |

## HIV therapy (continued)

| DRUG | MECHANISM | ADVERSE EFFECTS |
|------|-----------|-----------------|
| **Protease inhibitors** | | |
| Atazanavir<br>Darunavir<br>Lopinavir<br>Ritonavir | Prevents maturation of new virions. Maturation depends on HIV-1 protease (*pol* gene), which cleaves the polypeptide products of HIV mRNA into their functional parts.<br>All protease inhibitors require boosting with either ritonavir or cobicistat.<br>**Navir** (never) tease a protease. | Hyperglycemia, GI intolerance (nausea, diarrhea).<br>Rifampin (potent CYP/UGT inducer) ↓ protease inhibitor concentrations; use rifabutin instead.<br>Ritonavir (cytochrome P-450 inhibitor) is only used as a boosting agent. |
| **Entry inhibitors** | | |
| Enfuvirtide | Binds gp41, inhibiting viral entry.<br>**Enfuvirtide** inhibits **fusion.** | Skin reaction at injection sites. |
| Maraviroc | Binds CCR-5 on surface of T cells/monocytes, inhibiting interaction with gp120.<br>**Maraviroc** inhibits **docking.** | |

[a] All protease inhibitors require boosting with either ritonavir (protease inhibitor only used as a boosting agent) or cobicistat (cytochrome P450 inhibitor).

**Hepatitis C therapy**  Chronic HCV infection treated with multidrug therapy that targets specific steps within HCV replication cycle (HCV-encoded proteins). Examples of drugs are provided.

| DRUG | MECHANISM | TOXICITY |
|---|---|---|
| **NS5A inhibitors** | | |
| Elbasvir Ledipasvir Pibrentasvir Velpatasvir | Inhibits NS5A, a viral phosphoprotein that plays a key role in RNA replication Exact mechanism unknown | Headache, diarrhea |
| **NS5B inhibitors** | | |
| Sofosbuvir | Inhibits NS5B, an RNA-dependent RNA polymerase acting as a chain terminator Prevents viral RNA replication | Fatigue, headache |
| **NS3/4A inhibitors** | | |
| Glecaprevir Grazoprevir | Inhibits NS3/4A, a viral protease, preventing viral replication | Headache, fatigue |
| **Alternative drugs** | | |
| Ribavirin | Inhibits synthesis of guanine nucleotides by competitively inhibiting IMP dehydrogenase | Hemolytic anemia, severe teratogen |

**Disinfection and sterilization**  Goals include the reduction of pathogenic organism counts to safe levels (disinfection) and the inactivation of all microbes including spores (sterilization).

| | |
|---|---|
| **Autoclave**[a] | Pressurized steam at > 120°C. May not reliably inactivate prions. |
| **Alcohols** | Denature proteins and disrupt cell membranes. |
| **Chlorhexidine** | Disrupts cell membranes and coagulates intracellular components. |
| **Chlorine**[a] | Oxidizes and denatures proteins. |
| **Ethylene oxide**[a] | Alkylating agent. |
| **Hydrogen peroxide**[a] | Free radical oxidation. |
| **Iodine and iodophors** | Halogenation of DNA, RNA, and proteins. May be sporicidal. |
| **Quaternary amines** | Impair permeability of cell membranes. |

[a]Sporicidal.

**Antimicrobials to avoid in pregnancy**

| ANTIMICROBIAL | ADVERSE EFFECT |
|---|---|
| Sulfonamides | Kernicterus |
| Aminoglycosides | Ototoxicity |
| Fluoroquinolones | Cartilage damage |
| Clarithromycin | Embryotoxic |
| Tetracyclines | Discolored teeth, inhibition of bone growth |
| Ribavirin | Teratogenic |
| Griseofulvin | Teratogenic |
| Chloramphenicol | Gray baby syndrome |

Safe children take really good care.

# Pathology

*"Digressions, objections, delight in mockery, carefree mistrust are signs of health; everything unconditional belongs in pathology."*

—Friedrich Nietzsche

*"You cannot separate passion from pathology any more than you can separate a person's spirit from his body."*

—Richard Selzer

*"My business is not prognosis, but diagnosis. I am not engaged in therapeutics, but in pathology."*

—H.L. Mencken

The fundamental principles of pathology are key to understanding diseases in all organ systems. Major topics such as inflammation and neoplasia appear frequently in questions across different organ systems, and such topics are definitely high yield. For example, the concepts of cell injury and inflammation are key to understanding the inflammatory response that follows myocardial infarction, a very common subject of board questions. Similarly, a familiarity with the early cellular changes that culminate in the development of neoplasias—for example, esophageal or colon cancer—is critical. Make sure you recognize the major tumor-associated genes and are comfortable with key cancer concepts such as tumor staging and metastasis. Finally, take some time to learn about the major systemic changes that come with aging, and how these physiologic alterations differ from disease states.

## ▶ PATHOLOGY—CELLULAR INJURY

| | |
|---|---|
| **Cellular adaptations** | Reversible changes that can be physiologic (eg, uterine enlargement during pregnancy) or pathologic (eg, myocardial hypertrophy 2° to systemic HTN). If stress is excessive or persistent, adaptations can progress to cell injury (eg, significant LV hypertrophy → myocardial injury → HF). |
| **Hypertrophy** | ↑ structural proteins and organelles → ↑ in size of cells. Example: cardiac hypertrophy. |
| **Hyperplasia** | Controlled proliferation of stem cells and differentiated cells → ↑ in number of cells (eg, benign prostatic hyperplasia). Excessive stimulation → pathologic hyperplasia (eg, endometrial hyperplasia), which may progress to dysplasia and cancer. |
| **Atrophy** | ↓ in tissue mass due to ↓ in size (↑ cytoskeleton degradation via ubiquitin-proteasome pathway and autophagy; ↓ protein synthesis) and/or number of cells (apoptosis). Causes include disuse, denervation, loss of blood supply, loss of hormonal stimulation, poor nutrition. |
| **Metaplasia** | Reprogramming of stem cells → replacement of one cell type by another that can adapt to a new stressor. Usually due to exposure to an irritant, such as gastric acid (→ esophageal epithelium replaced by intestinal epithelium, called Barrett esophagus) or tobacco smoke (→ respiratory ciliated columnar epithelium replaced by stratified squamous epithelium). May progress to dysplasia → malignant transformation with persistent insult (eg, Barrett esophagus → esophageal adenocarcinoma). Metaplasia of connective tissue can also occur (eg, myositis ossificans, the formation of bone within muscle after trauma). |
| **Dysplasia** | Disordered, precancerous epithelial cell growth; not considered a true adaptive response. Characterized by loss of uniformity of cell size and shape (pleomorphism); loss of tissue orientation; nuclear changes (eg, ↑ nuclear:cytoplasmic ratio and clumped chromatin). Mild and moderate dysplasias (ie, do not involve entire thickness of epithelium) may regress with alleviation of inciting cause. Severe dysplasia often becomes irreversible and progresses to carcinoma in situ. Usually preceded by persistent metaplasia or pathologic hyperplasia. |

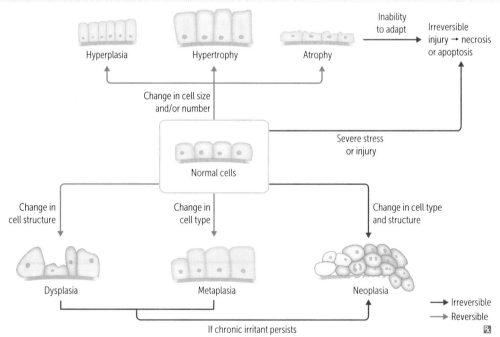

## Cell injury

| | |
|---|---|
| **Reversible cell injury** | ▪ ↓ ATP → ↓ activity of $Ca^{2+}$ and $Na^+/K^+$-ATPase pumps → cellular swelling (cytosol, mitochondria, endoplasmic reticulum/Golgi), which is the earliest morphologic manifestation<br>▪ Ribosomal/polysomal detachment → ↓ protein synthesis<br>▪ Plasma membrane changes (eg, blebbing)<br>▪ Nuclear changes (eg, chromatin clumping)<br>▪ Rapid loss of function (eg, myocardial cells are noncontractile after 1–2 minutes of ischemia)<br>▪ Myelin figures (aggregation of peroxidized lipids) |
| **Irreversible cell injury** | ▪ Breakdown of plasma membrane → cytosolic enzymes (eg, troponin) leak outside of cell, influx of $Ca^{2+}$ → activation of degradative enzymes<br>▪ Mitochondrial damage/dysfunction → loss of electron transport chain → ↓ ATP<br>▪ Rupture of lysosomes → autolysis<br>▪ Nuclear degradation: pyknosis (nuclear condensation) → karyorrhexis (nuclear fragmentation caused by endonuclease-mediated cleavage) → karyolysis (nuclear dissolution)<br>▪ Amorphous densities/inclusions in mitochondria |

| | |
|---|---|
| **Apoptosis** | ATP-dependent programmed cell death.<br>Intrinsic, extrinsic, and perforin/granzyme B pathways → activate caspases (cytosolic proteases) → cellular breakdown including cell shrinkage, chromatin condensation, membrane blebbing, and formation of apoptotic bodies, which are then phagocytosed.<br>Characterized by deeply eosinophilic cytoplasm and basophilic nucleus, pyknosis, and karyorrhexis.<br>Cell membrane typically remains intact without significant inflammation (unlike necrosis).<br>DNA laddering (fragments in multiples of 180 bp) is a sensitive indicator of apoptosis. |
| **Intrinsic (mitochondrial) pathway** | Involved in tissue remodeling in embryogenesis. Occurs when a regulating factor is withdrawn from a proliferating cell population (eg, ↓ IL-2 after a completed immunologic reaction → apoptosis of proliferating effector cells). Also occurs after exposure to injurious stimuli (eg, radiation, toxins, hypoxia).<br>Regulated by Bcl-2 family of proteins. **Ba**x and **Ba**k are proapoptotic (**Ba**d for survival), while **B**cl-2 and **B**cl-xL are antiapoptotic (**Be** clever, live).<br>BAX and BAK form pores in the mitochondrial membrane → release of cytochrome C from inner mitochondrial membrane into the cytoplasm → activation of caspases.<br>Bcl-2 keeps the mitochondrial membrane impermeable, thereby preventing cytochrome C release. Bcl-2 overexpression (eg, follicular lymphoma t[14;18]) → ↓ caspase activation → tumorigenesis. |
| **Extrinsic (death receptor) pathway** | Ligand receptor interactions: FasL binding to Fas (CD95) or TNF-α binding to its receptor.<br>Fas-FasL interaction is necessary in thymic medullary negative selection.<br>Autoimmune lymphoproliferative syndrome—caused by defective Fas-FasL interaction → failure of clonal deletion → ↑ numbers of self-reacting lymphocytes. Presents with lymphadenopathy, hepatosplenomegaly, autoimmune cytopenias. |
| **Perforin/granzyme B pathway** | Release of granules containing perforin and granzyme B by immune cells (cytotoxic T-cell and natural killer cell) → perforin forms a pore for granzyme B to enter the target cell. |

**Necrosis**    Exogenous injury → plasma membrane damage → intracellular components leak → cell undergoes enzymatic degradation and protein denaturation → local inflammatory reaction (unlike apoptosis).

| TYPE | SEEN IN | DUE TO | HISTOLOGY |
|------|---------|--------|-----------|
| **Coagulative** | Ischemia/infarcts in most tissues (except brain) | Ischemia or infarction; injury denatures enzymes → proteolysis blocked | Preserved cellular architecture (cell outlines seen), but nuclei disappear; ↑ cytoplasmic binding of eosin stain (→ ↑ eosinophilia; red/pink color) **A** |
| **Liquefactive** | Bacterial abscesses, CNS infarcts | Neutrophils release lysosomal enzymes that digest the tissue | Early: cellular debris and macrophages Late: cystic spaces and cavitation (CNS) **B** Neutrophils and cell debris seen with bacterial infection |
| **Caseous** | TB, systemic fungi (eg, *Histoplasma capsulatum*), *Nocardia* | Macrophages wall off the infecting microorganism → granular debris | Fragmented cells and debris surrounded by lymphocytes and macrophages (granuloma) Cheeselike gross appearance **C** |
| **Fat** | Enzymatic: acute pancreatitis (saponification of peripancreatic fat) Nonenzymatic: traumatic (eg, injury to breast tissue) | Damaged pancreatic cells release lipase, which breaks down triglycerides; liberated fatty acids bind calcium → saponification (chalky-white appearance) | Outlines of dead fat cells without peripheral nuclei; saponification of fat (combined with $Ca^{2+}$) appears dark blue on H&E stain **D** |
| **Fibrinoid** | Immune vascular reactions (eg, polyarteritis nodosa) Nonimmune vascular reactions (eg, hypertensive emergency, preeclampsia) | Immune complex deposition (type III hypersensitivity reaction) and/or plasma protein (eg, fibrin) leakage from damaged vessel | Vessel walls contain eosinophilic layer of proteinaceous material **E** |
| **Gangrenous** | Distal extremity and GI tract, after chronic ischemia | Dry: ischemia **F** | Coagulative |
| | | Wet: superinfection | Liquefactive superimposed on coagulative |

| | |
|---|---|
| **Ischemia**<br> | Inadequate blood supply to meet demand. Mechanisms include ↓ arterial perfusion (eg, atherosclerosis), ↓ venous drainage (eg, testicular torsion, Budd-Chiari syndrome), shock. Regions most vulnerable to hypoxia/ischemia and subsequent infarction: |

| ORGAN | SUSCEPTIBLE REGION |
|---|---|
| Brain | ACA/MCA/PCA boundary areas[a,b] |
| Heart | Subendocardium of LV (yellow lines in  outline a subendocardial infarction) |
| Kidney | Straight segment of proximal tubule (medulla)<br>Thick ascending limb (medulla) |
| Liver | Area around central vein (zone III) |
| Colon | Splenic flexure (Griffith point),[a] rectosigmoid junction (Sudeck point)[a] |

[a]Watershed areas (border zones) receive blood supply from most distal branches of 2 arteries with limited collateral vascularity. These areas are susceptible to ischemia from hypoperfusion.
[b]Neurons most vulnerable to hypoxic-ischemic insults include Purkinje cells of the cerebellum and pyramidal cells of the hippocampus and neocortex (layers 3, 5, 6).

## Types of infarcts

| | | |
|---|---|---|
| **Red infarct** | Occurs in venous occlusion and tissues with multiple blood supplies (eg, liver, lung , intestine, testes), and with reperfusion (eg, after angioplasty). **R**eperfusion injury is due to damage by free radicals. |  |
| **Pale infarct** | Occurs in solid organs with a single (end-arterial) blood supply (eg, heart **B**, kidney). | |

| | |
|---|---|
| **Free radical injury** | Free radicals damage cells via membrane lipid peroxidation, protein modification, DNA breakage. Initiated via radiation exposure (eg, cancer therapy), metabolism of drugs (phase I), redox reactions, nitric oxide (eg, inflammation), transition metals (eg, iron, copper; form free radicals via Fenton reaction), WBC (eg, neutrophils, macrophages) oxidative burst.<br>Free radicals can be eliminated by scavenging enzymes (eg, catalase, superoxide dismutase, glutathione peroxidase), spontaneous decay, antioxidants (eg, vitamins A, C, E), and certain metal carrier proteins (eg, transferrin, ceruloplasmin).<br>Examples:<br>• Oxygen toxicity: retinopathy of prematurity (abnormal vascularization), bronchopulmonary dysplasia, reperfusion injury after thrombolytic therapy<br>• Drug/chemical toxicity: acetaminophen overdose (hepatotoxicity), carbon tetrachloride (converted by cytochrome P-450 into $CCl_3$ free radical → fatty liver [cell injury → ↓ apolipoprotein synthesis → fatty change], centrilobular necrosis)<br>• Metal storage diseases: hemochromatosis (iron) and Wilson disease (copper) |

| | | |
|---|---|---|
| **Ionizing radiation toxicity** | Ionizing radiation causes DNA (eg, double strand breaks) and cellular damage both directly and indirectly through the production of free radicals. Complications usually arise when patient is exposed to significant doses (eg, radiotherapy, nuclear reactor accidents):<br>▪ Localized inflammation and fibrosis<br>▪ Neoplasia (eg, leukemia, thyroid cancer)<br>Acute radiation syndrome—develops after sudden whole-body exposure to high doses of ionizing radiation → nausea, vomiting, diarrhea, hair loss, erythema, cytopenias, headache, altered mental status. | Stem cells of rapidly regenerating tissues (eg, skin, bone marrow, GI tract, gonads) are the most susceptible to radiation injury. Radiotherapy damages cancer cells more than healthy cells because cancer cells have dysfunctional DNA repair mechanisms in addition to high replicative rates. |

**Types of calcification** — Calcium deposits appear deeply basophilic (arrow in **A**) on H&E stain.

| | Dystrophic calcification | Metastatic calcification |
|---|---|---|
| $Ca^{2+}$ DEPOSITION | In abnormal (diseased) tissues | In normal tissues |
| EXTENT | Tends to be localized (eg, calcific aortic stenosis) | Widespread (ie, diffuse, metastatic) |
| ASSOCIATED CONDITIONS | TB (lung and pericardium) and other granulomatous infections, liquefactive necrosis of chronic abscesses, fat necrosis, infarcts, thrombi, schistosomiasis, congenital CMV, toxoplasmosis, rubella, psammoma bodies, CREST syndrome, atherosclerotic plaques can become calcified | Predominantly in interstitial tissues of kidney, lung, and gastric mucosa (these tissues lose acid quickly; ↑ pH favors $Ca^{2+}$ deposition)<br>Nephrocalcinosis of collecting ducts may lead to nephrogenic diabetes insipidus and renal failure |
| ETIOLOGY | 2° to injury or necrosis | 2° to hyperphosphatemia (eg, chronic kidney disease) or hypercalcemia (eg, 1° hyperparathyroidism, sarcoidosis, hypervitaminosis D) |

| | | |
|---|---|---|
| **Psammoma bodies**<br> | Concentrically laminated calcified spherules **A**. Usually seen in certain types of tumors:<br>▪ Papillary thyroid carcinoma<br>▪ Meningioma<br>▪ Serous Ovarian carcinoma<br>▪ Mesothelioma<br>▪ Prolactinoma (Milk) | Please, MOM, don't forget the Milk! |

| Amyloidosis | Extracellular deposition of protein in abnormal fibrillar form (β-pleated sheet configuration) → cell injury and apoptosis. Manifestations vary depending on involved organ and include:<br>▪ Renal—nephrotic syndrome.<br>▪ Cardiac—restrictive cardiomyopathy.<br>▪ GI—hepatosplenomegaly.<br>▪ Neurologic—peripheral neuropathy.<br>▪ Musculoskeletal—muscle enlargement (eg, macroglossia), carpal tunnel syndrome.<br>▪ Skin—waxy thickening, easy bruising. | Amyloid deposits are visualized by Congo red stain (red/orange on nonpolarized light **A**, apple-green birefringence on polarized light **B**), and H&E stain (amorphous pink).<br> |

| COMMON TYPES | FIBRIL PROTEIN | NOTES |
| --- | --- | --- |
| **Systemic** | | |
| **Primary amyloidosis** | AL (from Ig Light chains) | Seen in plasma cell dyscrasias (eg, multiple myeloma) |
| **Secondary amyloidosis** | AA (serum Amyloid A) | Seen in chronic inflammatory conditions, (eg, rheumatoid arthritis, IBD, familial Mediterranean fever, protracted infection) |
| **Transthyretin amyloidosis** | Transthyretin | Sporadic (wild-type *TTR*)—slowly progressive, associated with aging; mainly affects the heart<br>Hereditary (mutated *TTR*)—familial amyloid polyneuropathy and/or cardiomyopathy |
| **Dialysis-related amyloidosis** | $\beta_2$-microglobulin | Seen in patients with ESRD on long-term dialysis |
| **Localized** | | |
| **Alzheimer disease** | β-amyloid protein | Cleaved from amyloid precursor protein |
| **Isolated atrial amyloidosis** | ANP | Common, associated with aging; ↑ risk for atrial fibrillation |
| **Type 2 diabetes mellitus** | Islet amyloid polypeptide | Caused by deposition of amylin in pancreatic islets |
| **Medullary thyroid cancer** | Calcitonin | Secreted from tumor cells |

## ▶ PATHOLOGY—INFLAMMATION

| | |
|---|---|
| **Inflammation** | Response to eliminate initial cause of cell injury, to remove necrotic cells resulting from the original insult, and to initiate tissue repair. Divided into acute and chronic. The inflammatory response itself can be harmful to the host if the reaction is excessive (eg, septic shock), prolonged (eg, persistent infections such as TB), or inappropriate (eg, autoimmune diseases such as SLE). |

| SIGN | MECHANISM |
|---|---|
| **Cardinal signs** | |
| **Rubor and calor** | Redness and warmth. Vasodilation (relaxation of arteriolar smooth muscle) → ↑ blood flow. Mediated by histamine, prostaglandins, bradykinin, NO. |
| **Tumor** | Swelling. Endothelial contraction/disruption (eg, from tissue damage) → ↑ vascular permeability → leakage of protein-rich fluid from postcapillary venules into interstitial space (exudate) → ↑ interstitial oncotic pressure. Endothelial cell contraction is mediated by leukotrienes ($C_4$, $D_4$, $E_4$), histamine, serotonin, bradykinin. |
| **Dolor** | Pain. Sensitization of sensory nerve endings. Mediated by bradykinin, $PGE_2$, histamine. |
| **Functio laesa** | Loss of function. Inflammation impairs function (eg, inability to make fist due to hand cellulitis). |
| **Systemic manifestations (acute-phase reaction)** | |
| **Fever** | Pyrogens (eg, LPS) induce macrophages to release IL-1 and TNF → ↑ COX activity in perivascular cells of anterior hypothalamus → ↑ $PGE_2$ → ↑ temperature set point. |
| **Leukocytosis** | ↑ WBC count; type of predominant cell depends on inciting agent or injury (eg, bacteria → ↑ neutrophils). |
| **↑ plasma acute-phase reactants** | Serum concentrations significantly change in response to acute and chronic inflammation. Produced by liver. Notably induced by IL-6. |

## Acute phase reactants

| POSITIVE (UPREGULATED) | |
|---|---|
| **C-reactive protein** | Opsonin; fixes complement and facilitates phagocytosis. Measured clinically as a nonspecific sign of ongoing inflammation. |
| **Ferritin** | Binds and sequesters iron to inhibit microbial iron scavenging. |
| **Fibrinogen** | Coagulation factor; promotes endothelial repair; correlates with ESR. |
| **Haptoglobin** | Binds extracellular hemoglobin, protects against oxidative stress. |
| **Hepcidin** | ↓ iron absorption (by degrading ferroportin) and ↓ iron release (from macrophages) → anemia of chronic disease. |
| **Procalcitonin** | Increases in bacterial infections; normal in viral infections. |
| **Serum amyloid A** | Prolonged elevation can lead to secondary amyloidosis. |
| NEGATIVE (DOWNREGULATED) | |
| **Albumin** | Reduction conserves amino acids for positive reactants. |
| **Transferrin** | Internalized by macrophages to sequester iron. |
| **Transthyretin** | Also called prealbumin. Reduction conserves amino acids for positive reactants. |

| **Erythrocyte sedimentation rate** | RBCs normally remain separated via ⊖ charges. Products of inflammation (eg, fibrinogen) coat RBCs → ↓ ⊖ charge → ↑ RBC aggregation. Denser RBC aggregates fall at a faster rate within a pipette tube → ↑ ESR. Often co-tested with CRP (more specific marker of inflammation). | |
|---|---|---|

| ↑ ESR | ↓ ESR[a] |
|---|---|
| Most anemias | Sickle cell anemia (altered shape) |
| Infections | Polycythemia (↑ RBCs "dilute" aggregation |
| Inflammation (eg, giant cell [temporal] arteritis, polymyalgia rheumatica) | factors) |
| | HF |
| Cancer (eg, metastases, multiple myeloma) | Microcytosis |
| Renal disease (end-stage or nephrotic syndrome) | Hypofibrinogenemia |
| Pregnancy | |

[a]Lower than expected.

| **Acute inflammation** | Transient and early response to injury or infection. Characterized by neutrophils in tissue , often with associated edema. Rapid onset (seconds to minutes) and short duration (minutes to days). Represents a reaction of the innate immune system (ie, less specific response than chronic inflammation). | |
|---|---|---|

| STIMULI | Infections, trauma, necrosis, foreign bodies. | |
|---|---|---|
| MEDIATORS | Toll-like receptors, arachidonic acid metabolites, neutrophils, eosinophils, antibodies (pre-existing), mast cells, basophils, complement, Hageman factor (factor XII). | Inflammasome—Cytoplasmic protein complex that recognizes products of dead cells, microbial products, and crystals (eg, uric acid crystals) → activation of IL-1 and inflammatory response. |
| COMPONENTS | ▪ Vascular: vasodilation (→ ↑ blood flow and stasis) and ↑ endothelial permeability (contraction of endothelial cells opens interendothelial junctions)<br>▪ Cellular: extravasation of leukocytes (mainly neutrophils) from postcapillary venules → accumulation of leukocytes in focus of injury → leukocyte activation | To bring cells and proteins to site of injury or infection.<br><br>Leukocyte extravasation has 4 steps: margination and rolling, adhesion, transmigration, and migration (chemoattraction). |
| OUTCOMES | ▪ Resolution and healing (IL-10, TGF-β)<br>▪ Persistent acute inflammation (IL-8)<br>▪ Abscess (acute inflammation walled off by fibrosis)<br>▪ Chronic inflammation (antigen presentation by macrophages and other APCs → activation of CD4+ Th cells)<br>▪ Scarring | Macrophages predominate in the late stages of acute inflammation (peak 2–3 days after onset) and influence outcome by secreting cytokines. |

**Leukocyte extravasation**

Extravasation predominantly occurs at postcapillary venules.

| STEP | VASCULATURE/STROMA | LEUKOCYTE |
|---|---|---|
| ❶ Margination and rolling—defective in leukocyte adhesion deficiency type 2 (↓ Sialyl Lewis$^X$) | E-selectin (upregulated by TNF and IL-1) | Sialyl Lewis$^X$ |
| | P-selectin (released from Weibel-Palade bodies) | Sialyl Lewis$^X$ |
| | GlyCAM-1, CD34 | L-selectin |
| ❷ Tight binding (adhesion)—defective in leukocyte adhesion deficiency type 1 (↓ CD18 integrin subunit) | ICAM-1 (CD54) | CD11/18 integrins (LFA-1, Mac-1) |
| | VCAM-1 (CD106) | VLA-4 integrin |
| ❸ DiaPEdesis (transmigration)—WBC travels between endothelial cells and exits blood vessel | PECAM-1 (CD31) | PECAM-1 (CD31) |
| ❹ Migration—WBC travels through interstitium to site of injury or infection guided by chemotactic signals | Chemotactic factors: C5a, IL-8, LTB$_4$, 5-HETE, kallikrein, platelet-activating factor, N-formylmethionyl peptides | Various |

| | |
|---|---|
| **Chronic inflammation** | Prolonged inflammation characterized by mononuclear infiltration (macrophages, lymphocytes, plasma cells), which leads to simultaneous tissue destruction and repair (including angiogenesis and fibrosis). May be preceded by acute inflammation. |
| STIMULI | Persistent infections (eg, TB, *T pallidum*, certain fungi and viruses) → type IV hypersensitivity, autoimmune diseases, prolonged exposure to toxic agents (eg, silica) and foreign material. |
| MEDIATORS | Macrophages are the dominant cells. Interaction of macrophages and T cells → chronic inflammation. <br> ▪ Th1 cells secrete IFN-γ → macrophage classical activation (proinflammatory) <br> ▪ Th2 cells secrete IL-4 and IL-13 → macrophage alternative activation (repair and anti-inflammatory) |
| OUTCOMES | Scarring, amyloidosis, and neoplastic transformation (eg, chronic HCV infection → chronic inflammation → hepatocellular carcinoma; *Helicobacter pylori* infection → chronic gastritis → gastric adenocarcinoma). |

## Wound healing

| **Tissue mediators** | MEDIATOR | ROLE |
|---|---|---|
| | FGF | Stimulates angiogenesis |
| | TGF-β | Angiogenesis, fibrosis |
| | VEGF | Stimulates angiogenesis |
| | PDGF | Secreted by activated platelets and macrophages <br> Induces vascular remodeling and smooth muscle cell migration <br> Stimulates fibroblast growth for collagen synthesis |
| | Metalloproteinases | Tissue remodeling |
| | EGF | Stimulates cell growth via tyrosine kinases (eg, EGFR/*ErbB1*) |

| PHASE OF WOUND HEALING | EFFECTOR CELLS | CHARACTERISTICS |
|---|---|---|
| **Inflammatory (up to 3 days after wound)** | Platelets, neutrophils, macrophages | Clot formation, ↑ vessel permeability and neutrophil migration into tissue; macrophages clear debris 2 days later |
| **Proliferative (day 3–weeks after wound)** | Fibroblasts, myofibroblasts, endothelial cells, keratinocytes, macrophages | Deposition of granulation tissue and type III collagen, angiogenesis, epithelial cell proliferation, dissolution of clot, and wound contraction (mediated by myofibroblasts) <br> Delayed second phase of wound healing in vitamin C and copper deficiency |
| **Remodeling (1 week–6+ months after wound)** | Fibroblasts | Type III collagen replaced by type I collagen, ↑ tensile strength of tissue <br> Collagenases (require zinc to function) break down type III collagen <br> Zinc deficiency → delayed wound healing |

| **Granulomatous inflammation** | A pattern of chronic inflammation. Can be induced by persistent T-cell response to certain infections (eg, TB), immune-mediated diseases, and foreign bodies. Granulomas "wall off" a resistant stimulus without completely eradicating or degrading it → persistent inflammation → fibrosis, organ damage. |

| HISTOLOGY | Focus of epithelioid cells (activated macrophages with abundant pink cytoplasm) surrounded by lymphocytes and multinucleated giant cells (formed by fusion of several activated macrophages). Two types:<br>Caseating: associated with central necrosis . Seen with infectious etiologies (eg, TB, fungal).<br>Noncaseating: no central necrosis. Seen with noninfectious etiologies (eg, sarcoidosis, Crohn disease). |

| MECHANISM | ❶ APCs present antigens to CD4+ Th cells and secrete IL-12 → CD4+ Th cells differentiate into Th1 cells<br>❷ Th1 secretes IFN-γ → macrophage activation<br>❸ Macrophages ↑ cytokine secretion (eg, TNF) → formation of epithelioid macrophages and giant cells<br>Anti-TNF therapy can cause sequestering granulomas to break down → disseminated disease. Always test for latent TB before starting anti-TNF therapy.<br>Associated with hypercalcemia due to ↑ 1α-hydroxylase activity in activated macrophages, resulting in ↑ vitamin D activity. |

| ETIOLOGIES | Infectious | Noninfectious |
|---|---|---|
| | Bacterial: *Mycobacteria* (tuberculosis, leprosy), *Bartonella henselae* (cat scratch disease; stellate necrotizing granulomas), *Listeria monocytogenes* (granulomatosis infantiseptica), *Treponema pallidum* (3° syphilis)<br>Fungal: endemic mycoses (eg, histoplasmosis)<br>Parasitic: schistosomiasis<br>Catalase ⊕ organisms in chronic granulomatous disease | Immune-mediated: sarcoidosis, Crohn disease, 1° biliary cholangitis, subacute (de Quervain/granulomatous) thyroiditis<br>Vasculitis: granulomatosis with polyangiitis, eosinophilic granulomatosis with polyangiitis, giant cell (temporal) arteritis, Takayasu arteritis<br>Foreign bodies: berylliosis, talcosis, hypersensitivity pneumonitis |

**Scar formation**

Occurs when repair cannot be accomplished by cell regeneration alone. Nonregenerated cells (2° to severe acute or chronic injury) are replaced by connective tissue. 70–80% of tensile strength regained at 3 months; little tensile strength regained thereafter. Excess TGF-β is associated with aberrant scarring, such as hypertrophic and keloid scars.

| | Hypertrophic scar A | Keloid scar B |
|---|---|---|
| COLLAGEN SYNTHESIS | ↑ (type III collagen) | ↑↑↑ (types I and III collagen) |
| COLLAGEN ORGANIZATION | Parallel | Disorganized |
| EXTENT OF SCAR | Confined to borders of original wound | Extends beyond borders of original wound with "clawlike" projections typically on earlobes, face, upper extremities |
| RECURRENCE | Infrequent | Frequent |
| PREDISPOSITION | None | ↑ incidence in people with darker skin |

## ▶ PATHOLOGY—NEOPLASIA

| | |
|---|---|
| **Neoplasia and neoplastic progression** | Uncontrolled, monoclonal proliferation of cells. Can be benign or malignant. Any neoplastic growth has two components: parenchyma (neoplastic cells) and supporting stroma (non-neoplastic; eg, blood vessels, connective tissue). |

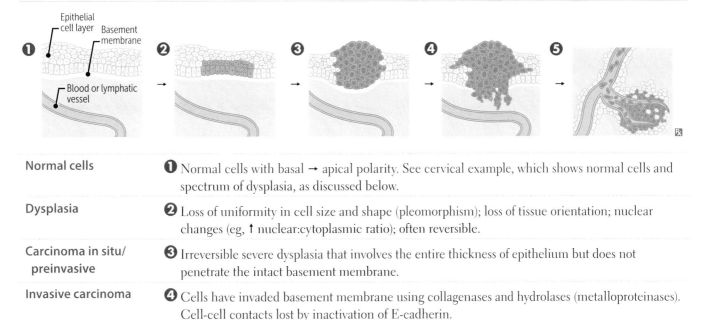

| | |
|---|---|
| **Normal cells** | ❶ Normal cells with basal → apical polarity. See cervical example, which shows normal cells and spectrum of dysplasia, as discussed below. |
| **Dysplasia** | ❷ Loss of uniformity in cell size and shape (pleomorphism); loss of tissue orientation; nuclear changes (eg, ↑ nuclear:cytoplasmic ratio); often reversible. |
| **Carcinoma in situ/ preinvasive** | ❸ Irreversible severe dysplasia that involves the entire thickness of epithelium but does not penetrate the intact basement membrane. |
| **Invasive carcinoma** | ❹ Cells have invaded basement membrane using collagenases and hydrolases (metalloproteinases). Cell-cell contacts lost by inactivation of E-cadherin. |
| **Metastasis** | ❺ Spread to distant organ(s) via lymphatics or blood. |

**Tumor nomenclature**

**Carcinoma** implies epithelial origin, whereas **sarcoma** denotes mesenchymal origin. Both terms generally imply malignancy.

**Benign** tumors are usually well-differentiated and well-demarcated, with low mitotic activity, no metastases, and no necrosis.

**Malignant** tumors (cancers) may show poor differentiation, erratic growth, local invasion, metastasis, and ↓ apoptosis.

Terms for non-neoplastic malformations include hamartoma (disorganized overgrowth of tissues in their native location, eg, Peutz-Jeghers polyps) and choristoma (normal tissue in a foreign location, eg, gastric tissue located in distal ileum in Meckel diverticulum).

| CELL TYPE | BENIGN | MALIGNANT |
|---|---|---|
| Epithelium | Adenoma, papilloma | Adenocarcinoma, papillary carcinoma |
| Mesenchyme | | |
| Blood cells | | Leukemia, lymphoma |
| Blood vessels | Hemangioma | Angiosarcoma |
| Smooth muscle | Leiomyoma | Leiomyosarcoma |
| Striated muscle | Rhabdomyoma | Rhabdomyosarcoma |
| Connective tissue | Fibroma | Fibrosarcoma |
| Bone | Osteoma | Osteosarcoma |
| Fat | Lipoma | Liposarcoma |
| Melanocyte | Nevus/mole | Melanoma |

**Tumor grade vs stage**

| | | |
|---|---|---|
| Grade | Degree of cell differentiation (tissue of origin resemblance) and mitotic activity on histology. Ranges from low-grade (well differentiated) to high-grade (poorly differentiated or undifferentiated [anaplastic]). Higher grade often correlates with higher aggressiveness. |   Low grade    High grade 🅁 |
| Stage | Degree of invasion and spread from initial site. Based on clinical (c) or pathologic (p) findings. **TNM** staging system (importance: M > N > T):<br> ▪ Primary tumor size/invasion.<br> ▪ Regional lymph node metastasis.<br> ▪ Distant metastasis.<br>Stage generally has more prognostic value than grade (eg, a high-stage yet low-grade tumor is usually worse than a low-stage yet high-grade tumor). Stage (spread) determines survival. | 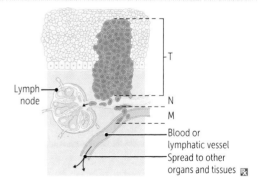 |

| Hallmarks of cancer | Cancer is caused by (mostly acquired) DNA mutations that affect fundamental cellular processes (eg, growth, DNA repair, survival). |
|---|---|

| HALLMARK | MECHANISM |
|---|---|
| Growth signal self-sufficiency | Mutations in genes encoding:<br>▪ Proto-oncogenes → ↑ growth factors → autocrine loop (eg, ↑ PDGF in brain tumors)<br>▪ Growth factor receptors → constitutive signaling (eg, *HER2* in breast cancer)<br>▪ Signaling molecules (eg, *RAS*)<br>▪ Transcription factors (eg, *MYC*)<br>▪ Cell cycle regulators (eg, cyclins, CDKs) |
| Anti-growth signal insensitivity | ▪ Mutations in tumor suppressor genes (eg, *Rb*)<br>▪ Loss of E-cadherin function → loss of contact inhibition (eg, *NF2* mutations) |
| Evasion of apoptosis | Mutations in genes that regulate apoptosis (eg, *TP53*, *BCL2* → follicular B cell lymphoma). |
| Limitless replicative potential | Reactivation of telomerase → maintenance and lengthening of telomeres → prevention of chromosome shortening and cell aging. |
| Sustained angiogenesis | ↑ pro-angiogenic factors (eg, VEGF) or ↓ inhibitory factors. Factors may be produced by tumor or stromal cells. Vessels can sprout from existing capillaries (neoangiogenesis) or endothelial cells are recruited from bone marrow (vasculogenesis). Vessels may be leaky and/or dilated. |
| Warburg effect | Shift of glucose metabolism away from mitochondrial oxidative phosphorylation toward glycolysis, even in the presence of oxygen. Aerobic glycolysis provides rapidly dividing cancer cells with the carbon needed for synthesis of cellular structures. |
| Immune evasion in cancer | Normally, immune cells can recognize and attack tumor cells. For successful tumorigenesis, tumor cells must evade the immune system. Multiple escape mechanisms exist:<br>▪ ↓ MHC class I expression by tumor cells → cytotoxic T cells are unable to recognize tumor cells.<br>▪ Tumor cells secrete immunosuppressive factors (eg, TGF-β) and recruit regulatory T cells to down regulate immune response.<br>▪ Tumor cells up regulate immune checkpoint molecules, which inhibit immune response. |
| Tissue invasion | Loss of E-cadherin function → loosening of intercellular junctions → metalloproteinases degrade basement membrane and ECM → cells attach to ECM proteins (eg, laminin, fibronectin) → cells migrate through degraded ECM ("locomotion") → vascular dissemination. |
| Metastasis | Tumor cells or emboli spread via lymphatics or blood → adhesion to endothelium → extravasation and homing. Site of metastasis can be predicted by site of 1° tumor, as the target organ is often the first-encountered capillary bed. Some cancers show organ tropism (eg, lung cancers commonly metastasize to adrenals). |

**Immune checkpoint interactions**

Signals that modulate T-cell activation and function → ↓ immune response against tumor cells. Targeted by several cancer immunotherapies. Examples:

- Interaction between PD-1 (on T cells) and PD-L1/2 (on tumor cells or immune cells in tumor microenvironment) → T-cell dysfunction (exhaustion). Inhibited by antibodies against PD-1 (eg, cemiplimab, nivolumab, pembrolizumab) or PD-L1 (eg, atezolizumab, durvalumab, avelumab).
- CTLA-4 on T cells outcompetes CD28 for B7 on APCs → loss of T-cell costimulatory signal. Inhibited by antibodies against CTLA-4 (eg, ipilimumab).

**Cancer epidemiology**

Skin cancer (basal > squamous >> melanoma) is the most common cancer (not included below).

| | MALES | FEMALES | CHILDREN (AGE 0–14) | NOTES |
|---|---|---|---|---|
| **Cancer incidence** | 1. Prostate<br>2. Lung<br>3. Colon/rectum | 1. Breast<br>2. Lung<br>3. Colon/rectum | 1. Leukemia<br>2. CNS<br>3. Neuroblastoma | Lung cancer incidence has ↓ in males, but has not changed significantly in females. |
| **Cancer mortality** | 1. Lung<br>2. Prostate<br>3. Colon/rectum | 1. Lung<br>2. Breast<br>3. Colon/rectum | 1. Leukemia<br>2. CNS<br>3. Neuroblastoma | Cancer is the 2nd leading cause of death in the United States (heart disease is 1st). |

| **Common metastases** | Most Carcinomas spread via Lymphatics; most Sarcomas spread Hematogenously (CLaSH). However, four carcinomas route hematogenously: follicular thyroid carcinoma, choriocarcinoma, renal cell carcinoma, and hepatocellular carcinoma. Metastasis to bone, liver, lung, and brain is more common than 1° malignancy in these organs. Metastases often appear as multiple lesions (vs 1° tumors which generally appear as solitary lesions). |
|---|---|

| SITE OF METASTASIS | 1° TUMOR | NOTES |
|---|---|---|
| **Bone** | Prostate, breast >> lung > kidney, colon | Predilection for axial skeleton<br>Bone metastasis can be:<br>  ▪ Blastic (eg, prostate, small cell lung cancer)<br>  ▪ Mixed (eg, breast)<br>  ▪ Lytic (eg, kidney, colon, non-small cell lung cancer) |
| **Liver** | Colon > breast >> pancreas, lung, prostate | Scattered throughout liver parenchyma |
| **Lung** | Colon, breast >> kidney, prostate | Typically involve both lungs |
| **Brain** | Lung > breast >> melanoma > colon, prostate | Usually seen at gray/white matter junction |

## Oncogenes

Gain of function mutation converts proto-oncogene (normal gene) to oncogene → ↑ cancer risk. Requires damage to only one allele of a proto-oncogene.

| GENE | GENE PRODUCT | ASSOCIATED NEOPLASM |
|---|---|---|
| ALK | Receptor tyrosine kinase | Lung adenocarcinoma |
| EGFR (ERBB1) | Receptor tyrosine kinase | Lung adenocarcinoma |
| HER2 (ERBB2) | Receptor tyrosine kinase | Breast and gastric carcinomas |
| RET | REceptor Tyrosine kinase | MEN2A and 2B, medullary and papillary thyroid carcinoma, pheochromocytoma |
| BCR-ABL | Non-receptor tyrosine kinase | CML, ALL |
| JAK2 | Non-receptor tyrosine kinase | Myeloproliferative neoplasms |
| BRAF | Serine/threonine kinase | Melanoma, non-Hodgkin lymphoma, colorectal carcinoma, papillary thyroid carcinoma, hairy cell leukemia |
| c-KIT | CytoKIne receptor (CD117) | Gastrointestinal stromal tumor (GIST), mastocytosis |
| MYCC (c-myc) | Transcription factor | Burkitt lymphoma |
| MYCN (N-myc) | Transcription factor | Neuroblastoma |
| KRAS | RAS GTPase | Pancreatic, colorectal, lung, endometrial cancers |
| BCL-2 | Antiapoptotic molecule (inhibits apoptosis) | Follicular and diffuse large B-Cell Lymphomas |

## Tumor suppressor genes

Loss of function → ↑ cancer risk; both (two) alleles of a tumor suppressor gene must be lost for expression of disease (the Knudson 2-hit hypothesis).

| GENE | GENE PRODUCT | ASSOCIATED CONDITION |
|---|---|---|
| APC | Negative regulator of β-catenin/WNT pathway | Colorectal cancer (associated with FAP) |
| BRCA1/BRCA2 | BRCA1/BRCA2 proteins | BReast, ovarian, prostate, pancreatic CAncers |
| CDKN2A | p16, blocks $G_1$ → S phase | Many cancers (eg, melanoma, lung, pancreatic) |
| DCC | DCC—Deleted in Colorectal Cancer | Colorectal cancer |
| SMAD4 (DPC4) | DPC—Deleted in Pancreatic Cancer | Pancreatic cancer, colorectal cancer |
| MEN1 | MENin | Multiple Endocrine Neoplasia type 1 |
| NF1 | Neurofibromin (Ras GTPase activating protein) | NeuroFibromatosis type 1 |
| NF2 | Merlin (schwannomin) protein | NeuroFibromatosis type 2 |
| PTEN | Negative regulator of PI3k/AKT pathway | Prostate, breasT, and ENdometrial cancers |
| RB1 | Inhibits E2F; blocks $G_1$ → S phase | Retinoblastoma, osteosarcoma (Bone cancer) |
| TP53 | p53, activates p21, blocks $G_1$ → S phase | Most cancers, Li-Fraumeni (SBLA) syndrome (multiple malignancies at early age; Sarcoma, Breast/Brain, Lung/Leukemia, Adrenal gland) |
| TSC1 | Hamartin protein | Tuberous sclerosis complex |
| TSC2 | Tuberin ("2berin") | Tuberous sclerosis complex |
| VHL | Inhibits hypoxia-inducible factor 1a | von Hippel-Lindau disease |
| WT1 | Urogenital development transcription factor | Wilms Tumor (nephroblastoma) |

## Carcinogens

| TOXIN | EXPOSURE | ORGAN | IMPACT |
|---|---|---|---|
| Aflatoxins (*Aspergillus*) | Stored grains and nuts | Liver | Hepatocellular carcinoma |
| Alkylating agents | Oncologic chemotherapy | Blood | Leukemia/lymphoma |
| Aromatic amines (eg, benzidine, 2-naphthylamine) | Textile industry (dyes), tobacco smoke (2-naphthylamine) | Bladder | Transitional cell carcinoma |
| Arsenic | Herbicides (vineyard workers), metal smelting, wood preservation | Liver<br>Lung<br>Skin | Hepatic angiosarcoma<br>Lung cancer<br>Squamous cell carcinoma |
| Asbestos | Old roofing material, shipyard workers | Lung | Bronchogenic carcinoma > mesothelioma |
| Tobacco smoke | | Bladder<br>Cervix<br>Esophagus<br><br>Kidney<br>Larynx<br>Lung<br><br>Oropharynx<br>Pancreas | Transitional cell carcinoma<br>Squamous cell carcinoma<br>Squamous cell carcinoma/ adenocarcinoma<br>Renal cell carcinoma<br>Squamous cell carcinoma<br>Squamous cell and small cell carcinoma<br>Squamous cell carcinoma<br>Pancreatic adenocarcinoma |
| Ethanol | | Esophagus<br>Liver<br>Breast | Squamous cell carcinoma<br>Hepatocellular carcinoma<br>Breast cancer |
| Ionizing radiation | | Blood<br>Thyroid | Leukemia<br>Papillary thyroid carcinoma |
| Nickel, chromium, beryllium, silica | Occupational exposure | Lung | Lung cancer |
| Nitrosamines | Smoked foods | Stomach | Gastric cancer (intestinal type) |
| Radon | Byproduct of uranium decay, accumulates in basements | Lung | Lung cancer (2nd leading cause after tobacco smoke) |
| Vinyl chloride | Used to make PVC pipes | LiVer | Hepatic angiosarcoma |

| | |
|---|---|
| **Field cancerization** | Replacement of a large area of normal cells by premalignant cells due to widespread carcinogen exposure. Affected area is at ↑ risk of developing multiple independent 1° malignancies. Involved in head and neck cancer (mucosal exposure to tobacco smoke), skin cancer (skin exposure to UV light), bladder cancer (urothelial exposure to urinary carcinogens). |

## Oncogenic microbes

| MICROBE | ASSOCIATED CANCER |
|---|---|
| EBV | Burkitt lymphoma, Hodgkin lymphoma, nasopharyngeal carcinoma, 1° CNS lymphoma (in immunocompromised patients) |
| HBV, HCV | Hepatocellular carcinoma |
| HHV-8 | Kaposi ("Ka∞si") sarcoma |
| HPV (usually types 16, 18) | Cervical and penile/anal carcinoma, head and neck cancer |
| *H pylori* | Gastric adenocarcinoma and MALT lymphoma |
| HTLV-1 | Adult T-cell Leukemia/Lymphoma |
| Liver fluke *(Clonorchis sinensis)* | Cholangiocarcinoma |
| *Schistosoma haematobium* | Squamous cell bladder cancer |

## Serum tumor markers

Tumor markers should not be used as the 1° tool for cancer diagnosis or screening. They may be used to monitor tumor recurrence and response to therapy, but definitive diagnosis is made via biopsy. Some can be associated with non-neoplastic conditions.

| MARKER | IMPORTANT ASSOCIATIONS | NOTES |
|---|---|---|
| **Alkaline phosphatase** | Metastases to bone or liver, Paget disease of bone, seminoma (PLAP). | Exclude hepatic origin by checking LFTs and GGT levels. |
| **α-fetoprotein** | Hepatocellular carcinoma, endodermal sinus (yolk sac) tumor, mixed germ cell tumor, ataxia-telangiectasia, neural tube defects. | Normally made by fetus. Transiently elevated in pregnancy. High levels associated with neural tube and abdominal wall defects, low levels associated with Down syndrome. |
| **hCG** | **H**ydatidiform moles and **C**horiocarcinomas (**G**estational trophoblastic disease), testicular cancer, mixed germ cell tumor. | Produced by syncytiotrophoblasts of the placenta. |
| **CA 15-3/CA 27-29** | Breast cancer. | |
| **CA 19-9** | Pancreatic adenocarcinoma. | |
| **CA 125** | Epithelial ovarian cancer. | |
| **Calcitonin** | Medullary thyroid carcinoma (alone and in MEN2A, MEN2B). | Calci2nin. |
| **CEA** | Colorectal and pancreatic cancers. Minor associations: gastric, breast, and medullary thyroid carcinomas. | CarcinoEmbryonic Antigen. Very nonspecific. |
| **Chromogranin** | Neuroendocrine tumors. | |
| **LDH** | Testicular germ cell tumors, ovarian dysgerminoma, other cancers. | Can be used as an indicator of tumor burden. |
| **Neuron-specific enolase** | Neuroendocrine tumors (eg, small cell lung cancer, carcinoid tumor, neuroblastoma). | |
| **PSA** | Prostate cancer. | Prostate-Specific Antigen. Also elevated in BPH and prostatitis. Questionable risk/benefit for screening. Marker for recurrence after treatment. |

| **Important immunohistochemical stains** | Determine primary site of origin for metastatic tumors and characterize tumors that are difficult to classify. Can have prognostic and predictive value. | |
|---|---|---|
| STAIN | TARGET | TUMORS IDENTIFIED |
| Chromogranin and synaptophysin | Neuroendocrine cells | Small cell carcinoma of the lung, carcinoid tumor, neuroblastoma |
| Cytokeratin | Epithelial cells | Epithelial tumors (eg, squamous cell carcinoma) |
| Desmin | Muscle | Muscle tumors (eg, rhabdomyosarcoma) |
| GFAP | NeuroGlia (eg, astrocytes, Schwann cells, oligodendrocytes) | Astrocytoma, Glioblastoma |
| Neurofilament | Neurons | Neuronal tumors (eg, neuroblastoma) |
| PSA | Prostatic epithelium | Prostate cancer |
| PECAM-1/CD-31 | Endothelial cells | Vascular tumors (eg, angiosarcoma) |
| S-100 | Neural crest cells | Melanoma, schwannoma, Langerhans cell histiocytosis |
| TRAP | Tartrate-resistant acid phosphatase | Hairy cell leukemia |
| Vimentin | Mesenchymal tissue (eg, fibroblasts, endothelial cells, macrophages) | Mesenchymal tumors (eg, sarcoma), but also many other tumors (eg, endometrial carcinoma, renal cell carcinoma, meningioma) |

| **P-glycoprotein** | ATP-dependent efflux pump also called multidrug resistance protein 1 (MDR1). Expressed in some cancer cells to pump out toxins, including chemotherapeutic agents (one mechanism of ↓ responsiveness or resistance to chemotherapy over time). |
|---|---|

**Paraneoplastic syndromes**

| MANIFESTATION | DESCRIPTION/MECHANISM | MOST COMMONLY ASSOCIATED TUMOR(S) |
|---|---|---|
| **Musculoskeletal and cutaneous** | | |
| Dermatomyositis | Progressive proximal muscle weakness, Gottron papules, heliotrope rash | Adenocarcinomas, especially ovarian |
| Acanthosis nigricans | Hyperpigmented velvety plaques in axilla and neck | Gastric adenocarcinoma and other visceral malignancies |
| Sign of Leser-Trélat | Sudden onset of multiple seborrheic keratoses | GI adenocarcinomas and other visceral malignancies |
| Hypertrophic osteoarthropathy | Abnormal proliferation of skin and bone at distal extremities → clubbing, arthralgia, joint effusions, periostosis of tubular bones | Adenocarcinoma of the lung |
| **Endocrine** | | |
| Hypercalcemia | PTHrP | SCa$^{2+}$mous cell carcinomas of lung, head, and neck; renal, bladder, breast, and ovarian carcinomas |
| | ↑ 1,25-$(OH)_2$ vitamin $D_3$ (calcitriol) | Lymphoma |
| Cushing syndrome | ↑ ACTH | Small cell lung cancer |
| Hyponatremia (SIADH) | ↑ ADH | |
| **Hematologic** | | |
| Polycythemia | ↑ Erythropoietin Paraneoplastic rise to High hematocrit levels | Pheochromocytoma, renal cell carcinoma, HCC, hemangioblastoma, leiomyoma |
| Pure red cell aplasia | Anemia with low reticulocytes | Thymoma |
| Good syndrome | Hypogammaglobulinemia | |
| Trousseau syndrome | Migratory superficial thrombophlebitis | |
| Nonbacterial thrombotic endocarditis | Deposition of sterile platelet thrombi on heart valves | Adenocarcinomas, especially pancreatic |
| **Neuromuscular** | | |
| Anti-NMDA receptor encephalitis | Psychiatric disturbance, memory deficits, seizures, dyskinesias, autonomic instability, language dysfunction | Ovarian teratoma |
| Opsoclonus-myoclonus ataxia syndrome | "Dancing eyes, dancing feet" | Neuroblastoma (children), small cell lung cancer (adults) |
| Paraneoplastic cerebellar degeneration | Antibodies against antigens in Purkinje cells | Small cell lung cancer (anti-Hu), gynecologic and breast cancers (anti-Yo), and Hodgkin lymphoma (anti-Tr) |
| Paraneoplastic encephalomyelitis | Antibodies against Hu antigens in neurons | Small cell lung cancer |
| Lambert-Eaton myasthenic syndrome | Antibodies against presynaptic (P/Q-type) $Ca^{2+}$ channels at NMJ | |
| Myasthenia gravis | Antibodies against postsynaptic ACh receptors at NMJ | Thymoma |

## ▶ PATHOLOGY—AGING

| | |
|---|---|
| **Normal aging** | Time-dependent progressive decline in organ function resulting in ↑ susceptibility to disease. Associated with genetic (eg, telomere shortening), epigenetic (eg, DNA methylation), and metabolic (eg, mitochondrial dysfunction) alterations. |
| Cardiovascular | ↓ arterial compliance (↑ stiffness), ↑ aortic diameter, ↓ left ventricular cavity size and sigmoid-shaped interventricular septum (due to myocardial hypertrophy), ↑ left atrial cavity size, aortic and mitral valve calcification, ↓ maximum heart rate. |
| Gastrointestinal | ↓ LES tone, ↓ gastric mucosal protection, ↓ colonic motility. |
| Hematopoietic | ↓ bone marrow mass, ↑ bone marrow fat; less vigorous response to stressors (eg, blood loss). |
| Immune | Predominant effect on adaptive immunity: ↓ naïve B cells and T cells, preserved memory B cells and T cells. Immunosenescence impairs response to new antigens (eg, pathogens, vaccines). |
| Musculoskeletal | ↓ skeletal muscle mass (sarcopenia), ↓ bone mass (osteopenia), joint cartilage thinning. |
| Nervous | ↓ brain volume (neuronal loss), ↓ cerebral blood flow; function is preserved despite mild cognitive decline. |
| Special senses | Impaired accommodation (presbyopia), ↓ hearing (presbycusis), ↓ smell and taste. |
| Skin | Atrophy with flattening of dermal-epidermal junction; ↓ dermal collagen and ↓ elastin (wrinkles, senile purpura), ↓ sweat glands (heat stroke), ↓ sebaceous glands (xerosis cutis).<br>▪ Intrinsic aging (chronological aging)—↓ biosynthetic capacity of dermal fibroblasts.<br>▪ Extrinsic aging (photoaging)—degradation of dermal collagen and elastin from sun exposure (UVA); degradation products accumulate in dermis (solar elastosis). |
| Renal | ↓ GFR (↓ nephrons), ↓ RBF, ↓ hormonal function. Voiding dysfunction (eg, urinary incontinence). |
| Reproductive | Males—testicular atrophy (↓ spermatogenesis), prostate enlargement, slower erection/ejaculation, longer refractory period. Less pronounced ↓ in libido as compared to females.<br>Females—vulvovaginal atrophy; vaginal shortening, thinning, dryness, ↑ pH. Due to ↓ estrogen from exhaustion of ovarian follicles (menopause). |
| Respiratory | ↑ lung compliance (↓ elastic recoil), ↓ chest wall compliance (↑ stiffness), ↓ respiratory muscle strength; ↓ $FEV_1$, ↓ FVC, ↑ RV (TLC is unchanged); ↑ A-a gradient, ↑ $\dot{V}/\dot{Q}$ mismatch. Ventilatory response to hypoxia/hypercapnia is blunted. Less vigorous cough, slower mucociliary clearance. |

| | |
|---|---|
| **Lipofuscin**<br> | A yellow-brown, "wear and tear" pigment **A** associated with normal aging.<br>Composed of polymers of lipids and phospholipids complexed with protein. May be derived through lipid peroxidation of polyunsaturated lipids of subcellular membranes.<br>Autopsy of older adult will reveal deposits in heart, colon, liver, kidney, eye, and other organs. |

▶ NOTES

# Pharmacology

*"Cure sometimes, treat often, and comfort always."*

—Hippocrates

*"One pill makes you larger, and one pill makes you small."*

—Jefferson Airplane, *White Rabbit*

*"For the chemistry that works on one patient may not work for the next, because even medicine has its own conditions."*

—Suzy Kassem

*"I wondher why ye can always read a doctor's bill an' ye niver can read his purscription."*

—Finley Peter Dunne

*"Love is the drug I'm thinking of."*

—The Bryan Ferry Orchestra

Preparation for pharmacology questions is not as straightforward as in years past. One major recent change is that the USMLE Step 1 has moved away from testing pharmacotherapeutics. That means you will generally not be required to identify medications indicated for a specific condition. You still need to know mechanisms and important adverse effects of key drugs and their major variants. Obscure derivatives are low-yield. Learn their classic and distinguishing toxicities as well as major drug-drug interactions.

Reviewing associated biochemistry, physiology, and microbiology concepts can be useful while studying pharmacology. The exam has a strong emphasis on ANS, CNS, antimicrobial, and cardiovascular agents as well as on NSAIDs, which are covered throughout the text. Specific drug dosages or trade names are generally not testable. The exam may use graphs to test various pharmacology content, so make sure you are comfortable interpreting them.

▸ PHARMACOLOGY—PHARMACOKINETICS AND PHARMACODYNAMICS

### Enzyme kinetics

| | | |
|---|---|---|
| **Michaelis-Menten kinetics** | $K_m$ is the substrate concentration needed for an enzyme to reach a rate of $1/2 V_{max}$ and is inversely related to the affinity of the enzyme for its substrate.<br><br>$V_{max}$ is directly proportional to the enzyme concentration.<br><br>Most enzymatic reactions follow a hyperbolic curve (ie, Michaelis-Menten kinetics); however, enzymatic reactions that exhibit a sigmoid curve usually indicate cooperative kinetics (eg, hemoglobin). | $[S]$ = concentration of substrate; $V$ = velocity.<br><br>Effects of enzyme inhibition<br>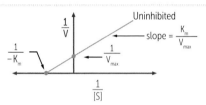 |
| **Lineweaver-Burk plot** | The closer to 0 on the Y-axis, the higher the $V_{max}$.<br>The closer to 0 on the X-axis, the higher the $K_m$.<br>The higher the $K_m$, the lower the affinity.<br><br>Competitive inhibitors cross each other, whereas noncompetitive inhibitors do not.<br><br>Kompetitive inhibitors increase $K_m$. | <br>Effects of enzyme inhibition<br> |

| | Competitive inhibitors, reversible | Competitive inhibitors, irreversible | Noncompetitive inhibitors |
|---|---|---|---|
| Resemble substrate | Yes | Yes | No |
| Overcome by ↑ [S] | Yes | No | No |
| Bind active site | Yes | Yes | No |
| Effect on $V_{max}$ | Unchanged | ↓ | ↓ |
| Effect on $K_m$ | ↑ | Unchanged | Unchanged |
| Pharmacodynamics | ↓ potency | ↓ efficacy | ↓ efficacy |

## Pharmacokinetics

| | | |
|---|---|---|
| **Bioavailability (F)** | Fraction of administered drug reaching systemic circulation. For an IV dose, F = 100%. Orally: F typically < 100% due to incomplete absorption and first-pass metabolism. Can be calculated from the area under the curve in a plot of plasma concentration over time. | 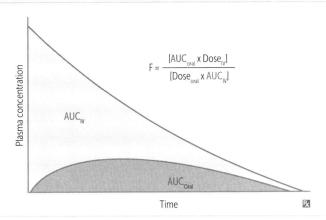 |

$$F = \frac{[AUC_{oral} \times Dose_{IV}]}{[Dose_{oral} \times AUC_{IV}]}$$

**Volume of distribution (V$_d$)**

Theoretical value that relates drug amount to plasma concentration. Liver and kidney disease increase V$_d$ (↓ protein binding, ↑ V$_d$). Drugs may distribute in more than one compartment. Hemodialysis is most effective for drugs with a low V$_d$.

$$V_d = \frac{\text{amount of drug in the body}}{\text{plasma drug concentration}}$$

| V$_d$ | COMPARTMENT | DRUG TYPES |
|---|---|---|
| Low | Intravascular | Large/charged molecules; plasma protein bound |
| Medium | ECF | Small hydrophilic molecules |
| High | All tissues including fat | Small lipophilic molecules, especially if bound to tissue protein |

**Clearance (CL)**

The volume of plasma cleared of drug per unit time. Clearance may be impaired with defects in cardiac, hepatic, or renal function.

$$CL = \frac{\text{rate of elimination of drug}}{\text{plasma drug concentration}} = V_d \times K_e \text{ (elimination constant)}$$

**Half-life (t$_{1/2}$)**

The time required to eliminate 1/2 of the drug from the body.

Steady state is a dynamic equilibrium in which drug concentration stays constant (ie, rate of drug elimination = rate of drug administration).

In first-order kinetics, a drug infused at a constant rate takes 4–5 half-lives to reach steady state. It takes 3.3 half-lives to reach 90% of the steady-state level.

$$t_{1/2} = \frac{0.7 \times V_d}{CL} \text{ in first-order elimination}$$

| # of half-lives | 1 | 2 | 3 | 4 |
|---|---|---|---|---|
| % remaining | 50% | 25% | 12.5% | 6.25% |

**Dosage calculations**

$$\text{Loading dose} = \frac{C_p \times V_d}{F}$$

$$\text{Maintenance dose} = \frac{C_p \times CL \times \tau}{F}$$

C$_p$ = target plasma concentration
τ = dosage interval (time between doses); does not apply for continuous infusions

In renal or liver disease, maintenance dose ↓ and loading dose is usually unchanged.

Time to steady state depends primarily on t$_{1/2}$ and is independent of dose and dosing frequency.

**Drug metabolism**

Drugs can be metabolized by either or both phase I and phase II reactions. These reactions serve to bioactivate or deactivate substances, and do not have to take place sequentially (eg, phase I can follow phase II, or take place as a single reaction).

Geriatric patients lose phase I first. Patients who are slow acetylators have ↑ adverse effects from certain drugs because of ↓ rate of metabolism (eg, isoniazid).

## Elimination of drugs

| | | |
|---|---|---|
| Zero-order elimination | Rate of elimination is constant regardless of $C_p$ (ie, constant **amount** of drug eliminated per unit time). $C_p$ ↓ linearly with time. Examples of drugs—Phenytoin, Ethanol, and Aspirin (at high or toxic concentrations). | Capacity-limited elimination. A PEA is round, shaped like the "0" in zero-order. |
| First-order elimination | Rate of first-order elimination is directly proportional to the drug concentration (ie, constant **fraction** of drug eliminated per unit time). $C_p$ ↓ exponentially with time. Applies to most drugs. | Flow-dependent elimination. |

| | |
|---|---|
| **Urine pH and drug elimination** | Ionized species are trapped in urine and cleared quickly. Neutral forms can be reabsorbed. |
| Weak acids | Examples: phenobarbital, methotrexate, aspirin (salicylates). Trapped in basic environments. Treat overdose with sodium bicarbonate to alkalinize urine. |

$$RCOOH \rightleftharpoons RCOO^- + H^+$$
$$\text{(lipid soluble)} \qquad \text{(trapped)}$$

| | |
|---|---|
| Weak bases | Examples: TCAs, amphetamines. Trapped in acidic environments. |

$$RNH_3^+ \rightleftharpoons RNH_2 + H^+$$
$$\text{(trapped)} \qquad \text{(lipid soluble)}$$

TCA toxicity is initially treated with sodium bicarbonate to overcome the sodium channel-blocking activity of TCAs. This treats cardiac toxicity, but does not accelerate drug elimination. For severe alkalosis, treat with ammonium chloride to acidify urine.

| | |
|---|---|
| pKa | pH at which drugs (weak acid or base) are 50% ionized and 50% nonionized. The pKa represents the strength of the weak acid or base. |

**Efficacy vs potency**

| | |
|---|---|
| **Efficacy** | Maximal effect a drug can produce (intrinsic activity). Represented by the y-value ($V_{max}$). ↑ y-value = ↑ $V_{max}$ = ↑ efficacy. Unrelated to potency (ie, efficacious drugs can have high or low potency). Partial agonists have less efficacy than full agonists. |

| | |
|---|---|
| **Potency** | Amount of drug needed for a given effect. Represented by the x-value ($EC_{50}$). Left shifting = ↓ $EC_{50}$ = ↑ potency = ↓ drug needed. Unrelated to efficacy (ie, potent drugs can have high or low efficacy). |

## Receptor binding

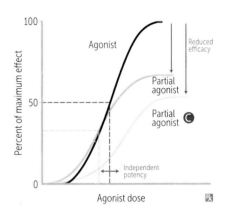

| AGONIST WITH | POTENCY | EFFICACY | REMARKS | EXAMPLE |
|---|---|---|---|---|
| **A** Competitive antagonist | ↓ | No change | **Can** be overcome by ↑ agonist concentration | Diazepam (agonist) + flumazenil (competitive antagonist) on GABA$_A$ receptor. |
| **B** Noncompetitive antagonist | No change | ↓ | **Cannot** be overcome by ↑ agonist concentration | Norepinephrine (agonist) + phenoxybenzamine (noncompetitive antagonist) on α-receptors. |
| **C** Partial agonist (alone) | Independent | ↓ | Acts at same site as full agonist | Morphine (full agonist) vs buprenorphine (partial agonist) at opioid μ-receptors. |

## Therapeutic index

Measurement of drug safety.

$$\frac{TD_{50}}{ED_{50}} = \frac{\text{median toxic dose}}{\text{median effective dose}}$$

Therapeutic window—range of drug concentrations that can safely and effectively treat disease.

TITE: Therapeutic Index = $TD_{50}$ / $ED_{50}$.
Safer drugs have higher TI values. Drugs with lower TI values frequently require monitoring (eg, warfarin, theophylline, digoxin, antiepileptic drugs, lithium; Warning! These drugs are lethal!).
$LD_{50}$ (lethal median dose) often replaces $TD_{50}$ in animal studies.

## Drug effect modifications

| TERM | DEFINITION | EXAMPLE |
| --- | --- | --- |
| Additive | Effect of substances A and B together is equal to the sum of their individual effects | Aspirin and acetaminophen "2 + 2 = 4" |
| Permissive | Presence of substance A is required for the full effects of substance B | Cortisol on catecholamine responsiveness |
| Synergistic | Effect of substances A and B together is greater than the sum of their individual effects | Clopidogrel with aspirin "2 + 2 > 4" |
| Potentiation | Similar to synergism, but drug B (with no therapeutic action alone) enhances the therapeutic action of drug A | Carbidopa only blocks enzyme to prevent peripheral conversion of levodopa "2 + 0 > 2" |
| Antagonistic | Effect of substances A and B together is less than the sum of their individual effects | Morphine with naloxone "2 + 2 < 4" |
| Tachyphylactic | Acute decrease in response to a drug after initial/repeated administration | Repeat use of intranasal decongestant (eg, oxymetazoline) → ↓ therapeutic response (with rebound congestion) |

▶ PHARMACOLOGY—AUTONOMIC DRUGS

### Autonomic receptors

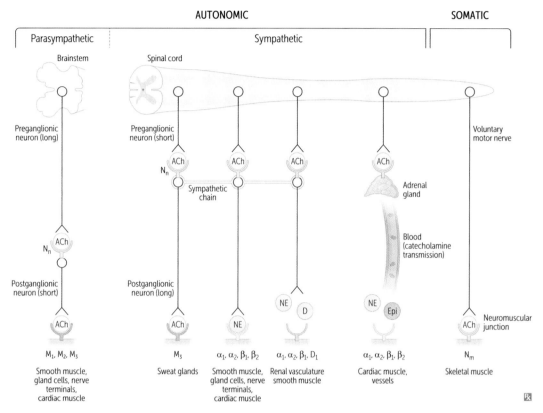

Pelvic splanchnic nerves and CNs III, VII, IX and X are part of the parasympathetic nervous system.
Adrenal medulla is directly innervated by preganglionic sympathetic fibers.
Sweat glands are part of the **sympathetic** pathway but are innervated by **chol**inergic fibers
(**sympathetic** nervous system results in a "**chold**" **sweat**).

| Acetylcholine receptors | Nicotinic ACh receptors are ligand-gated channels allowing efflux of $K^+$ and influx of $Na^+$ and in some cases $Ca^{2+}$. Two subtypes: $N_N$ (found in autonomic ganglia, adrenal medulla) and $N_M$ (found in neuromuscular junction of skeletal muscle). |
|---|---|
| | Muscarinic ACh receptors are G-protein–coupled receptors that usually act through 2nd messengers. 5 subtypes: $M_{1-5}$ found in heart, smooth muscle, brain, exocrine glands, and on sweat glands (cholinergic sympathetic). |

## Micturition control

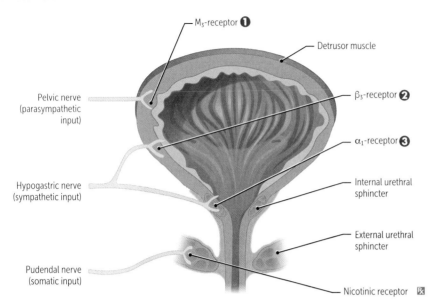

Micturition center in pons regulates involuntary bladder function via coordination of sympathetic and parasympathetic nervous systems.
⊕ sympathetic → ↑ urinary retention.
⊕ parasympathetic → ↑ urine voiding.
Some autonomic drugs act on smooth muscle receptors to treat bladder dysfunction.
Baby one more time.

| DRUGS | MECHANISM | APPLICATIONS |
|---|---|---|
| ❶ Muscarinic agonists (eg, bethanechol) | ⊕ $M_3$ receptor → contraction of detrusor smooth muscle → ↑ bladder emptying | Urinary retention |
| ❶ Muscarinic antagonists (eg, oxybutynin) | ⊖ $M_3$ receptor → relaxation of detrusor smooth muscle → ↓ detrusor overactivity | Urgency incontinence |
| ❷ Sympathomimetics (eg, mirabegron) | ⊕ $\beta_3$ receptor → relaxation of detrusor smooth muscle → ↑ bladder capacity | Urgency incontinence |
| ❸ $\alpha_1$-antagonists (eg, tamsulosin) | ⊖ $\alpha_1$-receptor → relaxation of smooth muscle (bladder neck, prostate) → ↓ urinary obstruction | BPH |

## Tissue distribution of adrenergic receptors

| RECEPTOR | TISSUE | EFFECT(S) |
|---|---|---|
| $\alpha_1$ | Vascular smooth muscle | Vasoconstriction |
| | Visceral smooth muscle | Smooth muscle contraction |
| $\alpha_2$ | Pancreas | Inhibition of insulin secretion |
| | Presynaptic terminals | Inhibition of neurotransmitter release |
| | Salivary glands | Inhibition of salivary secretion |
| $\beta_1$ | Heart | ↑ heart rate, contractility |
| | Kidney | ↑ renin secretion |
| $\beta_2$ | Bronchioles | Bronchodilation |
| | Cardiac muscle | ↑ heart rate, contractility |
| | Liver | Glycogenolysis, glucose release |
| | Arterial smooth muscle | Vasodilation |
| | Pancreas | Stimulation of insulin secretion |
| $\beta_3$ | Adipose | ↑ lipolysis |

## G-protein–linked second messengers

| RECEPTOR | G-PROTEIN CLASS | MAJOR FUNCTIONS |
|---|---|---|
| **Adrenergic** | | |
| $\alpha_1$ | q | ↑ vascular smooth muscle contraction, ↑ pupillary dilator muscle contraction (mydriasis), ↑ intestinal and bladder sphincter muscle contraction |
| $\alpha_2$ | i | ↓ sympathetic (adrenergic) outflow, ↓ insulin release, ↓ lipolysis, ↑ platelet aggregation, ↓ aqueous humor production |
| $\beta_1$ | s | ↑ heart rate, ↑ contractility (**one** heart), ↑ renin release, ↑ lipolysis |
| $\beta_2$ | s | Vasodilation, bronchodilation (**two** lungs), ↑ lipolysis, ↑ insulin release, ↑ glycogenolysis, ↓ uterine tone (tocolysis), ↑ aqueous humor production, ↑ cellular $K^+$ uptake |
| $\beta_3$ | s | ↑ lipolysis, ↑ thermogenesis in skeletal muscle, ↑ bladder relaxation |
| **Cholinergic** | | |
| $M_1$ | q | Mediates higher cognitive functions, stimulates enteric nervous system |
| $M_2$ | i | ↓ heart rate and contractility of atria |
| $M_3$ | q | ↑ exocrine gland secretions, gut peristalsis, bladder contraction, bronchoconstriction, vasodilation, ↑ pupillary sphincter muscle contraction (miosis), ciliary muscle contraction (accommodation) |
| **Dopamine** | | |
| $D_1$ | s | Relaxes renal vascular smooth muscle, activates direct pathway of striatum |
| $D_2$ | i | Modulates transmitter release, especially in brain, inhibits indirect pathway of striatum |
| **Histamine** | | |
| $H_1$ | q | ↑ bronchoconstriction, airway mucus production, ↑ vascular permeability/vasodilation, pruritus |
| $H_2$ | s | ↑ gastric acid secretion |
| **Vasopressin** | | |
| $V_1$ | q | ↑ vascular smooth muscle contraction |
| $V_2$ | s | ↑ $H_2O$ permeability and reabsorption via upregulating aquaporin-2 in collecting twobules (tubules) of kidney, ↑ release of vWF |

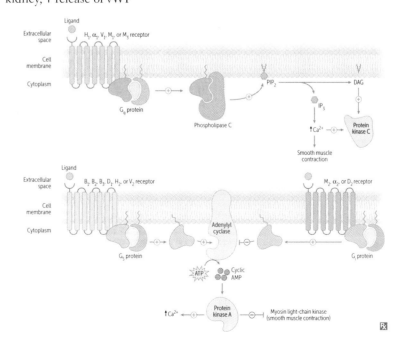

**Autonomic drugs**

Release of norepinephrine from a sympathetic nerve ending is modulated by NE itself, acting on presynaptic $\alpha_2$-autoreceptors → negative feedback.

Amphetamines use the NE transporter (NET) to enter the presynaptic terminal, where they utilize the vesicular monoamine transporter (VMAT) to enter neurosecretory vesicles. This displaces NE from the vesicles. Once NE reaches a concentration threshold within the presynaptic terminal, the action of NET is reversed, and NE is expelled into the synaptic cleft, contributing to the characteristics and effects of ↑ NE observed in patients taking amphetamines.

 represents transporters.

## Cholinomimetic agents

Watch for exacerbation of COPD, asthma, and peptic ulcers in susceptible patients.

| DRUG | ACTION | APPLICATIONS |
|---|---|---|
| **Direct agonists** | | |
| Bethanechol | Activates bladder smooth muscle; resistant to AChE. Acts on muscarinic receptors; no nicotinic activity. "Bethany, call me to activate your bladder." | Urinary retention. |
| Carbachol | Carbon copy of acetylcholine (but resistant to AChE). | Constricts pupil. Used for intraoperative miosis induction. |
| Methacholine | Stimulates muscarinic receptors in airway when inhaled. | Challenge test for diagnosis of asthma. |
| Pilocarpine | Contracts ciliary muscle of eye (open-angle glaucoma), pupillary sphincter (closed-angle glaucoma); resistant to AChE, can cross blood-brain barrier. "You cry, drool, and sweat on your 'pilow.'" | Potent stimulator of sweat, tears, and saliva Open-angle and closed-angle glaucoma, xerostomia (Sjögren syndrome). |
| **Indirect agonists (anticholinesterases)** | | |
| Donepezil, rivastigmine, galantamine | ↑ ACh. | 1st line for Alzheimer disease (Don Riva forgot the gala). |
| Neostigmine | ↑ ACh. Neo = no blood-brain barrier penetration due to positive charge. | Postoperative and neurogenic ileus and urinary retention, myasthenia gravis, reversal of neuromuscular junction blockade (postoperative). |
| Pyridostigmine | ↑ ACh; ↑ muscle strength. Does not penetrate CNS. Pyridostigmine gets rid of myasthenia gravis. | Myasthenia gravis (long acting). Used with glycopyrrolate or hyoscyamine to control pyridostigmine adverse effects. |
| Physostigmine | ↑ ACh. Phreely (freely) crosses blood-brain barrier as not charged → CNS. | Antidote for anticholinergic toxicity; physostigmine "phyxes" atropine overdose. |

## Anticholinesterase poisoning

Often due to organophosphates (eg, fenthion, parathion, malathion) that irreversibly inhibit AChE. Organophosphates commonly used as insecticides; poisoning usually seen in farmers.

| | | |
|---|---|---|
| Muscarinic effects | Diarrhea, Urination, Miosis, Bronchospasm, Bradycardia, Emesis, Lacrimation, Sweating, Salivation. | DUMBBELSS. Reversed by atropine, a competitive inhibitor. Atropine can cross BBB to relieve CNS symptoms. |
| Nicotinic effects | Neuromuscular blockade (mechanism similar to succinylcholine). | Reversed by pralidoxime, regenerates AChE via dephosphorylation if given early. Must be coadministered with atropine to prevent transient worsening of symptoms. Pralidoxime does not readily cross BBB. |
| CNS effects | Respiratory depression, lethargy, seizures, coma. | |

## Muscarinic antagonists

| DRUGS | ORGAN SYSTEMS | APPLICATIONS |
|---|---|---|
| Atropine, homatropine, tropicamide | Eye | Produce mydriasis and cycloplegia |
| Benztropine, trihexyphenidyl | CNS | Parkinson disease ("park my Benz") Acute dystonia |
| Glycopyrrolate | GI, respiratory | Parenteral: preoperative use to reduce airway secretions Oral: reduces drooling, peptic ulcer |
| Hyoscyamine, dicyclomine | GI | Antispasmodics for irritable bowel syndrome |
| Ipratropium, tiotropium | Respiratory | COPD, asthma Duration: tiotropium > ipratropium |
| Solifenacin, Oxybutynin, Flavoxate, Tolterodine | Genitourinary | Reduce bladder spasms and urge urinary incontinence (overactive bladder) Make bladder SOFT |
| Scopolamine | CNS | Motion sickness |

## Atropine

Muscarinic antagonist. Used to treat bradycardia and for ophthalmic applications.

| ORGAN SYSTEM | ACTION | NOTES |
|---|---|---|
| Eye | ↑ pupil dilation, cycloplegia | Blocks muscarinic effects (DUMBBELSS) of anticholinesterases, but not the nicotinic effects |
| Airway | Bronchodilation, ↓ secretions | |
| Heart | ↑ heart rate | |
| Stomach | ↓ acid secretion | |
| Gut | ↓ motility | |
| Bladder | ↓ urgency in cystitis | |
| ADVERSE EFFECTS | ↑ body **temperature** (due to ↓ sweating); ↑ **HR**; dry mouth; dry, flushed skin; cycloplegia; constipation; disorientation Can cause acute angle-closure glaucoma in older adults (due to mydriasis), **urinary retention** in men with prostatic hyperplasia, and hyperthermia in infants | Adverse effects: Hot as a hare Fast as a fiddle Dry as a bone Red as a beet Blind as a bat Mad as a hatter Full as a flask Jimson weed *(Datura)* → gardener's pupil (mydriasis) |

**ysiologic effects of npathomimetics**

NE ↑ systolic and diastolic pressures as a result of $\alpha_1$-mediated vasoconstriction → ↑ mean arterial pressure → reflex bradycardia. However, isoproterenol (rarely used) has little α effect but causes $\beta_2$-mediated vasodilation, resulting in ↓ mean arterial pressure and ↑ heart rate through $\beta_1$ and reflex activity.

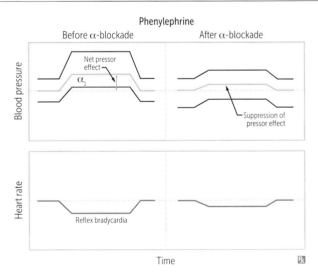

nephrine response exhibits reversal of mean arterial essure from a net increase (the α response) to a net crease (the $\beta_2$ response).

Phenylephrine response is suppressed but not reversed because it is a "pure" α-agonist (lacks β-agonist properties).

## Sympathomimetics

| DRUG | SITE | HEMODYNAMIC CHANGES | APPLICATIONS |
|---|---|---|---|
| **Direct sympathomimetics** | | | |
| **Albuterol, salmeterol, terbutaline** | $\beta_2 > \beta_1$ | ↑ HR (little effect) | Albuterol for acute asthma/COPD serial (long-term) asthma/COPD for acute bronchospasm in asthm |
| **Dobutamine** | $\beta_1 > \beta_2, \alpha$ | –/↓ BP, ↑ HR, ↑ CO | Cardiac stress testing, acute dec heart failure (HF) with cardiog (inotrope) |
| **Dopamine** | $D_1 = D_2 > \beta > \alpha$ | ↑ BP (high dose), ↑ HR, ↑ CO | Unstable bradycardia, shock; ino chronotropic effects at lower d vasoconstriction at high doses |
| **Epinephrine** | $\beta > \alpha$ | ↑ BP (high dose), ↑ HR, ↑ CO | Anaphylaxis, asthma, shock, op glaucoma; $\alpha$ effects predomin doses. Stronger effect at $\beta_2$-re norepinephrine. |
| **Fenoldopam** | $D_1$ | ↓ BP (vasodilation), ↑ HR, ↑ CO | Postoperative hypertension, hy Vasodilator (coronary, periph splanchnic). Promotes natriu hypotension, tachycardia, flu |
| **Isoproterenol** | $\beta_1 = \beta_2$ | ↓ BP (vasodilation), ↑ HR, ↑ CO | Electrophysiologic evaluation tachyarrhythmias. Can wors negligible $\alpha$ effect. |
| **Midodrine** | $\alpha_1$ | ↑ BP (vasoconstriction), ↓ HR, –/↓ CO | Autonomic insufficiency and hypotension. May exacerbat hypertension. |
| **Mirabegron** | $\beta_3$ | | Urinary urgency or incontine bladder. Think "mirab3gro |
| **Norepinephrine** | $\alpha_1 > \alpha_2 > \beta_1$ | ↑ BP, –/↓ HR (may have minor reflexive change in response to ↑ BP due to $\alpha_1$ agonism outweighing direct $\beta_1$ chronotropic effect), –/↑ CO | Hypotension, septic shock. |
| **Phenylephrine** | $\alpha_1 > \alpha_2$ | ↑ BP (vasoconstriction), ↓ HR, –/↓ CO | Hypotension (vasoconstrict (mydriatic), rhinitis (decor priapism. |
| **Indirect sympathomimetics** | | | |
| **Amphetamine** | Indirect general agonist, reuptake inhibitor, also releases stored catecholamines. | | Narcolepsy, obesity, ADHI |
| **Cocaine** | Indirect general agonist, reuptake inhibitor. Causes vasoconstriction and local anesthesia. Caution when giving $\beta$-blockers if cocaine intoxication is suspected (unopposed $\alpha_1$ activation → ↑↑↑ BP, coronary vasospasm). | | Causes mydriasis in eyes v innervation → used to c syndrome. |
| **Ephedrine** | Indirect general agonist, releases stored catecholamines. | | Nasal decongestion (pseu incontinence, hypotens |

## Sympatholytics ($\alpha_2$-agonists)

| DRUG | APPLICATIONS | ADVERSE EFFECTS |
|---|---|---|
| Clonidine, guanfacine | Hypertensive urgency (limited situations), ADHD, Tourette syndrome, symptom control in opioid withdrawal | CNS depression, bradycardia, hypotension, respiratory depression, miosis, rebound hypertension with abrupt cessation |
| $\alpha$-methyldopa | Hypertension in pregnancy | Direct Coombs ⊕ hemolysis, drug-induced lupus, hyperprolactinemia |
| Tizanidine | Relief of spasticity | Hypotension, weakness, xerostomia |

## $\alpha$-blockers

| DRUG | APPLICATIONS | ADVERSE EFFECTS |
|---|---|---|
| **Nonselective** | | |
| Phenoxybenzamine | Irreversible. Pheochromocytoma (used preoperatively) to prevent catecholamine (hypertensive) crisis. | Orthostatic hypotension, reflex tachycardia. |
| Phentolamine | Reversible. Given to patients on MAO inhibitors who eat tyramine-containing foods and for severe cocaine-induced hypertension (2nd line). Also used to treat norepinephrine extravasation. | |
| **$\alpha_1$ selective (-osin ending)** | | |
| Prazosin, terazosin, doxazosin, tamsulosin | Urinary symptoms of BPH; PTSD (prazosin); hypertension (except tamsulosin). | 1st-dose orthostatic hypotension, dizziness, headache. |
| **$\alpha_2$ selective** | | |
| Mirtazapine | Depression. | Sedation, ↑ serum cholesterol, ↑ appetite. |

## β-blockers

Atenolol, betaxolol, bisoprolol, carvedilol, esmolol, labetalol, metoprolol, nadolol, nebivolol, propranolol, timolol.

| APPLICATION | ACTIONS | NOTES/EXAMPLES |
|---|---|---|
| Angina pectoris | ↓ heart rate and contractility → ↓ $O_2$ consumption | |
| Glaucoma | ↓ production of aqueous humor | Timolol |
| Heart failure | Blockade of neurohormonal stress → prevention of deleterious cardiac remodeling → ↓ mortality | Bisoprolol, carvedilol, metoprolol (β-blockers curb mortality) |
| Hypertension | ↓ cardiac output, ↓ renin secretion (due to $\beta_1$-receptor blockade on JG cells) | |
| Hyperthyroidism/ thyroid storm | Symptom control (↓ heart rate, ↓ tremor) | Propranolol |
| Hypertrophic cardiomyopathy | ↓ heart rate → ↑ filling time, relieving obstruction | |
| Migraine | ↓ nitric oxide production | Effective for prevention |
| Myocardial infarction | ↓ $O_2$ demand (short-term), ↓ mortality (long-term) | |
| Supraventricular tachycardia | ↓ AV conduction velocity (class II antiarrhythmic) | Metoprolol, esmolol |
| Variceal bleeding | ↓ hepatic venous pressure gradient and portal hypertension (prophylactic use) | Nadolol, propranolol, carvedilol for no portal circulation |
| ADVERSE EFFECTS | Erectile dysfunction, cardiovascular (bradycardia, AV block, HF), CNS (seizures, sleep alterations), dyslipidemia (metoprolol), masked hypoglycemia, asthma/COPD exacerbations | Use of β-blockers for acute cocaine-associated chest pain remains controversial due to unsubstantiated concern for unopposed α-adrenergic stimulation |
| SELECTIVITY | $\beta_1$-selective antagonists ($\beta_1 > \beta_2$)—atenolol, betaxolol, bisoprolol, esmolol, metoprolol | Selective antagonists mostly go from **A** to **M** ($\beta_1$ with 1st half of alphabet) |
| | Nonselective antagonists ($\beta_1 = \beta_2$)—nadolol, propranolol, timolol | Non**Z**elective antagonists mostly go from **N** to **Z** ($\beta_2$ with 2nd half of alphabet) |
| | Nonselective α- and β-antagonists—carve**dilol**, labeta**lol** | Nonselective α- and β-antagonists have **modified suffixes** (instead of "-olol") |
| | Nebivolol combines cardiac-selective $\beta_1$-adrenergic blockade with stimulation of $\beta_3$-receptors (activate NO synthase in the vasculature and ↓ SVR) | Nebiv**O**lol increases **NO** |

**Phosphodiesterase inhibitors**

Phosphodiesterase (PDE) inhibitors inhibit PDE, which catalyzes the hydrolysis of cAMP and/or cGMP, and thereby increase cAMP and/or cGMP. These inhibitors have varying specificity for PDE isoforms and thus have different clinical uses.

| TYPE OF INHIBITOR | MECHANISM OF ACTION | CLINICAL USES | ADVERSE EFFECTS |
|---|---|---|---|
| **Nonspecific PDE inhibitor** Theophylline | ↓ cAMP hydrolysis → ↑ cAMP → bronchial smooth muscle relaxation → bronchodilation | COPD/asthma (rarely used) | Cardiotoxicity (eg, tachycardia, arrhythmia), neurotoxicity (eg, seizures, headache), abdominal pain |
| **PDE-5 inhibitors** Sildenafil, vardenafil, tadalafil, avanafil | ↓ hydrolysis of cGMP → ↑ cGMP → ↑ smooth muscle relaxation by enhancing NO activity → pulmonary vasodilation and ↑ blood flow in corpus cavernosum fills the penis | Erectile dysfunction Pulmonary hypertension Benign prostatic hyperplasia (tadalafil only) | Facial flushing, headache, dyspepsia, hypotension in patients taking nitrates; "hot and sweaty," then headache, heartburn, hypotension Sildenafil only: cyanopia (blue-tinted vision) via inhibition of PDE-6 (six) in retina |
| **PDE-4 inhibitor** Roflumilast | ↑ cAMP in neutrophils, granulocytes, and bronchial epithelium | Severe COPD | Abdominal pain, weight loss, depression, anxiety, insomnia |
| **PDE-3 inhibitor** Milrinone | In cardiomyocytes: ↑ cAMP → ↑ $Ca^{2+}$ influx → ↑ ionotropy and chronotropy In vascular smooth muscle: ↑ cAMP → MLCK inhibition → vasodilation → ↓ preload and afterload | Acute decompensated HF with cardiogenic shock (inotrope) | Tachycardia, ventricular arrhythmias, hypotension |
| **"Platelet inhibitors"** Cilostazol[a] Dipyridamole[b] | In platelets: ↑ cAMP → inhibition of platelet aggregation | Intermittent claudication Stroke or TIA prevention (with aspirin) Cardiac stress testing (dipyridamole only, due to coronary vasodilation) Prevention of coronary stent restenosis | Nausea, headache, facial flushing, hypotension, abdominal pain |

[a]Cilostazol is a PDE-3 inhibitor, but due to its indications is categorized as a platelet inhibitor together with dipyridamole.
[b]Dipyridamole is a nonspecific PDE inhibitor, leading to inhibition of platelet aggregation. It also prevents adenosine reuptake by platelets → ↑ extracellular adenosine → ↑ vasodilation.

▶ PHARMACOLOGY—TOXICITIES AND ADVERSE EFFECTS

**Ingested seafood toxins**

Toxin actions include histamine release, total block of $Na^+$ channels, or opening of $Na^+$ channels to cause depolarization.

| TOXIN | SOURCE | ACTION | SYMPTOMS | TREATMENT |
|---|---|---|---|---|
| Histamine (scombroid poisoning) | Spoiled dark-meat fish such as tuna, mahi-mahi, mackerel, and bonito | Bacterial histidine decarboxylase converts histidine to histamine Frequently misdiagnosed as fish allergy | Mimics anaphylaxis: oral burning sensation, facial flushing, erythema, urticaria, itching; may progress to bronchospasm, angioedema, hypotension | Antihistamines Albuterol +/– epinephrine |
| Tetrodotoxin | Pufferfish | Binds fast voltage-gated $Na^+$ channels in nerve tissue, preventing depolarization | Nausea, diarrhea, paresthesias, weakness, dizziness, loss of reflexes | Supportive |
| Ciguatoxin | Reef fish such as barracuda, snapper, and moray eel | Opens $Na^+$ channels, causing depolarization | Nausea, vomiting, diarrhea; perioral numbness; reversal of hot and cold sensations; bradycardia, heart block, hypotension | Supportive |

**Age-related changes in pharmacokinetics**

Aging alters the passage of drugs through the body and standard doses can result in ↑ plasma concentrations. Older patients often require reduced doses to prevent toxicity.

- Absorption—mostly unaffected.
- Distribution—↓ total body water (↓ $V_d$ of hydrophilic drugs → ↑ concentration), ↑ total body fat (↑ $V_d$ of lipophilic drugs → ↑ half-life).
- Metabolism—↓ hepatic mass and blood flow → ↓ first-pass metabolism, ↓ hepatic clearance. Phase I of drug metabolism is decreased; phase II is relatively preserved.
- Excretion—↓ renal mass and blood flow (↓ GFR) → ↓ renal clearance.

## Specific toxicity treatments

| TOXIN | TREATMENT |
|---|---|
| Acetaminophen | N-acetylcysteine (replenishes glutathione) |
| AChE inhibitors, organophosphates | Atropine > pralidoxime |
| Antimuscarinic, anticholinergic agents | Physostigmine (crosses BBB), control hyperthermia |
| Arsenic | Dimercaprol, succimer |
| Benzodiazepines | Flumazenil |
| β-blockers | Atropine, glucagon, saline |
| Carbon monoxide | 100% $O_2$, hyperbaric $O_2$ |
| Copper | "Penny"cillamine (penicillamine), trientine (3 copper pennies) |
| Cyanide | Hydroxocobalamin, nitrites + sodium thiosulfate |
| Dabigatran | Idarucizumab |
| Digoxin | Digoxin-specific antibody fragments |
| Direct factor Xa inhibitors (eg, apixaban) | Andexanet alfa |
| Heparin | Protamine sulfate |
| Iron (Fe) | Deferoxamine, deferasirox, deferiprone |
| Lead | Penicillamine, calcium disodium EDTA, Dimercaprol, Succimer, (correct lead poisoning in PEDS patients) |
| Mercury | Dimercaprol, succimer |
| Methanol, ethylene glycol (antifreeze) | Fomepizole > ethanol, dialysis |
| Methemoglobin | Methylene blue, vitamin C (reducing agent) |
| Methotrexate | Leucovorin |
| Opioids | Naloxone |
| Salicylates | $NaHCO_3$ (alkalinize urine), dialysis |
| TCAs | $NaHCO_3$ (stabilizes cardiac cell membrane) |
| Warfarin | Vitamin K (delayed effect), PCC (prothrombin complex concentrate)/FFP (immediate effect) |

## Drug reactions—cardiovascular

| DRUG REACTION | CAUSAL AGENTS |
|---|---|
| Coronary vasospasm | Cocaine, Amphetamines, Sumatriptan, Ergot alkaloids (CASE) |
| Cutaneous flushing | Vancomycin, Adenosine, Niacin, $Ca^{2+}$ channel blockers, Echinocandins, Nitrates (flushed from VANCEN [dancing]) |
| | Vancomycin infusion reaction (formerly called red man syndrome)—rate-dependent infusion reaction to vancomycin causing widespread pruritic erythema due to histamine release. Manage with diphenhydramine, slower infusion rate. |
| Dilated cardiomyopathy | Alcohol, anthracycline (eg, doxorubicin, daunorubicin; prevent with dexrazoxane), trastuzumab |
| Torsades de pointes | Agents that prolong QT interval: Methadone, antiArrhythmics (class IA, III), antiBiotics (eg, macrolides, fluoroquinolones), anti"C"ychotics (eg, ziprasidone), antiDepressants (eg, TCAs), antiEmetics (eg, ondansetron), antiFungals (eg, fluconazole) (Memorize your ABCDEF) |

## Drug reactions—endocrine/reproductive

| DRUG REACTION | CAUSAL AGENTS | NOTES |
|---|---|---|
| Adrenocortical insufficiency | HPA suppression secondary to chronic exogenous glucocorticoid use | Abrupt withdrawal of exogenous glucocorticoids leads to adrenal crisis |
| Diabetes insipidus | Lithium, demeclocycline | |
| Gynecomastia | Ketoconazole, cimetidine, spironolactone, GnRH analogs/antagonists, androgen receptor inhibitors, 5α-reductase inhibitors | |
| Hot flashes | SERMs (eg, tamoxifen, clomiphene, raloxifene) | |
| Hyperglycemia | Tacrolimus, protease inhibitors, niacin, HCTZ, glucocorticoids | The people need High glucose |
| Hyperprolactinemia | Typical antipsychotics (eg, haloperidol), atypical antipsychotics (eg, risperidone), metoclopramide, methyldopa, verapamil | Presents with hypogonadism (eg, infertility, amenorrhea, erectile dysfunction) and galactorrhea |
| Hyperthyroidism | Amiodarone, iodine, lithium | |
| Hypothyroidism | Amiodarone, lithium | I am lethargic |
| SIADH | Carbamazepine, Cyclophosphamide, SSRIs | Can't Concentrate Serum Sodium |

## Drug reactions—gastrointestinal

| DRUG REACTION | CAUSAL AGENTS | NOTES |
|---|---|---|
| Acute cholestatic hepatitis, jaundice | Macrolides (eg, erythromycin) | |
| Constipation | Antimuscarinics (eg, atropine), antipsychotics, opioids, non-dihydropyridine CCBs, ranolazine, amiodarone, aluminum hydroxide, loperamide, 5HT3 receptor antagonist (ondansetron), vincristine | |
| Diarrhea | Acamprosate, antidiabetic agents (acarbose, metformin, pramlintide), colchicine, cholinesterase inhibitors, lipid-lowering agents (eg, ezetimibe, orlistat), macrolides (eg, erythromycin), SSRIs, chemotherapy (eg, irinotecan) | |
| Focal to massive hepatic necrosis | *Amanita phalloides* (death cap mushroom), valproate, acetaminophen | |
| Hepatitis | Rifampin, isoniazid, pyrazinamide, statins, fibrates | |
| Pancreatitis | Diuretics (eg, furosemide, HCTZ), glucocorticoids, alcohol, valproate, azathioprine | Drugs generate a violent abdominal distress |
| Medication-induced esophagitis | Potassium chloride, NSAIDs, bisphosphonates, ferrous sulfate, tetracyclines **P**ills **N**ot beneficial for **f**ood **t**ube | Usually occurs at anatomic sites of esophageal narrowing (eg, near level of aortic arch); caustic effect minimized with upright posture and adequate water ingestion |
| Pseudomembranous colitis | Ampicillin, cephalosporins, clindamycin, fluoroquinolones, PPIs | Antibiotics predispose to superinfection by resistant *C difficile* |

## Drug reactions—hematologic

| DRUG REACTION | CAUSAL AGENTS | NOTES |
|---|---|---|
| Agranulocytosis | Dapsone, clozapine, carbamazepine, propylthiouracil, methimazole, ganciclovir, colchicine | Drugs can cause pretty major granulocytes collapse |
| Aplastic anemia | Carbamazepine, methimazole, NSAIDs, benzene, chloramphenicol, propylthiouracil | Can't make New blood cells properly |
| Direct Coombs ⊕ hemolytic anemia | Penicillin, methylDopa, Cephalosporins | P Diddy Coombs |
| Drug Reaction with Eosinophilia and Systemic Symptoms | Phenytoin, carbamazepine, minocycline, sulfa drugs, allopurinol, vancomycin | T cell-mediated hypersensitivity reaction. Also known as drug-induced hypersensitivity syndrome (DIHS)<br>DRESSes partially cover my skin and viscera |
| Hemolysis in G6PD deficiency | Sulfonamides, dapsone, primaquine, aspirin, nitrofurantoin | |
| Megaloblastic anemia | Hydroxyurea, Phenytoin, Methotrexate, Sulfa drugs | You're having a mega blast with PMS |
| Thrombocytopenia | Heparin, quinidine, ganciclovir, vancomycin, linezolid | |
| Thrombotic complications | Combined oral contraceptives, hormone replacement therapy, SERMs, epoetin alfa Testosterone supplements | Estrogen-mediated adverse effect<br>Increase blood viscosity and platelet accumulation |

## Drug reactions—musculoskeletal/skin/connective tissue

| DRUG REACTION | CAUSAL AGENTS | NOTES |
|---|---|---|
| Drug-induced lupus | Hydralazine, procainamide, quinidine | |
| Fat redistribution | Protease inhibitors, glucocorticoids | Fat protects glutes |
| Gingival hyperplasia | Cyclosporine, $Ca^{2+}$ channel blockers, phenytoin | Can Cause puffy gums |
| Hyperuricemia (gout) | Pyrazinamide, thiazides, furosemide, niacin, cyclosporine | Painful tophi and feet need care |
| Myopathy | Statins, fibrates, niacin, colchicine, daptomycin, hydroxychloroquine, interferon-$\alpha$, penicillamine, glucocorticoids | |
| Osteoporosis | Glucocorticoids, depot medroxyprogesterone acetate, GnRH agonists, aromatase inhibitors, anticonvulsants, heparin, PPIs | |
| Photosensitivity | Sulfonamides, amiodarone, tetracyclines, fluoroquinolones | Sat for photo |
| Rash (Stevens-Johnson syndrome) | Anti-epileptic drugs (especially lamotrigine), allopurinol, sulfa drugs, penicillin | Steven Johnson has epileptic allergy to sulfa drugs and penicillin |
| Teeth discoloration | Tetracyclines | Teethracyclines |
| Tendon/cartilage damage | Fluoroquinolones | |

## Drug reactions—neurologic

| DRUG REACTION | CAUSAL AGENTS | NOTES |
|---|---|---|
| Cinchonism | Quinidine, quinine | Can present with tinnitus, hearing/vision loss, psychosis, and cognitive impairment |
| Parkinson-like syndrome | Antipsychotics, metoclopramide | Cogwheel rigidity of arm |
| Peripheral neuropathy | Platinum agents (eg, cisplatin), isoniazid, vincristine, paclitaxtel, phenytoin | Cis, it's very painful peripherally |
| Idiopathic intracranial hypertension | Vitamin A, growth hormones, tetracyclines | Always grow head tension |
| Seizures | Isoniazid, bupropion, imipenem/cilastatin, tramadol | With seizures, I bit my tongue |
| Tardive dyskinesia | Antipsychotics, metoclopramide | |
| Visual disturbances | Topiramate (blurred vision/diplopia, haloes), hydroxychloroquine (↓ visual acuity, visual field defects), digoxin (yellow-tinged vision), isoniazid (optic neuritis), ivabradine (luminous phenomena), PDE-5 inhibitors (blue-tinged vision), ethambutol (color vision changes) | These horrible drugs iirritate Precious eyes |

## Drug reactions—renal/genitourinary

| DRUG REACTION | CAUSAL AGENTS | NOTES |
|---|---|---|
| Fanconi syndrome | Cisplatin, ifosfamide, expired tetracyclines, tenofovir | |
| Hemorrhagic cystitis | Cyclophosphamide, ifosfamide | Prevent by coadministering with mesna |
| Interstitial nephritis | Diuretics (Pee), NSAIDs (Pain-free), Penicillins and cephalosporins, PPIs, rifamPin, sulfa drugs | Remember the 5 P's |
| Nephrotoxicity | Cisplatin, aminoglycosides, amphotericin, vancomycin | |

## Drug reactions—respiratory

| DRUG REACTION | CAUSAL AGENTS | NOTES |
|---|---|---|
| Dry cough | ACE inhibitors | |
| Pulmonary fibrosis | Methotrexate, nitrofurantoin, carmustine, bleomycin, busulfan, amiodarone | My nose cannot breathe bad air |

## Drug reactions—multiorgan

| DRUG REACTION | CAUSAL AGENTS | NOTES |
|---|---|---|
| Antimuscarinic | Atropine, TCAs, $H_1$-blockers, antipsychotics | |
| Disulfiram-like reaction | 1st-generation sulfonylureas, procarbazine, certain cephalosporins, griseofulvin, metronidazole | Sorry pals, can't go mingle |

| **Drugs affecting pupil size** | ↑ pupil size (mydriasis) | ↓ pupil size (miosis) |
|---|---|---|
| | Anticholinergics (eg, atropine, TCAs, tropicamide, scopolamine, antihistamines) Indirect sympathomimetics (eg, amphetamines, cocaine, LSD), meperidine Direct sympathomimetics | Sympatholytics (eg, α₂-agonists) Opioids (except meperidine) Parasympathomimetics (eg, pilocarpine), organophosphates |

Radial muscle contraction
($\alpha_1$ receptor mediated)

Sphincter muscle contraction
($M_3$ receptor mediated)

---

**Cytochrome P-450 interactions (selected)**

| Inducers (+) | Substrates | Inhibitors (−) |
|---|---|---|
| St. John's wort Phenytoin Phenobarbital Modafinil Nevirapine Rifampin Griseofulvin Carbamazepine Chronic alcohol overuse | Theophylline OCPs Anti-epileptics Warfarin | Sodium valproate Isoniazid Cimetidine Ketoconazole Fluconazole Acute alcohol overuse Chloramphenicol Erythromycin/clarithromycin Sulfonamides Ciprofloxacin Omeprazole Amiodarone Ritonavir Grapefruit juice |
| St. John's funny funny (phen-phen) mom never refuses greasy **carbs** and **chronic alcohol** | The OCPs are anti-war | SICK FACES come when I am really drinking grapefruit juice |

---

**Sulfa drugs**

Sulfonamide antibiotics, Sulfasalazine, Probenecid, Furosemide, Acetazolamide, Celecoxib, Thiazides, Sulfonylureas. Patients with sulfa allergies may develop fever, urinary tract infection, Stevens-Johnson syndrome, hemolytic anemia, thrombocytopenia, agranulocytosis, acute interstitial nephritis, and urticaria (hives), and photosensitivity.

Scary Sulfa Pharm FACTS

## ▶ PHARMACOLOGY—MISCELLANEOUS

### Drug names

| ENDING | CATEGORY | EXAMPLE |
| --- | --- | --- |
| **Antimicrobial** | | |
| -asvir | NS5A inhibitor | Ledipasvir |
| -bendazole | Antiparasitic/antihelminthic | Mebendazole |
| -buvir | NS5B inhibitor | Sofosbuvir |
| -cillin | Transpeptidase inhibitor | Ampicillin |
| -conazole | Ergosterol synthesis inhibitor | Ketoconazole |
| -cycline | Protein synthesis inhibitor | Tetracycline |
| -floxacin | Fluoroquinolone | Ciprofloxacin |
| -mivir | Neuraminidase inhibitor | Oseltamivir |
| -navir | Protease inhibitor | Ritonavir |
| -ovir | Viral DNA polymerase inhibitor | Acyclovir |
| -previr | NS3/4A inhibitor | Grazoprevir |
| -tegravir | Integrase inhibitor | Dolutegravir |
| -thromycin | Macrolide | Azithromycin |
| **Antineoplastic** | | |
| -case | Recombinant uricase | Rasburicase |
| -mustine | Nitrosourea | Carmustine |
| -platin | Platinum compound | Cisplatin |
| -poside | Topoisomerase II inhibitor | Etoposide |
| -rubicin | Anthracycline | Doxorubicin |
| -taxel | Taxane | Paclitaxel |
| -tecan | Topoisomerase I inhibitor | Irinotecan |
| **CNS** | | |
| -flurane | Inhaled anesthetic | Sevoflurane |
| -apine, -idone | Atypical antipsychotic | Quetiapine, risperidone |
| -azine | Typical antipsychotic | Thioridazine |
| -barbital | Barbiturate | Phenobarbital |
| -benazine | VMAT inhibitor | Tetrabenazine |
| -caine | Local anesthetic | Lidocaine |
| -capone | COMT inhibitor | Entacapone |
| -curium, -curonium | Nondepolarizing neuromuscular blocker | Atracurium, pancuronium |
| -giline | MAO-B inhibitor | Selegiline |
| -ipramine, -triptyline | TCA | Imipramine, amitriptyline |
| -triptan | $5\text{-HT}_{1B/1D}$ agonist | Sumatriptan |
| -zepam, -zolam | Benzodiazepine | Diazepam, alprazolam |

**Drug names** *(continued)*

| ENDING | CATEGORY | EXAMPLE |
|---|---|---|
| **Autonomic** | | |
| -chol | Cholinergic agonist | Bethanechol |
| -olol | β-blocker | Propranolol |
| -stigmine | AChE inhibitor | Neostigmine |
| -terol | $\beta_2$-agonist | Albuterol |
| -zosin | $\alpha_1$-blocker | Prazosin |
| **Cardiovascular** | | |
| -afil | PDE-5 inhibitor | Sildenafil |
| -dipine | Dihydropyridine $Ca^{2+}$ channel blocker | Amlodipine |
| -parin | Low-molecular-weight heparin | Enoxaparin |
| -plase | Thrombolytic | Alteplase |
| -pril | ACE inhibitor | Captopril |
| -sartan | Angiotensin-II receptor blocker | Losartan |
| -xaban | Direct factor Xa inhibitor | Apixaban |
| **Metabolic** | | |
| -gliflozin | SGLT-2 inhibitor | Dapagliflozin |
| -glinide | Meglitinide | Repaglinide |
| -gliptin | DPP-4 inhibitor | Sitagliptin |
| -glitazone | PPAR-γ activator | Pioglitazone |
| -glutide | GLP-1 analog | Liraglutide |
| -statin | HMG-CoA reductase inhibitor | Lovastatin |
| **Other** | | |
| -caftor | CFTR modulator | Lumacaftor |
| -dronate | Bisphosphonate | Alendronate |
| -lukast | CysLT1 receptor blocker | Montelukast |
| -lutamide | Androgen receptor inhibitor | Flutamide |
| -pitant | $NK_1$ blocker | Aprepitant |
| -prazole | Proton pump inhibitor | Omeprazole |
| -prost | Prostaglandin analog | Latanoprost |
| -sentan | Endothelin receptor antagonist | Bosentan |
| -setron | $5-HT_3$ blocker | Ondansetron |
| -steride | 5α-reductase inhibitor | Finasteride |
| -tadine | $H_1$-antagonist | Loratadine |
| -tidine | $H_2$-antagonist | Cimetidine |
| -trozole | Aromatase inhibitor | Anastrozole |
| -vaptan | ADH antagonist | Tolvaptan |

**Biologic agents**

| ENDING | CATEGORY | EXAMPLE |
|---|---|---|
| **Monoclonal antibodies (-mab)—target overexpressed cell surface receptors** | | |
| -ximab | Chimeric human-mouse monoclonal antibody | Rituximab |
| -zumab | Humanized monoclonal antibody | Bevacizumab |
| -umab | Human monoclonal antibody | Denosumab |
| **Small molecule inhibitors (-ib)—target intracellular molecules** | | |
| -ciclib | Cyclin-dependent kinase inhibitor | Palbociclib |
| -coxib | COX-2 inhibitor | Celecoxib |
| -parib | Poly(ADP-ribose) polymerase inhibitor | Olaparib |
| -rafenib | BRAF inhibitor | Vemurafenib |
| -tinib | Tyrosine kinase inhibitor | Imatinib |
| -zomib | Proteasome inhibitor | Bortezomib |
| **Interleukin receptor modulators (-kin)—agonists and antagonists of interleukin receptors** | | |
| -leukin | Interleukin-2 agonist/analog | Aldesleukin |
| -kinra | Interleukin receptor antagonist | Anakinra |

# Public Health Sciences

"Medicine is a science of uncertainty and an art of probability."
—Sir William Osler

"People will forget what you said, people will forget what you did, but people will never forget how you made them feel."
—Maya Angelou

"On a long enough timeline, the survival rate for everyone drops to zero."
—Chuck Palahniuk, Fight Club

A heterogenous mix of epidemiology, biostatistics, ethics, law, healthcare delivery, patient safety, quality improvement, and more falls under the heading of public health sciences. Biostatistics and epidemiology are the foundations of evidence-based medicine and are very high yield. Make sure you can quickly apply biostatistical equations such as sensitivity, specificity, and predictive values in a problem-solving format. Also, know how to set up your own $2 \times 2$ tables, and beware questions that switch the columns. Quality improvement and patient safety topics were introduced a few years ago on the exam and represent trends in health system science. Medical ethics questions often require application of principles. Typically, you are presented with a patient scenario and then asked how you would respond. In this edition, we provide further details on communication skills and patient care given their growing emphasis on the exam. Effective communication is essential to the physician-patient partnership. Physicians must seek opportunities to connect with patients, understand their perspectives, express empathy, and form shared decisions and realistic goals.

▶ PUBLIC HEALTH SCIENCES—EPIDEMIOLOGY AND BIOSTATISTICS

## Observational studies

| STUDY TYPE | DESIGN | MEASURES/EXAMPLE |
|---|---|---|
| Case series | Describes several individual patients with the same diagnosis, treatment, or outcome. | Description of clinical findings and symptoms. Has no comparison group, thus cannot show risk factor association with disease. |
| Cross-sectional study | Frequency of disease and frequency of risk-related factors are assessed in the present. Asks, "What is happening?" | Disease prevalence. Can show risk factor association with disease, but does not establish causality. |
| Case-control study | Retrospectively compares a group of people with disease to a group without disease. Looks to see if odds of prior exposure or risk factor differ by disease state. Asks, "What happened?" | Odds ratio (OR). Control the case in the OR. Patients with COPD had higher odds of a smoking history than those without COPD. |
| Cohort study | Compares a group with a given exposure or risk factor to a group without such exposure. Looks to see if exposure or risk factor is associated with later development of disease. Can be prospective or retrospective, but risk factor has to be present prior to disease development. | Disease incidence. Relative risk (RR). People who smoke had a higher risk of developing COPD than people who do not. Cohort = relative risk. |
| Twin concordance study | Compares the frequency with which both monozygotic twins vs both dizygotic twins develop the same disease. | Measures heritability and influence of environmental factors ("nature vs nurture"). |
| Adoption study | Compares behavioral traits/genetics in siblings raised by biological vs adoptive parents. | Measures heritability and influence of environmental factors. |
| Ecological study | Compares frequency of disease and frequency of risk-related factors across populations. Measures population data not necessarily applicable to individuals (ecological fallacy). | Used to monitor population health. COPD prevalence was higher in more polluted cities. |

| | |
|---|---|
| **Clinical therapeutic trial** | Experimental study involving humans. Compares therapeutic benefits of ≥ 2 interventions (eg, treatment vs placebo, treatment vs treatment). Study quality improves when clinical trial is randomized, controlled, and double-blinded (ie, neither subject nor researcher knows whether the subject is in the treatment or control group). Triple-blind refers to additional blinding of the researchers analyzing the data. |

Crossover clinical trial—compares the effect of a series of ≥ 2 treatments on a subject. Order in which subjects receive treatments is randomized. Washout period occurs between treatments. Allows subjects to serve as their own controls.

Intention-to-treat analysis—all subjects are analyzed according to their original, randomly assigned treatment. No one is excluded, ie, once randomized, always analyzed. Attempts to avoid bias from attrition, crossover, and nonrandom noncompliance, but may dilute the true effects of intervention.

As-treated analysis—all subjects are analyzed according to the treatment they actually received. ↑ risk of bias.

Per-protocol analysis—subjects who fail to complete treatment as originally, randomly assigned are excluded. ↑ risk of bias.

Clinical trials occur after preclinical studies and consist of five phases ("Can **I SWIM**?").

| | Preclinical | Phase 0 | Phase 1 | Phase 2 | Phase 3 | Phase 4 |
|---|---|---|---|---|---|---|
| | Test drug in lab animals and in vitro experiments | Initial pharmacokinetic and pharmacodynamic assessment via microdosing. Often skipped. | Safety assessment via dose escalation. Determine maximum tolerable dose. | Efficacy assessment (does it Work?) Provides additional data on short-term adverse effects. | Effectiveness assessment via comparison with current standard of care/placebo (any Improvement?) | Provides data on long-term or rare adverse effects (can it stay on the Market?) |
| **Sample** | | Very small number of healthy volunteers or patients with disease of interest. Open label. | Small number of healthy volunteers or patients with disease of interest. Open label. | Moderate number of patients with disease of interest. Randomized, controlled, anonymized. | Large number of patients with disease of interest. Randomized, controlled, anonymized. | Postmarketing surveillance of patients with disease of interest. Open label. |

FDA approval

| | |
|---|---|
| **Off-label drug use** | Use of a drug to treat a disease in a form, population group, or dosage that is not specifically approved by the FDA. Reasons for off-label use include treatment of an illness with no approved pharmacologic treatment or exploring alternative treatments after failure of approved options. Example: use of tricyclic antidepressants for treating neuropathic/chronic pain. |

| | |
|---|---|
| **Bradford Hill criteria** | A group of principles that provide limited support (ie, necessary but not sufficient criteria) for establishing evidence of a causal relationship between presumed cause and effect. |
| Strength | Association does not necessarily imply causation, but the stronger the association, the more evidence for causation. |
| Consistency | Repeated observations of the findings in multiple distinct samples. |
| Specificity | The more specific the presumed cause is to the effect, the stronger the evidence for causation. |
| Temporality | The presumed cause precedes the effect by an expected amount of time. |
| Biological gradient | Greater effect observed with greater exposure to the presumed cause (dose-response relationship). |
| Plausibility | A conceivable mechanism exists by which the cause may lead to the effect. |
| Coherence | The presumed cause and effect do not conflict with existing scientific consensus. |
| Experiment | Empirical evidence supporting the presumed cause and effect (eg, animal studies, in vitro studies). |
| Analogy | The presumed cause and effect are comparable to a similar, established cause and effect. |

**Quantifying risk**

Definitions and formulas are based on the classic $2 \times 2$ or contingency table.

Disease or outcome

|  | ⊕ | ⊖ |
|---|---|---|
| Exposure or intervention ⊕ | a | b |
| ⊖ | c | d |

| TERM | DEFINITION | EXAMPLE | FORMULA |
|---|---|---|---|
| Odds ratio | Typically used in case-control studies. Represents the odds of exposure among cases (a/c) vs odds of exposure among controls (b/d). OR = 1 → odds of exposure are equal in cases and controls. OR > 1 → odds of exposure are greater in cases. OR < 1 → odds of exposure are greater in controls. | If in a case-control study, 20/30 patients with lung cancer and 5/25 healthy individuals report smoking, the **OR** is 8; so the patients with lung cancer are 8 times more likely to have a history of smoking. You take a **case** to the **OR**. | $OR = \dfrac{a/c}{b/d} = \dfrac{ad}{bc}$ <br><br> | a 20 | b 5 | <br> | c 10 | d 20 | |
| Relative risk | Typically used in cohort studies. Risk of developing disease in the exposed group divided by risk in the unexposed group. RR = 1 → no association between exposure and disease. RR > 1 → exposure associated with ↑ disease occurrence. RR < 1 → exposure associated with ↓ disease occurrence. | If 5/10 people exposed to radiation are diagnosed with cancer, and 1/10 people not exposed to radiation are diagnosed with cancer, the RR is 5; so people exposed to radiation have a 5 times greater risk of developing cancer. For rare diseases (low prevalence), OR approximates RR. | $RR = \dfrac{a/(a+b)}{c/(c+d)}$ <br><br> | a 5 | b 5 | <br> | c 1 | d 9 | |
| Relative risk reduction | The proportion of risk reduction attributable to the intervention/treatment (ART) as compared to a control (ARC). | If 2% of patients who receive a flu shot develop the flu, while 8% of unvaccinated patients develop the flu, then RR = 2/8 = 0.25, and RRR = 0.75. | $RRR = 1 - RR$ <br> $RRR = \dfrac{(ARC - ART)}{ARC}$ |
| Attributable risk | The difference in risk between exposed and unexposed groups. | If risk of lung cancer in people who smoke is 21% and risk in people who don't smoke is 1%, then the attributable risk is 20%. | $AR = \dfrac{a}{a+b} - \dfrac{c}{c+d}$ <br> $AR\% = \dfrac{RR - 1}{RR} \times 100$ |
| Absolute risk reduction | The difference in risk (not the proportion) attributable to the intervention as compared to a control. | If 8% of people who receive a placebo vaccine develop the flu vs 2% of people who receive a flu vaccine, then ARR = 8%–2% = 6% = 0.06. | $ARR = \dfrac{c}{c+d} - \dfrac{a}{a+b}$ |
| Number needed to treat | Number of patients who need to be treated for 1 patient to benefit. Lower number = better treatment. | | $NNT = 1/ARR$ |
| Number needed to harm | Number of patients who need to be exposed to a risk factor for 1 patient to be harmed. Higher number = safer exposure. | | $NNH = 1/AR$ |
| Case fatality rate | Percentage of deaths occurring among those with disease. | If 4 patients die among 10 cases of meningitis, case fatality rate is 40%. | $CFR\% = \dfrac{deaths}{cases} \times 100$ |

## Quantifying risk *(continued)*

| TERM | DEFINITION | EXAMPLE | FORMULA |
|---|---|---|---|
| Mortality rate | Number of deaths (in general or due to specific cause) within a population over a defined period. | If 80 people in a town of 10,000 die over 2 years, mortality rate is 4 per 1000 per year. | Deaths/1000 people per year. |
| Attack rate | Proportion of exposed people who become ill. | If 80 people in a town are exposed and 60 people become ill, attack rate is 75%. | $\dfrac{\text{People who become ill}}{\text{Total people exposed}}$ |

---

**Demographic transition**

As a country proceeds to higher levels of development, birth and mortality rates decline to varying degrees, changing the age composition of the population.

**Population pyramid**

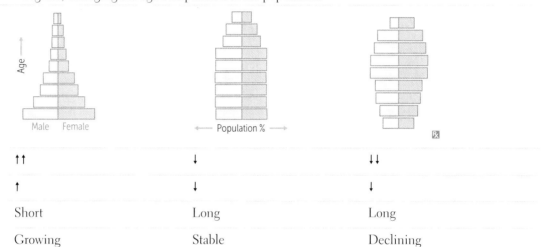

| | | | |
|---|---|---|---|
| Birth rate | ↑↑ | ↓ | ↓↓ |
| Mortality rate | ↑ | ↓ | ↓ |
| Life expectancy | Short | Long | Long |
| Population | Growing | Stable | Declining |

---

**Likelihood ratio**

$$LR^+ = \frac{\text{probability of positive result in patient with disorder}}{\text{probability of positive result in patient without disorder}} = \frac{\text{sensitivity}}{1 - \text{specificity}} = \frac{\text{TP rate}}{\text{FP rate}}$$

$$LR^- = \frac{\text{probability of negative result in patient with disorder}}{\text{probability of negative result in patient without disorder}} = \frac{1 - \text{sensitivity}}{\text{specificity}} = \frac{\text{FN rate}}{\text{TN rate}}$$

$LR^+ > 10$ indicates a highly specific test, while $LR^- < 0.1$ indicates a highly sensitive test.
Pretest odds × LR = posttest odds. Posttest probability = posttest odds / (posttest odds + 1).

---

**Kaplan-Meier curve**

Used to estimate probability of survival over time. Graphic representation shows the survival probabilities (y-axis) vs length of time (x-axis). Useful for displaying "time-to-event" data.

Outcomes examined may include any event, but frequently include mortality.

Survival probability = 1 – (event probability).

*P* value for the survival difference can be calculated using log rank test or Cox regression.

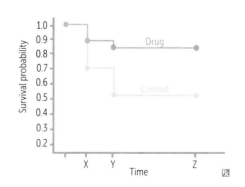

| | **Evaluation of diagnostic tests** | Sensitivity and specificity are fixed properties of a test. PPV and NPV vary depending on disease prevalence in population being tested.
Test efficiency =
$(TP + TN)/(TP + FN + FP + TN)$ |

| | | Disease |
| | | $\oplus$ | $\ominus$ | |
|---|---|---|---|---|
| Test | $\oplus$ | TP | FP | PPV $= TP/(TP + FP)$ |
| | $\ominus$ | FN | TN | NPV $= TN/(TN + FN)$ |
| | | Sensitivity $= TP/(TP + FN)$ | Specificity $= TN/(TN + FP)$ | Prevalence $\frac{TP + FN}{(TP + FN + FP + TN)}$ |

**Sensitivity (true-positive rate)**

Proportion of all people with disease who test positive, or the ability of a test to correctly identify those with the disease.
Value approaching 100% is desirable for **ruling out** disease and indicates a **low false-negative rate**.

$= TP / (TP + FN)$
$= 1 - FN$ rate
**SN-N-OUT** = highly **SeN**sitive test, when Negative, rules **OUT** disease
High sensitivity test used for screening

**Specificity (true-negative rate)**

Proportion of all people without disease who test negative, or the ability of a test to correctly identify those without the disease.
Value approaching 100% is desirable for **ruling in** disease and indicates a **low false-positive rate**.

$= TN / (TN + FP)$
$= 1 - FP$ rate
**SP-P-IN** = highly **SP**ecific test, when Positive, rules **IN** disease
High specificity test used for confirmation after a positive screening test

**Positive predictive value**

Probability that a person who has a positive test result actually has the disease.

$PPV = TP / (TP + FP)$
PPV varies directly with pretest probability (baseline risk, such as prevalence of disease): high pretest probability → high PPV

**Negative predictive value**

Probability that a person with a negative test result actually does not have the disease.

$NPV = TN / (TN + FN)$
NPV varies inversely with prevalence or pretest probability

Possible cutoff values for $\oplus$ vs $\ominus$ test result
**A** = 100% sensitivity cutoff value
**B** = practical compromise between specificity and sensitivity
**C** = 100% specificity cutoff value

| Lowering the cutoff value: **B → A** (↑ FP ↓ FN) | ↑ Sensitivity ↑ NPV ↓ Specificity ↓ PPV |
| Raising the cutoff value: **B → C** (↑ FN ↓ FP) | ↑ Specificity ↑ PPV ↓ Sensitivity ↓ NPV |

Note: In diseases where diagnosis is based on lower values (eg, anemia), the TP and TN are switched in the graph, ie, ↓ sensitivity and ↓ NPV, and vice-versa.

**Receiver operating characteristic curve**

ROC curve demonstrates how well a diagnostic test can distinguish between 2 groups (eg, disease vs healthy). Plots the true-positive rate (sensitivity) against the false-positive rate (1 − specificity).
The better performing test will have a higher area under the curve (AUC), with the curve closer to the upper left corner.

## Precision vs accuracy

| | | |
|---|---|---|
| **Precision (reliability)** | The consistency and **reproducibility** of a test. The absence of random variation in a test. | Random error ↓ precision in a test. ↑ precision → ↓ standard deviation. ↑ precision → ↑ statistical power (1 − β). |
| **Accuracy (validity)** | The closeness of test results to the true values. The absence of systematic error or bias in a test. | Systematic error ↓ accuracy in a test. |

## Incidence vs prevalence

$$\text{Incidence} = \frac{\text{\# of new cases}}{\text{\# of people at risk}} \quad \text{(per unit of time)}$$

$$\text{Prevalence} = \frac{\text{\# of existing cases}}{\text{Total \# of people in a population}} \quad \begin{array}{l}\text{(at a point in} \\ \text{time)}\end{array}$$

$$\frac{\text{Prevalence}}{1 - \text{prevalence}} = \text{Incidence rate} \times \begin{array}{l}\text{average duration} \\ \text{of disease}\end{array}$$

Prevalence ≈ incidence for short duration disease (eg, common cold).

Prevalence > incidence for chronic diseases, due to large # of existing cases (eg, diabetes).

**Incidence** looks at new cases (**incidents**).

Prevalence looks at **all** current cases.

Prevalence ~ pretest probability. ↑ prevalence → ↑ PPV and ↓ NPV.

| SITUATION | INCIDENCE | PREVALENCE |
|---|---|---|
| ↑ survival time | — | ↑ |
| ↑ mortality rate | — | ↓ |
| Faster recovery time | — | ↓ |
| Extensive vaccine administration | ↓ | ↓ |
| ↓ risk factors | ↓ | ↓ |
| ↑ diagnostic sensitivity | ↑ | ↑ |
| New effective treatment started | — | ↓ |
| ↓ contact between infected and noninfected patients with airborne infectious disease | ↓ | ↓ |

## Bias and study errors

| TYPE | DEFINITION | EXAMPLES | STRATEGIES TO REDUCE BIAS |
|------|-----------|----------|--------------------------|
| **Recruiting participants** | | | |
| **Selection bias** | Nonrandom sampling or treatment allocation of subjects such that study population is not representative of target population<br>Most commonly a sampling bias<br>Convenience sampling—patients are enrolled on basis of ease of contact | Berkson bias—cases and/or controls selected from hospitals (bedside bias) are less healthy and have different exposures<br>Attrition bias—participants lost to follow up have a different prognosis than those who complete the study | Randomization (creates groups with similar distributions of known and unknown variables)<br>Ensure the choice of the right comparison/reference group |
| **Performing study** | | | |
| **Recall bias** | Awareness of disorder alters recall by subjects; common in retrospective studies | Patients with disease recall exposure after learning of similar cases | Decrease time from exposure to follow-up; use medical records as sources |
| **Measurement bias** | Information is gathered in a systemically distorted manner | Using a faulty automatic sphygmomanometer<br>Hawthorne effect—participants change behavior upon awareness of being observed | Use objective, standardized, and previously tested methods of data collection that are planned ahead of time<br>Use placebo group |
| **Procedure bias** | Subjects in different groups are not treated the same | Patients in treatment group spend more time in highly specialized hospital units | Blinding (masking) and use of placebo reduce influence of participants and researchers on procedures and interpretation of outcomes as neither are aware of group assignments |
| **Observer-expectancy bias** | Researcher's belief in the efficacy of a treatment changes the outcome of that treatment (also called Pygmalion effect) | An observer expecting treatment group to show signs of recovery is more likely to document positive outcomes | |
| **Interpreting results** | | | |
| **Lead-time bias** | Early detection interpreted as ↑ survival, but the disease course has not changed | Breast cancer diagnosed early by mammography may appear to exaggerate survival time because patients are known to have the cancer for longer | Measure "back-end" survival (adjust survival according to the severity of disease at the time of diagnosis) |
| **Length-time bias** | Screening test detects diseases with long latency period, while those with shorter latency period become symptomatic earlier | A slowly progressive cancer is more likely detected by a screening test than a rapidly progressive cancer | A randomized controlled trial assigning subjects to the screening program or to no screening |

## Confounding vs effect modification

| TYPE | DEFINITION | EXAMPLES | STRATEGIES TO REDUCE BIAS |
|---|---|---|---|
| Confounding | Factor related to **both exposure and outcome** (but not on causal path) distorts effect on outcome<br>No true association exists between the outcome and the factor in some subgroups of the factor | An uncontrolled study shows association between drinking coffee and lung cancer; however, people who drink coffee may smoke more, which could account for the association | Crossover studies (with subject as their own controls)<br>Matching (patients with similar characteristics in both treatment and control groups)<br>Analytic techniques (eg, regression analysis when confounding variables are known and were measured) |
| Effect modification | Exposure leads to different outcomes in subgroups stratified by factor<br>True association exists | A study among women using OCPs showed significant risk of DVT, but when these data were stratified by smoking habits, there was a very strong association between OPC use and DVT among smokers, but there was no such association in people who do not smoke | Stratified analysis (eg, after testing for interaction between OCP and smoking, analyze risk among smokers and nonsmokers) |

### Confounding

Crude analysis

Drinking coffee ⟶ Lung cancer

Stratified analysis

Smokers    Drinking coffee ⟶ Lung cancer

Nonsmokers    Drinking coffee ----→ Lung cancer

Note: Association disappeared after stratification.

### Effect modification

Crude analysis

OCP use ⟶ DVT

Stratified analysis

Smokers    OCP use ⟶ DVT

Nonsmokers    OCP use ----→ DVT

Note: Association was strong in one subgroup with weak/no association in the other subgroup.

⟶ Strong association

⟶ Significant association

----→ Weak/no association

## Statistical distribution

| | | |
|---|---|---|
| **Measures of central tendency** | Mean = (sum of values)/(total number of values). | Most affected by outliers (extreme values). |
| | Median = middle value of a list of data sorted from least to greatest. | If there is an even number of values, the median will be the average of the middle two values. |
| | Mode = most common value. | Least affected by outliers. |
| **Measures of dispersion** | Standard deviation = how much variability exists in a set of values, around the mean of these values. | $\sigma$ = SD; n = sample size.<br>Variance = $(SD)^2$.<br>SE = $\sigma/\sqrt{n}$. |
| | Standard error = an estimate of how much variability exists in a (theoretical) set of sample means around the true population mean. | SE ↓ as n ↑. |
| **Normal distribution** | Gaussian, also called bell-shaped.<br>Mean = median = mode.<br>For normal distribution, mean is the best measure of central tendency.<br>For skewed data, median is a better measure of central tendency than mean. | 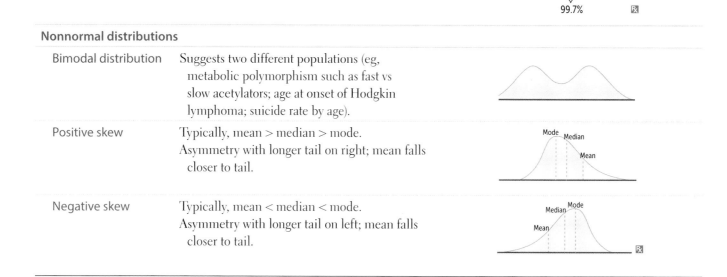 |

## Nonnormal distributions

| | |
|---|---|
| **Bimodal distribution** | Suggests two different populations (eg, metabolic polymorphism such as fast vs slow acetylators; age at onset of Hodgkin lymphoma; suicide rate by age). |
| **Positive skew** | Typically, mean > median > mode.<br>Asymmetry with longer tail on right; mean falls closer to tail. |
| **Negative skew** | Typically, mean < median < mode.<br>Asymmetry with longer tail on left; mean falls closer to tail. |

## Statistical hypothesis testing

| | |
|---|---|
| **Null hypothesis** | Also called $H_0$. Hypothesis of no difference or relationship (eg, there is no association between the disease and the risk factor in the population). |
| **Alternative hypothesis** | Also called $H_1$. Hypothesis of some difference or relationship (eg, there is some association between the disease and the risk factor in the population). |
| **P value** | Probability of obtaining test results at least as extreme as those observed during the test, assuming that $H_0$ is correct. Commonly accepted as 0.05 (< 5% of such repeated tests would show results that extreme just by chance alone). |

## Outcomes of statistical hypothesis testing

| Correct result | Stating that there is an effect or difference when one exists ($H_0$ rejected in favor of $H_1$). Stating that there is no effect or difference when none exists ($H_0$ not rejected). |
|---|---|

Reality

| | $H_1$ | $H_0$ |
|---|---|---|
| Study rejects $H_0$ | Power $(1 - \beta)$ | $\alpha$ Type I error |
| Study does not reject $H_0$ | $\beta$ Type II error | |

Blue shading = correct result.

### Testing errors

| Type I error ($\alpha$) | Stating that there is an effect or difference when none exists ($H_0$ incorrectly rejected in favor of $H_1$). $\alpha$ is the probability of making a type I error (usually 0.05 is chosen). If $P < \alpha$, then assuming $H_0$ is true, the probability of obtaining the test results would be less than the probability of making a type I error. $H_0$ is therefore rejected as false. Statistical significance ≠ clinical significance. | Also called false-positive error. 1st time boy cries wolf, the town believes there is a wolf, but there is not (false positive). You can never "prove" $H_1$, but you can reject the $H_0$ as being very unlikely. |
|---|---|---|
| Type II error ($\beta$) | Stating that there is not an effect or difference when one exists ($H_0$ is not rejected when it is in fact false). $\beta$ is the probability of making a type II error. $\beta$ is related to statistical power $(1 - \beta)$, which is the probability of rejecting $H_0$ when it is false. ↑ power and ↓ $\beta$ by: <br> ▪ ↑ sample size <br> ▪ ↑ expected effect size <br> ▪ ↑ precision of measurement <br> ▪ ↑ $\alpha$ level (↑ statistical significance level). | Also called false-negative error. 2nd time boy cries wolf, the town believes there is no wolf, but there is one. If you ↑ sample size, you ↑ power. There is power in numbers. Generally, when type I error increases, type II error decreases. |

| **Statistical vs clinical significance** | Statistical significance—defined by the likelihood of study results being due to chance. If there is a high statistical significance, then there is a low probability that the results are due to chance. Clinical significance—measure of effect on treatment outcomes. An intervention with high clinical significance is likely to have a large impact on patient outcomes/measures. Some studies have a very high statistical significance, but the proposed intervention may have limited clinical impact/significance, eg, a study might show a statistical significance of lowered blood sugar levels by 1 mg/dL correlated with better outcomes, but this may not be clinically as important. |
|---|---|

| **Confidence interval** | Range of values within which the true mean of the population is expected to fall, with a specified probability.<br>$CI = 1 - \alpha$. The 95% CI (corresponding to $\alpha = 0.05$) is often used. As sample size increases, CI narrows.<br>CI for sample mean = $\bar{x} \pm Z(SE)$<br>For the 95% CI, $Z = 1.96$.<br>For the 99% CI, $Z = 2.58$. | $H_0$ is rejected (and results are significant) when:<br>▪ 95% CI for mean difference excludes 0<br>▪ 95% CI OR or RR excludes 1<br>▪ CIs between two groups do not overlap<br>$H_0$ is not rejected (and results are not significant) when:<br>▪ 95% CI for mean difference includes 0<br>▪ 95% CI OR or RR includes 1<br>▪ CIs between two groups do overlap |
|---|---|---|
| **Meta-analysis** | A method of statistical analysis that pools summary data (eg, means, RRs) from multiple studies for a more precise estimate of the size of an effect. Also estimates heterogeneity of effect sizes between studies.<br>Improves power, strength of evidence, and generalizability (external validity) of study findings. Limited by quality of individual studies and bias in study selection. | |

### Common statistical tests

| *t*-test | Checks differences between **means** of 2 groups. | Tea is **meant** for **2**.<br>Example: comparing the mean blood pressure between men and women. |
|---|---|---|
| ANOVA | Checks differences between means of 3 or more groups. | 3 words: **AN**alysis **O**f **VA**riance.<br>Example: comparing the mean blood pressure between members of 3 different ethnic groups. |
| Chi-square ($\chi^2$) | Checks differences between 2 or more percentages or proportions of **categorical** outcomes (not mean values). | Pronounce **chi-tegorical**.<br>Example: comparing the proportion of members of 3 age groups who have essential hypertension. |
| Fisher's exact test | Checks differences between 2 percentages or proportions of categorical, nominal outcomes. Use instead of chi-square test with small samples. | Example: comparing the percentage of 20 men and 20 women with hypertension. |

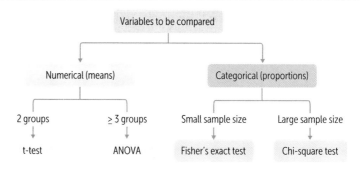

| **Pearson correlation coefficient** | A measure of the linear correlation between two variables. *r* is always between −1 and +1. The closer the absolute value of *r* is to 1, the stronger the linear correlation between the 2 variables. Variance is how much the measured values differ from the average value in a data set. |
| --- | --- |

Positive *r* value → positive correlation (as one variable ↑, the other variable ↑).
Negative *r* value → negative correlation (as one variable ↑, the other variable ↓).
Coefficient of determination = $r^2$ (amount of variance in one variable that can be explained by variance in the other variable). Correlation does not necessarily imply causation.

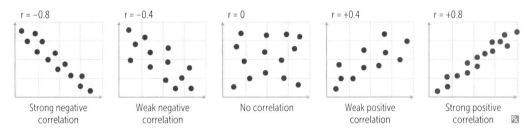

| r = −0.8 | r = −0.4 | r = 0 | r = +0.4 | r = +0.8 |
| --- | --- | --- | --- | --- |
| Strong negative correlation | Weak negative correlation | No correlation | Weak positive correlation | Strong positive correlation |

## ▶ PUBLIC HEALTH SCIENCES—ETHICS

### Core ethical principles

| **Autonomy** | Obligation to respect patients as individuals (truth-telling, confidentiality), to create conditions necessary for autonomous choice (informed consent), and to honor their preference in accepting or not accepting medical care. |
| --- | --- |
| **Beneficence** | "Do good." Physicians have a special ethical (fiduciary) duty to act in the patient's best interest. May conflict with autonomy (an informed patient has the right to decide) or what is best for society (eg, mandatory TB treatment). Traditionally, patient interest supersedes. Principle of double effect—facilitating comfort is prioritized over potential side effects (eg, respiratory depression with opioid use) for patients receiving end-of-life care. |
| **Nonmaleficence** | "Do no harm." Must be balanced against beneficence; if the benefits outweigh the risks, a patient may make an informed decision to proceed (most surgeries and medications fall into this category). |
| **Justice** | To treat persons fairly and equitably. This does not always imply equally (eg, triage). |

| **Decision-making capacity** | Physician must determine whether the patient is psychologically and legally capable of making a particular healthcare decision. Note that decisions made with capacity cannot be revoked simply if the patient later loses capacity. Intellectual disabilities and mental illnesses are not exclusion criteria unless the patient's condition presently impairs their ability to make healthcare decisions. Capacity is determined by a physician for a specific healthcare-related decision (eg, to refuse medical care). Competency is determined by a judge and usually refers to more global categories of decision-making (eg, legally unable to make any healthcare-related decision). | Four major components of decision-making: <br> ▪ Understanding (what do you know about your condition/proposed procedure/treatment?) <br> ▪ Appreciation (what does your condition mean to you? why do you think your doctor is recommending this course of treatment?) <br> ▪ Reasoning (how are you weighing your options?) <br> ▪ Expressing a choice (what would you like to do?) |
| --- | --- | --- |

| | | |
|---|---|---|
| **Informed consent** | A process (not just a document/signature) that requires:<br>▪ Disclosure: discussion of pertinent information, including risks/benefits (using medical interpreter, if needed)<br>▪ Understanding: ability to comprehend<br>▪ Capacity: ability to reason and make one's own decisions (distinct from competence, a legal determination)<br>▪ Voluntariness: freedom from coercion and manipulation<br>Patients must have a comprehensive understanding of their diagnosis and the risks/benefits of proposed treatment and alternative options, including no treatment.<br>Patients must be informed of their right to revoke written consent at any time, even orally. | Exceptions to informed consent (**WIPE** it away):<br>▪ **W**aiver—patient explicitly relinquishes the right of informed consent<br>▪ Legally **I**ncompetent—patient lacks decision-making capacity (obtain consent from legal surrogate)<br>▪ Therapeutic **P**rivilege—withholding information when disclosure would severely harm the patient or undermine informed decision-making capacity<br>▪ **E**mergency situation—implied consent may apply |
| **Consent for minors** | A minor is generally any person < 18 years old. Parental consent laws in relation to healthcare vary by state. In general, parental consent should be obtained, but exceptions exist for emergency treatment (eg, blood transfusions) or if minor is legally emancipated (eg, married, self-supporting, or in the military). | Situations in which parental consent is usually not required:<br>▪ **Sex** (contraception, STIs, prenatal care—usually not abortion)<br>▪ **Drugs** (substance use disorder treatment)<br>▪ **Rock and roll** (emergency/trauma)<br>Physicians should always encourage healthy minor-guardian communication.<br>Physician should seek a minor's assent (agreement of someone unable to legally consent) even if their consent is not required. |
| **Advance directives** | Instructions given by a patient in anticipation of the need for a medical decision. Details vary per state law. | |
| **Oral advance directive** | Incapacitated patient's prior oral statements commonly used as guide. Problems arise from variance in interpretation. If patient was informed, directive was specific, patient made a choice, and decision was repeated over time to multiple people, then the oral directive is more valid. | |
| **Written advance directive** | Delineates specific healthcare interventions that patient anticipates accepting or rejecting during treatment for a critical or life-threatening illness. A living will is an example. | |
| **Medical power of attorney** | Patient designates an agent to make medical decisions in the event that the patient loses decision-making capacity. Patient may also specify decisions in clinical situations. Can be revoked by patient if decision-making capacity is intact. More flexible than a living will. | |
| **Do not resuscitate order** | DNR order prohibits cardiopulmonary resuscitation (CPR). Patient may still consider other life-sustaining measures (eg, intubation, feeding tube, chemotherapy). | |

| | |
|---|---|
| **Ventilator-assisted life support** | Ideally, discussions with patients occur before ventilator support is necessary. However, information about patient preferences may be absent at the time patients require this intervention to survive. Medical decision-making frequently relies on surrogate decision-makers (patient identified or legally appointed) when discussing the continuation or withdrawal of ventilatory support, focusing on both the prognosis of the condition and the believed wishes of the patient. If surrogates indicate patient would not have wanted to receive life support with ventilation → withhold or withdraw life support regardless of what the surrogate prefers. If the decision is made to withhold or withdraw life support, involve palliative care, chaplain services, and the primary care physician in medical discussions with the family and provide emotional support. |
| **Surrogate decision-maker** | If a patient loses decision-making capacity and has not prepared an advance directive, individuals (surrogates) who know the patient must determine what the patient would have done. Priority of surrogates: **spouse** → adult **children** → **parents** → adult **siblings** → other relatives (the **spouse chips** in). |
| **Confidentiality** | Confidentiality respects patient privacy and autonomy. If the patient is incapacitated or the situation is emergent, disclosing information to family and friends should be guided by professional judgment of patient's best interest. The patient may voluntarily waive the right to confidentiality (eg, insurance company request).<br><br>General principles for exceptions to confidentiality:<br>▪ Potential physical harm to self or others is serious and imminent<br>▪ Alternative means to warn or protect those at risk is not possible<br>▪ Steps can be taken to prevent harm<br><br>Examples of exceptions to patient confidentiality (many are state specific) include the following ("The physician's good judgment **SAVED** the day"):<br>▪ Patients with active **S**uicidal/homicidal ideation<br>▪ **A**buse (children, older adults, and/or prisoners)<br>▪ Duty to protect—state-specific laws that sometimes allow physician to inform or somehow protect potential **V**ictim from harm<br>▪ Patients with **E**pilepsy and other impaired automobile drivers<br>▪ Reportable **D**iseases (eg, STIs, hepatitis, food poisoning); physicians may have a duty to warn public officials, who will then notify people at risk. Dangerous communicable diseases, such as TB or Ebola, may require involuntary treatment. |
| **Accepting gifts from patients** | A complex subject without definitive regulations. Some argue that the patient-physician relationship is strengthened through accepting a gift from a patient, while others argue that negative consequences outweigh the benefits of accepting any gift.<br><br>In practice, patients often present items such as cards, baked goods, and inexpensive gifts to physicians. The physician's decision to accept or decline is based on an individual assessment of whether or not the risk of harm outweighs the potential benefit.<br>▪ Physicians should not accept gifts that are inappropriately large or valuable.<br>▪ Gifts should not be accepted if the physician identifies that the gift could detrimentally affect patient care.<br>▪ Gifts that may cause emotional or financial stress for the patient should not be accepted.<br><br>If a gift violates any of the guidelines above, the best practice is to thank the patient for offering a kind gift, but politely indicate that it must be declined. During this conversation it should be emphasized that the incident does not influence the physician-patient relationship in any way. |

## ▶ PUBLIC HEALTH SCIENCES—COMMUNICATION SKILLS

### Patient-centered interviewing techniques

| | |
|---|---|
| Introduction | Introduce yourself and ask the patient their name and how they would like to be addressed. Address the patient by the name and pronouns given. Avoid making gender assumptions. Sit at eye level, near the patient, while facing them directly. |
| Agenda setting | Identify concerns and set goals by developing joint agenda between the physician and the patient. |
| Reflection | Actively listen and synthesize information offered by the patient, particularly with respect to primary concern(s). |
| Validation | Legitimize or affirm the patient's perspectives. |
| Recapitulation | Summarize what the patient has said so far to ensure correct interpretation. |
| Facilitation | Encourage the patient to speak freely without guiding responses or leading questions. Allow the patient to ask questions throughout the encounter. |

### Establishing rapport — PEARLS

| | |
|---|---|
| Partnership | Work together with patient to identify primary concerns and develop preferred solutions. |
| Empathy | Acknowledge the emotions displayed and demonstrate understanding of why the patient is feeling that way. |
| Apology | Take personal responsibility when appropriate. |
| Respect | Commend the patient for coming in to discuss a problem, pushing through challenging circumstances, keeping a positive attitude, or other constructive behaviors. |
| Legitimization | Assure patient that emotional responses are understandable or common. |
| Support | Reassure patient that you will work together through difficult times and offer appropriate resources. |

### Delivering bad news — SPIKES

| | |
|---|---|
| Setting | Offer in advance for the patient to bring support. Eliminate distractions, ensure privacy, and sit down with the patient to talk. |
| Perception | Determine the patient's understanding and expectations of the situation. |
| Invitation | Obtain the patient's permission to disclose the news and what level of detail is desired. |
| Knowledge | Share the information in small pieces without medical jargon, allowing time to process. Assess the patient's understanding. |
| Emotions | Acknowledge the patient's emotions, and provide opportunity to express them. Listen and offer empathetic responses. |
| Strategy | If the patient feels ready, discuss treatment options and goals of care. Offer an agenda for the next appointment. Giving control to the patient may be empowering. Ask how they feel a problem might be solved and what they would like to do about the plan of action. |

| | |
|---|---|
| **Gender- and sexuality-inclusive history taking** | Avoid making assumptions about sexual orientation, gender identity, gender expression, and behavior (eg, a patient who identifies as heterosexual may engage in same-sex sexual activity). |
| | Use gender-neutral terms when referring to the patient or the patient's family (eg, "partner" rather than "husband" or "wife") upon first meeting the patient until the patient instructs otherwise or uses specific pronouns. A patient's assigned sex at birth and gender identity may differ. Do not bring up gender or sexuality if it is not relevant to the visit (eg, a gender-nonconforming patient seeking care for a hand laceration). |
| | Consider stating what pronouns you use when you introduce yourself (eg, "I'm Dr. Smith, and I use she/her pronouns") and asking patients how they would like to be addressed. Also consider ways of being inclusive (eg, ensuring correct name and pronouns are in the EMR). |
| | Reassure them about the confidentiality of their visits and be sensitive to the fact that patients may not be open about their sexual orientation or gender identity to others in their life. |
| | Remember: trust is built over time, and listening to and learning from patients about how they would like to approach the topics discussed above is key. |
| **Cultural formulation interview** | Identify the problem through the patient's perspective. Ask the patient to describe the problem in their own words, or how the patient would describe the problem to their family and friends. |
| | Identify cultural perceptions of factors leading to a problem. Ask the patient to explain why they think they are experiencing their problem. |
| | Identify how the patient's background influences their problem. Ask the patient about what makes their problem better or worse. Investigate roles of family, community, and spirituality. |
| | Identify how culture may impact current and future interventions. Ask the patient if they have any concerns or suggestions about the current plan of treatment. If they do not want to follow medical advice, investigate if there is a way to combine their plans with the standard medical regimen. |
| | Identify possible barriers to care based on culture. Ask the patient if there is anything that would prevent them from seeking care in a standard medical institution. Probe for explanations and what may increase the chance of maintaining a good patient-physician relationship. |
| **Motivational interviewing** | Counseling technique to facilitate behavior modification by helping patients resolve ambivalence about change. Useful for many conditions (eg, nicotine dependence, obesity). Helpful when patient has some desire to change, but it does not require that the patient be committed to making the change. May involve asking patients to examine how their behavior interferes with their life or why they might want to change it. Assess barriers (eg, food access, untreated trauma) that may make behavior change difficult. |
| | Assessing a patient's readiness for change is also important for guiding physician-suggested goals. These goals should be Specific, Measurable, Achievable, Relevant, and Time bound (SMART). |
| **Trauma-informed care** | Patients with history of psychological trauma should receive thorough behavioral health screenings. Regularly assess mood, substance use, social supports, and suicide risk. |
| | Focus assessments on trauma-related symptoms that interfere with social and occupational function. Always be empathetic. Do not ask invasive questions requiring the patient to describe trauma in detail. Ask permission prior to discussion. |
| | Before the physical exam, reassure patients that they may signal to end it immediately if they experience too much physical or emotional discomfort. Offer the presence of additional staff for support. Psychological counseling may be indicated. Follow-up counseling is offered (or advised) as appropriate. Remember 4 R's: Realize, Recognize, Respond, Resist retraumatization. |

## Challenging patient and ethical scenarios

The most appropriate response is usually one that acknowledges the issues, validates emotions, and is open ended, empathetic, and patient centered. It often honors one or more of the principles of autonomy, beneficence, nonmaleficence, and justice. Appropriate responses are respectful of patients and other members of the healthcare team.

| SITUATION | APPROPRIATE RESPONSE |
| --- | --- |
| Patient does not follow the medical plan. | Determine whether there are financial, logistical, or other obstacles preventing the patient's adherence. Do not coerce the patient into adhering or refer the patient to another physician. Schedule regular follow-up visits to track patient progress. |
| Patient desires an unnecessary procedure. | Attempt to understand why the patient wants the procedure and address underlying concerns. Do not refuse to see the patient or refer to another physician. Avoid performing unnecessary procedures. |
| Patient has difficulty taking medications. | Determine what factors are involved in the patient's difficulties. If comprehension or memory are issues, use techniques such as providing written instructions, using the teach-back method, or simplifying treatment regimens. |
| Family members ask for information about patient's prognosis. | Avoid discussing issues with relatives without the patient's permission. |
| A patient's family member asks you not to disclose the results of a test if the prognosis is poor because the patient will be "unable to handle it." | Explore why the family member believes this would be detrimental, including possible cultural factors. Explain that if the patient would like to know information concerning care, it will not be withheld. However, if you believe the patient might seriously harm self or others if informed, you may invoke therapeutic privilege and withhold the information. |
| A 17-year-old is pregnant and requests an abortion. | Many states require parental notification or consent for minors for an abortion. Unless there are specific medical risks associated with pregnancy, a physician should not sway the patient's decision for, or against, an elective abortion (regardless of patient's age or fetal condition). Discuss options for terminating the pregnancy and refer to abortion care, if needed. |
| A 15-year-old is pregnant and wants to raise the child. The patient's parents want you to tell the patient to give the child up for adoption. | The patient retains the right to make decisions regarding the child, even if the patient's parents disagree. Provide information to the teenager about the practical aspects of caring for a baby. Discuss options for terminating the pregnancy, if requested. Encourage discussion between the patient and parents to reach the best decision. |
| A terminally ill patient requests physician-assisted dying. | The overwhelming majority of states prohibit most forms of physician-assisted dying. Physicians may, however, prescribe medically appropriate analgesics even if they potentially shorten the patient's life. |
| Patient is suicidal. | Assess the seriousness of the threat. If patient is actively suicidal with a plan, suggest remaining in the hospital voluntarily; patient may be hospitalized involuntarily if needed. |
| Patient states that you are attractive and asks if you would go on a date. | Use a chaperone if necessary. Romantic relationships with patients are never appropriate. Set firm professional boundaries with direct communication. Transition care to another physician if necessary. |
| A woman who had a mastectomy says she now feels "ugly." | Find out why the patient feels this way. Do not offer falsely reassuring statements (eg, "You still look good"). |
| Patient is angry about the long time spent in the waiting room. | Acknowledge the patient's anger, but do not take a patient's anger personally. Thank the patient for being patient and apologize for any inconvenience. Stay away from efforts to explain the delay. |
| Patient is upset with treatment received from another physician. | Suggest that the patient speak directly to that physician regarding the concern. If the problem is with a member of the office staff, reassure the patient you will speak to that person. |

## Challenging patient and ethical scenarios *(continued)*

| SITUATION | APPROPRIATE RESPONSE |
|---|---|
| An invasive test is performed on the wrong patient. | Regardless of the outcome, a physician is ethically obligated to inform a patient that a mistake has been made. |
| A patient requires a treatment not covered by insurance. | Discuss all treatment options with patients, even if some are not covered by their insurance companies. Inform patient of financial assistance programs. |
| A 7-year-old boy loses a sister to cancer and now feels responsible. | At ages 5–7, children begin to understand that death is permanent, all life functions end completely at death, and everything that is alive eventually dies. Provide a direct, concrete description of his sister's death. Avoid clichés and euphemisms. Reassure the boy that he is not responsible. Identify and normalize fears and feelings. Encourage play and healthy coping behaviors (eg, remembering her in his own way). |
| Patient is victim of intimate partner violence. | Ask if patient is safe and help devise an emergency plan if there isn't one. Ask patient direct, open-ended questions about exam findings and summarize patient's answers back to them. Ask if patient has any questions. Do not necessarily pressure patient to leave a partner or disclose the incident to the authorities (unless required by state law). |
| Patient wants to try alternative or holistic medicine. | Explore any underlying reasons with the patient in a supportive, nonjudgmental manner. Advise the patient of known benefits and risks of treatment, including adverse effects, contraindications, and medication interactions. Consider referral to an appropriate complementary or alternative medicine provider. |
| Physician colleague presents to work impaired. | This presents a potential risk to patient safety. You have an ethical and usually a legal obligation to report impaired colleagues so they can cease patient care and receive appropriate assistance in a timely manner. Seek guidance in reporting as procedures and applicable law vary by institution and state. |
| Patient's family insists on maintaining life support after brain death has occurred, citing patient's movements when touched. | Gently explain to family that there is no chance of recovery, and that brain death is equivalent to death. Movement is due to spinal arc reflex and is not voluntary. Bring case to appropriate ethics board regarding futility of care and withdrawal of life support. |
| A pharmaceutical company offers you a sponsorship in exchange for advertising its new drug. | Reject this offer. Generally, decline gifts and sponsorships to avoid any conflict of interest. The AMA Code of Ethics does make exceptions for gifts directly benefitting patients; special funding for medical education of students, residents, fellows; grants whose recipients are chosen by independent institutional criteria; and funds that are distributed without attribution to sponsors. |
| Patient requests a nonemergent procedure that is against your personal or religious beliefs. | Provide accurate and unbiased information so patients can make an informed decision. In a neutral, nonjudgmental manner, explain to the patient that you do not perform the procedure but offer to refer to another physician. |
| Mother and 15-year-old daughter are unresponsive and bleeding heavily, but father refuses transfusion because they are Jehovah's Witnesses. | Transfuse daughter, but do not transfuse mother. Emergent care can be refused by the healthcare proxy for an adult, particularly when patient preferences are known or reasonably inferred, but not for a minor based solely on faith. |
| A dependent patient presents with injuries inconsistent with caretaker's story. | Document detailed history and physical. If possible and appropriate, interview the patient alone. Provide any necessary medical care. If suspicion remains, contact the appropriate agencies or authorities (eg, child or adult protective services) for an evaluation. Inform the caretaker of your obligation to report. Physicians are required by law to report any reasonable suspicion of abuse, neglect, or endangerment. |
| A pediatrician recommends standard vaccinations for a patient, but the child's parent refuses. | Address any concerns the parent has. Explain the risks and benefits of vaccinations and why they are recommended. Do not administer routine vaccinations without the parent's consent. |

**Communicating with patients with disabilities**

Patients may identify with person-first (ie, "a person with a disability") or identity-first (ie, "a disabled person") language. Ask patients what terms they use.

Under most circumstances, talk directly to the patient. Do not assume that nonverbal patients do not understand. Accompanying caregivers can add information to any discussion as needed.

Ask if assistance is desired rather than assuming the patient cannot do something alone. Most people, including people with disabilities, value their independence.

For patients with speech difficulties, provide extra time for the interview. If their speech is difficult to understand, consider asking them to write down a few words or ask them to rephrase their sentence. Repeat what they said to ensure you understood it correctly.

For patients with a cognitive impairment, use concrete, specific language. Ask simple, direct questions. Eliminate background noise and distractions. Do not assume the patient can read. Adjust to how the patient understands best (eg, use hand gestures or ask them to demonstrate a task).

Ask patients who are deaf or hard of hearing their preferred mode of communication. Use light touch or waving to get their attention. For patients who prefer to speak and lipread, eliminate background noise, face the patient, and do not change your mode of speaking. Consider using an interpreter when necessary.

As with other parts of a medical history, do not bring up a disability if it is not relevant to a visit (eg, a patient in a wheelchair with an ear infection). Do not skip relevant parts of the physical exam even if the disability makes the exam challenging.

---

**Use of interpreters**

Visits with a patient who speaks little English should utilize a professionally trained medical interpreter unless the physician is conversationally fluent in the patient's preferred language. If an interpreter is unavailable in person, interpretation services may be provided by telephone or video call. If the patient prefers to utilize a family member, this should be recorded in the chart.

Do not assume that a patient is a poor English speaker because of name, skin tone, or accent. Ask the patient what language is preferred.

The physician should make eye contact with the patient and speak to them directly, without use of third-person statements such as "tell him."

Allow extra time for the interview, and ask one question at a time.

For in-person spoken language interpretation, the interpreter should ideally be next to or slightly behind the patient. For sign language interpretation, the interpreter should be next to or slightly behind the physician.

In cases of emergency, facilitate communication by any tools available (eg, friends, family, sketches, interpreter apps) even though they do not comprise standard procedure otherwise.

▶ PUBLIC HEALTH SCIENCES—HEALTHCARE DELIVERY

### Disease prevention

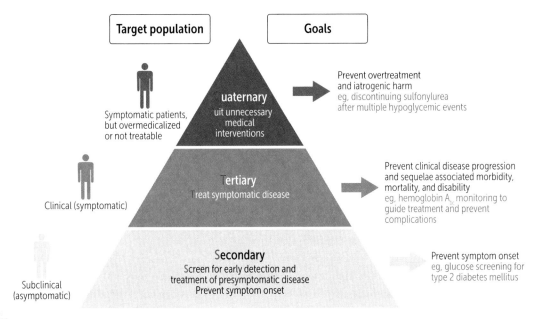

| Target population | Goals |

**uaternary**
uit unnecessary medical interventions

Symptomatic patients, but overmedicalized or not treatable

Prevent overtreatment and iatrogenic harm
eg, discontinuing sulfonylurea after multiple hypoglycemic events

**Tertiary**
Treat symptomatic disease

Clinical (symptomatic)

Prevent clinical disease progression and sequelae associated morbidity, mortality, and disability
eg, hemoglobin A$_{1c}$ monitoring to guide treatment and prevent complications

**Secondary**
Screen for early detection and treatment of presymptomatic disease
Prevent symptom onset

Subclinical (asymptomatic)

Prevent symptom onset
eg, glucose screening for type 2 diabetes mellitus

**Primary**
Prevent disease onset by reducing risks or increasing immunity

Susceptible/general population

Prevent disease onset
eg, healthy diet and exercise to prevent diabetes

### Major medical insurance plans

| PLAN | PROVIDERS | PAYMENTS | SPECIALIST CARE |
| --- | --- | --- | --- |
| Exclusive provider organization | Restricted to limited panel (except emergencies) | | No referral required |
| Health maintenance organization | Restricted to limited panel (except emergencies) | Most affordable | Requires referral from primary care provider |
| Point of service | Patient can see providers outside network | Higher copays and deductibles for out-of-network services | Requires referral from primary care provider |
| Preferred provider organization | Patient can see providers outside network | Higher copays and deductibles for all services | No referral required |
| Accountable care organization | Providers voluntarily enroll | Medicare | Specialists voluntarily enroll |

## Healthcare payment models

| | |
|---|---|
| **Bundled payment** | Healthcare organization receives a set amount per service, regardless of ultimate cost, to be divided among all providers and facilities involved. |
| **Capitation** | Physicians receive a set amount per patient assigned to them per period of time, regardless of how much the patient uses the healthcare system. Used by some HMOs. |
| **Discounted fee-for-service** | Insurer and/or patient pays for each individual service at a discounted rate predetermined by providers and payers (eg, PPOs). |
| **Fee-for-service** | Insurer and/or patient pays for each individual service. |
| **Global payment** | Insurer and/or patient pays for all expenses associated with a single incident of care with a single payment. Most commonly used during elective surgeries, as it covers the cost of surgery as well as the necessary pre- and postoperative visits. |

| | | |
|---|---|---|
| **Medicare and Medicaid** | Medicare and Medicaid—federal social healthcare programs that originated from amendments to the Social Security Act.<br>Medicare is available to patients ≥ 65 years old, < 65 with certain disabilities, and those with end-stage renal disease.<br>Medicaid is joint federal and state health assistance for people with limited income and/ or resources. | MedicarE is for Elderly.<br>MedicaiD is for Disadvantaged.<br><br>The 4 parts of Medicare:<br>▪ Part A: hospital Admissions, including hospice, skilled nursing<br>▪ Part B: Basic medical bills (eg, physician fees, diagnostic testing)<br>▪ Part C: (parts A + B = Combo) delivered by approved private companies<br>▪ Part D: prescription Drugs |

| | |
|---|---|
| **Palliative care** | Medical care aiming to provide comfort, relieve suffering, and improve quality of life in patients with serious illness regardless of their diagnosis or prognosis. Often concurrent with curative or life-prolonging treatment.<br>Delivered by interdisciplinary team (eg, physicians, nurses, social workers) in hospitals, outpatient clinics, or at home.<br>Hospice care (end-of-life care)—form of palliative care for patients with prognosis ≤ 6 months when curative or life-prolonging treatment is no longer beneficial. |

## Common causes of death (US) by age

| | < 1 YR | 1–14 YR | 15–34 YR | 35–44 YR | 45–64 YR | 65+ YR[a] |
|---|---|---|---|---|---|---|
| #1 | Congenital malformations | Unintentional injury | Unintentional injury | Unintentional injury | Cancer | Heart disease |
| #2 | Preterm birth | Cancer | Suicide | Cancer | Heart disease | Cancer |
| #3 | Sudden unexpected infant death | Congenital malformations | Homicide | Heart disease | Unintentional injury | Chronic lower respiratory disease |

[a]With the ongoing pandemic, COVID-19 has been included as one of the most common causes of death among people 65+ years old.

| | | |
|---|---|---|
| **Types of medical errors** | May involve patient identification, diagnosis, monitoring, healthcare-associated infection, medications, procedures, devices, documentation, handoffs. Medical errors should be disclosed to patients, independent of immediate outcome (harmful or not).<br>Burnout—prolonged, excessive stress → medical errors due to reduced professional efficacy.<br>Fatigue—sleep/rest deprivation → medical errors due to cognitive impairment. | |
| **Active error** | Occurs at level of frontline operator (eg, wrong IV pump dose programmed). | Immediate impact. |
| **Latent error** | Occurs in processes indirect from operator but impacts patient care (eg, different types of IV pumps used within same hospital). | Accident waiting to happen. |
| **Never event** | Adverse event that is identifiable, serious, and usually preventable (eg, scalpel retained in a surgical patient's abdomen). | Major error that should never occur.<br>Sentinel event—a never event that leads to death, permanent harm, or severe temporary harm. |
| **Near miss** | Unplanned event that does not result in harm but has the potential to do so (eg, pharmacist recognizes a medication interaction and cancels the order). | Narrow prevention of harm that exposes dangers. |

**Medical error analysis**

| | DESIGN | METHODS |
|---|---|---|
| **Root cause analysis** | Retrospective approach. Applied after failure event to prevent recurrence. | Uses records and participant interviews (eg, 5 whys approach, fishbone/cause-and-effect diagrams, process maps) to identify all the underlying problems (eg, process, people, environment, equipment, materials, management) that led to an error. |
| **Failure mode and effects analysis** | Forward-looking approach. Applied before process implementation to prevent failure occurrence. | Uses inductive reasoning to identify all the ways a process might fail and prioritizes them by their probability of occurrence and impact on patients. |

# SECTION III

# High-Yield Organ Systems

"Symptoms, then, are in reality nothing but the cry from suffering organs."
—Jean-Martin Charcot

"Man is an intelligence in servitude to his organs."
—Aldous Huxley

"When every part of the machine is correctly adjusted and in perfect harmony, health will hold dominion over the human organism by laws as natural and immutable as the laws of gravity."
—Andrew T. Still

## ▶ APPROACHING THE ORGAN SYSTEMS

In this section, we have divided the High-Yield Facts into the major **Organ Systems**. Within each Organ System are several subsections, including **Embryology, Anatomy, Physiology, Pathology,** and **Pharmacology.** As you progress through each Organ System, refer back to information in the previous subsections to organize these basic science subsections into a "vertically integrated" framework for learning. Below is some general advice for studying the organ systems by these subsections.

### Embryology

Relevant embryology is included in each organ system subsection. Embryology tends to correspond well with the relevant anatomy, especially with regard to congenital malformations.

### Anatomy

Several topics fall under this heading, including gross anatomy, histology, and neuroanatomy. Do not memorize all the small details; however, do not ignore anatomy altogether. Review what you have already learned and what you wish you had learned. Many questions require two or more steps. The first step is to identify a structure on anatomic cross section, electron micrograph, or photomicrograph. The second step may require an understanding of the clinical significance of the structure.

While studying, emphasize clinically relevant material. For example, be familiar with gross anatomy and radiologic anatomy related to specific diseases (eg, Pancoast tumor, Horner syndrome), traumatic injuries (eg, fractures, sensory and motor nerve deficits), procedures (eg, lumbar puncture), and common surgeries (eg, cholecystectomy). There are also many questions on the exam involving x-rays, CT scans, and neuro MRI scans. Many students suggest browsing through a general radiology atlas, pathology atlas, and histology atlas. Focus on learning basic anatomy at key levels in the body (eg, sagittal brain MRI; axial CT of the midthorax, abdomen, and pelvis). Basic neuroanatomy (especially pathways, blood supply, and functional anatomy), associated neuropathology, and neurophysiology have good yield. Please note that many of the photographic images in this book are for illustrative purposes and are not necessarily reflective of Step 1 emphasis.

### Physiology

The portion of the examination dealing with physiology is broad and concept oriented and thus does not lend itself as well to fact-based review. Diagrams are often the best study aids, especially given the increasing number of questions requiring the interpretation of diagrams. Learn to apply basic physiologic relationships in a variety of ways (eg, the Fick equation, clearance equations). You are seldom asked to perform complex calculations. Hormones are the focus of many questions; learn where and how they are synthesized, their regulatory mechanisms and sites of action.

A large portion of the physiology tested on the USMLE Step 1 is clinically relevant and involves understanding physiologic changes associated with pathologic processes (eg, changes in pulmonary function with COPD). Thus, it is worthwhile to review the physiologic changes that are found with common pathologies of the major organ systems (eg, heart, lungs, kidneys, GI tract) and endocrine glands.

## Pathology

Questions dealing with this discipline are difficult to prepare for because of the sheer volume of material involved. Review the basic principles and hallmark characteristics of the key diseases. Given the clinical orientation of Step 1, it is no longer sufficient to know only the "buzzword" associations of certain diseases (eg, café-au-lait macules and neurofibromatosis); you must also recognize the clinical descriptions of these high-yield physical exam findings.

Given the clinical slant of the USMLE Step 1, it is also important to review the classic presenting signs and symptoms of diseases as well as their associated laboratory findings. Delve into the signs, symptoms, and pathophysiology of major diseases that have a high prevalence in the United States (eg, alcohol use disorder, diabetes, hypertension, heart failure, ischemic heart disease, infectious disease). Be prepared to think one step beyond the simple diagnosis to treatment or complications.

The examination includes a number of color photomicrographs and photographs of gross specimens that are presented in the setting of a brief clinical history. However, read the question and the choices carefully before looking at the illustration, because the history will help you identify the pathologic process. Flip through an illustrated pathology textbook, color atlases, and appropriate Web sites in order to look at the pictures in the days before the exam. Pay attention to potential clues such as age, sex, ethnicity, occupation, recent activities and exposures, and specialized lab tests.

## Pharmacology

Preparation for questions on pharmacology is straightforward. Learning all the key drugs and their characteristics (eg, mechanisms, clinical use, and important adverse effects) is high yield. Focus on understanding the prototype drugs in each class. Avoid memorizing obscure derivatives. Learn the "classic" and distinguishing toxicities of the major drugs. Do not bother with drug dosages or brand names. Reviewing associated biochemistry, physiology, and microbiology can be useful while studying pharmacology. There is a strong emphasis on ANS, CNS, antimicrobial, and cardiovascular agents as well as NSAIDs. Much of the material is clinically relevant. Newer drugs on the market are also fair game.

▶ NOTES

# Cardiovascular

*"As for me, except for an occasional heart attack, I feel as young as I ever did."*

—Robert Benchley

*"Hearts will never be practical until they are made unbreakable."*
—The Wizard of Oz

*"As the arteries grow hard, the heart grows soft."*

—H. L. Mencken

*"Nobody has ever measured, not even poets, how much the heart can hold."*

—Zelda Fitzgerald

*"The art of medicine has its roots in the heart."*

—Paracelsus

*"It is not the size of the man but the size of his heart that matters."*
—Evander Holyfield

The cardiovascular system is one of the highest yield areas for the boards and, for some students, may be the most challenging. Focusing on understanding the mechanisms instead of memorizing the details can make a big difference. Pathophysiology of atherosclerosis and heart failure, mechanism of action of drugs (particularly, their interplay with cardiac physiology) and their adverse effects, ECGs of heart blocks, the cardiac cycle, and the Starling curve are some of the more high-yield topics. Differentiating between systolic and diastolic dysfunction is also very important. Heart murmurs and maneuvers that affect these murmurs have also been high yield and may be asked in a multimedia format.

| | |
|---|---|
| **Heart morphogenesis** | First functional organ in vertebrate embryos; beats spontaneously by week 4 of development. |
| **Cardiac looping** | Primary heart tube loops to establish left-right polarity; begins in week 4 of development. | Defect in left-right dynein (involved in left-right asymmetry) can lead to dextrocardia, as seen in Kartagener syndrome. |

**Septation of the chambers**

Atria

❶ Septum primum grows toward endocardial cushions, narrowing ostium primum.
❷ Ostium secundum forms in septum primum due to cell death (ostium primum regresses).
❸ Septum secundum develops on the right side of septum primum, as ostium secundum maintains right-to-left shunt.
❹ Septum secundum expands and covers most of ostium secundum. The residual foramen is the foramen ovale.
❺ Remaining portion of septum primum forms the one-way valve of the foramen ovale.

6. Septum primum closes against septum secundum, sealing the foramen ovale soon after birth because of ↑ LA pressure and ↓ RA pressure.
7. Septum secundum and septum primum fuse during infancy/early childhood, forming the atrial septum.

Patent foramen ovale—failure of septum primum and septum secundum to fuse after birth; seen in 25% of population. Most are asymptomatic and remain undetected. Can lead to paradoxical emboli (venous thromboemboli entering the systemic arterial circulation through right-to-left shunt) as can occur in atrial septal defect (ASD).

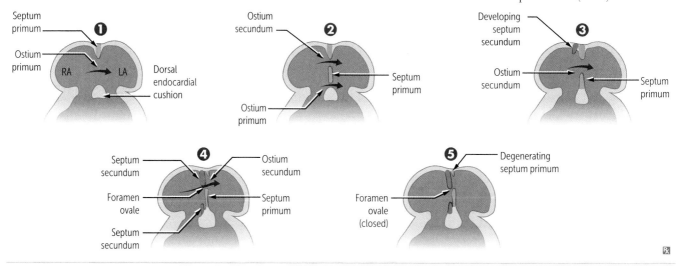

### Heart morphogenesis *(continued)*

| | | |
|---|---|---|
| Ventricles | ❶ Muscular interventricular septum forms. Opening is called interventricular foramen.<br>❷ Aorticopulmonary septum rotates and fuses with muscular ventricular septum to form membranous interventricular septum, closing interventricular foramen.<br>❸ Growth of endocardial cushions separates atria from ventricles and contributes to both atrial septation and membranous portion of the interventricular septum. | Ventricular septal defect—most common congenital cardiac anomaly, usually occurs in membranous septum. |

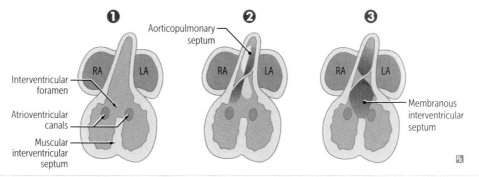

| | | |
|---|---|---|
| **Outflow tract formation** | Neural crest cell migrations → truncal and bulbar ridges that spiral and fuse to form aorticopulmonary septum → ascending aorta and pulmonary trunk. | Conotruncal abnormalities associated with failure of neural crest cells to migrate:<br>▪ Transposition of great arteries.<br>▪ Tetralogy of Fallot.<br>▪ Persistent truncus arteriosus. |
| **Valve development** | Aortic/pulmonary: derived from endocardial cushions of outflow tract.<br>Mitral/tricuspid: derived from fused endocardial cushions of the AV canal. | Valvular anomalies may be stenotic, regurgitant, atretic (eg, tricuspid atresia), or displaced (eg, Ebstein anomaly). |

**Heart embryology**

| EMBRYONIC STRUCTURE | GIVES RISE TO |
| --- | --- |
| Right common cardinal vein and right anterior cardinal vein | Superior vena cava (SVC) |
| Posterior cardinal, subcardinal, and supracardinal veins | Inferior vena cava (IVC) |
| Right horn of sinus venosus | Smooth part of right atrium (sinus venarum) |
| Left horn of sinus venosus | Coronary sinus |
| Primitive pulmonary vein | Smooth part of left atrium |
| Primitive atrium | Trabeculated part of left and right atria |
| Endocardial cushion | Atrial septum, membranous interventricular septum; AV and semilunar valves |
| Primitive ventricle | Trabeculated part of left and right ventricles |
| Bulbus cordis | Smooth parts (outflow tract) of left and right ventricles |
| Truncus arteriosus | Ascending aorta and pulmonary trunk |

## Fetal circulation

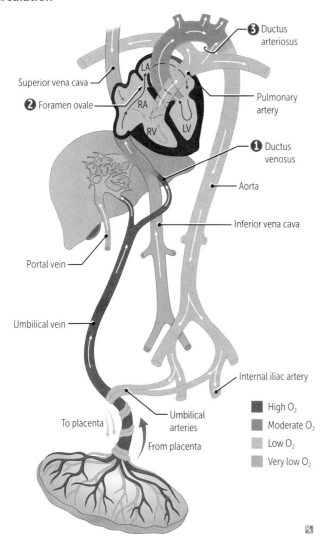

Superior vena cava

❷ Foramen ovale

RA

LA

RV

LV

❸ Ductus arteriosus

Pulmonary artery

❶ Ductus venosus

Aorta

Inferior vena cava

Portal vein

Internal iliac artery

Umbilical vein

Umbilical arteries

To placenta

From placenta

■ High $O_2$
■ Moderate $O_2$
■ Low $O_2$
■ Very low $O_2$

Blood in umbilical vein has a $Po_2$ of ≈ 30 mm Hg and is ≈ 80% saturated with $O_2$. Umbilical arteries have low $O_2$ saturation.

3 important shunts:

❶ Blood entering fetus through the umbilical vein is conducted via the **ductus venosus** into the IVC, bypassing hepatic circulation.

❷ Most of the highly oxygenated blood reaching the heart via the IVC is directed through the **foramen ovale** into the left atrium.

❸ Deoxygenated blood from the SVC passes through the RA → RV → main pulmonary artery → **ductus arteriosus** → descending aorta; shunt is due to high fetal pulmonary artery resistance.

At birth, infant takes a breath → ↓ resistance in pulmonary vasculature → ↑ left atrial pressure vs right atrial pressure→ foramen ovale closes (now called fossa ovalis); ↑ in $O_2$ (from respiration) and ↓ in prostaglandins (from placental separation) → closure of ductus arteriosus.

NSAIDs (eg, indomethacin, ibuprofen) or acetaminophen help close the patent ductus arteriosus → ligamentum arteriosum (remnant of ductus arteriosus). "Endomethacin" ends the PDA.

Prostaglandins $E_1$ and $E_2$ kEEp PDA open.

## Fetal-postnatal derivatives

| FETAL STRUCTURE | POSTNATAL DERIVATIVE | NOTES |
| --- | --- | --- |
| **Ductus arteriosus** | Ligamentum arteriosum | Near the left recurrent laryngeal nerve |
| **Ductus venosus** | Ligamentum venosum | |
| **Foramen ovale** | Fossa ovalis | |
| **Allantois → urachus** | Median umbilical ligament | Urachus is part of allantois between bladder and umbilicus |
| **Umbilical arteries** | Medial umbilical ligaments | |
| **Umbilical vein** | Ligamentum teres hepatis (round ligament) | Contained in falciform ligament |

▶ CARDIOVASCULAR—ANATOMY

### Heart anatomy

LA is the most posterior part of the heart ; LA enlargement (eg, in mitral stenosis) can lead to:
- Dysphagia; compression of esophagus
- Hoarseness; compression of left recurrent laryngeal nerve, a branch of vagus nerve (Ortner syndrome)

RV is the most anterior part of the heart and most commonly injured in trauma. LV is about 2/3 and RV is about 1/3 of the inferior (diaphragmatic) cardiac surface **B**.

### Pericardium

Consists of 3 layers (from outer to inner):
- Fibrous pericardium
- Parietal pericardium
- Epicardium (visceral pericardium)

Pericardial space lies between parietal pericardium and epicardium.

Pericardium innervated by phrenic nerve.

Pericarditis can cause referred pain to the neck, arms, or one or both shoulders (often left).

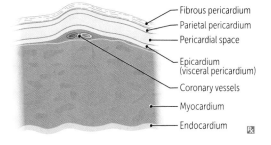

### Coronary blood supply

LAD and its branches supply anterior 2/3 of interventricular septum, anterolateral papillary muscle, and anterior surface of LV. Most commonly occluded.

PDA supplies posterior 1/3 of interventricular septum, posterior 2/3 walls of ventricles, and posteromedial papillary muscle.

RCA supplies AV node and SA node. Infarct may cause nodal dysfunction (bradycardia or heart block). Right (acute) marginal artery supplies RV.

Dominance:
- Right-dominant circulation (most common) = PDA arises from RCA
- Left-dominant circulation = PDA arises from LCX
- Codominant circulation = PDA arises from both LCX and RCA

Coronary blood flow to LV and interventricular septum peaks in early diastole.

Coronary sinus runs in the left AV groove and drains into the RA.

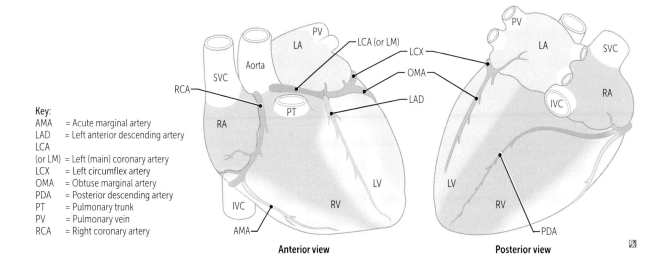

Key:
AMA = Acute marginal artery
LAD = Left anterior descending artery
LCA
(or LM) = Left (main) coronary artery
LCX = Left circumflex artery
OMA = Obtuse marginal artery
PDA = Posterior descending artery
PT = Pulmonary trunk
PV = Pulmonary vein
RCA = Right coronary artery

**Anterior view**　　　**Posterior view**

▶ **CARDIOVASCULAR—PHYSIOLOGY**

## Cardiac output variables

| | | |
|---|---|---|
| **Stroke volume** | Stroke Volume affected by Contractility, Afterload, and Preload.<br>↑ SV with:<br>  ▪ ↑ Contractility (eg, anxiety, exercise)<br>  ▪ ↑ Preload (eg, early pregnancy)<br>  ▪ ↓ Afterload | SV CAP.<br>Stroke work (SW) is work done by ventricle to eject SV.<br>$SW \propto SV \times MAP$<br>A failing heart has ↓ SV (systolic and/or diastolic dysfunction). |
| **Contractility** | Contractility (and SV) ↑ with:<br>  ▪ Catecholamine stimulation via $\beta_1$ receptor:<br>    ▪ Activated protein kinase A<br>      → phospholamban phosphorylation<br>      → active $Ca^{2+}$ ATPase → ↑ $Ca^{2+}$ storage in sarcoplasmic reticulum<br>    ▪ Activated protein kinase A → $Ca^{2+}$ channel phosphorylation → ↑ $Ca^{2+}$ entry → ↑ $Ca^{2+}$-induced $Ca^{2+}$ release<br>  ▪ ↑ intracellular $Ca^{2+}$<br>  ▪ ↓ extracellular $Na^+$ (↓ activity of $Na^+/Ca^{2+}$ exchanger)<br>  ▪ Digoxin (blocks $Na^+/K^+$ pump → ↑ intracellular $Na^+$ → ↓ $Na^+/Ca^{2+}$ exchanger activity → ↑ intracellular $Ca^{2+}$) | Contractility (and SV) ↓ with:<br>  ▪ $\beta_1$-blockade (↓ cAMP)<br>  ▪ Heart failure (HF) with systolic dysfunction<br>  ▪ Acidosis<br>  ▪ Hypoxia/hypercapnia (↓ $P_{O_2}$/↑ $P_{CO_2}$)<br>  ▪ Nondihydropyridine $Ca^{2+}$ channel blockers |
| **Preload** | Preload approximated by ventricular end-diastolic volume (EDV); depends on venous tone and circulating blood volume. | Venous vasodilators (eg, nitroglycerin) ↓ preload. |
| **Afterload** | Afterload approximated by MAP.<br>↑ wall tension per Laplace's law → ↑ pressure → ↑ afterload.<br><br>LV compensates for ↑ afterload by thickening (hypertrophy) in order to ↓ wall stress. | Arterial vasodilators (eg, hydralazine) ↓ afterload.<br>ACE inhibitors and ARBs ↓ both preload and afterload.<br>Chronic hypertension (↑ MAP) → LV hypertrophy. |
| **Cardiac oxygen demand** | Myocardial $O_2$ demand is ↑ by:<br>  ▪ ↑ contractility<br>  ▪ ↑ afterload (proportional to arterial pressure)<br>  ▪ ↑ heart rate<br>  ▪ ↑ diameter of ventricle (↑ wall tension)<br>Coronary sinus contains most deoxygenated blood in body. | Wall tension follows Laplace's law:<br>Wall tension = pressure × radius<br>$$\text{Wall stress} = \frac{\text{pressure} \times \text{radius}}{2 \times \text{wall thickness}}$$ |

## Cardiac output equations

| | EQUATION | NOTES |
|---|---|---|
| Stroke volume | $SV = EDV - ESV$ | ESV = end-systolic volume. |
| Ejection fraction | $EF = \dfrac{SV}{EDV} = \dfrac{EDV - ESV}{EDV}$ | EF is an index of ventricular contractility (↓ in systolic HF; usually normal in diastolic HF). Normal EF is 50%–70%. |
| Cardiac output | $CO = \dot{Q} = SV \times HR$<br><br>Fick principle:<br>$CO = \dfrac{\text{rate of } O_2 \text{ consumption}}{(\text{arterial } O_2 \text{ content} - \text{venous } O_2 \text{ content})}$ | In early stages of exercise, CO maintained by ↑ HR and ↑ SV. In later stages, CO maintained by ↑ HR only (SV plateaus).<br>Diastole is shortened with ↑↑ HR (eg, ventricular tachycardia) → ↓ diastolic filling time → ↓ SV → ↓ CO. |
| Pulse pressure | PP = systolic blood pressure (SBP) – diastolic blood pressure (DBP) | PP directly proportional to SV and inversely proportional to arterial compliance.<br>↑ PP in aortic regurgitation, aortic stiffening (isolated systolic hypertension in older adults), obstructive sleep apnea (↑ sympathetic tone), high-output state (eg, anemia, hyperthyroidism), exercise (transient).<br>↓ PP in aortic stenosis, cardiogenic shock, cardiac tamponade, advanced HF. |
| Mean arterial pressure | MAP = CO × total peripheral resistance (TPR) | MAP (at resting HR) = 2/3 DBP + 1/3 SBP = DBP + 1/3 PP. |

## Starling curves

Force of contraction is proportional to end-diastolic length of cardiac muscle fiber (preload).

↑ contractility with catecholamines, positive inotropes (eg, dobutamine, milrinone, digoxin).

↓ contractility with loss of functional myocardium (eg, MI), β-blockers (acutely), nondihydropyridine $Ca^{2+}$ channel blockers, HF.

**Resistance, pressure, flow**

Volumetric flow rate ($\dot{Q}$) = flow velocity (v) × cross-sectional area (A)

$$\text{Resistance} = \frac{\text{driving pressure }(\Delta P)}{\dot{Q}} = \frac{8\eta\text{ (viscosity)} \times \text{length}}{\pi r^4}$$

Total resistance of vessels in series:

$$R_T = R_1 + R_2 + R_3 \ldots$$

Total resistance of vessels in parallel:

$$\frac{1}{R_T} = \frac{1}{R_1} + \frac{1}{R_2} + \frac{1}{R_3} \ldots$$

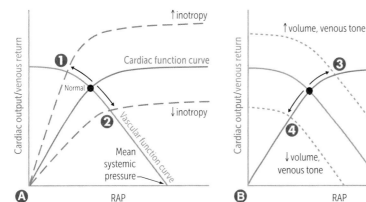

$Q \propto r^4$
$R \propto 1/r^4$

Capillaries have highest total cross-sectional area and lowest flow velocity.

Pressure gradient drives flow from high pressure to low pressure.

Arterioles account for most of TPR. Veins provide most of blood storage capacity.

Viscosity depends mostly on hematocrit.

Viscosity ↑ in hyperproteinemic states (eg, multiple myeloma), polycythemia.

Viscosity ↓ in anemia.

---

**Cardiac and vascular function curves**

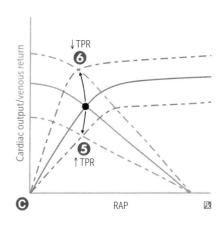

Intersection of curves = operating point of heart (ie, venous return and CO are equal, as circulatory system is a closed system).

| GRAPH | EFFECT | EXAMPLES |
|---|---|---|
| **Ⓐ Inotropy** | Changes in contractility → altered SV → altered CO/VR and RA pressure (RAP) | ❶ Catecholamines, dobutamine, digoxin, exercise ⊕<br>❷ HF with reduced EF, narcotic overdose, sympathetic inhibition ⊖ |
| **Ⓑ Venous return** | Changes in circulating volume → altered RAP → altered SV → change in CO | ❸ Fluid infusion, sympathetic activity, arteriovenous shunt ⊕<br>❹ Acute hemorrhage, spinal anesthesia ⊖ |
| **Ⓒ Total peripheral resistance** | Changes in TPR → altered CO<br>Change in RAP unpredictable | ❺ Vasopressors ⊕<br>❻ Exercise, arteriovenous shunt ⊖ |

Changes often occur in tandem, and may be reinforcing (eg, exercise ↑ inotropy and ↓ TPR to maximize CO) or compensatory (eg, HF ↓ inotropy → fluid retention to ↑ preload to maintain CO).

## Pressure-volume loops and cardiac cycle

The black loop represents normal cardiac physiology.

Phases—left ventricle:

❶ Isovolumetric contraction—period between mitral valve closing and aortic valve opening; period of highest $O_2$ consumption

❷ Systolic ejection—period between aortic valve opening and closing

❸ Isovolumetric relaxation—period between aortic valve closing and mitral valve opening

❹ Rapid filling—period just after mitral valve opening

❺ Reduced filling—period just before mitral valve closing

Heart sounds:

S1—mitral and tricuspid valve closure. Loudest at mitral area.

S2—aortic and pulmonary valve closure. Loudest at left upper sternal border.

S3—in early diastole during rapid ventricular filling phase. Best heard at apex with patient in left lateral decubitus position. Associated with ↑ filling pressures (eg, MR, AR, HF, thyrotoxicosis) and more common in dilated ventricles (but can be normal in children, young adults, athletes, and pregnancy). Turbulence caused by blood from LA mixing with ↑ ESV.

S4—in late diastole ("atrial kick"). Turbulence caused by blood entering stiffened LV. Best heard at apex with patient in left lateral decubitus position. High atrial pressure. Associated with ventricular noncompliance (eg, hypertrophy). Considered abnormal if palpable. Common in older adults.

Jugular venous pulse (JVP):

a wave—atrial contraction. Prominent in AV dissociation (cannon a wave), absent in atrial fibrillation.

c wave—RV contraction (closed tricuspid valve bulging into atrium).

x descent—atrial relaxation and downward displacement of closed tricuspid valve during rapid ventricular ejection phase. Reduced or absent in tricuspid regurgitation and right HF because pressure gradients are reduced.

v wave—↑ RA pressure due to ↑ volume against closed tricuspid valve.

y descent—RA emptying into RV. Prominent in constrictive pericarditis, absent in cardiac tamponade.

## Jugular venous pressure tracings

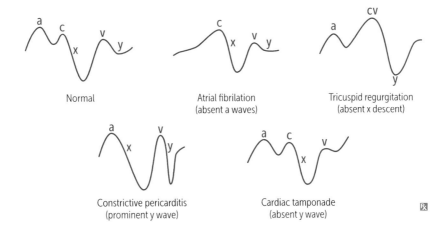

Normal

Atrial fibrilation
(absent a waves)

Tricuspid regurgitation
(absent x descent)

Constrictive pericarditis
(prominent y wave)

Cardiac tamponade
(absent y wave)

## Pressure-volume loops and valvular disease

### Aortic stenosis

↑ LV pressure

↑ ESV

No change in EDV (if mild)

↓ SV

Ventricular hypertrophy → ↓ ventricular compliance → ↑ EDP for given EDV

### Aortic regurgitation

No true isovolumetric phase

↑ EDV

↑ SV

Loss of dicrotic notch

### Mitral stenosis

↑ LA pressure

↓ EDV because of impaired ventricular filling

↓ ESV

↓ SV

### Mitral regurgitation

No true isovolumetric phase

↓ ESV due to ↓ resistance and ↑ regurgitation into LA during systole

↑ EDV due to ↑ LA volume/pressure from regurgitation → ↑ ventricular filling

↑ SV (forward flow into systemic circulation plus backflow into LA)

## Splitting of S2

| | | |
|---|---|---|
| **Physiologic splitting** | Inspiration → drop in intrathoracic pressure → ↑ venous return → ↑ RV filling → ↑ RV stroke volume → ↑ RV ejection time → delayed closure of pulmonic valve. ↓ pulmonary impedance (↑ capacity of the pulmonary circulation) also occurs during inspiration, which contributes to delayed closure of pulmonic valve. | E    S1    A2 P2 <br> I    Normal delay Rx <br><br> **E** = Expiration <br> **I** = Inspiration |
| **Wide splitting** | Seen in conditions that delay RV emptying (eg, pulmonic stenosis, right bundle branch block). Causes delayed pulmonic sound (especially on inspiration). An exaggeration of normal splitting. | E    S1    A2    P2 <br> I    Abnormal delay Rx |
| **Fixed splitting** | Heard in ASD. ASD → left-to-right shunt → ↑ RA and RV volumes → ↑ flow through pulmonic valve → delayed pulmonic valve closure (independent of respiration). | E    = <br> S1    A2    P2 <br> I    =    Rx |
| **Paradoxical splitting** | Heard in conditions that delay aortic valve closure (eg, aortic stenosis, left bundle branch block). Normal order of semilunar valve closure is reversed: in paradoxical splitting **P2** occurs before A2. On inspiration, P2 closes later and moves closer to A2, "paradoxically" eliminating the split. On expiration, the split can be heard (opposite to physiologic splitting). | E    S1    P2    A2 <br> I    Rx |

## Auscultation of the heart

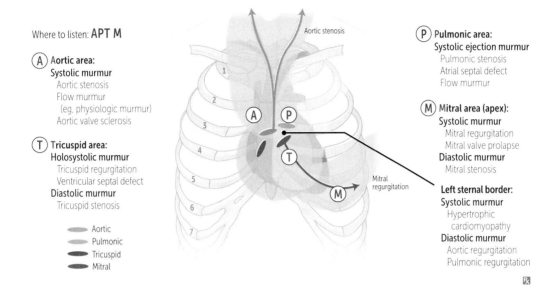

Where to listen: **APT M**

(A) **Aortic area:**
Systolic murmur
Aortic stenosis
Flow murmur
 (eg, physiologic murmur)
Aortic valve sclerosis

(T) **Tricuspid area:**
Holosystolic murmur
Tricuspid regurgitation
Ventricular septal defect
Diastolic murmur
Tricuspid stenosis

━━ Aortic
━━ Pulmonic
━━ Tricuspid
━━ Mitral

Aortic stenosis

(P) **Pulmonic area:**
Systolic ejection murmur
Pulmonic stenosis
Atrial septal defect
Flow murmur

(M) **Mitral area (apex):**
Systolic murmur
Mitral regurgitation
Mitral valve prolapse
Diastolic murmur
Mitral stenosis

**Left sternal border:**
Systolic murmur
Hypertrophic
 cardiomyopathy
Diastolic murmur
Aortic regurgitation
Pulmonic regurgitation

Mitral regurgitation

| MANEUVER | CARDIOVASCULAR CHANGES | MURMURS THAT INCREASE WITH MANEUVER | MURMURS THAT DECREASE WITH MANEUVER |
|---|---|---|---|
| Standing, Valsalva (strain phase) | ↓ preload (↓ LV volume) | MVP (↓ LV volume) with earlier midsystolic click HCM (↓ LV volume) | Most murmurs (↓ flow through stenotic or regurgitant valve) |
| Passive leg raise | ↑ preload (↑ LV volume) | Most murmurs (↑ flow through stenotic or regurgitant valve) | MVP (↑ LV volume) with later midsystolic click HCM (↑ LV volume) |
| Squatting | ↑ preload, ↑ afterload (↑ LV volume) | | |
| Hand grip | ↑↑ afterload → ↑ reverse flow across aortic valve (↑ LV volume) | Most other left-sided murmurs (AR, MR, VSD) | AS (↓ transaortic valve pressure gradient) HCM (↑ LV volume) |
| Inspiration | ↑ venous return to right heart, ↓ venous return to left heart | Most right-sided murmurs | Most left-sided murmurs |

## Heart murmurs

| | AUSCULTATION | CLINICAL ASSOCIATIONS | NOTES |
|---|---|---|---|
| **Systolic** | | | |
| **Aortic stenosis** | Crescendo-decrescendo ejection murmur, loudest at heart base, radiates to carotids. Soft S2 +/− ejection click "Pulsus parvus et tardus"— weak pulses with delayed peak | In older (>60 years old) patients, most commonly due to age-related calcification. In younger patients, most commonly due to early-onset calcification of bicuspid aortic valve | Can lead to Syncope, Angina, Dyspnea on exertion (SAD). LV pressure > aortic pressure during systole |
| **Mitral/tricuspid regurgitation** | Holosystolic, high-pitched "blowing" murmur. MR: loudest at apex, radiates toward axilla. TR: loudest at tricuspid area | MR: often due to ischemic heart disease (post-MI), MVP, LV dilatation, rheumatic fever. TR: often due to RV dilatation. Either MR or TR: infective endocarditis | |
| **Mitral valve prolapse** | Late crescendo murmur with midsystolic click (MC) that occurs after carotid pulse. Best heard over apex. Loudest just before S2 | Usually benign, but can predispose to infective endocarditis. Can be caused by rheumatic fever, chordae rupture, or myxomatous degeneration (1° or 2° to connective tissue disease) | MC due to sudden tensing of chordae tendineae as mitral leaflets prolapse into LA (chordae cause crescendo with click) |
| **Ventricular septal defect** | Holosystolic, harsh-sounding murmur. Loudest at tricuspid area | Congenital | Larger VSDs have lower intensity murmur than smaller VSDs |
| **Diastolic** | | | |
| **Aortic regurgitation** | Early diastolic, decrescendo, high-pitched "blowing" murmur best heard at base (aortic root dilation) or left sternal border (valvular disease) | Causes include **BEAR**: ▪ Bicuspid aortic valve ▪ Endocarditis ▪ Aortic root dilation ▪ Rheumatic fever. Wide pulse pressure, pistol shot femoral pulse, pulsing nail bed (Quincke pulse) | Hyperdynamic pulse and head bobbing when severe and chronic. Can progress to left HF |
| **Mitral stenosis** | Follows opening snap (OS). Delayed rumbling mid-to-late murmur (↓ interval between S2 and OS correlates with ↑ severity) | Late and highly specific sequelae of rheumatic fever. Chronic MS can result in LA dilation and pulmonary congestion, atrial fibrillation, Ortner syndrome, hemoptysis, right HF | OS due to abrupt halt in leaflet motion in diastole after rapid opening due to fusion at leaflet tips. LA >> LV pressure during diastole |
| **Continuous** | | | |
| **Patent ductus arteriosus** | Continuous machinelike murmur, best heard at left infraclavicular area. ℞ Loudest at S2 | Often due to congenital rubella or prematurity | You need a patent for that machine. |

**Myocardial action potential**

**Phase 0** = rapid upstroke and depolarization—voltage-gated $Na^+$ channels open.

**Phase 1** = initial repolarization—inactivation of voltage-gated $Na^+$ channels. Voltage-gated $K^+$ channels begin to open.

**Phase 2** = plateau ("platwo")—$Ca^{2+}$ influx through voltage-gated $Ca^{2+}$ channels balances $K^+$ efflux. $Ca^{2+}$ influx triggers $Ca^{2+}$ release from sarcoplasmic reticulum and myocyte contraction (excitation-contraction coupling).

**Phase 3** = rapid repolarization—massive $K^+$ efflux due to opening of voltage-gated slow delayed-rectifier $K^+$ channels and closure of voltage-gated $Ca^{2+}$ channels.

**Phase 4** = resting potential—high $K^+$ permeability through $K^+$ channels.

In contrast to skeletal muscle:

- Cardiac muscle action potential has a plateau due to $Ca^{2+}$ influx and $K^+$ efflux.
- Cardiac muscle contraction requires $Ca^{2+}$ influx from ECF to induce $Ca^{2+}$ release from sarcoplasmic reticulum ($Ca^{2+}$-induced $Ca^{2+}$ release).
- Cardiac myocytes are electrically coupled to each other by gap junctions.

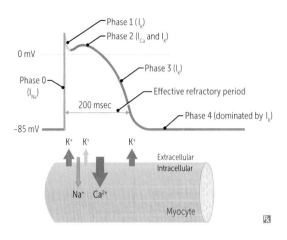

Occurs in all cardiac myocytes except for those in the SA and AV nodes.

**Pacemaker action potential**

Occurs in the SA and AV nodes. Key differences from the ventricular action potential include:

**Phase 0** = upstroke—opening of voltage-gated $Ca^{2+}$ channels. Fast voltage-gated $Na^+$ channels are permanently inactivated because of the less negative resting potential of these cells. Results in a slow conduction velocity that is used by the AV node to prolong transmission from the atria to ventricles. Phases 1 and 2 are absent.

**Phase 3** = repolarization—inactivation of the $Ca^{2+}$ channels and ↑ activation of $K^+$ channels → ↑ $K^+$ efflux.

**Phase 4** = slow spontaneous diastolic depolarization due to $I_f$ ("funny current"). $I_f$ channels responsible for a slow, mixed $Na^+$ inward/$K^+$ outward current; different from $I_{Na}$ in phase 0 of ventricular action potential. Accounts for automaticity of SA and AV nodes. The slope of phase 4 in the SA node determines HR. ACh/adenosine ↓ the rate of diastolic depolarization and ↓ HR, while catecholamines ↑ depolarization and ↑ HR. Sympathetic stimulation ↑ the chance that $I_f$ channels are open and thus ↑ HR.

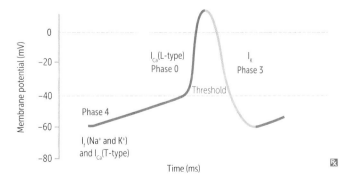

**Electrocardiogram**

Conduction pathway: SA node → atria → AV node → bundle of His → right and left bundle branches → Purkinje fibers → ventricles; left bundle branch divides into left anterior and posterior fascicles.

SA node—located in upper part of crista terminalis near SVC opening; "pacemaker" inherent dominance with slow phase of upstroke.

AV node—located in interatrial septum near coronary sinus opening. Blood supply usually from RCA. 100-msec delay allows time for ventricular filling.

Pacemaker rates: SA > AV > bundle of His/Purkinje/ventricles.

Speed of conduction: His-Purkinje > Atria > Ventricles > AV node. He Parks At Ventura AVenue.

P wave—atrial depolarization.

PR interval—time from start of atrial depolarization to start of ventricular depolarization (normally 120-200 msec).

QRS complex—ventricular depolarization (normally < 100 msec).

QT interval—ventricular depolarization, mechanical contraction of the ventricles, ventricular repolarization.

T wave—ventricular repolarization. T-wave inversion may indicate ischemia or recent MI.

J point—junction between end of QRS complex and start of ST segment.

ST segment—isoelectric, ventricles depolarized.

U wave—prominent in hypokalemia (think hyp"U"kalemia), bradycardia.

| **Atrial natriuretic peptide** | Released from **atrial myocytes** in response to ↑ blood volume and atrial pressure. Acts via cGMP. Causes vasodilation and ↓ $Na^+$ reabsorption at the renal collecting tubule. Dilates afferent renal arterioles and constricts efferent arterioles, promoting diuresis and contributing to "aldosterone escape" mechanism. |
|---|---|

| **B-type (brain) natriuretic peptide** | Released from **ventricular myocytes** in response to ↑ tension. Similar physiologic action to ANP, with longer half-life. BNP blood test used for diagnosing HF (very good negative predictive value). |
|---|---|

### Baroreceptors and chemoreceptors

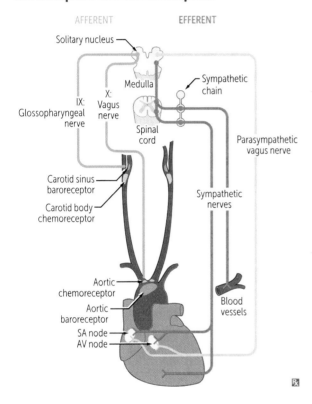

**Receptors:**
- Aortic arch transmits via vagus nerve to nucleus tractus solitarius of medulla (responds to changes in BP).
- Carotid sinus (dilated region superior to bifurcation of carotid arteries) transmits via glossopharyngeal nerve to nucleus tractus solitarius of medulla (responds to changes in BP).

**Chemoreceptors:**
- Peripheral—carotid and aortic bodies are stimulated by ↑ $Pco_2$, ↓ pH of blood, and ↓ $Po_2$ (< 60 mm Hg).
- Central—are stimulated by changes in pH and $Pco_2$ of brain interstitial fluid, which in turn are influenced by arterial $CO_2$ as $H^+$ cannot cross the blood-brain barrier. Do not directly respond to $Po_2$. Central chemoreceptors become less responsive with chronically ↑ $Pco_2$ (eg, COPD) → ↑ dependence on peripheral chemoreceptors to detect ↓ $O_2$ to drive respiration.

**Baroreceptors:**
- Hypotension—↓ arterial pressure → ↓ stretch → ↓ afferent baroreceptor firing → ↑ efferent sympathetic firing and ↓ efferent parasympathetic stimulation → vasoconstriction, ↑ HR, ↑ contractility, ↑ BP. Important in the response to hypovolemic shock.
- Carotid massage—↑ carotid sinus pressure → ↑ afferent baroreceptor firing → ↑ AV node refractory period → ↓ HR → ↓ CO. Also leads to peripheral vasodilation. Can cause presyncope/syncope. Exaggerated in underlying atherosclerosis, prior neck surgery, older age.
- Component of Cushing reflex (triad of hypertension, bradycardia, and respiratory depression)—↑ intracranial pressure constricts arterioles → cerebral ischemia → ↑ $pCO_2$ and ↓ pH → central reflex sympathetic ↑ in perfusion pressure (hypertension) → ↑ stretch → peripheral reflex baroreceptor–induced bradycardia.

**Normal resting cardiac pressures**

Pulmonary capillary wedge pressure (PCWP; in mm Hg) is a good approximation of left atrial pressure, except in mitral stenosis when PCWP > LV end diastolic pressure. PCWP is measured with pulmonary artery catheter (Swan-Ganz catheter).

| **Autoregulation** | How blood flow to an organ remains constant over a wide range of perfusion pressures. | |
|---|---|---|
| ORGAN | FACTORS DETERMINING AUTOREGULATION | |
| Lungs | Hypoxia causes vasoconstriction | The pulmonary vasculature is unique in that alveolar hypoxia causes vasoconstriction so that only well-ventilated areas are perfused. In other organs, hypoxia causes vasodilation |
| Heart | Local metabolites (vasodilatory): NO, $CO_2$, ↓ $O_2$ | |
| Brain | Local metabolites (vasodilatory): $CO_2$ (pH) | |
| Kidneys | Myogenic (stretch-dependent response of afferent arteriole) and tubuloglomerular feedback | |
| Skeletal muscle | Local metabolites during exercise (vasodilatory): **C**$O_2$, **H**$^+$, **A**denosine, **L**actate, **K**$^+$<br>At rest: sympathetic tone in arteries | **CHALK** |
| Skin | Sympathetic vasoconstriction most important mechanism for temperature control | |

**Capillary fluid exchange**

Starling forces determine fluid movement through capillary membranes:
- $P_c$ = capillary hydrostatic pressure—pushes fluid out of capillary
- $P_i$ = interstitial hydrostatic pressure—pushes fluid into capillary
- $\pi_c$ = plasma oncotic pressure—pulls fluid into capillary
- $\pi_i$ = interstitial fluid oncotic pressure—pulls fluid out of capillary

$J_v$ = net fluid flow = $K_f [(P_c - P_i) - \sigma(\pi_c - \pi_i)]$

$K_f$ = capillary permeability to fluid

$\sigma$ = reflection coefficient (measure of capillary impermeability to protein)

Edema—excess fluid outflow into interstitium commonly caused by:
- ↑ capillary pressure (↑ $P_c$; eg, HF)
- ↑ capillary permeability (↑ $K_f$; eg, toxins, infections, burns)
- ↑ interstitial fluid oncotic pressure (↑ $\pi_i$; eg, lymphatic blockage)
- ↓ plasma proteins (↓ $\pi_c$; eg, nephrotic syndrome, liver failure, protein malnutrition)

Net fluid flow = $K_f [(P_c - P_i) - \sigma(\pi_c - \pi_i)]$

## ▶ CARDIOVASCULAR—PATHOLOGY

### Congenital heart diseases

| | | |
|---|---|---|
| RIGHT-TO-LEFT SHUNTS | Early cyanosis—"blue babies." Often diagnosed prenatally or become evident immediately after birth. Usually require urgent surgical treatment and/or maintenance of a PDA. | The 5 T's:<br>1. Truncus arteriosus (1 vessel)<br>2. Transposition (2 switched vessels)<br>3. Tricuspid atresia (3 = Tri)<br>4. Tetralogy of Fallot (4 = Tetra)<br>5. TAPVR (5 letters in the name) |
| **Persistent truncus arteriosus** | Truncus arteriosus fails to divide into pulmonary trunk and aorta due to failure of aorticopulmonary septum formation; most patients have accompanying VSD. | |
| **D-transposition of great arteries**<br> | Aorta leaves RV (anterior) and pulmonary trunk leaves LV (posterior) → separation of systemic and pulmonary circulations A. Not compatible with life unless a shunt is present to allow mixing of blood (eg, VSD, PDA, or patent foramen ovale).<br>Due to failure of the aorticopulmonary septum to spiral (narrow superior mediastinum causes "egg on a string" appearance on CXR).<br>Without surgical intervention, most infants die within the first few months of life. |  |
| **Tricuspid atresia** | Absence of tricuspid valve, hypoplastic RV; requires both ASD and VSD/PDA for viability. | ECG shows hypertrophy of RA (tall P-waves) and LV (left axis deviation). |
| **Tetralogy of Fallot**<br> | Caused by anterosuperior displacement of the infundibular septum. Most common cause of early childhood cyanosis.<br>❶ Pulmonary infundibular stenosis (most important determinant for prognosis)<br>❷ Right ventricular hypertrophy (RVH)—boot-shaped heart on CXR B<br>❸ Overriding aorta—straddles VSD receiving blood from both LV and RV<br>❹ VSD<br>Pulmonary stenosis forces right-to-left flow across VSD → RVH, "tet spells" (often caused by crying, fever, and exercise due to exacerbation of RV outflow obstruction). | PROVe.<br>Squatting: ↑ SVR, ↓ right-to-left shunt, improves cyanosis.<br>Associated with 22q11 syndromes. |
| **Total anomalous pulmonary venous return** | Pulmonary veins drain into right heart circulation (SVC, coronary sinus, etc); associated with ASD and sometimes PDA to allow for right-to-left shunting to maintain CO. | |
| **Ebstein anomaly** | Displacement of tricuspid valve leaflets downward into RV, artificially "atrializing" the ventricle. Associated with tricuspid regurgitation, accessory conduction pathways, right-sided HF. | Rare. Can be caused by lithium exposure in utero. |

## Congenital heart diseases *(continued)*

| LEFT-TO-RIGHT SHUNTS | Acyanotic at presentation; cyanosis may occur years later. Frequency: VSD > ASD > PDA. | Right-to-left shunts: early cyanosis.<br>Left-to-right shunts: "later" cyanosis. |
|---|---|---|
| **Ventricular septal defect** | Asymptomatic at birth, may manifest weeks later or remain asymptomatic throughout life. Most smaller defects self-resolve; larger defects, if left surgically untreated, cause ↑ pulmonary blood flow and LV overload, which may progress to HF. | $O_2$ saturation ↑ in RV and pulmonary artery. |
| **Atrial septal defect**  | Defect in interatrial septum **C**; systolic ejection murmur with wide, fixed split S2. Ostium secundum defects most common and usually an isolated finding; ostium primum defects rarer and usually occur with other cardiac anomalies. Symptoms range from none to HF. Distinct from patent foramen ovale, which is due to failed fusion. | $O_2$ saturation ↑ in RA, RV, and pulmonary artery. May lead to paradoxical emboli (systemic venous emboli use ASD to bypass lungs and become systemic arterial emboli). Associated with Down syndrome. |
| **Patent ductus arteriosus**  | In fetal period, shunt is right to left (normal). In neonatal period, ↓ pulmonary vascular resistance → shunt becomes left to right → progressive RVH and/or LVH and HF. Associated with a continuous, "machinelike" murmur. Patency is maintained by PGE synthesis and low $O_2$ tension. Uncorrected PDA **D** can eventually result in late cyanosis in the lower extremities (differential cyanosis). | PDA is normal in utero and normally closes soon after birth.<br>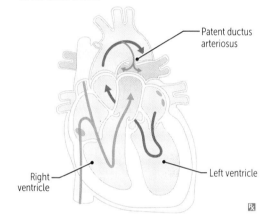 |
| **Eisenmenger syndrome** | Uncorrected left-to-right shunt (VSD, ASD, PDA) → ↑ pulmonary blood flow → pathologic remodeling of vasculature → pulmonary arterial hypertension. RVH occurs to compensate → shunt becomes right to left when RV > LV pressure (see illustration). Causes late cyanosis, clubbing, and polycythemia. Age of onset varies depending on size and severity of initial left-to-right shunt. |  |

| | |
|---|---|
| **Coarctation of the aorta**<br> | Aortic narrowing  near insertion of ductus arteriosus ("juxtaductal"). Associated with bicuspid aortic valve, other heart defects, and Turner syndrome. Hypertension in upper extremities. Lower extremities are cold with weak, delayed pulses (brachiofemoral delay). With age, intercostal arteries enlarge due to collateral circulation.<br>Complications include HF, ↑ risk of cerebral hemorrhage (berry aneurysms), aortic rupture, and possible infective endocarditis. |
| **Persistent pulmonary hypertension of the newborn** | Persistence of ↑ pulmonary vascular resistance after birth. Associated with abnormal development and postpartum adaptation of pulmonary vasculature. Risk factors include aspiration of meconium-stained amniotic fluid and neonatal pneumonia. Leads to right-to-left shunt through foramen ovale and ductus arteriosus. Newborn presents with signs of respiratory distress (eg, tachypnea) and cyanosis. Preductal O₂ saturation is often higher than postductal. Equal pulses (no delay). |

**Congenital cardiac defect associations**

| ASSOCIATION | DEFECT |
|---|---|
| Prenatal alcohol exposure (fetal alcohol syndrome) | VSD, PDA, ASD, tetralogy of Fallot |
| Congenital rubella | PDA, pulmonary artery stenosis, septal defects |
| Down syndrome | AV septal defect (endocardial cushion defect), VSD, ASD |
| Infant of patient with diabetes during pregnancy | Transposition of great arteries, truncus arteriosus, tricuspid atresia, VSD |
| Marfan syndrome | MVP, thoracic aortic aneurysm and dissection, aortic regurgitation |
| Prenatal lithium exposure | Ebstein anomaly |
| Turner syndrome | Bicuspid aortic valve, coarctation of aorta |
| Williams syndrome | Supravalvular aortic stenosis |
| 22q11 syndromes | Truncus arteriosus, tetralogy of Fallot |

| | |
|---|---|
| **Hypertension** | Persistent systolic BP ≥ 130 mm Hg and/or diastolic BP ≥ 80 mm Hg. |
| RISK FACTORS | ↑ age, obesity, diabetes, physical inactivity, high-sodium diet, excess alcohol intake, tobacco smoking, family history; incidence greatest in Black > White > Asian populations. |
| FEATURES<br> | 90% of hypertension is 1° (essential) and related to ↑ CO or ↑ TPR. Remaining 10% mostly 2° to renal/renovascular diseases such as fibromuscular dysplasia (characteristic "string of beads" appearance of renal artery , usually seen in adult females) and atherosclerotic renal artery stenosis, 1° hyperaldosteronism, or obstructive sleep apnea.<br>**Hypertensive urgency**—severe (≥ 180/≥ 120 mm Hg) hypertension without acute end-organ damage.<br>**Hypertensive emergency**—formerly called malignant hypertension. Severe hypertension with evidence of acute end-organ damage (eg, encephalopathy, stroke, retinal hemorrhages and exudates, papilledema, MI, HF, aortic dissection, kidney injury, microangiopathic hemolytic anemia, eclampsia). Arterioles may show fibrinoid necrosis. |
| PREDISPOSES TO | CAD, LVH, HF, atrial fibrillation; aortic dissection, aortic aneurysm; stroke; CKD (hypertensive nephropathy); retinopathy. |

## Hyperlipidemia signs

| | |
|---|---|
| Xanthomas | Plaques or nodules composed of lipid-laden histiocytes in skin **A**, especially the eyelids (xanthelasma **B**). |
| Tendinous xanthoma | Lipid deposit in tendon **C**, especially Achilles tendon and finger extensors. Associated with familial hypercholesterolemia. |
| Corneal arcus | Lipid deposit in cornea. Common in older adults (arcus senilis **D**), but appears earlier in life with hypercholesterolemia. |

| | |
|---|---|
| **Atherosclerosis** | Very common form of arteriosclerosis (hardening of arteries). Disease of elastic arteries and large- and medium-sized muscular arteries; caused by buildup of cholesterol plaques in tunica intima. |
| LOCATION | Abdominal aorta > coronary artery > popliteal artery > carotid artery > circle of Willis. A copy cat named Willis. |
| RISK FACTORS | Modifiable: hypertension, tobacco smoking, dyslipidemia (↑ LDL, ↓ HDL), diabetes. Non-modifiable: age, male sex, postmenopausal status, family history. |
| SYMPTOMS | Angina, claudication, but can be asymptomatic. |
| PROGRESSION | Inflammation important in pathogenesis: endothelial cell dysfunction → macrophage and LDL accumulation → foam cell formation → fatty streaks → smooth muscle cell migration (involves PDGF and FGF), proliferation, and extracellular matrix deposition → fibrous plaque → complex atheromas **A** → calcification (calcium content correlates with risk of complications). |
| COMPLICATIONS | Ischemia, infarction, aneurysm formation, peripheral vascular disease, thrombosis, embolism. |

| | |
|---|---|
| **Cholesterol emboli syndrome** | Microembolization of cholesterol displaced from atherosclerotic plaques in large arteries (usually the aorta). Results in end-organ damage due to small artery emboli and an inflammatory response (eg, livedo reticularis, digital ischemia [blue toe syndrome], acute renal failure, cerebrovascular accident, gut ischemia). Pulses remain palpable because larger arteries are unaffected. May follow invasive vascular procedures (angiography, angioplasty, endovascular grafting). |

**Arteriolosclerosis**

Common form of arteriosclerosis. Affects small arteries and arterioles. Two types:
- **Hyaline**—vessel wall thickening 2° to plasma protein leak into subendothelium in hypertension or diabetes mellitus **A**.
- **Hyperplastic**—"onion skinning" **B** in severe hypertension with proliferation of smooth muscle cells.

**Aortic aneurysm**

Localized pathologic dilation of the aorta. May cause abdominal and/or back pain, which is a sign of leaking, dissection, or imminent rupture.

**Thoracic aortic aneurysm**

Associated with cystic medial degeneration. Risk factors include hypertension, bicuspid aortic valve, connective tissue disease (eg, Marfan syndrome). Also associated with 3° syphilis (obliterative endarteritis of the vasa vasorum). Aortic root dilatation may lead to aortic valve regurgitation.

**Abdominal aortic aneurysm**

Associated with transmural (all 3 layers) inflammation and extracellular matrix degradation. Risk factors include tobacco smoking (strongest risk factor), ↑ age, male sex, family history. May present as palpable pulsatile abdominal mass (arrows in **A** point to outer dilated aortic wall). Rupture may present as triad of pulsatile abdominal mass, acute abdominal/back pain, and resistant hypotension. Most often infrarenal (distribution of vasa vasorum is reduced).

● Ascending thoracic aorta
◐ Aortic arch
○ Descending thoracic aorta
○ Abdominal aorta

**Traumatic aortic rupture**

Due to trauma and/or deceleration injury, most commonly at aortic isthmus (proximal descending aorta just distal to origin of left subclavian artery). X-ray may reveal widened mediastinum.

**Aortic dissection**

Longitudinal intimal tear forming a false lumen. Associated with hypertension (strongest risk factor), bicuspid aortic valve, inherited connective tissue disorders (eg, Marfan syndrome). Can present with tearing, sudden-onset chest pain radiating to the back +/− markedly unequal BP in arms. CXR can show mediastinal widening. Can result in organ ischemia, aortic rupture, death.

Stanford type **A** (proximal): involves Ascending aorta (red arrow in A). May extend to aortic arch or descending aorta (blue arrow in A). May result in acute aortic regurgitation or cardiac tamponade. Treatment: surgery.

Stanford type **B** (distal): involves only descending aorta (**B**elow left subclavian artery). Treatment: β-blockers, then vasodilators.

Stanford classification
Type A            Type B

Ascending
Descending

Type I    Type II    Type III
DeBakey classification

**Subclavian steal syndrome**

Stenosis of subclavian artery proximal to origin of vertebral artery → hypoperfusion distal to stenosis → reversed blood flow in ipsilateral vertebral artery → reduced cerebral perfusion on exertion of affected arm. Causes arm ischemia, pain, paresthesia, vertebrobasilar insufficiency (dizziness, vertigo), > 15 mm Hg difference in systolic BP between arms. Associated with atherosclerosis, Takayasu arteritis, heart surgery.

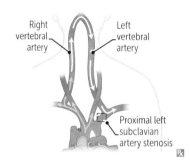

Right vertebral artery          Left vertebral artery

Proximal left subclavian artery stenosis

## Coronary artery disease

| | |
|---|---|
| **Angina** | Chest pain due to ischemic myocardium 2° to coronary artery narrowing or spasm; no necrosis.<br>▪ Stable—usually 2° to atherosclerosis (≥ 70% occlusion); exertional chest pain in classic distribution resolving with rest or nitroglycerin.<br>▪ Unstable—thrombosis with incomplete coronary artery occlusion; ↑ in frequency or intensity of chest pain or any chest pain at rest. No cardiac biomarker elevation (vs non–ST-segment elevation MI [NSTEMI]).<br>▪ Vasospastic (formerly Prinzmetal or variant)—occurs at rest 2° to coronary artery spasm; transient ischemic ST changes on ECG. Tobacco smoking is a major risk factor. Triggers include cocaine, amphetamines, alcohol, triptans. Treat with $Ca^{2+}$ channel blockers, nitrates, and smoking cessation (if applicable). |
| **Myocardial infarction** | Most often due to rupture of coronary artery atherosclerotic plaque → acute thrombosis. ↑ cardiac biomarkers (CK-MB, troponins) are diagnostic. |

| | Stable angina | Unstable angina | NSTEMI | STEMI |
|---|---|---|---|---|
| PAIN | On exertion | Mild exertion or at rest | At rest | At rest |
| TROPONIN LEVEL | No elevation | No elevation | Elevated | Elevated |
| INFARCTION | None | None | Subendocardial | Transmural |
| ECG CHANGES | Possible ST depression and/or T-wave inversion | Possible ST depression and/or T-wave inversion | ST depression and/or T-wave inversion | ST elevation, pathologic Q waves |

## Ischemic heart disease manifestations

| | |
|---|---|
| **Coronary steal syndrome** | Distal to coronary stenosis, vessels are maximally dilated at baseline. Administration of vasodilators (eg, dipyridamole, regadenoson) dilates normal vessels → blood is shunted toward well-perfused areas → ischemia in myocardium perfused by stenosed vessels. Vasodilator stress tests rely on differential flow to detect potential ischemia. Rarely, they can cause coronary steal and true ischemia. |
| **Sudden cardiac death** | Unexpected death due to cardiac causes within 1 hour of symptom onset, most commonly due to lethal arrhythmia (eg, ventricular fibrillation). Associated with CAD (up to 70% of cases), cardiomyopathy (hypertrophic, dilated), and hereditary channelopathies (eg, long QT syndrome, Brugada syndrome). Prevent with implantable cardioverter-defibrillator. |
| **Chronic ischemic heart disease** | Progressive onset of HF over many years due to chronic ischemic myocardial damage.<br>Myocardial hibernation—potentially reversible LV systolic dysfunction in the setting of chronic ischemia. Contrast with myocardial stunning, a transient LV systolic dysfunction after a brief episode of acute ischemia. |

| **Evolution of myocardial infarction** | Commonly occluded coronary arteries: LAD > RCA > circumflex. |
|---|---|
| | Symptoms: diaphoresis, nausea, vomiting, severe retrosternal pain, pain in left arm and/or jaw, shortness of breath, fatigue. |

| TIME | GROSS | LIGHT MICROSCOPE | COMPLICATIONS |
|---|---|---|---|
| 0–24 hours | Occluded artery; Dark mottling; pale with tetrazolium stain | Wavy fibers (0–4 hr), early coagulative necrosis (4–24 hr) **A** → cell content released into blood; edema, hemorrhage<br>Reperfusion injury → free radicals and ↑ $Ca^{2+}$ influx → hypercontraction of myofibrils (dark eosinophilic stripes)<br> | Ventricular arrhythmia, HF, cardiogenic shock |
| 1–3 days | Hyperemia | Extensive coagulative necrosis Tissue surrounding infarct shows acute inflammation with neutrophils **B**<br> | Postinfarction fibrinous pericarditis |
| 3–14 days | Hyperemic border; central yellow-brown softening | Macrophages, then granulation tissue at margins **C**<br> | Free wall rupture → tamponade; papillary muscle rupture → mitral regurgitation; interventricular septal rupture due to macrophage-mediated structural degradation → left-to-right shunt<br>LV pseudoaneurysm (risk of rupture) |
| 2 weeks to several months | Gray-white scar | Contracted scar complete **D**<br> | Postcardiac injury syndrome, HF, arrhythmias, true ventricular aneurysm (risk of mural thrombus) |

**Diagnosis of myocardial infarction**

In the first 6 hours, ECG is the gold standard. Cardiac troponin I rises after 4 hours (peaks at 24 hr) and is ↑ for 7–10 days; more specific than other protein markers.

CK-MB increases after 6–12 hours (peaks at 16–24 hr) and is predominantly found in myocardium but can also be released from skeletal muscle. Useful in diagnosing reinfarction following acute MI because levels return to normal after 48 hours.

ECG changes can include ST elevation (STEMI, transmural infarct), ST depression (NSTEMI, subendocardial infarct), hyperacute (peaked) T waves, T-wave inversion, and pathologic Q waves or poor R wave progression (evolving or old transmural infarct).

**ECG localization of STEMI**

| INFARCT LOCATION | LEADS WITH ST-SEGMENT ELEVATIONS OR Q WAVES |
|---|---|
| Anteroseptal (LAD) | $V_1$–$V_2$ |
| Anteroapical (distal LAD) | $V_3$–$V_4$ |
| Anterolateral (LAD or LCX) | $V_5$–$V_6$ |
| Lateral (LCX) | I, aVL |
| Inferior (RCA) | II, III, aVF |
| Posterior (PDA) | $V_7$–$V_9$,  ST depression in $V_1$–$V_3$ with tall R waves |

| Narrow complex tachycardias | Narrow QRS complex < 120 msec, rapid ventricular activation via normal ventricular conduction system, tachycardia originates within or above AV node (supraventricular arrhythmia). | |
|---|---|---|
| **ARRHYTHMIA** | **DESCRIPTION** | **ECG FINDINGS** |
| **Atrial fibrillation** | Irregularly irregular rate and rhythm with no discrete P waves. Arrhythmogenic activity usually originates from automatic foci near pulmonary vein ostia in left atrium. Common risk factors include hypertension and CAD. May predispose to thromboembolic events due to LA blood stasis, particularly stroke. Management: rate and rhythm control, cardioversion. Definitive treatment is ablation of pulmonary vein ostia. Consider anticoagulation based on stroke risk. | $RR_1 \neq RR_2 \neq RR_3 \neq RR_4$ Irregular baseline (absent P waves) |
| **Multifocal atrial tachycardia** | Irregularly irregular rate and rhythm with at least 3 distinct P wave morphologies, due to multiple ectopic foci in atria. Associated with underlying conditions such as COPD, pneumonia, HF. | |
| **Atrial flutter** | Rapid succession of identical, consecutive atrial depolarization waves causing "sawtooth" appearance of P waves. Arrhythmogenic activity usually originates from reentry circuit around tricuspid annulus in right atrium. Treat like atrial fibrillation +/– catheter ablation of region between tricuspid annulus and IVC. | $RR_1 = RR_2 = RR_3$ 4:1 sawtooth pattern |
| **Paroxysmal supraventricular tachycardia** | Most often due to a reentrant tract between atrium and ventricle, most commonly in AV node. Commonly presents with sudden-onset palpitations, lightheadedness, diaphoresis. Treatment: terminate reentry rhythm by slowing AV node conduction (eg, vagal maneuvers, IV adenosine), electrical cardioversion if hemodynamically unstable. Definitive treatment is catheter ablation of reentry tract. | |

| Wolff-Parkinson-White syndrome | Most common type of ventricular preexcitation syndrome. Abnormal fast accessory conduction pathway from atria to ventricle (bundle of Kent) bypasses rate-slowing AV node → ventricles partially depolarize earlier → characteristic delta wave with widened QRS complex and shortened PR interval. May result in reentry circuit → supraventricular tachycardia. Treatment: procainamide, ibutilide. Avoid AV nodal–blocking drugs (eg, adenosine, calcium channel blockers, β-blockers). | Delta wave PR interval Shortened PR interval Normal PR interval |

| | | |
|---|---|---|
| **Wide complex tachycardias** | Wide QRS complex ≥ 120 msec, slow ventricular activation outside normal ventricular conduction system, tachycardia originates below AV node (ventricular arrhythmia). | |

| ARRHYTHMIA | DESCRIPTION | ECG FINDINGS |
|---|---|---|
| Ventricular tachycardia | Typically regular rhythm, rate > 100. Most commonly due to structural heart disease (eg, cardiomyopathy, scarring after myocardial infarction). High risk of sudden cardiac death. | |
| Torsades de pointes | Polymorphic ventricular tachycardia. Shifting sinusoidal waveforms. May progress to ventricular fibrillation. Long QT interval predisposes to torsades de pointes. Caused by drugs, ↓ $K^+$, ↓ $Mg^{2+}$, ↓ $Ca^{2+}$.<br>Torsades de pointes = twisting of the points<br>Treatment: defibrillation for unstable patients, magnesium sulfate for stable patients.<br>Drug-induced long QT (ABCDEF+NO):<br>▪ anti-Arrhythmics (Ia and III), Arsenic<br>▪ anti-Biotics (macrolides, fluoroquinolones)<br>▪ anti-Cychotics (haloperidol), Chloroquine<br>▪ anti-Depressants (TCAs), Diuretics (thiazides)<br>▪ anti-Emetics (ondansetron)<br>▪ anti-Fungals (Fluconazole)<br>▪ Navir (protease inhibitors)<br>▪ Opioids (methadone) | |
| Ventricular fibrillation | Disorganized rhythm with no identifiable waves.<br>Treatment: fatal without immediate CPR and defibrillation. | <br>No discernible rhythm |

| | | |
|---|---|---|
| **Hereditary channelopathies** | Inherited mutations of cardiac ion channels → abnormal myocardial action potential → ↑ risk of ventricular tachyarrhythmias and sudden cardiac death (SCD). | |
| Brugada syndrome | Autosomal dominant; most commonly due to loss of function mutation of $Na^+$ channels. ↑ prevalence in Asian males. ECG pattern of pseudo-right bundle branch block and ST-segment elevations in leads $V_1$–$V_2$. Prevent SCD with ICD. | |
| Congenital long QT syndrome | Most commonly due to loss of function mutation of $K^+$ channels (affects repolarization). Includes:<br>▪ Romano-Ward syndrome—autosomal dominant, pure cardiac phenotype (no deafness).<br>▪ Jervell and Lange-Nielsen syndrome—autosomal recessive, sensorineural deafness. | |

| | | |
|---|---|---|
| **Sick sinus syndrome** | Age-related degeneration of SA node. ECG can show bradycardia, sinus pauses, sinus arrest, junctional escape beats. | <br>sinus pause |

## Conduction blocks

| ARRHYTHMIA | DESCRIPTION | ECG FINDINGS |
| --- | --- | --- |
| First-degree AV block | Prolonged PR interval (>200 msec). Treatment: none required (benign and asymptomatic). | |

### Second-degree AV block

| ARRHYTHMIA | DESCRIPTION | ECG FINDINGS |
| --- | --- | --- |
| Mobitz type I (Wenckebach) | Progressive lengthening of PR interval until a beat is "dropped" (P wave not followed by QRS complex). Variable RR interval with a pattern (regularly irregular). Treatment: none required (usually asymptomatic) | |
| Mobitz type II | Dropped beats that are not preceded by a change in PR interval. May progress to 3rd-degree block, as it usually indicates a structural abnormality such as ischemia or fibrosis. Treatment: usually a pacemaker. | |
| Third-degree (complete) AV block | P waves and QRS complexes rhythmically dissociated. Atria and ventricles beat independently of each other. Atrial rate > ventricular rate. May be caused by Lyme disease. Treatment: pacemaker. | |
| Bundle branch block | Interruption of conduction of normal left or right bundle branches. Affected ventricle depolarizes via slower myocyte-to-myocyte conduction from the unaffected ventricle, which depolarizes via the faster His-Purkinje system. Commonly due to degenerative changes (eg, cardiomyopathy, infiltrative disease). | |

## Premature beats

| ARRHYTHMIA | DESCRIPTION | ECG FINDINGS |
| --- | --- | --- |
| Premature atrial contraction | Extra beats arising from ectopic foci in atria instead of the SA node. Often $2°$ to ↑ adrenergic drive (eg, caffeine consumption). Benign, but may increase risk for atrial fibrillation and flutter. Narrow QRS complex with preceding P wave on ECG. | |
| Premature ventricular contraction | Ectopic beats arising from ventricle instead of the SA node. Shortened diastolic filling time → ↓ SV compared to a normal beat. Prognosis is largely influenced by underlying heart disease. Wide QRS complex with no preceding P wave on ECG. | |

## Myocardial infarction complications

| COMPLICATION | TIMEFRAME | FINDINGS | NOTES |
|---|---|---|---|
| Cardiac arrhythmia | First few days to several months | Can be supraventricular arrhythmias, ventricular arrhythmias, or conduction blocks. | Due to myocardial death and scarring. Important cause of death before reaching the hospital and within the first 48 hours post-MI. |
| Peri-infarction pericarditis | 1–3 days | Pleuritic chest pain, pericardial friction rub, ECG changes, and/or small pericardial effusion. | Usually self-limited. |
| Papillary muscle rupture | 2–7 days | Can result in acute mitral regurgitation → cardiogenic shock, severe pulmonary edema. | Posteromedial >> anterolateral papillary muscle rupture , as the posteromedial has single artery blood supply (PDA) whereas anterolateral has dual (LAD, LCX). |
| Interventricular septal rupture | 3–5 days | Symptoms can range from mild to severe with cardiogenic shock and pulmonary edema. | Macrophage-mediated degradation → VSD → ↑ $O_2$ saturation and ↑ pressure in RV. |
| Ventricular pseudoaneurysm | 3–14 days | May be asymptomatic. Symptoms may include chest pain, murmur, arrhythmia, syncope, HF, embolus from mural thrombus. Rupture → cardiac tamponade. | Free wall rupture contained by adherent pericardium or scar tissue—does not contain endocardium or myocardium. More likely to rupture than true aneurysm. |
| Ventricular free wall rupture | 5–14 days | Free wall rupture  → cardiac tamponade; acute form usually leads to sudden death. | LV hypertrophy and previous MI protect against free wall rupture. |
| True ventricular aneurysm | 2 weeks to several months | Similar to pseudoaneurysm. | Outward bulge with contraction ("dyskinesia"). Associated with fibrosis. |
| Postcardiac injury syndrome | Weeks to several months | Fibrinous pericarditis due to autoimmune reaction. | Also called Dressler syndrome. Cardiac antigens released after injury → deposition of immune complexes in pericardium → inflammation. |

Ventricular aneurysm

Pseudoaneurysm ℞

| | | |
|---|---|---|
| **Acute coronary syndrome treatments** | **Unstable angina/NSTEMI**—Anticoagulation (eg, heparin), antiplatelet therapy (eg, aspirin) + ADP receptor inhibitors (eg, clopidogrel), β-blockers, ACE inhibitors, statins. Symptom control with nitroglycerin +/– morphine. **STEMI**—In addition to above, reperfusion therapy most important (percutaneous coronary intervention preferred over fibrinolysis). If RV affected (eg, RCA occlusion), support venous return/preload to maintain cardiac output (eg, IV fluids, avoiding nitroglycerin). | |

## Cardiomyopathies

| | | |
|---|---|---|
| **Dilated cardiomyopathy**  | Most common cardiomyopathy (90% of cases). Often idiopathic or familial (eg, due to mutation of *TTN* gene encoding the sarcomeric protein titin). Other etiologies include drugs (eg, alcohol, cocaine, doxorubicin), infection (eg, coxsackie B virus, Chagas disease), ischemia (eg, CAD), systemic conditions (eg, hemochromatosis, sarcoidosis, thyrotoxicosis, wet beriberi), peripartum cardiomyopathy. Findings: HF, S3, systolic regurgitant murmur, dilated heart on echocardiogram, balloon appearance of heart on CXR. Treatment: $Na^+$ restriction, ACE inhibitors/ARBs, β-blockers, sacubitril, diuretics, mineralocorticoid receptor blockers (eg, spironolactone), ICD, heart transplant. | Leads to systolic dysfunction. Displays eccentric hypertrophy Ⓐ (sarcomeres added in series). Compare to athlete's heart, where LV and RV enlargement facilitates ↑ SV and ↑ CO. Stress cardiomyopathy (also called takotsubo cardiomyopathy, broken heart syndrome)—ventricular apical ballooning likely due to ↑ sympathetic stimulation (eg, stressful situations). |
| **Hypertrophic cardiomyopathy**  | 60–70% of cases are familial, autosomal dominant (most commonly due to mutations in genes encoding sarcomeric proteins, such as myosin binding protein C and β-myosin heavy chain). Causes syncope during exercise and may lead to sudden death (eg, in young athletes) due to ventricular arrhythmia. Findings: S4, systolic murmur. May see mitral regurgitation due to impaired mitral valve closure. Treatment: cessation of high-intensity athletics, use of β-blocker or nondihydropyridine $Ca^{2+}$ channel blockers (eg, verapamil). ICD if high risk. Avoid drugs that decrease preload (eg, diuretics, vasodilators). | Diastolic dysfunction ensues. Displays ventricular concentric hypertrophy (sarcomeres added in parallel) Ⓑ, often septal predominance. Myofibrillar disarray and fibrosis. Classified as hypertrophic obstructive cardiomyopathy when LV outflow tract is obstructed. Asymmetric septal hypertrophy and systolic anterior motion of mitral valve → outflow obstruction → dyspnea, possible syncope. Other causes of concentric LV hypertrophy: chronic HTN, Friedreich ataxia. |
| **Restrictive/infiltrative cardiomyopathy** | Postradiation fibrosis, Löffler endocarditis, Endocardial fibroelastosis (thick fibroelastic tissue in endocardium of young children), Amyloidosis, Sarcoidosis, Hemochromatosis (**PLEASe Help!**). | Diastolic dysfunction ensues. Can have low-voltage ECG despite thick myocardium (especially in amyloidosis). Löffler endocarditis—associated with hypereosinophilic syndrome; histology shows eosinophilic infiltrates in myocardium. |

## Heart failure

Clinical syndrome of cardiac pump dysfunction → congestion and low perfusion. Symptoms include dyspnea, orthopnea, fatigue; signs include S3 heart sound, rales, jugular venous distention (JVD), pitting edema .

Systolic dysfunction—heart failure with reduced ejection fraction (HFrEF), ↑ EDV; ↓ contractility often 2° to ischemia/MI or dilated cardiomyopathy.

Diastolic dysfunction—heart failure with preserved ejection fraction (HFpEF), normal EDV; ↓ compliance (↑ EDP) often 2° to myocardial hypertrophy.

Right HF most often results from left HF. Cor pulmonale refers to isolated right HF due to pulmonary cause.

ACE inhibitors, ARBs, angiotensin receptor–neprilysin inhibitors, β-blockers (except in acute decompensated HF), and aldosterone receptor antagonists ↓ mortality in HFrEF. Loop and thiazide diuretics are used mainly for symptomatic relief. Hydralazine with nitrate therapy and SGLT2 inhibitors improve both symptoms and mortality in select patients.

### Left heart failure

| | |
|---|---|
| Orthopnea | Shortness of breath when supine: ↑ venous return from redistribution of blood (immediate gravity effect) exacerbates pulmonary vascular congestion. |
| Paroxysmal nocturnal dyspnea | Breathless awakening from sleep: ↑ venous return from redistribution of blood, reabsorption of peripheral edema, etc. |
| Pulmonary edema | ↑ pulmonary venous pressure → pulmonary venous distention and transudation of fluid. Presence of hemosiderin-laden macrophages ("HF" cells) in lungs. |

### Right heart failure

| | |
|---|---|
| Congestive hepatomegaly | ↑ central venous pressure → ↑ resistance to portal flow. Rarely, leads to "cardiac cirrhosis." Associated with nutmeg liver (mottled appearance) on gross exam. |
| Jugular venous distention | ↑ venous pressure. |
| Peripheral edema | ↑ venous pressure → fluid transudation. |

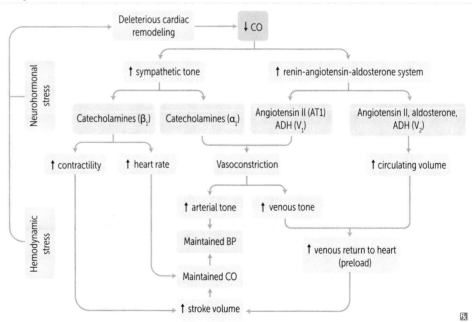

| | |
|---|---|
| **High-output heart failure** | Uncommon form of HF characterized by ↑ CO. High-output state is due to ↓ SVR from either vasodilation or arteriovenous shunting. Causes include severe obesity, advanced cirrhosis, severe anemia, hyperthyroidism, wet beriberi, Paget disease of bone.<br>Presents with symptoms and signs of pulmonary and/or systemic venous congestion. |

**Shock** — Inadequate organ perfusion and delivery of nutrients necessary for normal tissue and cellular function. Initially may be reversible but life threatening if not treated promptly.

| TYPE | CAUSED BY | MECHANISM | SKIN | CVP | PCWP | CO | SVR | SVO$_2$ |
|---|---|---|---|---|---|---|---|---|
| **Hypovolemic shock** | Hemorrhage, dehydration, burns | Volume depletion | | ↓ | ↓ | ↓ | ↑ | ↓ |
| **Cardiogenic shock** | MI, HF, valvular dysfunction, arrhythmia | Left heart dysfunction | Cold, clammy | ↑ | ↑ | ↓ | ↑ | ↓ |
| **Obstructive shock** | PE, tension pneumothorax | Impeded cardiopulmonary blood flow | | ↑ | ↓ | ↓ | ↑ | ↓ |
| | Cardiac tamponade | | | ↑ | ↑ | ↓ | ↑ | ↓ |
| **Distributive shock** | Sepsis (early), anaphylaxis | Systemic vasodilation | Warm, dry | ↓ | ↓ | ↑ | ↓ | ↑ |
| | CNS injury | | | ↓ | ↓ | ↓ | ↓ | normal/↑ |

↓ = 1° disturbance driving the shock.

| | |
|---|---|
| **Cardiac tamponade**<br> | Compression of the heart by fluid (eg, blood, effusions) → ↓ CO. Equilibration of diastolic pressures in all 4 chambers.<br>Findings: Beck triad (hypotension, distended neck veins, distant heart sounds), ↑ HR, pulsus paradoxus. ECG shows low-voltage QRS and electrical alternans **A** (due to "swinging" movement of heart in large effusion). Echocardiogram shows pericardial effusion (arrows in **B**), systolic RA collapse, diastolic RV collapse, and IVC plethora.<br>Treatment: pericardiocentesis or surgical drainage.<br><br>**Pulsus paradoxus**—↓ in amplitude of systolic BP by > 10 mm Hg during inspiration. ↑ venous return during inspiration → ↑ RV filling → interventricular septum bows toward LV (due to ↓ pericardial compliance) → ↓ LV ejection volume → ↓ systolic BP. Seen in constrictive pericarditis, obstructive pulmonary disease (eg, Croup, OSA, Asthma, COPD), cardiac Tamponade (pca COAT). |

| | |
|---|---|
| **Syncope** | Transient loss of consciousness caused by a period of ↓ cerebral blood flow. Types:<br>▪ Reflex (most common)—vasovagal (common faint), situational (eg, coughing/sneezing, swallowing, defecation, micturition), carotid sinus hypersensitivity (eg, wearing tight collar).<br>▪ Orthostatic—hypovolemia, drugs (eg, antihypertensives), autonomic dysfunction. Orthostatic hypotension is defined as a drop in systolic BP > 20 mm Hg and/or diastolic BP > 10 mm Hg upon standing.<br>▪ Cardiac—arrhythmias, structural (eg, aortic stenosis, HCM). |

**Infective endocarditis**

Infection of the endocardial surface of the heart, typically involving ≥1 heart valves. Caused by bacteria >> fungi. Forms:
- Acute—classically *S aureus* (high virulence). Large destructive vegetations **A** on previously normal valves. Rapid onset.
- Subacute—classically viridans streptococci (low virulence). Smaller vegetations on congenitally abnormal or diseased valves. Sequela of dental procedures. Gradual onset.

Presents with fever (most common), new murmur, vascular and immunologic phenomena.

Vascular phenomena—septic embolism, petechiae, splinter hemorrhages (linear hemorrhagic lesions on nail bed **B**), Janeway lesions (painless, flat, erythematous lesions on palms or soles).

Immunologic phenomena—immune complex deposition, glomerulonephritis, **O**sler nodes (painful ["**O**uchy"], raised, violaceous lesions on finger or toe pads **C**), **R**oth spots (**R**etinal hemorrhagic lesions with pale centers **D**).

Mitral valve (most common) > aortic valve. Tricuspid valve involvement is associated with injection **drug** use (don't "**tri**" drugs). Common associations:
- Prosthetic valves—*S epidermidis*
- GI/GU procedures—*Enterococcus*
- Colon cancer—*S gallolyticus*
- Gram ⊖—**HACEK** organisms (*Haemophilus, Aggregatibacter* [formerly *Actinobacillus*], *Cardiobacterium, Eikenella, Kingella*)
- Culture ⊖—*Coxiella, Bartonella*
- Injection drug use—*S aureus, Pseudomonas, Candida*

Endothelial injury → formation of vegetations consisting of platelets, fibrin, and microbes on heart valves → valve regurgitation, septic embolism (systemic circulation in left-sided endocarditis, pulmonary in right-sided).

Diagnosis requires multiple blood cultures and echocardiography.

| | | |
|---|---|---|
| **Nonbacterial thrombotic endocarditis** | Also called marantic endocarditis. Rare, noninfective. Vegetations typically arise on mitral or aortic valve and consist of sterile, platelet-rich thrombi that dislodge easily. Usually asymptomatic until embolism occurs. | Associated with the hypercoagulable state seen in advanced malignancy (especially pancreatic adenocarcinoma) or SLE (called Libman-Sacks endocarditis in this setting). |

**Rheumatic fever**

A consequence of pharyngeal infection with group A β-hemolytic streptococci. Late sequelae include rheumatic heart disease, which affects heart valves—mitral > aortic >> tricuspid (high-pressure valves affected most). Early valvular regurgitation, late valvular stenosis.

Associated with Aschoff bodies (granuloma with giant cells, Anitschkow cells (enlarged macrophages with ovoid, wavy, rodlike nucleus), ↑ anti-streptolysin O (ASO) and ↑ anti-DNase B titers.

Immune mediated (type II hypersensitivity); not a direct effect of bacteria. Antibodies to M protein cross-react with self antigens, often myosin (molecular mimicry).

Treatment/prophylaxis: penicillin.

J♥NES (major criteria):
Joint (migratory polyarthritis)
♥ (carditis)
Nodules in skin (subcutaneous)
Erythema marginatum (evanescent rash with ring margin)
Sydenham chorea (involuntary irregular movements of limbs and face)

**Syphilitic heart disease**

3° syphilis disrupts the vasa vasorum of the aorta with consequent atrophy of vessel wall and dilation of aorta and valve ring.

May see calcification of aortic root, ascending aortic arch, and thoracic aorta. Leads to "tree bark" appearance of aorta.

Can result in aneurysm of ascending aorta or aortic arch, aortic insufficiency.

**Acute pericarditis**

Inflammation of the pericardium (red arrows in A). Commonly presents with sharp pain, aggravated by inspiration, and relieved by sitting up and leaning forward. Often complicated by pericardial effusion (between yellow arrows in A). Presents with friction rub. ECG changes include widespread/diffuse ST-segment elevation and/or PR depression.

Usually idiopathic, but may be due to viral infections (eg, coxsackievirus B), malignancy (metastasis), cardiac surgery, thoracic radiotherapy (early), MI (eg, postcardiac injury syndrome), autoimmune diseases (eg, SLE, rheumatoid arthritis), renal failure (uremia).

Treatment: NSAIDs, colchicine, glucocorticoids, dialysis (uremia).

**Constrictive pericarditis**

Chronic inflammation of pericardium → pericardial fibrosis +/– calcification → limited space for expansion → ↓ ventricular filling. Usually idiopathic, but may be due to viral infections, cardiac surgery, thoracic radiotherapy (late). TB is the most common cause in resource-limited countries. ↓ EDV → ↓ CO → ↓ venous return. Presents with dyspnea, peripheral edema, jugular venous distention, Kussmaul sign, pulsus paradoxus, pericardial knock.

| | |
|---|---|
| **Kussmaul sign** | Paradoxical ↑ in JVP on inspiration (normally, inspiration → negative intrathoracic pressure → ↑ venous return → ↓ JVP). Impaired RV filling → RV cannot accommodate ↑ venous return during inspiration → blood backs up into vena cava → Kussmaul sign. May be seen with constrictive pericarditis, restrictive cardiomyopathy, right HF, massive pulmonary embolism, right atrial or ventricular tumors. |

| | |
|---|---|
| **Myocarditis** | Inflammation of myocardium. Major cause of SCD in adults < 40 years old.<br>Presentation highly variable, can include dyspnea, chest pain, fever, arrhythmias (persistent tachycardia out of proportion to fever is characteristic).<br>Multiple causes:<br>▪ Viral (eg, adenovirus, coxsackie B, parvovirus B19, HIV, HHV-6, COVID-19); lymphocytic infiltrate with focal necrosis highly indicative of viral myocarditis<br>▪ Parasitic (eg, *Trypanosoma cruzi*, *Toxoplasma gondii*)<br>▪ Bacterial (eg, *Borrelia burgdorferi*, *Mycoplasma pneumoniae*, *Corynebacterium diphtheriae*)<br>▪ Toxins (eg, carbon monoxide, black widow venom)<br>▪ Rheumatic fever<br>▪ Drugs (eg, doxorubicin, cocaine)<br>▪ Autoimmune (eg, Kawasaki disease, sarcoidosis, SLE, polymyositis/dermatomyositis)<br>Complications include sudden death, arrhythmias, heart block, dilated cardiomyopathy, HF, mural thrombus with systemic emboli. |

| | |
|---|---|
| **Hereditary hemorrhagic telangiectasia** | Also called Osler-Weber-Rendu syndrome. Autosomal dominant disorder of blood vessels. Findings: blanching lesions (telangiectasias) on skin and mucous membranes, recurrent epistaxis, AVMs (eg, brain, lung, liver), GI bleeding, hematuria.<br>**Arteriovenous malformation**—abnormal, high-flow connection between artery and vein. |

| | |
|---|---|
| **Cardiac tumors** | Most common cardiac tumor is a metastasis (eg, melanoma). |
| **Myxomas**<br> | Most common 1° cardiac tumor in **adults** (arrows in A). 90% occur in the atria (mostly left atrium). Myxomas are usually described as a "ball valve" obstruction in the left atrium (associated with multiple syncopal episodes). IL-6 production by tumor → constitutional symptoms (eg, fever, weight loss). May auscultate early diastolic "tumor plop" sound (mimics mitral stenosis). Histology: gelatinous material, myxoma cells immersed in glycosaminoglycans.<br>**Adults** make 6 **myxed** drinks. |
| **Rhabdomyomas** | Most frequent 1° cardiac tumor in children (associated with tuberous sclerosis). Histology: hamartomatous growths. More common in the ventricles. |

▶ CARDIOVASCULAR—PHARMACOLOGY

**Hypertension treatment**

| | | |
|---|---|---|
| Primary (essential) hypertension | Thiazide diuretics, ACE inhibitors, angiotensin II receptor blockers (ARBs), dihydropyridine $Ca^{2+}$ channel blockers. | |
| Hypertension with heart failure | Diuretics, ACE inhibitors/ARBs, β-blockers (compensated HF), aldosterone antagonists. | β-blockers must be used cautiously in decompensated HF and are contraindicated in cardiogenic shock. In HF, ARBs may be combined with the neprilysin inhibitor sacubitril. |
| Hypertension with diabetes mellitus | ACE inhibitors/ARBs, $Ca^{2+}$ channel blockers, β-blockers. | ACE inhibitors/ARBs are protective against diabetic nephropathy. β-blockers can mask hypoglycemia symptoms. |
| Hypertension in asthma | ARBs, $Ca^{2+}$ channel blockers, thiazide diuretics, cardioselective β-blockers. | Avoid nonselective β-blockers to prevent $\beta_2$-receptor–induced bronchoconstriction. Avoid ACE inhibitors to prevent confusion between drug or asthma-related cough. |
| Hypertension in pregnancy | Nifedipine, methyldopa, labetalol, hydralazine. | New moms love hugs. |

## Cardiovascular agents and molecular targets

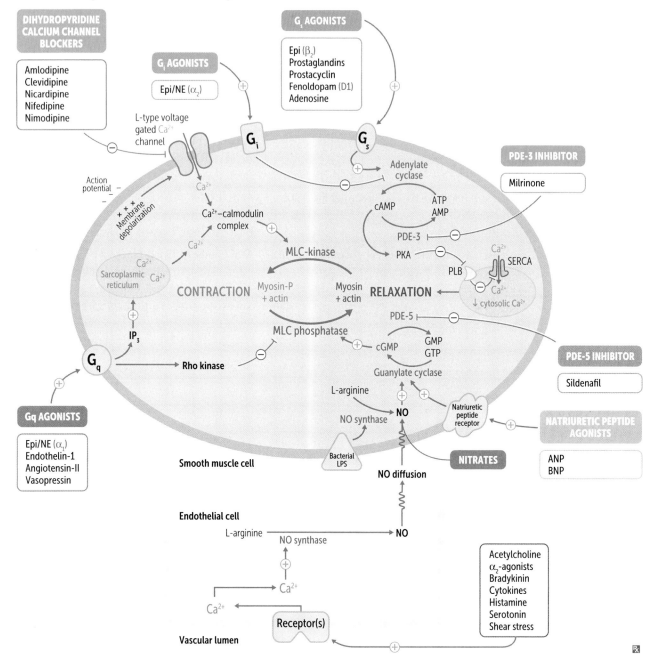

| Nitrates | Nitroglycerin, isosorbide dinitrate, isosorbide mononitrate. |
|---|---|
| MECHANISM | Vasodilate by ↑ NO in vascular smooth muscle → ↑ in cGMP and smooth muscle relaxation. Dilate veins >> arteries. ↓ preload. |
| CLINICAL USE | Angina, acute coronary syndrome, pulmonary edema. |
| ADVERSE EFFECTS | Reflex tachycardia (treat with β-blockers), methemoglobinemia, hypotension, flushing, headache, "Monday disease" in industrial nitrate exposure: development of tolerance for the vasodilating action during the work week and loss of tolerance over the weekend → tachycardia, dizziness, headache upon reexposure. Contraindicated in right ventricular infarction, hypertrophic cardiomyopathy, and with concurrent PDE-5 inhibitor use. |

| | |
|---|---|
| **Calcium channel blockers** | Amlodipine, clevidipine, nicardipine, nifedipine, nimodipine (dihydropyridines, act on vascular smooth muscle); diltiazem, verapamil (nondihydropyridines, act on heart). |
| MECHANISM | Block voltage-dependent L-type calcium channels of cardiac and smooth muscle → ↓ muscle contractility.<br>Vascular smooth muscle—amlodipine = nifedipine > diltiazem > verapamil.<br>Heart—verapamil > diltiazem > amlodipine = nifedipine. |
| CLINICAL USE | Dihydropyridines (except nimodipine): hypertension, angina (including vasospastic type), Raynaud phenomenon. Dihydropyridine mainly dilates arteries.<br>Nimodipine: subarachnoid hemorrhage (prevents delayed ischemia).<br>Nicardipine, clevidipine: hypertensive urgency or emergency.<br>Nondihydropyridines: hypertension, angina, atrial fibrillation/flutter. |
| ADVERSE EFFECTS | Gingival hyperplasia.<br>Dihydropyridine: peripheral edema, flushing, dizziness.<br>Nondihydropyridine: cardiac depression, AV block, hyperprolactinemia (verapamil), constipation. |

| | |
|---|---|
| **Hydralazine** | |
| MECHANISM | ↑ cGMP → smooth muscle relaxation. Hydralazine vasodilates arterioles > veins; afterload reduction. |
| CLINICAL USE | Severe hypertension (particularly acute), HF (with organic nitrate). Safe to use during pregnancy. Frequently coadministered with a β-blocker to prevent reflex tachycardia. |
| ADVERSE EFFECTS | Compensatory tachycardia (contraindicated in angina/CAD), fluid retention, headache, angina, drug-induced lupus. |

| | |
|---|---|
| **Hypertensive emergency** | Treat with labetalol, clevidipine, fenoldopam, nicardipine, nitroprusside. |
| Nitroprusside | Short acting vasodilator (arteries = veins); ↑ cGMP via direct release of NO. Can cause cyanide toxicity (releases cyanide). |
| Fenoldopam | Dopamine $D_1$ receptor agonist—coronary, peripheral, renal, and splanchnic vasodilation.<br>↓ BP, ↑ natriuresis. Also used postoperatively as an antihypertensive. Can cause hypotension, tachycardia, flushing, headache, nausea. |

| | |
|---|---|
| **Antianginal therapy** | Goal is reduction of myocardial $O_2$ consumption ($MVO_2$) by ↓ 1 or more of the determinants of $MVO_2$: end-diastolic volume, BP, HR, contractility. |

| COMPONENT | NITRATES | β-BLOCKERS | NITRATES + β-BLOCKERS |
|---|---|---|---|
| End-diastolic volume | ↓ | No effect or ↑ | No effect or ↓ |
| Blood pressure | ↓ | ↓ | ↓ |
| Contractility | ↑ (reflex response) | ↓ | Little/no effect |
| Heart rate | ↑ (reflex response) | ↓ | No effect or ↓ |
| Ejection time | ↓ | ↑ | Little/no effect |
| $MVO_2$ | ↓ | ↓ | ↓↓ |

Nondihydropyridine calcium channel blockers (verapamil, diltiazem) are similar to β-blockers in effect.

## Ranolazine

| | |
|---|---|
| MECHANISM | Inhibits the late phase of inward sodium current thereby reducing diastolic wall tension and oxygen consumption. Does not affect heart rate or blood pressure. |
| CLINICAL USE | Refractory angina. |
| ADVERSE EFFECTS | Constipation, dizziness, headache, nausea. |

## Sacubitril

| | |
|---|---|
| MECHANISM | A neprilysin inhibitor; prevents degradation of bradykinin, natriuretic peptides, angiotensin II, and substance P → ↑ vasodilation, ↓ ECF volume. |
| CLINICAL USE | Used in combination with valsartan (an ARB) to treat HFrEF. |
| ADVERSE EFFECTS | Hypotension, hyperkalemia, cough, dizziness; contraindicated with ACE inhibitors due to angioedema (both drugs ↑ bradykinin). |

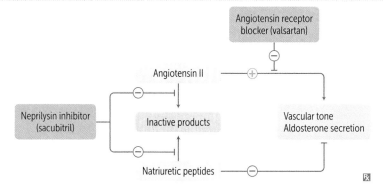

## Lipid-lowering agents

| DRUG | LDL | HDL | TRIGLYCERIDES | MECHANISM | ADVERSE EFFECTS |
|---|---|---|---|---|---|
| **Statins** Atorvastatin, lovastatin, pravastatin, rosuvastatin, simvastatin | ↓↓↓ | ↑ | ↓ | Inhibit HMG-CoA reductase → ↓ cholesterol synthesis; → ↓ intrahepatic cholesterol → ↑ LDL receptor recycling → ↑ LDL catabolism ↓ in mortality in patients with CAD | Hepatotoxicity (↑ LFTs), myopathy (especially when used with fibrates or niacin) |
| **Bile acid resins** Cholestyramine, colesevelam, colestipol | ↓↓ | ↑ slightly | ↑ slightly | Disrupt enterohepatic bile acid circulation → compensatory ↑ conversion of cholesterol to bile → ↓ intrahepatic cholesterol → ↑ LDL receptor recycling | GI upset, ↓ absorption of other drugs and fat-soluble vitamins |
| **Ezetimibe** | ↓↓ | ↑/— | ↓/— | Prevents cholesterol absorption at small intestine brush border | Rare ↑ LFTs, diarrhea |

## Lipid-lowering agents (continued)

| DRUG | LDL | HDL | TRIGLYCERIDES | MECHANISM | ADVERSE EFFECTS |
|------|-----|-----|---------------|-----------|-----------------|
| **Fibrates**<br>Fenofibrate,<br>gemfibrozil | ↓ | ↑ | ↓↓↓ | Activate PPAR-α<br>→ upregulate LPL → ↑ TG<br>clearance<br>Activate PPAR-α → induce<br>HDL synthesis | Myopathy (↑ risk with<br>statins), cholesterol<br>gallstones (via<br>inhibition of cholesterol<br>7α-hydroxylase) |
| **Niacin** | ↓↓ | ↑↑ | ↓ | Inhibits lipolysis (hormone-<br>sensitive lipase) in adipose<br>tissue; reduces hepatic<br>VLDL synthesis | Flushed face<br>(prostaglandin mediated;<br>↓ by NSAIDs or long-<br>term use)<br>Hyperglycemia<br>Hyperuricemia |
| **PCSK9 inhibitors**<br>Alirocumab,<br>evolocumab | ↓↓↓ | ↑ | ↓ | Inactivation of LDL-receptor<br>degradation → ↑ removal of<br>LDL from bloodstream | Myalgias, delirium,<br>dementia, other<br>neurocognitive effects |
| **Fish oil and marine<br>omega-3 fatty acids** | ↑ slightly | ↑ slightly | ↓ at high<br>doses | Believed to decrease FFA<br>delivery to liver and decrease<br>activity of TG-synthesizing<br>enzymes | Nausea, fishlike taste |

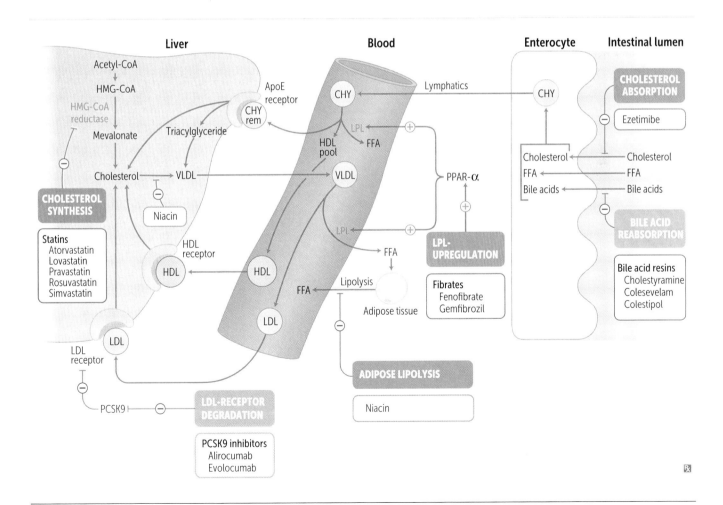

## Digoxin

| | |
|---|---|
| MECHANISM | Direct inhibition of $Na^+/K^+$-ATPase.<br>→ indirect inhibition of $Na^+/Ca^{2+}$ exchanger.<br>$\uparrow [Ca^{2+}]_i$ → positive inotropy. Stimulates vagus nerve → $\downarrow$ HR. |

Na⁺/Ca²⁺ exchanger — Digoxin — Na⁺/K⁺-ATPase

$Ca^{2+}$ — $Na^+$ — $K^+$

$SR \longrightarrow \uparrow\uparrow Ca^{2+} \rightarrow \uparrow TnC\ Ca^{2+}$ binding $\rightarrow \uparrow$ cardiac contraction

| | |
|---|---|
| CLINICAL USE | HF ($\uparrow$ contractility); atrial fibrillation ($\downarrow$ conduction at AV node and depression of SA node). |
| ADVERSE EFFECTS | Cholinergic effects (nausea, vomiting, diarrhea), blurry yellow vision ("van Glow"), arrhythmias, atrial tachycardia with AV block.<br>Can lead to hyperkalemia, which indicates poor prognosis.<br>Factors predisposing to toxicity: renal failure ($\downarrow$ excretion), hypokalemia (permissive for digoxin binding at $K^+$-binding site on $Na^+/K^+$-ATPase), drugs that displace digoxin from tissue-binding sites, and $\downarrow$ clearance (eg, verapamil, amiodarone, quinidine). |
| ANTIDOTE | Slowly normalize $K^+$, cardiac pacer, anti-digoxin Fab fragments, $Mg^{2+}$. |

## Antiarrhythmics— sodium channel blockers (class I)

Slow or block conduction (especially in depolarized cells). $\downarrow$ slope of phase 0 depolarization. $\uparrow$ action at faster HR. State dependent $\uparrow$ HR → shorter diastole, $Na^+$ channels spend less time in resting state (drugs dissociate during this state) → less time for drug to dissociate from receptor. Effect most pronounced in IC>IA>IB due to relative binding strength. **Fast taxi CAB.**

| | |
|---|---|
| **Class IA** | Quinidine, procainamide, disopyramide.<br>"The queen proclaims Diso's pyramid." |
| MECHANISM | Moderate $Na^+$ channel blockade.<br>$\uparrow$ AP duration, $\uparrow$ effective refractory period (ERP) in ventricular action potential, $\uparrow$ QT interval, some $K^+$ channel blocking effects. |
| CLINICAL USE | Both atrial and ventricular arrhythmias, especially reentrant and ectopic SVT and VT. |
| ADVERSE EFFECTS | Cinchonism (headache, tinnitus with quinidine), reversible SLE-like syndrome (procainamide), HF (disopyramide), thrombocytopenia, torsades de pointes due to $\uparrow$ QT interval. |

0 mV
Slope of phase 0 $I_{Na}$

| | |
|---|---|
| **Class IB** | Lidocaine, mexiletine.<br>"I'd Buy Liddy's Mexican tacos." |
| MECHANISM | Weak $Na^+$ channel blockade.<br>$\downarrow$ AP duration. Preferentially affect ischemic or depolarized Purkinje and ventricular tissue. |
| CLINICAL USE | Acute ventricular arrhythmias (especially post-MI), digitalis-induced arrhythmias.<br>IB is Best post-MI. |
| ADVERSE EFFECTS | CNS stimulation/depression, cardiovascular depression. |

0 mV
Slope of phase 0 $I_{Na}$

**Antiarrhythmics—sodium channel blockers (class I)** *(continued)*

| | | |
|---|---|---|
| **Class IC** | Flecainide, propafenone. "Can I have fries, please?" |  |
| MECHANISM | Strong Na⁺ channel blockade. Significantly prolongs ERP in AV node and accessory bypass tracts. No effect on ERP in Purkinje and ventricular tissue. Minimal effect on AP duration. | |
| CLINICAL USE | SVTs, including atrial fibrillation. Only as a last resort in refractory VT. | |
| ADVERSE EFFECTS | Proarrhythmic, especially post-MI (contraindicated). IC is Contraindicated in structural and ischemic heart disease. | |

| | |
|---|---|
| **Antiarrhythmics— β-blockers (class II)** | Metoprolol, propranolol, esmolol, atenolol, timolol, carvedilol. |
| MECHANISM | Decrease SA and AV nodal activity by ↓ cAMP, ↓ $Ca^{2+}$ currents. Suppress abnormal pacemakers by ↓ slope of phase 4. AV node particularly sensitive—↑ PR interval. Esmolol very short acting. |
| CLINICAL USE | SVT, ventricular rate control for atrial fibrillation and atrial flutter, prevent ventricular arrhythmia post-MI. |
| ADVERSE EFFECTS | Impotence, exacerbation of COPD and asthma, cardiovascular effects (bradycardia, AV block, HF), CNS effects (sedation, sleep alterations). May mask the signs of hypoglycemia. Metoprolol can cause dyslipidemia. Propranolol can exacerbate vasospasm in vasospastic angina. β-blockers (except the nonselective α- and β-antagonists carvedilol and labetalol) cause unopposed $α_1$-agonism if given alone for pheochromocytoma or for cocaine toxicity (unsubstantiated). Treat β-blocker overdose with saline, atropine, glucagon. |

For the β-blockers graph:
- Membrane potential (mv) on y-axis (60, 30, 0, −30, −60, −90)
- Time (ms) on x-axis (0, 100, 200, 300, 400, 500, 600, 700, 800)
- Decrease slope of phase 4 depolarization
- Prolonged repolarization (at AV node)
- Threshold potential
- Pacemaker cell action potential

**Antiarrhythmics— potassium channel blockers (class III)**

Amiodarone, Ibutilide, Dofetilide, Sotalol.

AIDS.

| | |
|---|---|
| MECHANISM | ↑ AP duration, ↑ ERP, ↑ QT interval. |
| CLINICAL USE | Atrial fibrillation, atrial flutter; ventricular tachycardia (amiodarone, sotalol). |

ADVERSE EFFECTS

Sotalol—torsades de pointes, excessive β blockade.
Ibutilide—torsades de pointes.
Amiodarone—pulmonary fibrosis, hepatotoxicity, hypothyroidism or hyperthyroidism (amiodarone is 40% iodine by weight), acts as hapten (corneal deposits, blue/gray skin deposits resulting in photodermatitis), neurologic effects, constipation, cardiovascular effects (bradycardia, heart block, HF).

Remember to check PFTs, LFTs, and TFTs when using amiodarone.
Amiodarone is lipophilic and has class I, II, III, and IV effects.

Cell action potential

**Antiarrhythmics— calcium channel blockers (class IV)**

Diltiazem, verapamil.

| | |
|---|---|
| MECHANISM | Decrease conduction velocity, ↑ ERP, ↑ PR interval. |
| CLINICAL USE | Prevention of nodal arrhythmias (eg, SVT), rate control in atrial fibrillation. |
| ADVERSE EFFECTS | Constipation, gingival hyperplasia, flushing, edema, cardiovascular effects (HF, AV block, sinus node depression). |

**Other antiarrhythmics**

| | |
|---|---|
| Adenosine | ↑ K⁺ out of cells → hyperpolarizing the cell and ↓ $I_{Ca}$, decreasing AV node conduction. Drug of choice in diagnosing/terminating certain forms of SVT. Very short acting (~ 15 sec). Effects blunted by theophylline and caffeine (both are adenosine receptor antagonists). Adverse effects include flushing, hypotension, chest pain, sense of impending doom, bronchospasm. |
| Magnesium | Effective in torsades de pointes and digoxin toxicity. |

**Ivabradine**

| | |
|---|---|
| MECHANISM | IVabradine prolongs slow depolarization (phase "IV") by selectively inhibiting "funny" sodium channels ($I_f$). |
| CLINICAL USE | Chronic HFrEF. |
| ADVERSE EFFECTS | Luminous phenomena/visual brightness, hypertension, bradycardia. |

# Endocrine

*"If you skew the endocrine system, you lose the pathways to self."*
—Hilary Mantel

*"Sometimes you need a little crisis to get your adrenaline flowing and help you realize your potential."*
—Jeannette Walls, *The Glass Castle*

*"Chocolate causes certain endocrine glands to secrete hormones that affect your feelings and behavior by making you happy."*
—Elaine Sherman, *Book of Divine Indulgences*

The endocrine system comprises widely distributed organs that work in a highly integrated manner to orchestrate a state of hormonal equilibrium within the body. Generally speaking, endocrine diseases can be classified either as diseases of underproduction or overproduction, or as conditions involving the development of mass lesions—which themselves may be associated with underproduction or overproduction of hormones. Therefore, study the endocrine system first by learning the glands, their hormones, and their regulation, and then by integrating disease manifestations with diagnosis and management. Take time to learn the multisystem connections.

▶ **ENDOCRINE—EMBRYOLOGY**

**Thyroid development**

Thyroid diverticulum arises from floor of primitive pharynx and descends into neck. Connected to tongue by thyroglossal duct, which normally disappears but may persist as cysts or the pyramidal lobe of thyroid. Foramen cecum is normal remnant of thyroglossal duct.

Most common ectopic thyroid tissue site is the tongue (lingual thyroid). Removal may result in hypothyroidism if it is the only thyroid tissue present.

Thyroglossal duct cyst **A** presents as an anterior midline neck mass that moves with swallowing or protrusion of the tongue (vs persistent cervical sinus leading to pharyngeal cleft cyst in lateral neck).

Thyroid follicular cells **B** derived from endoderm.

Parafollicular cells arise from 4th pharyngeal pouch.

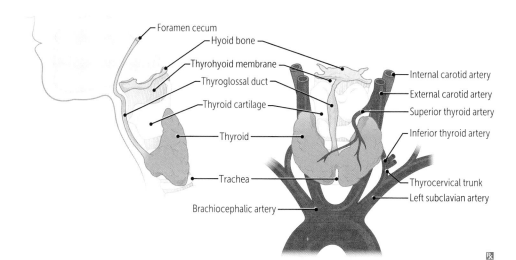

## ▶ ENDOCRINE—ANATOMY

### Pituitary gland

| | | |
|---|---|---|
| Anterior pituitary (adenohypophysis) | Secretes FSH, LH, ACTH, TSH, prolactin, GH, and β-endorphin. Melanotropin (MSH) secreted from intermediate lobe of pituitary. Derived from oral ectoderm (Rathke pouch).<br>  ▪ α subunit—hormone subunit common to TSH, LH, FSH, and hCG.<br>  ▪ β subunit—determines hormone specificity. | Proopiomelanocortin derivatives—β-endorphin, ACTH, and MSH. Go **pro** with a **BAM!**<br>**FLAT PeG**: FSH, LH, ACTH, TSH, PRL, GH.<br>**B-FLAT**: Basophils—FSH, LH, ACTH, TSH.<br>**Acid PiG**: Acidophils — PRL, GH. |
| Posterior pituitary (neurohypophysis) | Stores and releases vasopressin (antidiuretic hormone, or ADH) and oxytocin, both made in the hypothalamus (supraoptic and paraventricular nuclei) and transported to posterior pituitary via neurophysins (carrier proteins). Derived from **neuro**ectoderm. | |

### Adrenal cortex and medulla

Adrenal cortex (derived from mesoderm) and medulla (derived from neural crest).

| ANATOMY | HISTOLOGY | | | 1° REGULATION BY | HORMONE CLASS | 1° HORMONE PRODUCED |
|---|---|---|---|---|---|---|
| | Zona **G**lomerulosa | | | Angiotensin II | Mineralocorticoids | Aldosterone |
| | Zona **F**asciculata | CORTEX | | ACTH, CRH | Glucocorticoids | Cortisol |
| | Zona **R**eticularis | | | ACTH, CRH | Androgens | DHEA |
| | Chromaffin cells | MEDULLA | | Preganglionic sympathetic fibers | Catecholamines | Epi, NE |

**GFR** corresponds with **s**alt (mineralocorticoids), **s**ugar (glucocorticoids), and **s**ex (androgens).

### Endocrine pancreas cell types

Islets of Langerhans are collections of α, β, and δ endocrine cells. Islets arise from pancreatic buds.

α = gluc**α**gon (peripheral)
β = insulin (central)
δ = somatostatin (interspersed)

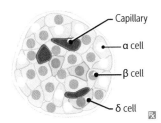

▶ **ENDOCRINE—PHYSIOLOGY**

### Hypothalamic-pituitary hormones

| HORMONE | FUNCTION | CLINICAL NOTES |
|---|---|---|
| ADH | ↑ water permeability of distal convoluted tubule and collecting duct cells in kidney to ↑ water reabsorption | Alcohol consumption → ↓ ADH secretion → polyuria and dehydration |
| CRH | ↑ ACTH, ↑ MSH, ↑ β-endorphin | ↓ in chronic glucocorticoid use |
| Dopamine | ↓ prolactin, ↓ TSH | Also called prolactin-inhibiting factor<br>Dopamine antagonists (eg, antipsychotics) can cause galactorrhea due to hyperprolactinemia |
| GHRH | ↑ GH | Analog (tesamorelin) used to treat HIV-associated lipodystrophy |
| GnRH | ↑ FSH, ↑ LH | Suppressed by hyperprolactinemia<br>Tonic GnRH analog (eg, leuprolide) suppresses hypothalamic–pituitary–gonadal axis.<br>Pulsatile GnRH leads to puberty, fertility |
| MSH | ↑ melanogenesis by melanocytes | Causes hyperpigmentation in Cushing disease, as MSH and ACTH share the same precursor molecule, proopiomelanocortin |
| Oxytocin | Causes uterine contractions during labor. Responsible for milk letdown reflex in response to suckling. | Modulates fear, anxiety, social bonding, mood, and depression |
| Prolactin | ↓ GnRH<br>Stimulates lactogenesis. | Pituitary prolactinoma → amenorrhea, osteoporosis, hypogonadism, galactorrhea<br>Breastfeeding → ↑ prolactin → ↓ GnRH → delayed postpartum ovulation (natural contraception) |
| Somatostatin | ↓ GH, ↓ TSH | Also called growth hormone inhibiting hormone (GHIH) |
| TRH | ↑ TSH, ↑ prolactin | ↑ TRH (eg, in 1°/2° hypothyroidism) may increase prolactin secretion → galactorrhea |

## Growth hormone

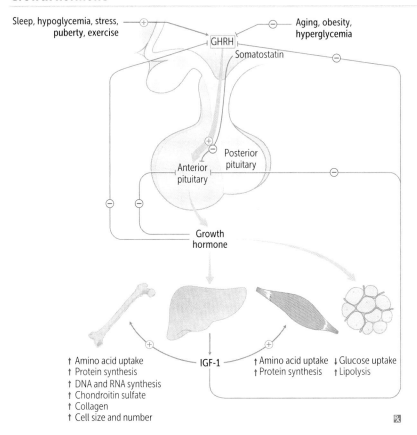

Also called somatotropin. Secreted by anterior pituitary.

Stimulates linear growth and muscle mass through IGF-1 (somatomedin C) secretion by liver. ↑ insulin resistance (diabetogenic).

Released in pulses in response to growth hormone–releasing hormone (GHRH).

Secretion ↑ during sleep, hypoglycemia, stress, puberty, exercise.

Secretion ↓ with aging, obesity, hyperglycemia, somatostatin, somatomedin (regulatory molecule secreted by liver in response to GH acting on target tissues).

Excess secretion of GH (eg, pituitary adenoma) may cause acromegaly (adults) or gigantism (children). Treatment: somatostatin analogs (eg, octreotide) or surgery.

| Antidiuretic hormone | Also called vasopressin. |
|---|---|
| SOURCE | Synthesized in hypothalamus (supraoptic and paraventricular nuclei), stored and secreted by posterior pituitary. |
| FUNCTION | Regulates blood pressure ($V_1$-receptors) and serum osmolality ($V_2$-receptors). Primary function is serum osmolality regulation (ADH ↓ serum osmolality, ↑ urine osmolality) via regulation of aquaporin channel insertion in principal cells of renal collecting duct. — ADH level is ↓ in central diabetes insipidus (DI), normal or ↑ in nephrogenic DI. Desmopressin (ADH analog) is a treatment for central DI and nocturnal enuresis. Vasopressin is a potent vasopressor that can be used to increase organ perfusion in septic shock. |
| REGULATION | Plasma osmolality (1°); hypovolemia. |

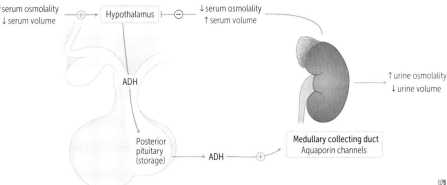

## Prolactin

SOURCE
Secreted mainly by anterior pituitary.

Structurally homologous to growth hormone.

FUNCTION
Stimulates milk production in breast; inhibits ovulation in females and spermatogenesis in males by inhibiting GnRH synthesis and release.

Excessive amounts of prolactin associated with ↓ libido.

REGULATION
Prolactin secretion from anterior pituitary is tonically inhibited by dopamine from tuberoinfundibular pathway of hypothalamus. Prolactin in turn inhibits its own secretion by ↑ dopamine synthesis and secretion from hypothalamus. TRH ↑ prolactin secretion (eg, in 1° or 2° hypothyroidism). Dopamine has stronger effect on prolactin regulation than TRH does.

Dopamine agonists (eg, bromocriptine, cabergoline) inhibit prolactin secretion and can be used in treatment of prolactinoma. Dopamine antagonists (eg, most antipsychotics, metoclopramide) and estrogens (eg, OCPs, pregnancy) stimulate prolactin secretion.

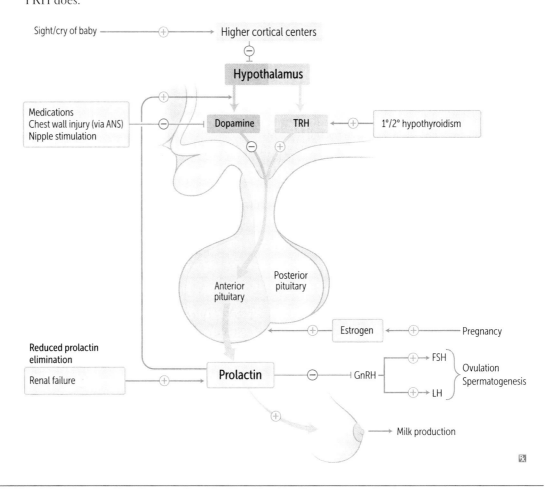

| | |
|---|---|
| **Thyroid hormones** | Thyroid produces triiodothyronine ($T_3$) and thyroxine ($T_4$), iodine-containing hormones that control the body's metabolic rate. |
| SOURCE | Follicles of thyroid. 5′-deiodinase converts $T_4$ (the major thyroid product) to $T_3$ in peripheral tissue (5, 4, 3). Peripheral conversion is inhibited by glucocorticoids, β-blockers, and propylthiouracil (PTU). Reverse $T_3$ ($rT_3$) is a metabolically inactive byproduct of the peripheral conversion of $T_4$ and its production is increased by growth hormone and glucocorticoids. Functions of thyroid peroxidase include oxidation, organification of iodine, and coupling of monoiodotyrosine (MIT) and diiodotyrosine (DIT). Inhibited by PTU and methimazole. DIT + DIT = $T_4$. DIT + MIT = $T_3$. Wolff-Chaikoff effect—protective autoregulation; sudden exposure to excess iodine temporarily turns off thyroid peroxidase → ↓ $T_3/T_4$ production. |
| FUNCTION | Only free hormone is active. $T_3$ binds nuclear receptor with greater affinity than $T_4$. $T_3$ functions —7 B's:<br>▪ Brain maturation<br>▪ Bone growth (synergism with GH and IGF-1)<br>▪ β-adrenergic effects. ↑ $\beta_1$ receptors in heart → ↑ CO, HR, SV, contractility; β-blockers alleviate adrenergic symptoms in thyrotoxicosis<br>▪ Basal metabolic rate ↑ (via ↑ $Na^+/K^+$-ATPase → ↑ $O_2$ consumption, RR, body temperature)<br>▪ Blood sugar (↑ glycogenolysis, gluconeogenesis)<br>▪ Break down lipids (↑ lipolysis)<br>▪ Stimulates surfactant synthesis in Babies |
| REGULATION | TRH → ⊕ TSH release → ⊕ follicular cells. Thyroid-stimulating immunoglobulin (TSI) may ⊕ follicular cells in Graves disease.<br>Negative feedback primarily by free $T_3/T_4$:<br>▪ Anterior pituitary → ↓ sensitivity to TRH<br>▪ Hypothalamus → ↓ TRH secretion<br>Thyroxine-binding globulin (TBG) binds most $T_3/T_4$ in blood. Bound $T_3/T_4$ = inactive.<br>▪ ↑ TBG in pregnancy, OCP use (estrogen → ↑ TBG) → ↑ total $T_3/T_4$<br>▪ ↓ TBG in steroid use, nephrotic syndrome<br>$T_3$ and $T_4$ are the only lipophilic hormones with charged amino acids and require specific transporters to diffuse into the cell (facilitated diffusion). |

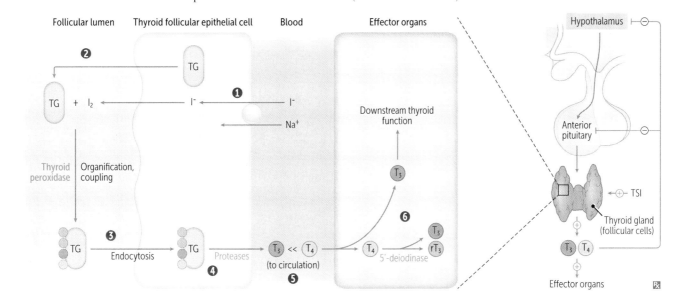

## Parathyroid hormone

| | |
|---|---|
| SOURCE | Chief cells of parathyroid |
| FUNCTION | ↑ free $Ca^{2+}$ in the blood (1° function)<br>↑ $Ca^{2+}$ and $PO_4^{3-}$ absorption in GI system<br>↑ $Ca^{2+}$ and $PO_4^{3-}$ from bone resorption<br>↑ $Ca^{2+}$ reabsorption from DCT<br>↓ $PO_4^{3-}$ reabsorption in PCT<br>↑ 1,25-$(OH)_2D_3$ (calcitriol) production by activating 1α-hydroxylase in PCT (**tri** to make $D_3$ in the PCT) | PTH ↑ serum $Ca^{2+}$, ↓ serum $PO_4^{3-}$, ↑ urine $PO_4^{3-}$, ↑ urine cAMP<br>↑ RANK-L (receptor activator of NF-κB ligand) secreted by osteoblasts and osteocytes; binds RANK (receptor) on osteoclasts and their precursors to stimulate osteoclasts and ↑ $Ca^{2+}$ → bone resorption (intermittent PTH release can also stimulate bone formation)<br>PTH = Phosphate-Trashing Hormone<br>PTH-related peptide (PTHrP) functions like PTH and is commonly increased in malignancies (eg, squamous cell carcinoma of the lung, renal cell carcinoma) |
| REGULATION | ↓ serum $Ca^{2+}$ → ↑ PTH secretion<br>↑ serum $PO_4^{3-}$ → ↑ PTH secretion<br>↓ serum $Mg^{2+}$ → ↑ PTH secretion<br>↓↓ serum $Mg^{2+}$ → ↓ PTH secretion<br>Common causes of ↓ $Mg^{2+}$ include diarrhea, aminoglycosides, diuretics, alcohol use disorder | $Ca^{2+}$ is the major regulator of PTH release |

**PTH activity**

↓ ionized $Ca^{2+}$, ↑ $PO_4^{3-}$, or ↓ 1,25-$(OH)_2 D_3$

⊕

Four parathyroid glands

⊖ Feedback inhibition of PTH synthesis

PTH released into circulation

↑ 1,25-$(OH)_2 D_3$

Renal tubular cells

↑ 1,25-$(OH)_2 D_3$ synthesis
Reabsorption: ↑ $Ca^{2+}$, ↓ $PO_4^{3-}$
Urine ↓ $Ca^{2+}$, ↑ $PO_4^{3-}$

↑ $Ca^{2+}$ and ↓ $PO_4^{3-}$

**Vitamin D activity**

25-OH $D_3$

⊕    ⊕    ↓ $PO_4^{3-}$

1α-hydroxylase

1,25-$(OH)_2 D_3$

Bone          Intestines

↑ $Ca^{2+}$ and ↑ $PO_4^{3-}$ released from bone

↑ absorption of $Ca^{2+}$ and $PO_4^{3-}$

↑ $Ca^{2+}$ and ↑ $PO_4^{3-}$

| | | |
|---|---|---|
| **Calcium homeostasis** | Plasma $Ca^{2+}$ exists in three forms: <br> ▪ Ionized/free (~ 45%, active form) <br> ▪ Bound to albumin (~ 40%) <br> ▪ Bound to anions (~ 15%) <br> Ionized/free $Ca^{2+}$ is 1° regulator of PTH; changes in pH alter PTH secretion, whereas changes in albumin concentration do not | $Ca^{2+}$ competes with $H^+$ to bind to albumin <br> ↑ pH (less $H^+$) → albumin binds more $Ca^{2+}$ → ↓ ionized $Ca^{2+}$ (eg, cramps, pain, paresthesias, carpopedal spasm) → ↑ PTH <br> ↓ pH (more $H^+$) → albumin binds less $Ca^{2+}$ → ↑ ionized $Ca^{2+}$ → ↓ PTH |

## Calcitonin

| | | |
|---|---|---|
| SOURCE | Parafollicular cells (C cells) of thyroid. | Calcitonin opposes actions of PTH. Not important in normal $Ca^{2+}$ homeostasis |
| FUNCTION | ↓ bone resorption. | Calcitonin tones down serum $Ca^{2+}$ levels and keeps it in bones |
| REGULATION | ↑ serum $Ca^{2+}$ → ↑ calcitonin secretion. | |

Parafollicular cells (C cells) of thyroid

↑ serum $Ca^{2+}$ → ↑ calcitonin

Peripheral blood

Osteoclast — Decreased resorption

Calcitonin lowers serum $Ca^{2+}$ by inhibiting osteoclastic bone resorption

## Glucagon

| | |
|---|---|
| SOURCE | Made by $\alpha$ cells of pancreas. |
| FUNCTION | Promotes glycogenolysis, gluconeogenesis, lipolysis, ketogenesis. Elevates blood sugar levels to maintain homeostasis when bloodstream glucose levels fall too low (ie, fasting state). |
| REGULATION | Secreted in response to hypoglycemia. Inhibited by insulin, amylin, somatostatin, hyperglycemia. |

## Insulin

| | |
|---|---|
| SYNTHESIS | Preproinsulin (synthesized in RER of pancreatic β cells) → cleavage of "presignal" → proinsulin (stored in secretory granules) → cleavage of proinsulin → exocytosis of insulin and C-peptide equally. Both insulin and C-peptide are ↑ in endogenous insulin secretion (eg, type 2 DM, insulin secretagogues, insulinoma), whereas exogenous insulin lacks C-peptide. |

☐ Insulin  ■ C-peptide
Proinsulin

Insulin is synthesized in pancreas and cleared by both liver and kidneys.

FUNCTION

Binds insulin receptors (tyrosine kinase activity ❶), inducing glucose uptake (carrier-mediated transport) into insulin-dependent tissue ❷ and gene transcription.

Anabolic effects of insulin:
- ↑ glucose transport in skeletal muscle and adipose tissue
- ↑ glycogen synthesis and storage
- ↑ triglyceride synthesis
- ↑ Na⁺ retention (kidneys)
- ↑ protein synthesis (muscles)
- ↑ cellular uptake of K⁺ and amino acids
- ↓ glucagon release
- ↓ lipolysis in adipose tissue

Unlike glucose, insulin does not cross placenta. In mothers with diabetes, excess glucose can cross placenta and ↑↑ fetal insulin.

Insulin-dependent glucose transporters:
- GLUT4: adipose tissue, striated muscle (exercise can also ↑ GLUT4 expression)

Insulin-independent transporters:
- GLUT1: RBCs, brain, cornea, placenta
- GLUT2 (bidirectional): β islet cells, liver, kidney, GI tract (think 2-way street)
- GLUT3: brain, placenta
- GLUT5 (fructose): spermatocytes, GI tract
- SGLT1/SGLT2 (Na⁺-glucose cotransporters): kidney, small intestine

Brain prefers glucose, but may use ketone bodies during starvation. RBCs utilize only glucose, as they lack mitochondria for aerobic metabolism.

**BRICK LIPS** (insulin-independent glucose uptake): Brain, RBCs, Intestine, Cornea, Kidney, Liver, Islet (β) cells, Placenta, Spermatocytes.

REGULATION

Glucose is the major regulator of insulin release. ↑ insulin response with oral vs IV glucose due to incretins (eg, glucagonlike peptide 1 [GLP-1], glucose-dependent insulinotropic polypeptide [GIP]), which are released after meals and ↑ β cell sensitivity to glucose. Release ↓ by α₂, ↑ by β₂ stimulation (2 = regulates insulin).

Glucose enters β cells ❸ → ↑ ATP generated from glucose metabolism ❹ closes K⁺ channels (target of sulfonylureas) ❺ and depolarizes β cell membrane ❻. Voltage-gated Ca²⁺ channels open → Ca²⁺ influx ❼ and stimulation of insulin exocytosis ❽.

Insulin-dependent glucose uptake          Insulin secretion by pancreatic β cells

## Adrenal steroids and congenital adrenal hyperplasias

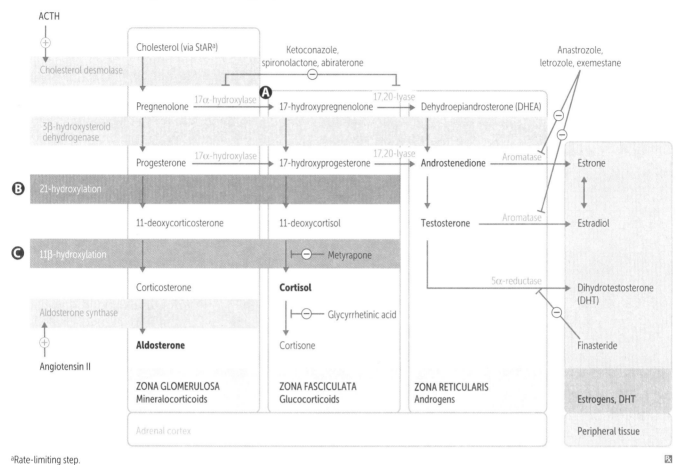

[a]Rate-limiting step.

| ENZYME DEFICIENCY | MINERALOCORTICOIDS | [K⁺] | BP | CORTISOL | SEX HORMONES | LABS | PRESENTATION |
|---|---|---|---|---|---|---|---|
| **A 17α-hydroxylase[a]** | ↑ | ↓ | ↑ | ↓ | ↓ | ↓ androstenedione | XY: atypical genitalia, undescended testes<br>XX: lacks 2° sexual development |
| **B 21-hydroxylase[a]** | ↓ | ↑ | ↓ | ↓ | ↑ | ↑ renin activity<br>↑ 17-hydroxy-progesterone | Most common<br>Presents in infancy (salt wasting) or childhood (precocious puberty)<br>XX: virilization |
| **C 11β-hydroxylase[a]** | ↓ aldosterone<br>↑ 11-deoxycorti-costerone<br>(results in ↑ BP) | ↓ | ↑ | ↓ | ↑ | ↓ renin activity | Presents in infancy (severe hypertension) or childhood (precocious puberty)<br>XX: virilization |

[a]All congenital adrenal enzyme deficiencies are autosomal recessive disorders and most are characterized by skin hyperpigmentation (due to ↑ MSH production, which is coproduced and secreted with ACTH) and bilateral adrenal gland enlargement (due to ↑ ACTH stimulation).

If deficient enzyme starts with 1, it causes hypertension; if deficient enzyme ends with 1, it causes virilization in females.

## Cortisol

| | | |
|---|---|---|
| SOURCE | Adrenal zona fasciculata. | Bound to corticosteroid-binding globulin. |
| FUNCTION | ↑ Appetite<br>↑ Blood pressure:<br>  ▪ Upregulates $\alpha_1$-receptors on arterioles → ↑ sensitivity to norepinephrine and epinephrine (permissive action)<br>  ▪ At high concentrations, can bind to mineralocorticoid (aldosterone) receptors<br>↑ Insulin resistance (diabetogenic)<br>↑ Gluconeogenesis, lipolysis, and proteolysis (↓ glucose utilization)<br>↓ Fibroblast activity (poor wound healing, ↓ collagen synthesis, ↑ striae)<br>↓ Inflammatory and Immune responses:<br>  ▪ Inhibits production of leukotrienes and prostaglandins<br>  ▪ Inhibits WBC adhesion → neutrophilia<br>  ▪ Blocks histamine release from mast cells<br>  ▪ Eosinopenia, lymphopenia<br>  ▪ Blocks IL-2 production<br>↓ Bone formation (↓ osteoblast activity) | Cortisol is **A BIG FIB**.<br>Exogenous glucocorticoids can cause reactivation of TB and candidiasis (blocks IL-2 production).<br><br> |
| REGULATION | CRH (hypothalamus) stimulates ACTH release (pituitary) → cortisol production in adrenal zona fasciculata. Excess cortisol ↓ CRH, ACTH, and cortisol secretion. | Chronic stress may induce prolonged cortisol secretion, cortisol resistance, impaired immunocompetency, and dysregulation of HPA axis. |

## Appetite regulation

| | |
|---|---|
| **Ghrelin** | Stimulates hunger (orexigenic effect) and GH release (via GH secretagog receptor). Produced by stomach. Sleep deprivation, fasting, or Prader-Willi syndrome → ↑ ghrelin production.<br>Ghrelin makes you ghrow hunghry. Acts on lateral area of hypothalamus (hunger center) to ↑ appetite. |
| **Leptin** | Satiety hormone. Produced by adipose tissue. Mutation of leptin gene → severe obesity. Obese people have ↑ leptin due to ↑ adipose tissue but are tolerant or resistant to leptin's anorexigenic effect. Sleep deprivation or starvation → ↓ leptin production.<br>Leptin keeps you thin. Acts on ventromedial area of hypothalamus (satiety center) to ↓ appetite. |
| **Endocannabinoids** | Act at cannabinoid receptors in hypothalamus and nucleus accumbens, two key brain areas for the homeostatic and hedonic control of food intake → ↑ appetite.<br>Exogenous cannabinoids cause "the munchies." |

## Signaling pathways of endocrine hormones

| cAMP | FSH, LH, ACTH, TSH, CRH, hCG, ADH ($V_2$-receptor), MSH, PTH, Calcitonin, Histamine ($H_2$-receptor), Glucagon, GHRH | FLAT ChAMPs CHuGG |
|---|---|---|
| cGMP | BNP, ANP, EDRF (NO) | BAD GraMPa<br>Think vasodilation and diuresis |
| $IP_3$ | GnRH, Oxytocin, ADH ($V_1$-receptor), TRH, Histamine ($H_1$-receptor), Angiotensin II, Gastrin | GOAT HAG |
| Intracellular receptor | Progesterone, Estrogen, Testosterone, Cortisol, Aldosterone, $T_3$/$T_4$, Vitamin D | PET CAT in TV |
| Receptor tyrosine kinase | IGF-1, FGF, PDGF, EGF, Insulin | MAP kinase pathway<br>Get Found In the MAP |
| Nonreceptor tyrosine kinase | G-CSF, Erythropoietin, Thrombopoietin Prolactin, Immunomodulators (eg, cytokines IL-2, IL-6, IFN), GH | JAK/STAT pathway<br>Think acidophils and cytokines<br>GET a JAKed PIG |

## Signaling pathways of steroid hormones

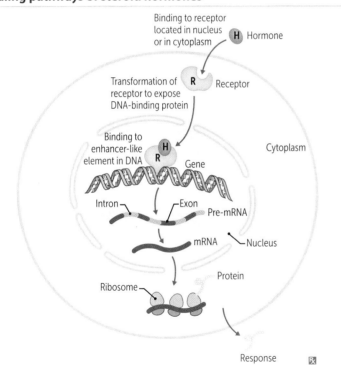

Steroid hormones are lipophilic and therefore must circulate bound to specific binding globulins, which ↑ their solubility.

In males, ↑ sex hormone–binding globulin (SHBG) lowers free testosterone → gynecomastia.

In females, ↓ SHBG raises free testosterone → hirsutism.

↑ estrogen (eg, OCPs, pregnancy) → ↑ SHBG.

## ▶ ENDOCRINE—PATHOLOGY

### Syndrome of inappropriate antidiuretic hormone secretion

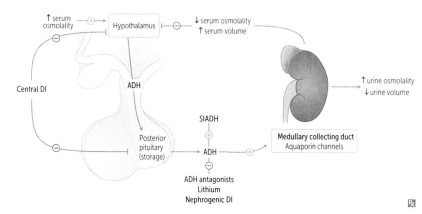

Characterized by excessive free water retention, euvolemic hyponatremia with continued urinary $Na^+$ excretion, urine osmolality > serum osmolality.

Body responds to water retention with ↓ aldosterone and ↑ ANP and BNP → ↑ urinary $Na^+$ secretion → normalization of extracellular fluid volume → euvolemic hyponatremia.

Treatment: fluid restriction (first line), salt tablets, IV hypertonic saline, diuretics, ADH antagonists (eg, conivaptan, tolvaptan, demeclocycline).

SIADH causes include (**HEELD**-up water):
- Head trauma/CNS disorders
- Ectopic ADH (eg, small cell lung cancer)
- Exogenous hormones (eg, vasopressin, desmopressin, oxytocin)
- Lung disease
- Drugs (eg, SSRIs, carbamazepine, cyclophosphamide)

### Primary polydipsia and diabetes insipidus

Characterized by the production of large amounts of dilute urine +/– thirst. Urine specific gravity < 1.006. Urine osmolality usually < 300 mOsm/kg. Central DI may be transient if damage is below hypothalamic median eminence or in the posterior pituitary (ADH in hypothalamus can still be secreted systemically via portal capillaries in median eminence).

| | Primary polydipsia | Central DI | Nephrogenic DI |
|---|---|---|---|
| DEFINITION | Excessive water intake | ↓ ADH release | ADH resistance |
| CAUSES | Psychiatric illnesses, hypothalamic lesions affecting thirst center | Idiopathic, brain injury (trauma, hypoxia, tumor, surgery, infiltrative diseases) | Hereditary (ADH receptor mutation), drugs (eg, lithium, demeclocycline), hypercalcemia, hypokalemia |
| SERUM OSMOLALITY | ↓ | ↑ | ↑ |
| ADH LEVEL | ↓ or normal | ↓ | Normal or ↑ |
| WATER RESTRICTION[a] | Significant ↑ in urine osmolality (> 700 mOsm/kg) | No change or slight ↑ in urine osmolality | No change or slight ↑ in urine osmolality |
| DESMOPRESSIN ADMINISTRATION[b] | — | Significant ↑ in urine osmolality (> 50%) | Minimal change in urine osmolality |
| TREATMENT | Water restriction | Desmopressin (DDAVP) | Manage the underlying cause; low-solute diet, HCTZ, amiloride, indomethacin |

[a]No water intake for 2–3 hours followed by hourly measurements of urine volume and osmolality as well as plasma $Na^+$ concentration and osmolality.

[b]Desmopressin (ADH analog) is administered if serum osmolality > 295–300 mOsm/kg, plasma $Na^+$ ≥ 145 mEq/L, or urine osmolality does not increase despite ↑ plasma osmolality.

| | |
|---|---|
| **Hypopituitarism** | Undersecretion of pituitary hormones due to |
| | ▪ Nonsecreting pituitary adenoma, craniopharyngioma |
| | ▪ Sheehan syndrome—ischemic infarct of pituitary following severe postpartum hemorrhage; pregnancy-induced pituitary growth → ↑ susceptibility to hypoperfusion. Usually presents with failure to lactate, amenorrhea, cold intolerance (anterior pituitary hormones mainly affected). |
| | ▪ Pituitary apoplexy—sudden hemorrhage of pituitary gland, often in the presence of an existing pituitary adenoma. Usually presents with sudden onset severe headache, visual impairment (eg, bitemporal hemianopia, diplopia due to CN III palsy), and features of hypopituitarism |
| | ▪ Brain injury |
| | ▪ Radiation |
| | Treatment: hormone replacement therapy (glucocorticoids, thyroxine, sex steroids, human growth hormone) |

| | |
|---|---|
| **Acromegaly** | Excess GH in adults. Typically caused by pituitary adenoma. |

| | | |
|---|---|---|
| FINDINGS | Large tongue with deep furrows, frontal bossing, coarsening of facial features with aging , deep voice, diaphoresis (excessive sweating), hypertrophic arthropathy, impaired glucose tolerance (insulin resistance), HTN, LVH, HFpEF (most common cause of death). | ↑ GH in children → gigantism (↑ linear bone growth due to unfused epiphysis). Acromegaly in adults, gigantism in j(g)uniors. |
| DIAGNOSIS | ↑ serum IGF-1 (GH levels unreliable as they fluctuate throughout the day); failure to suppress serum GH following oral glucose tolerance test; pituitary mass seen on brain MRI. | Baseline RU |
| TREATMENT | Pituitary adenoma resection. If not cured, treat with octreotide (somatostatin analog), pegvisomant (GH receptor antagonist), or dopamine agonists (eg, cabergoline). | |

## Hypothyroidism vs hyperthyroidism

| | Hypothyroidism | Hyperthyroidism |
|---|---|---|
| METABOLIC | Cold intolerance, ↓ sweating, weight gain (↓ basal metabolic rate → ↓ calorigenesis), hyponatremia (↓ free water clearance) | Heat intolerance, ↑ sweating, weight loss (↑ synthesis of $Na^+/K^+$-ATPase → ↑ basal metabolic rate → ↑ calorigenesis) |
| SKIN/HAIR | Dry, cool skin (due to ↓ blood flow); coarse, brittle hair; diffuse alopecia; brittle nails; puffy facies and generalized nonpitting edema (myxedema) due to ↑ GAGs in interstitial spaces → ↑ osmotic pressure → water retention | Warm, moist skin (due to vasodilation); fine hair; onycholysis (); pretibial myxedema in Graves disease  |
| OCULAR | Periorbital edema  | Ophthalmopathy in Graves disease (including periorbital edema, exophthalmos), lid lag/retraction (↑ sympathetic stimulation of superior tarsal muscle) |
| GASTROINTESTINAL | Constipation (↓ GI motility), ↓ appetite | Hyperdefecation/diarrhea (↑ GI motility), ↑ appetite |
| MUSCULOSKELETAL | Hypothyroid myopathy (proximal weakness, ↑ CK), carpal tunnel syndrome, myoedema (small lump rising on the surface of a muscle when struck with a hammer) | Thyrotoxic myopathy (proximal weakness, normal CK), osteoporosis/↑ fracture rate ($T_3$ directly stimulates bone resorption) |
| REPRODUCTIVE | Abnormal uterine bleeding, ↓ libido, infertility | Abnormal uterine bleeding, gynecomastia, ↓ libido, infertility |
| NEUROPSYCHIATRIC | Hypoactivity, lethargy, fatigue, weakness, depressed mood, ↓ reflexes (delayed/slow relaxing) | Hyperactivity, restlessness, anxiety, insomnia, fine tremors (due to ↑ β-adrenergic activity), ↑ reflexes (brisk) |
| CARDIOVASCULAR | Bradycardia, dyspnea on exertion (↓ cardiac output) | Tachycardia, palpitations, dyspnea, arrhythmias (eg, atrial fibrillation), chest pain and systolic HTN due to ↑ number and sensitivity of β-adrenergic receptors, ↑ expression of cardiac sarcolemmal ATPase and ↓ expression of phospholamban |
| LABS | ↑ TSH (if 1°)<br>↓ free $T_4$<br>Hypercholesterolemia (due to ↓ LDL receptor expression) | ↓ TSH (if 1°)<br>↑ free $T_3$ and $T_4$<br>↓ LDL, HDL, and total cholesterol |

## Hypothyroidism

| | |
|---|---|
| **Hashimoto thyroiditis** | Also called chronic autoimmune thyroiditis. Most common cause of hypothyroidism in iodine-sufficient regions. Associated with HLA-DR3 (differs by ethnicity), ↑ risk of primary thyroid lymphoma (typically diffuse large B-cell lymphoma). <br> Findings: moderately enlarged, **nontender** thyroid. May be preceded by transient hyperthyroid state ("Hashitoxicosis") due to follicular rupture and thyroid hormone release. <br> Serology: ⊕ antithyroid peroxidase (antimicrosomal) and antithyroglobulin antibodies. <br> Histology: Hürthle cells A, lymphoid aggregates with germinal centers B. <br> Postpartum thyroiditis—mild, self-limited variant of Hashimoto thyroiditis arising < 1 year after delivery. |
| **Subacute granulomatous thyroiditis** | Also called de Quervain thyroiditis. Usually, a self-limited disease. Natural history: transient hyperthyroidism → euthyroid state → hypothyroidism → euthyroid state. Often preceded by viral infection. <br> Findings: ↑ ESR, jaw pain, very **tender** thyroid (de Quervain is associated with **pain**). <br> Histology: granulomatous inflammation C. |
| **Riedel thyroiditis** | Also called invasive fibrous thyroiditis. May occur as part of IgG₄-related disease spectrum (eg, autoimmune pancreatitis, retroperitoneal fibrosis, noninfectious aortitis). Hypothyroidism occurs in ⅓ of patients. Fibrosis may extend to local structures (eg, trachea, esophagus), mimicking anaplastic carcinoma. <br> Findings: slowly enlarging, hard (rocklike), fixed, **nontender** thyroid. <br> Histology: thyroid replaced by fibrous tissue and inflammatory infiltrate D. |
| **Congenital hypothyroidism** | Formerly called cretinism. Most commonly caused by thyroid dysgenesis (abnormal thyroid gland development; eg, agenesis, hypoplasia, ectopy) or dyshormonogenesis (abnormal thyroid hormone synthesis; eg, mutations in thyroid peroxidase) in iodine-sufficient regions. <br> Findings (6 P's): pot-bellied, pale, puffy-faced child E with protruding umbilicus, protuberant tongue F, and poor brain development. |
| **Other causes** | Iodine deficiency (most common cause worldwide; typically presents with goiter G), iodine excess (Wolff-Chaikoff effect), drugs (eg, amiodarone, lithium), nonthyroidal illness syndrome (also called euthyroid sick syndrome; ↓ $T_3$ with normal/↓ $T_4$ and TSH in critically ill patients). |

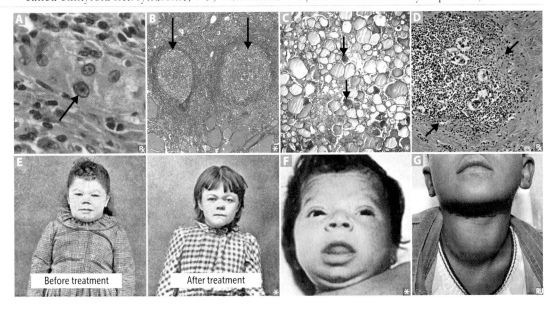

Before treatment

After treatment

## Hyperthyroidism

| | |
|---|---|
| **Graves disease**  | Most common cause of hyperthyroidism. Thyroid-stimulating immunoglobulin (IgG, can cause transient neonatal hyperthyroidism; type II hypersensitivity) stimulates TSH receptors on thyroid (hyperthyroidism, diffuse goiter), dermal fibroblasts (pretibial myxedema), and orbital fibroblasts (Graves orbitopathy; treat with glucocorticoids). Activation of T-cells → lymphocytic infiltration of retroorbital space → ↑ cytokines (eg, TNF-α, IFN-γ) → ↑ fibroblast secretion of hydrophilic GAGs → ↑ osmotic muscle swelling, muscle inflammation, and adipocyte count → exophthalmos A. Often presents during stress (eg, pregnancy). Associated with HLA-DR3 and HLA-B8. Histology: tall, crowded follicular epithelial cells; scalloped colloid. |
| **Toxic multinodular goiter** | Focal patches of hyperfunctioning follicular cells distended with colloid working independently of TSH (due to TSH receptor mutations in 60% of cases). ↑ release of $T_3$ and $T_4$. Hot nodules (hyperfunctioning nodules visualized on radioactive iodine scan) are rarely malignant. |
| **Thyroid storm** | Uncommon but serious complication that occurs when hyperthyroidism is incompletely treated/ untreated and then significantly worsens in the setting of acute stress such as infection, trauma, surgery. Presents with agitation, delirium, fever, diarrhea, coma, and tachyarrhythmia (cause of death). May see ↑ LFTs. Treat with the 4 P's: β-blockers (eg, propranolol), propylthiouracil, glucocorticoids (eg, prednisolone), potassium iodide (Lugol iodine). Iodide load → ↓ $T_4$ synthesis → Wolff-Chaikoff effect. |
| **Other causes** | Exogenous thyrotoxicosis (excessive intake of thyroid hormone; suspect in patient trying to lose weight), ectopic thyroid production (struma ovarii), contrast-induced thyroiditis (Jod-Basedow phenomenon), drug-induced thyroiditis (amiodarone, lithium). |

| | |
|---|---|
| **Causes of goiter** | Smooth/diffuse: Graves disease, Hashimoto thyroiditis, iodine deficiency, TSH-secreting pituitary adenoma.<br>Nodular: toxic multinodular goiter, thyroid adenoma, thyroid cancer, thyroid cyst. |

| | |
|---|---|
| **Thyroid adenoma**  | Benign solitary growth of the thyroid. Most are nonfunctional ("cold" on radioactive iodine scan), can rarely cause hyperthyroidism via autonomous thyroid hormone production ("hot" or "toxic"). Most common histology is follicular (arrows in A); absence of capsular or vascular invasion (unlike follicular carcinoma). |

| | |
|---|---|
| **Thyroid cancer** | Typically diagnosed with fine needle aspiration; treated with thyroidectomy. Complications of surgery include hypocalcemia (due to removal of parathyroid glands), transection of recurrent laryngeal nerve during ligation of inferior thyroid artery (leads to dysphagia and dysphonia [hoarseness]), and injury to the external branch of the superior laryngeal nerve during ligation of superior thyroid vascular pedicle (may lead to loss of tenor usually noticeable in professional voice users). |
| **Papillary carcinoma**<br> | Most common. Empty-appearing nuclei with central clearing ("Orphan Annie" eyes) $\blacksquare$, psam**Moma** bodies, nuclear grooves (**Papi** and **Moma** adopted Orphan Annie). ↑ risk with *RET/PTC* rearrangements and *BRAF* mutations, childhood irradiation.<br>Papillary carcinoma: most prevalent, palpable lymph nodes. Good prognosis. |
| **Follicular carcinoma** | Good prognosis. Invades tumor capsule and vasculature (unlike follicular adenoma), uniform follicles; hematogenous spread is common. Associated with *RAS* mutation and *PAX8-PPAR-γ* translocations. Fine needle aspiration cytology may not be able to distinguish between follicular adenoma and carcinoma. |
| **Medullary carcinoma**<br> | From parafollicular "C cells"; produces calcitonin, sheets of polygonal cells in an amyloid stroma $\blacksquare$ (stains with Congo red). Associated with MEN 2A and 2B (*RET* mutations). |
| **Undifferentiated/ anaplastic carcinoma** | Older patients; presents with rapidly enlarging neck mass → compressive symptoms (eg, dyspnea, dysphagia, hoarseness); very poor prognosis. Associated with *TP53* mutation. |

**Diagnosing parathyroid disease**

**Hypoparathyroidism**

Due to injury to parathyroid glands or their blood supply (usually during thyroid surgery), autoimmune destruction, or DiGeorge syndrome. Findings: tetany, hypocalcemia, hyperphosphatemia.

Chvostek sign—tapping of facial nerve (tap the Cheek) → contraction of facial muscles.

Trousseau sign—occlusion of brachial artery with BP cuff (cuff the Triceps) → carpal spasm.

**Pseudohypoparathyroidism type 1A**—autosomal dominant, maternally transmitted mutations (imprinted GNAS gene). GNASl-inactivating mutation (coupled to PTH receptor) that encodes the $G_s$ protein α subunit → inactivation of adenylate cyclase when PTH binds to its receptor → end-organ resistance (kidney and bone) to PTH.

Physical findings: Albright hereditary osteodystrophy (shortened 4th/5th digits , short stature, round face, subcutaneous calcifications, developmental delay).

Labs: ↑ PTH, ↓ $Ca^{2+}$, ↑ $PO_4^{3-}$.

**Pseudopseudohypoparathyroidism**—autosomal dominant, paternally transmitted mutations (imprinted GNAS gene) but without end-organ resistance to PTH due to normal maternal allele maintaining renal responsiveness to PTH.

Physical findings: same as Albright hereditary osteodystrophy.

Labs: normal PTH, $Ca^{2+}$, $PO_4^{3-}$.

**Lab values in hypocalcemic disorders**

| DISORDER | $Ca^{2+}$ | $PO_4^{3-}$ | PTH | ALP | 25(OH) VITAMIN D | 1,25(OH)₂ VITAMIN D |
|---|---|---|---|---|---|---|
| Vitamin D deficiency | —/↓ | —/↓ | ↑ | ↑ | ↓ | —/↑ |
| 2° hyperparathyroidism (CKD) | ↓ | ↑ | ↑ | ↑ | — | ↓ |
| Hypoparathyroidism | ↓ | ↑ | ↓ | — | — | —/↓ |
| Pseudohypoparathyroidism | ↓ | ↑ | ↑ | ↑ | — | —/↓ |

## Hyperparathyroidism

| | | |
|---|---|---|
| **Primary hyperparathyroidism**  | Usually due to parathyroid adenoma or hyperplasia. **Hypercalcemia**, hypercalciuria (renal **stones**), polyuria (**thrones**), hypophosphatemia, ↑ PTH, ↑ ALP, ↑ urinary cAMP. Most often asymptomatic. May present with **bone** pain, weakness, constipation ("**groans**"), abdominal/flank pain (kidney stones, acute pancreatitis), neuropsychiatric disturbances ("**psychiatric overtones**"). | Osteitis fibrosa cystica—cystic bone spaces filled with brown fibrous tissue **A** ("brown tumor" consisting of osteoclasts and deposited hemosiderin from hemorrhages; causes bone pain). Due to ↑ PTH, classically associated with 1° (but also seen with 2°) hyperparathyroidism. "Stones, thrones, bones, groans, and psychiatric overtones." |
| **Secondary hyperparathyroidism** | 2° hyperplasia due to ↓ $Ca^{2+}$ absorption and/or ↑ $PO_4^{3-}$, most often in chronic kidney disease (causes hypovitaminosis D and hyperphosphatemia → ↓ $Ca^{2+}$). **Hypocalcemia**, hyperphosphatemia in chronic kidney disease (vs hypophosphatemia with most other causes), ↑ ALP, ↑ PTH. | Renal osteodystrophy—renal disease → 2° and 3° hyperparathyroidism → bone lesions. |
| **Tertiary hyperparathyroidism** | Refractory (autonomous) hyperparathyroidism resulting from end-stage renal disease. ↑↑ PTH, ↑ $Ca^{2+}$. | |

| | |
|---|---|
| **Familial hypocalciuric hypercalcemia** | Autosomal dominant. Defective G-coupled $Ca^{2+}$-sensing receptors in multiple tissues (eg, parathyroids, kidneys). Higher than normal $Ca^{2+}$ levels required to suppress PTH. Excessive renal $Ca^{2+}$ reabsorption → mild hypercalcemia and hypocalciuria with normal to ↑ PTH levels. |

## Diabetes mellitus

| | |
|---|---|
| ACUTE MANIFESTATIONS | Polydipsia, polyuria, polyphagia (**3 P's**), weight loss, DKA (type 1), hyperosmolar hyperglycemic state (type 2).<br><br>Rarely, can be caused by unopposed secretion of GH and epinephrine. Also seen in patients on glucocorticoid therapy (steroid diabetes). |
| CHRONIC COMPLICATIONS | Nonenzymatic glycation:<br>  ▪ Small vessel disease (hyaline arteriolosclerosis) → retinopathy, neuropathy, nephropathy.<br>  ▪ Large vessel disease (atherosclerosis) → CAD, cerebrovascular disease, peripheral vascular disease. MI is the most common cause of death.<br>Osmotic damage (sorbitol accumulation in organs with aldose reductase and ↓ or absent sorbitol dehydrogenase):<br>  ▪ Neuropathy: motor, sensory (glove and stocking distribution), autonomic degeneration (eg, GERD, gastroparesis, diabetic diarrhea).<br>  ▪ Cataracts. |

| DIAGNOSIS | TEST | DIAGNOSTIC CUTOFF | NOTES |
|---|---|---|---|
| | HbA$_{1c}$ | ≥ 6.5% | Reflects average blood glucose over prior 3 months (influenced by RBC turnover) |
| | Fasting plasma glucose | ≥ 126 mg/dL | Fasting for > 8 hours |
| | 2-hour oral glucose tolerance test | ≥ 200 mg/dL | 2 hours after consumption of 75 g of glucose in water |
| | Random plasma glucose | ≥ 200 mg/dL | Presence of hyperglycemic symptoms is required |

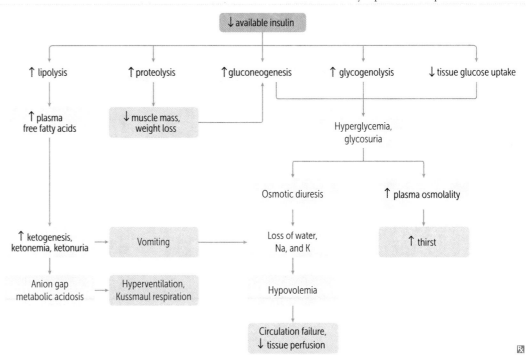

## Type 1 vs type 2 diabetes mellitus

|  | Type 1 | Type 2 |
|---|---|---|
| 1° DEFECT | Autoimmune T-cell–mediated destruction of β cells | ↑ resistance to insulin, progressive pancreatic β-cell failure |
| INSULIN NECESSARY IN TREATMENT | Always | Sometimes |
| AGE (EXCEPTIONS COMMON) | < 30 yr | > 40 yr |
| ASSOCIATION WITH OBESITY | No | Yes |
| GENETIC PREDISPOSITION | Relatively weak (50% concordance in identical twins), polygenic | Relatively strong (90% concordance in identical twins), polygenic |
| ASSOCIATION WITH HLA SYSTEM | Yes, HLA-DR4 and -DR3 (4 – 3 = type 1) | No |
| GLUCOSE INTOLERANCE | Severe | Mild to moderate |
| INSULIN SENSITIVITY | High | Low |
| KETOACIDOSIS | Common | Rare |
| β-CELL NUMBERS IN THE ISLETS | ↓ | Variable (with amyloid deposits) |
| SERUM INSULIN LEVEL | ↓ | ↑ initially, but ↓ in advanced disease |
| CLASSIC SYMPTOMS OF POLYURIA, POLYDIPSIA, POLYPHAGIA, WEIGHT LOSS | Common | Sometimes |
| HISTOLOGY | Islet leukocytic infiltrate | Islet amyloid polypeptide deposits |

## Hyperglycemic emergencies

|  | Diabetic ketoacidosis | Hyperosmolar hyperglycemic state |
|---|---|---|
| PATHOGENESIS | Insulin noncompliance or ↑ requirements due to ↑ stress (eg, infection) → lipolysis and oxidation of free fatty acids → ↑ ketone bodies (β-hydroxybutyrate > acetoacetate). **Insulin deficient, ketones present.** | Profound hyperglycemia → excessive osmotic diuresis → dehydration and ↑ serum osmolality → HHS. Classically seen in older patients with type 2 DM and limited ability to drink. **Insulin present, ketones deficient.** |
| SIGNS/SYMPTOMS | DKA is Deadly: Delirium/psychosis, Kussmaul respirations (rapid, deep breathing), Abdominal pain/nausea/vomiting, Dehydration. Fruity breath odor due to exhaled acetone. | Thirst, polyuria, lethargy, focal neurologic deficits, seizures. |
| LABS | Hyperglycemia, ↑ H$^+$, ↓ HCO$_3^-$ (↑ anion gap metabolic acidosis), ↑ urine and blood ketone levels, leukocytosis. Normal/↑ serum K$^+$, but depleted intracellular K$^+$ due to transcellular shift from ↓ insulin and acidosis. Osmotic diuresis → ↑ K$^+$ loss in urine → total body K$^+$ depletion. | Hyperglycemia (often > 600 mg/dL), ↑ serum osmolality (> 320 mOsm/kg), normal pH (no acidosis), no ketones. Normal/↑ serum K$^+$, ↓ intracellular K$^+$. |
| COMPLICATIONS | Life-threatening mucormycosis, cerebral edema, cardiac arrhythmias. | Can progress to coma and death if untreated. |
| TREATMENT | IV fluids, IV insulin, and K$^+$ (to replete intracellular stores). Glucose may be required to prevent hypoglycemia from insulin therapy. | |

| | |
|---|---|
| **Hypoglycemia in diabetes mellitus** | Usually occurs in patients treated with insulin or insulin secretagogues (eg, sulfonylureas, meglitinides) in the setting of high-dose treatment, inadequate food intake, and/or exercise. |

- Neurogenic (autonomic) symptoms: diaphoresis, tachycardia, tremor, anxiety, hunger. Allow perception of ↓ glucose (hypoglycemia awareness).
- Neuroglycopenic symptoms: altered mental status, seizures, death due to insufficient glucose in CNS. May occur in the absence of preceding neurogenic symptoms in patients with attenuated autonomic response (hypoglycemia unawareness).

Treatment: simple carbohydrates (eg, glucose tablets, fruit juice), IM glucagon, IV dextrose.

## Cushing syndrome

| | |
|---|---|
| ETIOLOGY | ↑ cortisol due to a variety of causes: |

- Exogenous glucocorticoids → ↓ ACTH → bilateral adrenal atrophy. Most common cause.
- Primary adrenal adenoma, hyperplasia, or carcinoma → ↓ ACTH → atrophy of uninvolved adrenal gland.
- ACTH-secreting pituitary adenoma (Cushing disease); paraneoplastic ACTH secretion (eg, small cell lung cancer, bronchial carcinoids) → bilateral adrenal hyperplasia. Cushing disease is responsible for the majority of endogenous cases of Cushing syndrome.

| | |
|---|---|
| FINDINGS | **MOON FACIES**: Metabolic syndrome (hypertension, hyperglycemia, hyperlipidemia), Obesity (truncal weight gain with wasting of extremities, round "moon" facies , dorsocervical fat pad "buffalo hump"), Osteoporosis, Neuropsychiatric (depression, anxiety, irritability), Facial plethora, Androgen excess (acne, hirsutism), Cataract, Immunosuppression, Ecchymoses (easy bruising), Skin changes (thinning, striae , hyperpigmentation). |
| DIAGNOSIS | Screening tests include: ↑ free cortisol on 24-hr urinalysis, ↑ late night salivary cortisol, and no suppression with overnight low-dose dexamethasone test. |

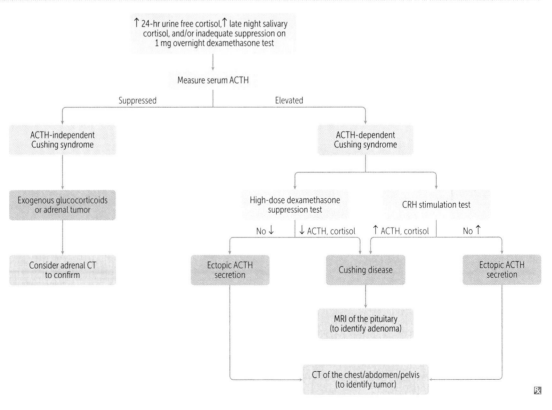

| | |
|---|---|
| **Adrenal insufficiency** | Inability of adrenal glands to generate enough glucocorticoids +/− mineralocorticoids for the body's needs. Can be acute or chronic. Symptoms include weakness, fatigue, orthostatic hypotension, muscle aches, weight loss, GI disturbances, sugar and/or salt cravings. Treatment: glucocorticoid +/− mineralocorticoid replacement. |
| **Primary adrenal insufficiency**  | ↓ gland function → ↓ cortisol, ↓ aldosterone → hypotension (hyponatremic volume contraction), hyperkalemia, metabolic acidosis, skin/mucosal hyperpigmentation  (↑ melanin synthesis due to ↑ MSH, a byproduct of POMC cleavage). Primary pigments the skin/mucosa. Addison disease—chronic 1° adrenal insufficiency; caused by adrenal atrophy or destruction. Most commonly due to autoimmune adrenalitis (high-income countries) or TB (low-income countries). |
| **Secondary and tertiary adrenal insufficiency** | ↓ pituitary ACTH secretion (secondary) or ↓ hypothalamic CRH secretion (tertiary). No hyperkalemia (aldosterone synthesis preserved due to functioning adrenal gland, intact RAAS), no hyperpigmentation. 2° adrenal insufficiency is due to pituitary pathologies, 3° adrenal insufficiency is most commonly due to abrupt cessation of chronic glucocorticoid therapy (HPA suppression). Tertiary from treatment. |
| **Acute adrenal insufficiency** | Also called adrenal (addisonian) crisis; often precipitated by acute stressors that ↑ glucocorticoid requirements (eg, infection) in patients with pre-existing adrenal insufficiency or on glucocorticoid therapy. May present with acute abdominal pain, nausea, vomiting, altered mental status, shock. Waterhouse-Friderichsen syndrome—bilateral adrenal hemorrhage in the setting of sepsis (eg, meningococcemia) → acute 1° adrenal insufficiency. |

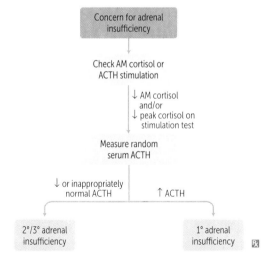

Concern for adrenal insufficiency

Check AM cortisol or ACTH stimulation

↓ AM cortisol and/or ↓ peak cortisol on stimulation test

Measure random serum ACTH

↓ or inappropriately normal ACTH → 2°/3° adrenal insufficiency

↑ ACTH → 1° adrenal insufficiency

| | |
|---|---|
| **Hyperaldosteronism** | Increased secretion of aldosterone from adrenal gland. Clinical features include hypertension, ↓ or normal K⁺, metabolic alkalosis. 1° hyperaldosteronism does not directly cause edema due to aldosterone escape mechanism. However, certain 2° causes of hyperaldosteronism (eg, heart failure) impair the aldosterone escape mechanism, leading to worsening of edema. |
| **Primary hyperaldosteronism** | Seen in patients with bilateral adrenal hyperplasia or adrenal adenoma (Conn syndrome). ↑ aldosterone, ↓ renin. Leads to treatment-resistant hypertension. |
| **Secondary hyperaldosteronism** | Seen in patients with renovascular hypertension, juxtaglomerular cell tumors (renin-producing), and edema (eg, cirrhosis, heart failure, nephrotic syndrome). ↑ aldosterone, ↑ renin. |

| | |
|---|---|
| **Neuroendocrine tumors** | Heterogeneous group of neoplasms originating from neuroendocrine cells (which have traits similar to nerve cells and hormone-producing cells). |
| | Most neoplasms occur in the GI system (eg, carcinoid, gastrinoma), pancreas (eg, insulinoma, glucagonoma), and lungs (eg, small cell carcinoma). Also in thyroid (eg, medullary carcinoma) and adrenals (eg, pheochromocytoma). |
| | Neuroendocrine cells (eg, pancreatic β cells, enterochromaffin cells) share a common biologic function through amine precursor uptake decarboxylase (APUD) despite differences in embryologic origin, anatomic site, and secretory products (eg, chromogranin A, neuron-specific enolase [NSE], synaptophysin, serotonin, histamine, calcitonin). Treatment: surgical resection, somatostatin analogs. |

| | |
|---|---|
| **Neuroblastoma**<br> | Most common solid extracranial tumor in children (typically < 4 years old). Usually arises in adrenal medulla, but may occur anywhere along the sympathetic chain. Originates from neural crest cells. |
| | Most common presentation is abdominal distension and a firm, irregular mass that can cross the midline (vs Wilms tumor, which is smooth and unilateral). Less likely to develop hypertension than with pheochromocytoma (neuroblastoma is normotensive). Can also present with opsoclonus-myoclonus syndrome ("dancing eyes-dancing feet"). |
| | ↑ HVA and VMA (catecholamine metabolites) in urine. Homer-Wright rosettes (neuroblasts surrounding a central area of neuropil A) characteristic of neuroblastoma and medulloblastoma. Bombesin and NSE ⊕. Associated with amplification of N-*myc* oncogene. |

## Pheochromocytoma

| | | |
|---|---|---|
| ETIOLOGY | Most common tumor of the adrenal medulla in adults (black arrow in **A**; red arrow points to bone metastases). Derived from chromaffin cells (arise from neural crest). Rare. May be associated with germline mutations (eg, *NF-1, VHL, RET* [MEN 2A, 2B]). | Rule of 10's:<br>    10% malignant<br>    10% bilateral<br>    10% extra-adrenal (paraganglioma;<br>        eg, bladder wall, organ of Zuckerkandl)<br>    10% calcify<br>    10% kids |
| SYMPTOMS | Most tumors secrete epinephrine, norepinephrine, and dopamine, which can cause episodic hypertension. May also secrete EPO → polycythemia.<br>Symptoms occur in "spells"—relapse and remit. | Episodic hyperadrenergic symptoms (5 P's):<br>    Pressure (↑ BP)<br>    Pain (headache)<br>    Perspiration<br>    Palpitations (tachycardia)<br>    Pallor |
| FINDINGS | ↑ catecholamines and metanephrines (eg, homovanillic acid, vanillylmandelic acid) in urine and plasma. | Chromogranin, synaptophysin and NSE ⊕. |
| TREATMENT | Irreversible α-antagonists (eg, phenoxybenzamine) followed by β-blockers prior to tumor resection. α-blockade must be achieved before giving β-blockers to avoid a hypertensive crisis. **A** before **B**. | Phenoxybenzamine for **pheochromocytoma**. |

| Multiple endocrine neoplasias | All **MEN** syndromes have autosomal **d**ominant inheritance. The X-MEN are **d**ominant over villains. |
|---|---|
| SUBTYPE | CHARACTERISTICS |
| MEN1 | Pituitary tumors (prolactin or GH) Pancreatic endocrine tumors—Zollinger-Ellison syndrome, insulinomas, VIPomas, glucagonomas (rare) Parathyroid adenomas Associated with mutation of *MEN1* (tumor suppressor, codes for menin, chromosome 11), angiofibromas, collagenomas, meningiomas |
| MEN2A | Parathyroid hyperplasia Medullary thyroid carcinoma—neoplasm of parafollicular C cells; secretes calcitonin; prophylactic thyroidectomy required Pheochromocytoma (secretes catecholamines) Associated with mutation in *RET* (protooncogene, codes for receptor tyrosine kinase, chromosome 10) |
| MEN2B | Medullary thyroid carcinoma Pheochromocytoma Mucosal neuromas **A** (oral/intestinal ganglioneuromatosis) Associated with marfanoid habitus; mutation in *RET* gene |

MEN1 = 3 P's  MEN2A = 2 P's, 1 M  MEN2B = 1 P, 2 M's

Pituitary
Parathyroid
Medullary thyroid carcinoma
Mucosal neuromas
Pancreas
Pheochromocytoma

## Pancreatic islet cell tumors

| | |
|---|---|
| **Insulinoma** | Tumor of pancreatic β cells → overproduction of insulin → hypoglycemia. May see Whipple triad: low blood glucose, symptoms of hypoglycemia (eg, lethargy, syncope, diplopia), and resolution of symptoms after normalization of plasma glucose levels. Symptomatic patients have ↓ blood glucose and ↑ C-peptide levels (vs exogenous insulin use). ~ 10% of cases associated with MEN1 syndrome. Treatment: surgical resection. |
| **Glucagonoma** | Tumor of pancreatic α cells → overproduction of glucagon. Presents with 6 D's: dermatitis (necrolytic migratory erythema), diabetes (hyperglycemia), DVT, declining weight, depression, diarrhea. Treatment: octreotide, surgical resection. |
| **Somatostatinoma** | Tumor of pancreatic δ cells → overproduction of somatostatin → ↓ secretion of secretin, cholecystokinin, glucagon, insulin, gastrin, gastric inhibitory peptide (GIP). May present with diabetes/glucose intolerance, steatorrhea, gallstones, achlorhydria. Treatment: surgical resection; somatostatin analogs (eg, octreotide) for symptom control. |

| | |
|---|---|
| **Carcinoid tumors**<br> | Carcinoid tumors arise from neuroendocrine cells, most commonly in the intestine or lung. Neuroendocrine cells secrete 5-HT, which undergoes hepatic first-pass metabolism and enzymatic breakdown by MAO in the lung. If 5-HT reaches the systemic circulation (eg, after liver metastasis), carcinoid tumor may present with **carcinoid syndrome**—episodic flushing, diarrhea, wheezing, right-sided valvular heart disease (eg, tricuspid regurgitation, pulmonic stenosis), niacin deficiency (pellagra), ↑ urinary 5-HIAA.<br>Histology: rosettes **A**, chromogranin A ⊕, synaptophysin ⊕.<br>Treatment: surgical resection, somatostatin analog (eg, octreotide) or tryptophan hydroxylase inhibitor (eg, telotristat) for symptom control.<br>Rule of thirds:<br>    1/3 metastasize<br>    1/3 present with 2nd malignancy<br>    1/3 are multiple |

| | |
|---|---|
| **Zollinger-Ellison syndrome** | Constellation of symptoms due to acid hypersecretion resulting from gastrin-secreting tumor (gastrinoma) in duodenum or pancreas → multiple, recurrent ulcers in duodenum/jejunum (often refractory to proton pump inhibitors) and malabsorption. Presents with abdominal pain, heartburn, steatorrhea, weight loss. Positive secretin stimulation test (↑ gastrin levels after secretin administration, which normally inhibits gastrin release). Chromogranin A ⊕. May be associated with MEN1. |

## ▶ ENDOCRINE—PHARMACOLOGY

**Diabetes mellitus therapy**

All patients with diabetes mellitus should receive education on diet, exercise, blood glucose monitoring, and complication management. Treatment differs based on the type of diabetes and glycemic control:

- Type 1 DM—insulin replacement
- Type 2 DM—oral agents (metformin is first line), non-insulin injectables, insulin replacement; weight loss particularly helpful in lowering blood glucose
- Gestational DM—insulin replacement if nutrition therapy and exercise alone fail

Regular (short-acting) insulin is preferred for DKA (IV), hyperkalemia (+ glucose), stress hyperglycemia.

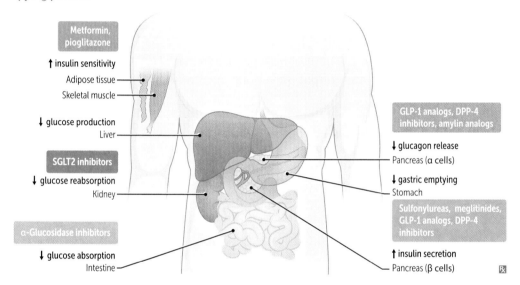

| DRUG | MECHANISM | ADVERSE EFFECTS |
|---|---|---|
| **Insulin preparations** | | |
| Rapid acting (no **lag**): lispro, aspart, glulisine<br>Short acting: regular<br>Intermediate acting: NPH<br>Long acting: detemir, glargine<br>Very long acting: degludec | Bind insulin receptor (tyrosine kinase activity)<br>Liver: ↑ glucose storage as glycogen<br>Muscle: ↑ glycogen, protein synthesis<br>Fat: ↑ TG storage<br>Cell membrane: ↑ K$^+$ uptake | Hypoglycemia, lipodystrophy, hypersensitivity reactions (rare), weight gain |

## Diabetes mellitus therapy *(continued)*

| DRUG | MECHANISM | ADVERSE EFFECTS |
|------|-----------|-----------------|
| **Increase insulin sensitivity** | | |
| **Metformin** | Inhibits mitochondrial glycerol-3-phosphate dehydrogenase (mGPD) → inhibition of hepatic gluconeogenesis and the action of glucagon.<br>↑ glycolysis, peripheral glucose uptake (↑ insulin sensitivity). | GI upset, lactic acidosis (use with caution in renal insufficiency), vitamin $B_{12}$ deficiency. Weight loss (often desired). |
| **Pioglitazone** | Activate PPAR-γ (a nuclear receptor) → ↑ insulin sensitivity and levels of adiponectin → regulation of glucose metabolism and fatty acid storage. | Weight gain, edema, HF, ↑ risk of fractures. Delayed onset of action (several weeks). |
| **Increase insulin secretion** | | |
| **Sulfonylureas (1st gen)**<br> Chlorpropamide, tolbutamide<br>**Sulfonylureas (2nd gen)**<br> Glipizide, glyburide<br>**Meglitinides**<br> Nateglinide, repaglinide | Close $K^+$ channels in pancreatic B cell membrane → cell depolarizes → insulin release via ↑ $Ca^{2+}$ influx. | Disulfiram-like reaction with first-generation sulfonylureas only (rarely used). Hypoglycemia (↑ risk in renal insufficiency), weight gain. |
| **Increase glucose-induced insulin secretion** | | |
| **GLP-1 analogs**<br> Exenatide, liraglutide, semaglutide | ↓ glucagon release, ↓ gastric emptying, ↑ glucose-dependent insulin release. | Nausea, vomiting, pancreatitis. Weight loss (often desired). ↑ satiety (often desired). |
| **DPP-4 inhibitors**<br> Linagliptin, saxagliptin, sitagliptin | Inhibit DPP-4 enzyme that deactivates GLP-1 → ↓ glucagon release, ↓ gastric emptying. ↑ glucose-dependent insulin release. | Respiratory and urinary infections, weight neutral. ↑ satiety (often desired). |
| **Decrease glucose absorption** | | |
| **Sodium-glucose co-transporter 2 inhibitors**<br> Canagliflozin, dapagliflozin, empagliflozin | Block reabsorption of glucose in proximal convoluted tubule. | Glucosuria (UTIs, vulvovaginal candidiasis), dehydration (orthostatic hypotension), weight loss. Glucose flows in urine. Use with caution in renal insufficiency (↓ efficacy with ↓ GFR). |
| **α-glucosidase inhibitors**<br> Acarbose, miglitol | Inhibit intestinal brush-border α-glucosidases → delayed carbohydrate hydrolysis and glucose absorption → ↓ postprandial hyperglycemia. | GI upset, bloating. Not recommended in renal insufficiency. |
| **Others** | | |
| **Amylin analogs**<br> Pramlintide | ↓ glucagon release, ↓ gastric emptying. | Hypoglycemia, nausea. ↑ satiety (often desired). |

| Thionamides | Propylthiouracil, methimazole. |
|---|---|
| MECHANISM | Block thyroid peroxidase, inhibiting the oxidation of iodide as well as the organification and coupling of iodine → inhibition of thyroid hormone synthesis. PTU also blocks 5'-deiodinase → ↓ Peripheral conversion of $T_4$ to $T_3$. |
| CLINICAL USE | Hyperthyroidism. PTU used in Primary (first) trimester of pregnancy (due to methimazole teratogenicity); methimazole used in second and third trimesters of pregnancy (due to risk of PTU-induced hepatotoxicity). Not used to treat Graves ophthalmopathy (treated with glucocorticoids). |
| ADVERSE EFFECTS | Skin rash, agranulocytosis (rare), aplastic anemia, hepatotoxicity. PTU use has been associated with ANCA-positive vasculitis. Methimazole is a possible teratogen (can cause aplasia cutis). |

### Levothyroxine, liothyronine

| | |
|---|---|
| MECHANISM | Hormone replacement for $T_4$ (levothyroxine; levo = 4 letters) or $T_3$ (liothyronine; lio = 3 letters). Avoid levothyroxine with antacids, bile acid resins, or ferrous sulfate (↓ absorption). |
| CLINICAL USE | Hypothyroidism, myxedema. May be misused for weight loss. Distinguish exogenous hyperthyroidism from endogenous hyperthyroidism by using a combination of TSH receptor antibodies, radioactive iodine uptake, and/or measurement of thyroid blood flow on ultrasound. |
| ADVERSE EFFECTS | Tachycardia, heat intolerance, tremors, arrhythmias. |

### Hypothalamic/pituitary drugs

| DRUG | CLINICAL USE |
|---|---|
| **Conivaptan, tolvaptan** | ADH antagonists<br>SIADH (block action of ADH at $V_2$-receptor) |
| **Demeclocycline** | ADH antagonist, a tetracycline<br>SIADH (interferes with ADH signaling) |
| **Desmopressin** | ADH analog<br>Central DI, von Willebrand disease, sleep enuresis, hemophilia A |
| **GH** | GH deficiency, Turner syndrome |
| **Oxytocin** | Induction of labor (stimulates uterine contractions), control uterine hemorrhage |
| **Octreotide** | Somatostatin analog<br>Acromegaly, carcinoid syndrome, gastrinoma, glucagonoma, esophageal varices |

### Fludrocortisone

| | |
|---|---|
| MECHANISM | Synthetic analog of aldosterone with glucocorticoid effects. Fluidrocortisone retains fluid. |
| CLINICAL USE | Mineralocorticoid replacement in 1° adrenal insufficiency. |
| ADVERSE EFFECTS | Similar to glucocorticoids; also edema, exacerbation of heart failure, hyperpigmentation. |

## Cinacalcet

| | |
|---|---|
| MECHANISM | Sensitizes calcium-sensing receptor (CaSR) in parathyroid gland to circulating $Ca^{2+} \rightarrow \downarrow$ PTH. Pronounce "Senacalcet." |
| CLINICAL USE | 2° hyperparathyroidism in patients with CKD receiving hemodialysis, hypercalcemia in 1° hyperparathyroidism (if parathyroidectomy fails), or in parathyroid carcinoma. |
| ADVERSE EFFECTS | Hypocalcemia. |

## Sevelamer

| | |
|---|---|
| MECHANISM | Nonabsorbable phosphate binder that prevents phosphate absorption from the GI tract. |
| CLINICAL USE | Hyperphosphatemia in CKD. |
| ADVERSE EFFECTS | Hypophosphatemia, GI upset. |

## Cation exchange resins — Patiromer, sodium polystyrene sulfonate, zirconium cyclosilicate.

| | |
|---|---|
| MECHANISM | Bind $K^+$ in colon in exchange for other cations (eg, $Na^+$, $Ca^{2+}$) $\rightarrow K^+$ excreted in feces. |
| CLINICAL USE | Hyperkalemia. |
| ADVERSE EFFECTS | Hypokalemia, GI upset. |

# Gastrointestinal

"A good set of bowels is worth more to a man than any quantity of brains."
—Josh Billings

"Man should strive to have his intestines relaxed all the days of his life."
—Moses Maimonides

"All right, let's not panic. I'll make the money by selling one of my livers. I can get by with one."
—Homer Simpson, *The Simpsons*

"The truth does not change according to our ability to stomach it emotionally."
—Flannery O'Connor

When studying the gastrointestinal system, be sure to understand the normal embryology, anatomy, and physiology and how the system is affected by various pathologies. Study not only disease pathophysiology, but also its specific findings, so that you can differentiate between two similar diseases. For example, what specifically makes ulcerative colitis different from Crohn disease? Also, be comfortable with basic interpretation of abdominal x-rays, CT scans, and endoscopic images.

## ▶ GASTROINTESTINAL—EMBRYOLOGY

### Tongue development

1st pharyngeal arch forms anterior 2/3 of tongue (sensation via CN $V_3$, taste via CN VII).

3rd and 4th pharyngeal arches form posterior 1/3 of tongue (sensation and taste mainly via CN IX, extreme posterior via CN X).

Motor innervation is via CN XII to hyoglossus (retracts and depresses tongue), **geni**oglossus (**protrudes** tongue), and **sty**loglossus (draws sides of tongue upward to create a trough for swallowing).

Motor innervation is via CN X to palatoglossus (elevates posterior tongue during swallowing).

Taste—CN VII, IX, X (nucleus tractus solitarius [NTS]).

Pain—CN $V_3$, IX, X.

Motor—CN X, XII.

The **geni**e comes **out** of the lamp in **sty**le.

CN 10 innervates pala**ten**glossus.

### Normal gastrointestinal embryology

Foregut—esophagus to duodenum at level of pancreatic duct and common bile duct insertion (ampulla of Vater).
- 4th-6th week of development—stomach rotates 90° clockwise.
- Left vagus becomes anteriorly positioned, and right vagus becomes posteriorly positioned.

Midgut—lower duodenum to proximal 2/3 of transverse colon.
- 6th week of development—physiologic herniation of midgut through umbilical ring.
- 10th week of development—returns to abdominal cavity rotating around superior mesenteric artery (SMA), 270° counterclockwise (~90° before 10th week, remaining ~180° in 10th week when contents retract back into abdominal cavity).

Hindgut—distal 1/3 of transverse colon to anal canal above pectinate line.

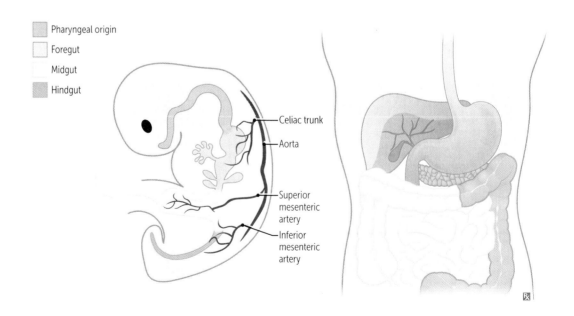

| **Ventral wall defects** | Developmental defects due to failure of rostral fold closure (eg, sternal defects [ectopia cordis]), lateral fold closure (eg, omphalocele, gastroschisis), or caudal fold closure (eg, bladder exstrophy). | |
| --- | --- | --- |
| | **Gastroschisis** | **Omphalocele** |
| PRESENTATION | Paraumbilical herniation of abdominal contents through abdominal wall defect | Herniation of abdominal contents through umbilicus |
| COVERAGE | Not covered by peritoneum or amnion ; right sided/paraumbilical | Covered by peritoneum and amnion  (light gray shiny sac); midline, membrane covered |
| ASSOCIATIONS | Not associated with chromosome abnormalities; good prognosis | Associated with congenital anomalies (eg, trisomies 13 and 18, Beckwith-Wiedemann syndrome) and other structural abnormalities (eg, cardiac, GU, neural tube) |

**Congenital umbilical hernia**

Delay of umbilical ring to close spontaneously following physiological herniation of midgut → patent umbilical orifice. Covered by skin C. Protrudes with ↑ intra-abdominal pressure (eg, crying). May be associated with congenital disorders (eg, Down syndrome, congenital hypothyroidism). Small defects usually close spontaneously.

**Tracheoesophageal anomalies**

Esophageal atresia (EA) with distal tracheoesophageal fistula (TEF) is the most common (85%) and often presents as polyhydramnios in utero (due to inability of fetus to swallow amniotic fluid). Neonates drool, choke, and vomit with first feeding. TEFs allow air to enter stomach (visible on CXR). Cyanosis is 2° to laryngospasm (to avoid reflux-related aspiration). Clinical test: failure to pass nasogastric tube into stomach. Associated with VATER/VACTERL defects.

In H-type, the fistula resembles the letter H. In pure EA, CXR shows gasless abdomen.

Normal anatomy

Pure EA (atresia or stenosis)

Pure TEF (H-type)

EA with distal TEF (most common)

Normal — Gastric bubble

Gasless stomach

Prominent gastric bubble

**Hypertrophic pyloric stenosis**

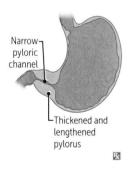

Narrow pyloric channel

Thickened and lengthened pylorus

Most common cause of gastric outlet obstruction in infants. Palpable olive-shaped mass (due to hypertrophy and hyperplasia of pyloric sphincter muscle) in epigastric region, visible peristaltic waves, and nonbilious projectile vomiting at ~ 2–6 weeks old. More common in firstborn males; associated with exposure to macrolides.

Results in hypokalemic hypochloremic metabolic alkalosis (2° to vomiting of gastric acid and subsequent volume contraction).

Ultrasound shows thickened and lengthened pylorus.

Treatment: surgical incision of pyloric muscles (pyloromyotomy).

**Intestinal atresia**

Presents with bilious vomiting and abdominal distension within first 1–2 days of life.

**Duodenal atresia**—failure to recanalize lumen from solid cord stage. X-ray A shows "double bubble" (dilated stomach, proximal duodenum). Associated with Down syndrome.

**Jejunal and ileal atresia**—disruption of mesenteric vessels (typically SMA) → ischemic necrosis of fetal intestine → segmental resorption: bowel becomes discontinuous. X-ray may show "triple bubble" (dilated stomach, duodenum, proximal jejunum) and gasless colon. Associated with cystic fibrosis and gastroschisis. May be caused by maternal tobacco smoking or use of vasoconstrictive drugs (eg, cocaine) during pregnancy.

## Pancreas and spleen embryology

Pancreas—derived from foregut. Ventral pancreatic bud contributes to uncinate process. Both ventral and dorsal buds contribute to pancreatic head and main pancreatic duct.

**Annular pancreas**—abnormal rotation of ventral pancreatic bud forms a ring of pancreatic tissue → encircles 2nd part of duodenum; may cause duodenal narrowing (arrows in ) and vomiting. Associated with Down syndrome.

**Pancreas divisum**—ventral and dorsal parts fail to fuse at 7 weeks of development. Common anomaly; mostly asymptomatic, but may cause chronic abdominal pain and/or pancreatitis.

Spleen—arises in mesentery of the stomach (dorsal mesogastrium, hence, mesodermal), but has foregut supply (celiac trunk → splenic artery).

Gallbladder
Accessory pancreatic duct
Minor papilla
Major papilla
Ventral pancreatic bud
Dorsal pancreatic bud
Uncinate process
Main pancreatic duct
Annular pancreas
Main pancreatic duct
Ventral pancreatic duct

---

## ▶ GASTROINTESTINAL—ANATOMY

### Retroperitoneal structures

Retroperitoneal structures  are posterior to (and outside of) the peritoneal cavity. Injuries to retroperitoneal structures can cause blood or gas accumulation in retroperitoneal space.

SAD PUCKER:
Suprarenal (adrenal) glands [not shown]
Aorta and IVC
Duodenum (2nd through 4th parts)
Pancreas (except tail)
Ureters [not shown]
Colon (descending and ascending)
Kidneys
Esophagus (thoracic portion) [not shown]
Rectum (partially) [not shown]

Duodenum
Ascending colon
Peritoneum
Duodenum/jejunum
Descending colon
Right
Pancreas
Left
Liver
IVC
Aorta
Kidney

Asc Colon
Desc Colon
IVC   Ao
R. Kid
L. Kid

## Important gastrointestinal ligaments

| LIGAMENT | CONNECTS | STRUCTURES CONTAINED | NOTES |
|---|---|---|---|
| **Falciform ligament** | Liver to anterior abdominal wall | Ligamentum teres hepatis (derivative of fetal umbilical vein), patent paraumbilical veins | Derivative of ventral mesentery |
| **Hepatoduodenal ligament** | Liver to duodenum | Portal triad: proper hepatic artery, portal vein, common bile duct | Derivative of ventral mesentery<br>Pringle maneuver—ligament is compressed manually or with a vascular clamp in omental foramen to control bleeding from hepatic inflow source (portal vein, hepatic artery) vs outflow (hepatic veins, IVC)<br>Borders the omental foramen, which connects the greater and lesser sacs<br>Part of lesser omentum |
| **Hepatogastric ligament** | Liver to lesser curvature of stomach | Gastric vessels | Derivative of ventral mesentery<br>Separates greater and lesser sacs on the right<br>May be cut during surgery to access lesser sac<br>Part of lesser omentum |
| **Gastrocolic ligament** | Greater curvature and transverse colon | Gastroepiploic arteries | Derivative of dorsal mesentery<br>Part of greater omentum |
| **Gastrosplenic ligament** | Greater curvature and spleen | Short gastrics, left gastroepiploic vessels | Derivative of dorsal mesentery<br>Separates greater and lesser sacs on the left<br>Part of greater omentum |
| **Splenorenal ligament** | Spleen to left pararenal space | Splenic artery and vein, tail of pancreas | Derivative of dorsal mesentery |

**Digestive tract anatomy**

Layers of gut wall 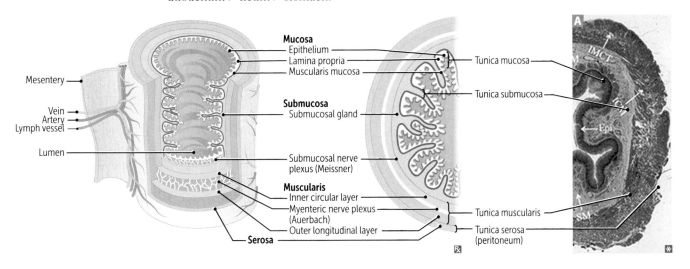 (inside to outside—MSMS):

- Mucosa—epithelium, lamina propria, muscularis mucosa
- Submucosa—includes submucosal nerve plexus (Meissner), secretes fluid
- Muscularis externa—includes myenteric nerve plexus (Auerbach), motility
- Serosa (when intraperitoneal), adventitia (when retroperitoneal)

Ulcers can extend into submucosa, inner or outer muscular layer. Erosions are in mucosa only.

Frequency of basal electric rhythm (slow waves), which originate in the interstitial cells of Cajal: duodenum > ileum > stomach.

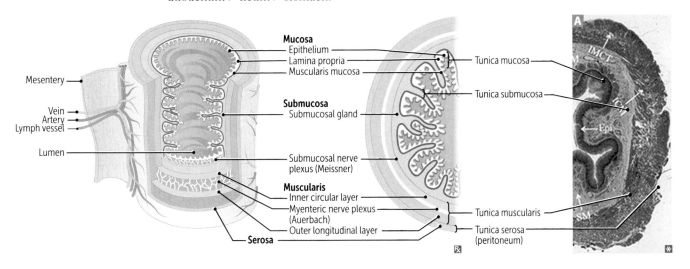

### Digestive tract histology

| | |
|---|---|
| **Esophagus** | Nonkeratinized stratified squamous epithelium. Upper 1/3, striated muscle; middle and lower 2/3 smooth muscle, with some overlap at the transition. |
| **Stomach** | Gastric glands A. Parietal cells are eosinophilic (pink), chief cells are basophilic. |
| **Duodenum** | Villi B and microvilli ↑ absorptive surface. Brunner glands (bicarbonate-secreting cells of submucosa), crypts of Lieberkühn (contain stem cells that replace enterocytes/goblet cells and Paneth cells that secrete defensins, lysozyme, and TNF), and plicae circulares (distal duodenum). |
| **Jejunum** | Villi, crypts of Lieberkühn, and plicae circulares (taller, more prominent, numerous [vs ileum]) → feathered appearance with oral contrast and ↑ surface area. |
| **Ileum** | Villi, Peyer patches (arrow in C; lymphoid aggregates in lamina propria, submucosa), plicae circulares (proximal ileum), crypts of Lieberkühn. Largest number of goblet cells in small intestine. |
| **Colon** | Crypts of Lieberkühn with abundant goblet cells, but no villi D. |

## Abdominal aorta and branches

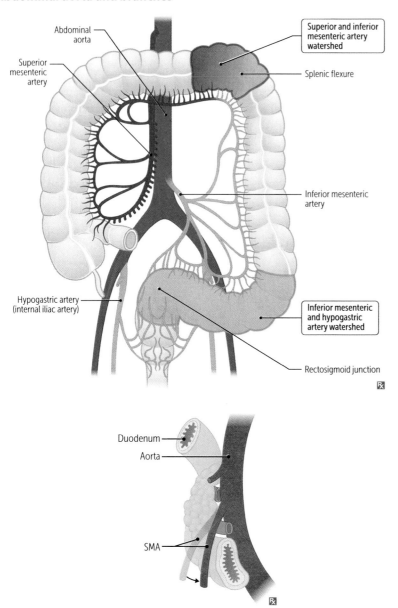

Abdominal aorta

Superior mesenteric artery

Superior and inferior mesenteric artery watershed

Splenic flexure

Inferior mesenteric artery

Hypogastric artery (internal iliac artery)

Inferior mesenteric and hypogastric artery watershed

Rectosigmoid junction

Duodenum

Aorta

SMA

Arteries supplying GI structures are single and branch anteriorly.

Arteries supplying non-GI structures are paired and branch laterally and posteriorly.

Two areas of the colon have dual blood supply from distal arterial branches ("watershed areas") → susceptible in colonic ischemia (hypotensive states, thromboemboli, or atheroemboli):

- Splenic flexure—SMA and IMA
- Rectosigmoid junction—IMA branches (last sigmoid arterial branch and superior rectal artery)

**Nutcracker syndrome**—compression of left renal vein between superior mesenteric artery and aorta. May cause abdominal (flank) pain, gross hematuria (from rupture of thin-walled renal varicosities), left-sided varicocele.

**Superior mesenteric artery syndrome**—characterized by intermittent intestinal obstruction symptoms (primarily postprandial pain) when SMA and aorta compress transverse (third) portion of duodenum. Typically occurs in conditions associated with diminished mesenteric fat (eg, rapid weight loss, low body weight, malnutrition, gastric bypass surgeries).

## Gastrointestinal blood supply and innervation

| EMBRYONIC GUT REGION | ARTERY | PARASYMPATHETIC INNERVATION | VERTEBRAL LEVEL | STRUCTURES SUPPLIED |
|---|---|---|---|---|
| **Foregut** | Celiac | Vagus | T12/L1 | Pharynx (vagus nerve only) and lower esophagus (celiac artery only) to proximal duodenum; liver, gallbladder, pancreas, spleen (mesoderm) |
| **Midgut** | SMA | Vagus | L1 | Distal duodenum to proximal 2/3 of transverse colon |
| **Hindgut** | IMA | Pelvic splanchnic | L3 | Distal 1/3 of transverse colon to upper portion of anal canal |

Sympathetic innervation arises from abdominal prevertebral ganglia: celiac, superior mesenteric, and inferior mesenteric.

**Celiac trunk**

Branches of celiac trunk: common hepatic, splenic, and left gastric. These constitute the main blood supply of the foregut.

Strong anastomoses exist between:
- Left and right gastroepiploics
- Left and right gastrics

## Portosystemic anastomoses

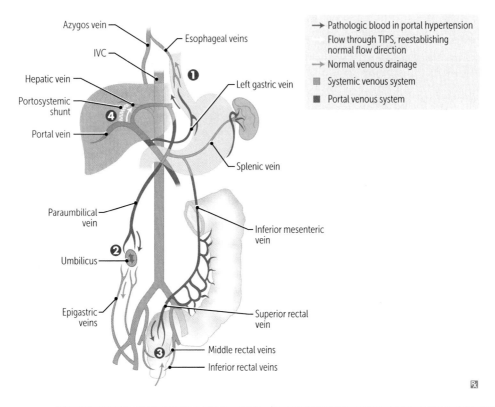

| SITE OF ANASTOMOSIS | CLINICAL SIGN | PORTAL ↔ SYSTEMIC |
|---|---|---|
| ❶ Esophagus | Esophageal varices | Left gastric ↔ esophageal (drains into azygos) |
| ❷ Umbilicus | Caput medusae | Paraumbilical ↔ small epigastric veins (branches of inferior and superficial epigastric veins) of the anterior abdominal wall |
| ❸ Rectum | Anorectal varices | Superior rectal ↔ middle and inferior rectal |

Varices of **gut, butt**, and **caput** (medusae) are commonly seen with portal hypertension.

❹ Transjugular Intrahepatic Portosystemic Shunt (**TIPS**) treatment creates an anastomosis between portal vein and hepatic vein, relieving portal hypertension by shunting blood to the systemic circulation, bypassing the liver. TIPS can precipitate hepatic encephalopathy due to ↓ clearance of ammonia from shunting.

**Pectinate line**

Also called dentate line. Formed where endoderm (hindgut) meets ectoderm.

**Internal hemorrhoids**—abnormal distention of anal venous plexus 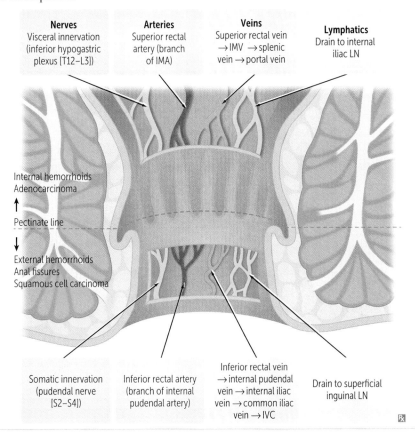. Risk factors include older age and chronic constipation. Receive visceral innervation and are therefore **not painful**.

**External hemorrhoids**—receive somatic innervation (inferior rectal branch of pudendal nerve) and are therefore **painful** if thrombosed.

**Anal fissure**—tear in anoderm below pectinate line. Pain while pooping; blood on toilet paper. Located in the posterior midline because this area is poorly perfused. Associated with low-fiber diets and constipation.

**Nerves**
Visceral innervation
(inferior hypogastric
plexus [T12–L3])

**Arteries**
Superior rectal
artery (branch
of IMA)

**Veins**
Superior rectal vein
→ IMV → splenic
vein → portal vein

**Lymphatics**
Drain to internal
iliac LN

Internal hemorrhoids
Adenocarcinoma

↑

Pectinate line

↓

External hemorrhoids
Anal fissures
Squamous cell carcinoma

**Somatic innervation**
(pudendal nerve
[S2–S4])

**Inferior rectal artery**
(branch of internal
pudendal artery)

**Inferior rectal vein**
→ internal pudendal
vein → internal iliac
vein → common iliac
vein → IVC

Drain to superficial
inguinal LN

## Liver tissue architecture

The functional unit of the liver is made up of hexagonally arranged lobules surrounding the central vein with portal triads on the edges (consisting of a portal vein, hepatic artery, bile ducts, as well as lymphatics) **A**.

Apical surface of hepatocytes faces bile canaliculi. Basolateral surface faces sinusoids.

Kupffer cells (specialized macrophages) located in sinusoids clear bacteria and damaged or senescent RBCs.

Hepatic stellate (Ito) cells in space of Disse store vitamin A (when quiescent) and produce extracellular matrix (when activated). Responsible for hepatic fibrosis.

Dual blood supply to liver: portal vein (~80%) and hepatic artery (~20%).

Zone I—periportal zone:
- Affected 1st by viral hepatitis
- Best oxygenated, most resistant to circulatory compromise
- Ingested toxins (eg, cocaine)

Zone II—intermediate zone:
- Yellow fever

Zone III—pericentral (centrilobular) zone:
- Affected 1st by ischemia as least oxygenated (eg, congestive hepatopathy)
- High concentration of cytochrome P-450
- Most sensitive to metabolic toxins (eg, ethanol, $CCl_4$, rifampin, acetaminophen)
- Site of alcoholic hepatitis

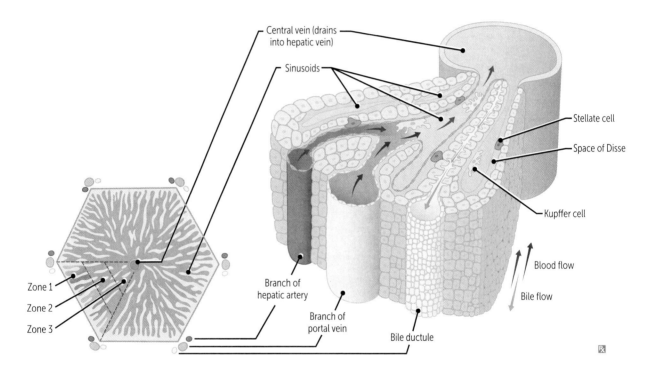

Central vein (drains into hepatic vein)
Sinusoids
Stellate cell
Space of Disse
Kupffer cell
Blood flow
Bile flow
Branch of hepatic artery
Branch of portal vein
Bile ductule
Zone 1
Zone 2
Zone 3

## Biliary structures

Cholangiography shows filling defects in gallbladder (blue arrow in **A**) and common bile duct (red arrow in **A**).

Gallstones that reach the confluence of the common bile and pancreatic ducts at the ampulla of Vater can block both the common bile and pancreatic ducts (double duct sign), causing both cholangitis and pancreatitis, respectively.

Tumors that arise in head of pancreas (usually ductal adenocarcinoma) can cause obstruction of common bile duct → enlarged nontender gallbladder with jaundice (Courvoisier sign).

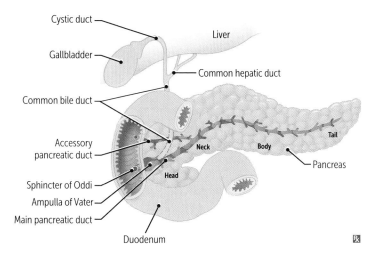

## Femoral region

| ORGANIZATION | Lateral to medial: nerve-artery-vein-lymphatics. | You go from lateral to medial to find your navel. |
|---|---|---|
| **Femoral triangle** | Contains femoral nerve, artery, vein. | Venous near the penis. |
| **Femoral sheath** | Fascial tube 3–4 cm below inguinal ligament. Contains femoral vein, artery, and canal (deep inguinal lymph nodes) but not femoral nerve. | |

## Inguinal canal

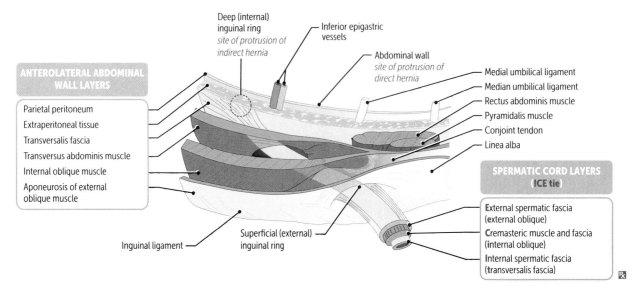

Deep (internal) inguinal ring
*site of protrusion of indirect hernia*

Inferior epigastric vessels

Abdominal wall
*site of protrusion of direct hernia*

**ANTEROLATERAL ABDOMINAL WALL LAYERS**

Parietal peritoneum
Extraperitoneal tissue
Transversalis fascia
Transversus abdominis muscle
Internal oblique muscle
Aponeurosis of external oblique muscle

Medial umbilical ligament
Median umbilical ligament
Rectus abdominis muscle
Pyramidalis muscle
Conjoint tendon
Linea alba

**SPERMATIC CORD LAYERS (ICE tie)**

External spermatic fascia (external oblique)
Cremasteric muscle and fascia (internal oblique)
Internal spermatic fascia (transversalis fascia)

Inguinal ligament

Superficial (external) inguinal ring

## Myopectineal orifice

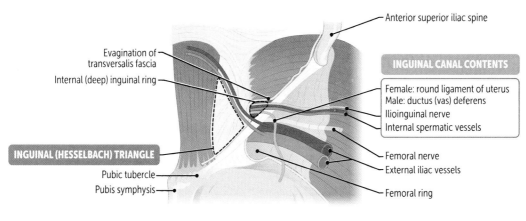

Anterior superior iliac spine

Evagination of transversalis fascia
Internal (deep) inguinal ring

**INGUINAL CANAL CONTENTS**

Female: round ligament of uterus
Male: ductus (vas) deferens
Ilioinguinal nerve
Internal spermatic vessels

**INGUINAL (HESSELBACH) TRIANGLE**

Pubic tubercle
Pubis symphysis

Femoral nerve
External iliac vessels

Femoral ring

**Anterior abdominal wall**
(viewed from inside)

| Hernias | Protrusion of peritoneum through an opening, usually at a site of weakness. Contents may be at risk for incarceration (not reducible back into abdomen/pelvis) and strangulation (ischemia and necrosis). Complicated hernias can present with tenderness, erythema, fever. |
|---|---|
| Spigelian hernia | Also called spontaneous lateral ventral hernia or hernia of semilunar line. Occurs through defects between the rectus abdominis and the semilunar line in the Spigelian aponeurosis.<br>Most occur in the lower abdomen due to lack of the posterior rectus sheath.<br>Presentation is variable but may include abdominal pain and a palpable lump along the Spigelian fascia.<br>Diagnosis: ultrasound and CT scan. |

## Hernias (continued)

### Diaphragmatic hernia

Abdominal structures enter the thorax. Bowel sounds may be heard on chest auscultation. Most common causes:

- Infants—congenital defect of pleuroperitoneal membrane → left-sided herniation (right hemidiaphragm is relatively protected by liver) **A**.
- Adults—laxity/defect of phrenoesophageal membrane → hiatal hernia (herniation of stomach through esophageal hiatus).

Sliding hiatal hernia—gastroesophageal junction is displaced upward as gastric cardia slides into hiatus; "hourglass stomach." Most common type. Associated with GERD.

Paraesophageal hiatal hernia—gastroesophageal junction is usually normal but gastric fundus protrudes into the thorax.

### Indirect inguinal hernia

Protrudes through the internal (deep) inguinal ring, external (superficial) inguinal ring, and into the groin. Enters internal inguinal ring lateral to inferior epigastric vessels. Caused by failure of processus vaginalis to close (can form hydrocele). May be noticed in infants or discovered in adulthood. Much more common in males **B**.

Follows the pathway of testicular descent. Covered by all 3 layers of spermatic fascia.

### Direct inguinal hernia

Protrudes through inguinal (Hesselbach) triangle. Bulges directly through parietal peritoneum medial to the inferior epigastric vessels but lateral to the rectus abdominis. Goes through external (superficial) inguinal ring only. Covered by external spermatic fascia. Usually occurs in older males due to acquired weakness of transversalis fascia.

MDs don't lie:

Medial to inferior epigastric vessels = Direct hernia.

Lateral to inferior epigastric vessels = indirect hernia.

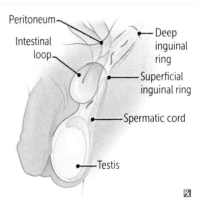

### Femoral hernia

Protrudes below inguinal ligament through femoral canal below and lateral to pubic tubercle. More common in females, but overall inguinal hernias are the most common. More likely to present with incarceration or strangulation (vs inguinal hernia).

## Gastrointestinal regulatory substances

| REGULATORY SUBSTANCE | SOURCE | ACTION | REGULATION | NOTES |
|---|---|---|---|---|
| **Gastrin** | G cells (antrum of stomach, duodenum) | ↑ gastric H⁺ secretion<br>↑ growth of gastric mucosa<br>↑ gastric motility | ↑ by stomach distention/alkalinization, amino acids, peptides, vagal stimulation via gastrin-releasing peptide (GRP)<br>↓ by pH < 1.5 | ↑ by chronic PPI use<br>↑ in chronic atrophic gastritis (eg, *H pylori*)<br>↑↑ in Zollinger-Ellison syndrome (gastrinoma) |
| **Somatostatin** | D cells (pancreatic islets, GI mucosa) | ↓ gastric acid and pepsinogen secretion<br>↓ pancreatic and small intestine fluid secretion<br>↓ gallbladder contraction<br>↓ insulin and glucagon release | ↑ by acid<br>↓ by vagal stimulation | Inhibits secretion of various hormones (encourages somato-stasis)<br>Octreotide is an analog used to treat acromegaly, carcinoid syndrome, VIPoma, and variceal bleeding |
| **Cholecystokinin** | I cells (duodenum, jejunum) | ↑ pancreatic secretion<br>↑ gallbladder contraction<br>↓ gastric emptying<br>↑ sphincter of Oddi relaxation | ↑ by fatty acids, amino acids | Acts on neural muscarinic pathways to cause pancreatic secretion |
| **Secretin** | S cells (duodenum) | ↑ pancreatic $HCO_3^-$ secretion<br>↓ gastric acid secretion<br>↑ bile secretion | ↑ by acid, fatty acids in lumen of duodenum | ↑ $HCO_3^-$ neutralizes gastric acid in duodenum, allowing pancreatic enzymes to function |
| **Glucose-dependent insulinotropic peptide** | K cells (duodenum, jejunum) | Exocrine:<br>↓ gastric H⁺ secretion<br>Endocrine:<br>↑ insulin release | ↑ by fatty acids, amino acids, oral glucose | Also called gastric inhibitory peptide (GIP)<br>Oral glucose load ↑ insulin compared to IV equivalent due to GIP secretion |
| **Motilin** | Small intestine | Produces migrating motor complexes (MMCs) | ↑ in fasting state | Motilin receptor agonists (eg, erythromycin) are used to stimulate intestinal peristalsis. |
| **Vasoactive intestinal polypeptide** | Parasympathetic ganglia in sphincters, gallbladder, small intestine | ↑ intestinal water and electrolyte secretion<br>↑ relaxation of intestinal smooth muscle and sphincters | ↑ by distention and vagal stimulation<br>↓ by adrenergic input | VIPoma—non-α, non-β islet cell pancreatic tumor that secretes VIP; associated with Watery Diarrhea, Hypokalemia, Achlorhydria (WDHA syndrome) |
| **Nitric oxide** | | ↑ smooth muscle relaxation, including lower esophageal sphincter (LES) | | Loss of NO secretion is implicated in ↑ LES tone of achalasia |
| **Ghrelin** | Stomach | ↑ appetite ("ghrowlin' stomach") | ↑ in fasting state<br>↓ by food | ↑ in Prader-Willi syndrome<br>↓ after gastric bypass surgery |

### Gastrointestinal secretory products

| PRODUCT | SOURCE | ACTION | REGULATION | NOTES |
|---|---|---|---|---|
| **Gastric acid** | Parietal cells (stomach 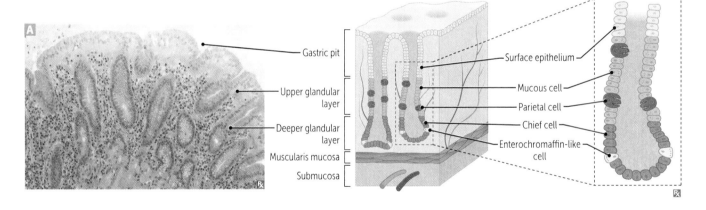) | ↓ stomach pH | ↑ by histamine, vagal stimulation (ACh), gastrin ↓ by somatostatin, GIP, prostaglandin, secretin | Autoimmune destruction of parietal cells (pink/ eosinophilic histology) → chronic gastritis and pernicious anemia |
| **Intrinsic factor** | Parietal cells (stomach) | Vitamin $B_{12}$–binding protein (required for $B_{12}$ uptake in terminal ileum) | | |
| **Pepsin** | Chief cells (stomach) | Protein digestion | ↑ by vagal stimulation (ACh), local acid | Pepsinogen (inactive) is converted to pepsin (active) in the presence of $H^+$ |
| **Bicarbonate** | Mucosal cells (stomach, duodenum, salivary glands, pancreas) and Brunner glands (duodenum) | Neutralizes acid | ↑ by pancreatic and biliary secretion with secretin | Trapped in mucus that covers the gastric epithelium |

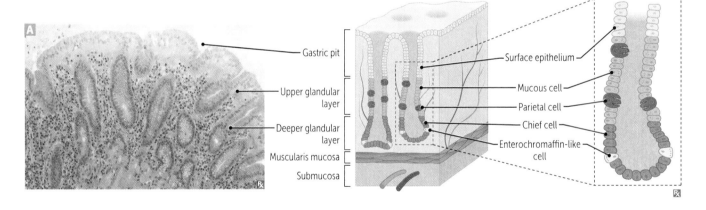

A

Gastric pit
Upper glandular layer
Deeper glandular layer
Muscularis mucosa
Submucosa

Surface epithelium
Mucous cell
Parietal cell
Chief cell
Enterochromaffin-like cell

**Locations of gastrointestinal secretory cells**

Gastrin ↑ acid secretion primarily through its effects on enterochromaffin-like (ECL) cells (leading to histamine release) rather than through its direct effect on parietal cells.

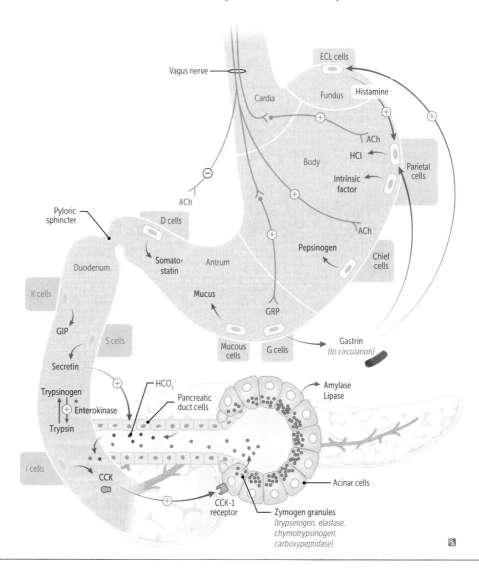

---

**Pancreatic secretions**

Isotonic fluid; low flow → high Cl⁻, high flow → high $HCO_3^-$.

| ENZYME | ROLE | NOTES |
|---|---|---|
| α-amylase | Starch digestion | Secreted in active form |
| Lipases | Lipid digestion | |
| Proteases | Protein digestion | Includes trypsin, chymotrypsin, elastase, carboxypeptidases<br>Secreted as proenzymes also called zymogens<br>Dipeptides and tripeptides degraded within intestinal mucosa via intracellular process |
| Trypsinogen | Converted to active enzyme trypsin → activation of other proenzymes and cleaving of additional trypsinogen molecules into active trypsin (positive feedback loop) | Converted to trypsin by enterokinase/enteropeptidase, a brush-border enzyme on duodenal and jejunal mucosa |

## Carbohydrate absorption

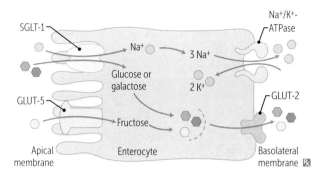

Only monosaccharides (glucose, galactose, fructose) are absorbed by enterocytes. Glucose and galactose are taken up by SGLT1 (Na⁺ dependent). Fructose is taken up via facilitated diffusion by GLUT5. All are transported to blood by GLUT2.

D-xylose test: simple sugar that is passively absorbed in proximal small intestine; blood and urine levels ↓ with mucosal damage, normal in pancreatic insufficiency.

## Vitamin and mineral absorption

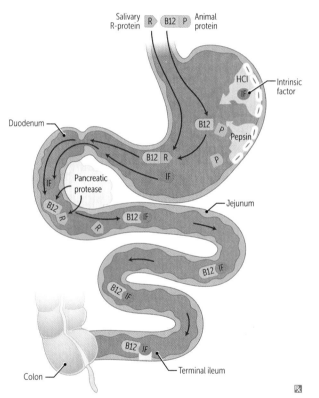

Vitamin and mineral deficiencies may develop in patients with small bowel disease, bowel resection, intestinal failure (also called short bowel syndrome), or bariatric surgery (eg, vitamin $B_{12}$ deficiency after terminal ileum resection).

Iron absorbed as $Fe^{2+}$ in duodenum.
Folate absorbed in small bowel.
Vitamin $B_{12}$ absorbed in terminal ileum along with bile salts, requires intrinsic factor.
Iron fist, Bro

## Peyer patches

Unencapsulated lymphoid tissue **A** found in lamina propria and submucosa of ileum. Contain specialized Microfold (M) cells that sample and present antigens to iMmune cells. B cells stimulated in germinal centers of Peyer patches differentiate into IgA-secreting plasma cells, which ultimately reside in lamina propria. IgA receives protective secretory component and is then transported across the epithelium to the gut to deal with intraluminal antigen.

Think of IgA, the Intra-gut Antibody

**Bile**

Composed of bile salts (bile acids conjugated to glycine or taurine, making them water soluble), phospholipids, cholesterol, bilirubin, water, and ions. Cholesterol 7α-hydroxylase catalyzes rate-limiting step of bile acid synthesis.

Functions:
- Digestion and absorption of lipids and fat-soluble vitamins
- Bilirubin and cholesterol excretion (body's 1° means of elimination)
- Antimicrobial activity (via membrane disruption)

↓ absorption of enteric bile salts at distal ileum (as in short bowel syndrome, Crohn disease) prevents normal fat absorption and may cause bile acid diarrhea.

Calcium, which normally binds oxalate, binds fat instead, so free oxalate is absorbed by gut → ↑ frequency of calcium oxalate kidney stones.

---

**Bilirubin**

Heme is metabolized by heme oxygenase to biliverdin (green), which is subsequently reduced to bilirubin (yellow-brown). Unconjugated bilirubin is removed from blood by liver, conjugated with glucuronate, and excreted in bile.

Direct bilirubin: conjugated with glucuronic acid; water soluble (dissolves in water).

Indirect bilirubin: unconjugated; water insoluble.

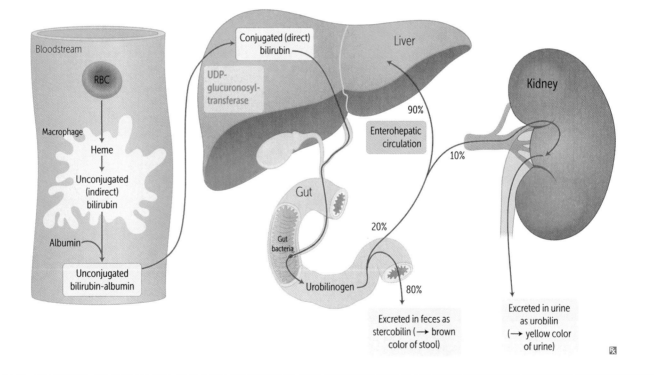

## Oral pathologies

| | |
|---|---|
| **Aphthous ulcers** | Also called canker sores. Common oral lesions that appear as painful, shallow, round to oval ulcers covered by yellowish exudate A. Recurrent aphthous stomatitis is associated with celiac disease, IBD, SLE, Behçet syndrome, HIV infection. |
| **Squamous cell carcinoma** | Most common malignancy of oral cavity. Usually affects the tongue. Associated with tobacco, alcohol, HPV-16. Presents as nonhealing ulcer with irregular margins and raised borders. Leukoplakia (white patch B) and erythroplakia (red patch) are precursor lesions. |
| **Sialolithiasis** | Stone formation in major salivary gland ducts (parotid C, submandibular, or sublingual). Associated with salivary stasis (eg, dehydration) and trauma. Presents as recurrent pre-/periprandial pain and swelling in affected gland. |
| **Sialadenitis** | Inflammation of salivary gland due to obstruction, infection (eg, S aureus, mumps virus), or immune-mediated mechanisms (eg, Sjögren syndrome). |
| **Salivary gland tumors** | Usually benign and most commonly affect the parotid gland. Submandibular, sublingual, and minor salivary gland tumors are more likely to be malignant. Typically present as painless mass/swelling. Facial paralysis or pain suggests malignant involvement.<br>■ Pleomorphic adenoma (benign mixed tumor)—most common salivary gland tumor D. Composed of chondromyxoid stroma and epithelium and recurs if incompletely excised or ruptured intraoperatively. May undergo malignant transformation.<br>■ **War**thin tumor (papillary cystadenoma lymphomatosum)—benign cystic tumor with germinal centers. May be bilateral or multifocal. Typically found in people who smoke. "Warriors from Germany love smoking."<br>■ Mucoepidermoid carcinoma—most common malignant tumor. Mucinous and squamous components. |

| | |
|---|---|
| **Achalasia**<br> | Failure of LES to relax due to degeneration of inhibitory neurons (containing NO and VIP) in the myenteric (Auerbach) plexus of esophageal wall.<br>1° idiopathic. 2° from Chagas disease (*T cruzi* infection) or extraesophageal malignancies (mass effect or paraneoplastic). Chagas disease can cause achalasia.<br>Presents with progressive dysphagia to solids and liquids (vs obstruction—primarily solids).<br>Associated with ↑ risk of esophageal cancer. | Manometry findings include uncoordinated or absent peristalsis with ↑ LES resting pressure.<br>Barium swallow shows dilated esophagus with area of distal stenosis ("bird's beak" A).<br>Treatment: surgery, endoscopic procedures (eg, botulinum toxin injection). |

## Other esophageal pathologies

| | |
|---|---|
| **Gastroesophageal reflux disease** | Transient decreases in LES tone. Commonly presents as heartburn, regurgitation, dysphagia. May also present as chronic cough, hoarseness (laryngopharyngeal reflux). Associated with asthma. Complications include erosive esophagitis, strictures, and Barrett esophagus. |
| **Esophagitis** | Inflammation of esophageal mucosa. Presents with odynophagia and/or dysphagia. Types:<br> ▪ Reflux (erosive) esophagitis—most common type. 2° to GERD.<br> ▪ Medication-induced esophagitis—2° to bisphosphonates, tetracyclines, NSAIDs, ferrous sulfate, potassium chloride.<br> ▪ Eosinophilic esophagitis—chronic, immune-mediated, eosinophil-predominant. Associated with atopic disorders (eg, asthma). Esophageal rings and linear furrows on endoscopy.<br> ▪ Infectious esophagitis—*Candida* (most common; white pseudomembranes ), HSV-1 (punched-out ulcers), CMV (linear ulcers). Associated with immunosuppression.<br> ▪ Corrosive esophagitis—2° to caustic ingestion. |
| **Plummer-Vinson syndrome** | Triad of dysphagia, iron deficiency anemia, esophageal webs. ↑ risk of esophageal squamous cell carcinoma ("Plumber dies"). May be associated with glossitis. |
| **Mallory-Weiss syndrome** | Partial thickness, longitudinal lacerations of gastroesophageal junction, confined to mucosa/submucosa, due to severe vomiting. Often presents with hematemesis +/– abdominal/back pain. Usually found in patients with alcohol use disorder, bulimia nervosa. |
| **Esophageal varices** | Dilated submucosal veins (red arrows in B) in lower 1/3 of esophagus 2° to portal hypertension. Common in patients with cirrhosis, may be source of life-threatening hematemesis. |
| **Distal esophageal spasm** | Formerly called diffuse esophageal spasm. Spontaneous, nonperistaltic (uncoordinated) contractions of the esophagus with normal LES pressure. Presents with dysphagia and anginalike chest pain. Barium swallow may reveal "corkscrew" esophagus. Manometry is diagnostic. Treatment includes nitrates and CCBs. |
| **Scleroderma esophageal involvement** | Esophageal smooth muscle atrophy → ↓ LES pressure and distal esophageal dysmotility → acid reflux and dysphagia → stricture, Barrett esophagus, and aspiration. Part of CREST syndrome. |
| **Esophageal perforation** | Most commonly iatrogenic following esophageal instrumentation. Noniatrogenic causes include spontaneous rupture, foreign body ingestion, trauma, malignancy.<br> Pneumomediastinum (arrows in C) and subcutaneous emphysema (signs include crepitus in the neck region or chest wall) can indicate dissecting air.<br> Boerhaave syndrome—transmural, usually distal esophageal rupture due to violent retching. |

**Barrett esophagus**

Specialized intestinal metaplasia (arrow in 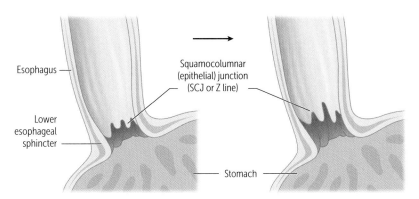A)—replacement of nonkeratinized stratified squamous epithelium with intestinal epithelium (nonciliated columnar with goblet cells [arrows in B]) in distal esophagus. Due to chronic gastroesophageal reflux disease (GERD). Associated with ↑ risk of esophageal adenocarcinoma.

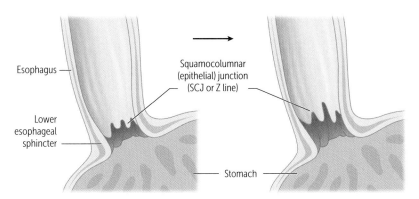

Esophagus —

Lower esophageal sphincter —

Squamocolumnar (epithelial) junction (SCJ or Z line)

Stomach —

---

**Esophageal cancer**

Typically presents with progressive dysphagia (first solids, then liquids) and weight loss. Aggressive course due to lack of serosa in esophageal wall, allowing rapid extension. Poor prognosis due to advanced disease at presentation.

| CANCER | PART OF ESOPHAGUS AFFECTED | RISK FACTORS | PREVALENCE |
|---|---|---|---|
| Squamous cell carcinoma | Upper 2/3 | Alcohol, hot liquids, caustic strictures, smoking, achalasia, nitrosamine-rich foods | More common worldwide |
| Adenocarcinoma | Lower 1/3 | Chronic GERD, Barrett esophagus, obesity, tobacco smoking | More common in America |

## Gastritis

| | | |
|---|---|---|
| **Acute gastritis** | Erosions can be caused by:<br>■ NSAIDs—↓ PGE$_2$ → ↓ gastric mucosa protection<br>■ Burns (Curling ulcer)—hypovolemia → mucosal ischemia<br>■ Brain injury (Cushing ulcer)—↑ vagal stimulation → ↑ ACh → ↑ H$^+$ production | Especially common among patients with alcohol use disorder and those taking daily NSAIDs (eg, for rheumatoid arthritis)<br>Burned by the Curling iron<br><br>Always Cushion the brain |
| **Chronic gastritis** | Mucosal inflammation, often leading to atrophy (hypochlorhydria → hypergastrinemia) and intestinal metaplasia (↑ risk of gastric cancers) | |
| *H pylori* | Most common. ↑ risk of peptic ulcer disease, MALT lymphoma | Affects antrum first and spreads to body of stomach |
| Autoimmune | Autoantibodies (T-cell induced) to the H$^+$/K$^+$-ATPase on parietal cells and to intrinsic factor. ↑ risk of pernicious anemia | Affects body/fundus of stomach |

---

**Ménétrier disease**

Hyperplasia of gastric mucosa → hypertrophied rugae ("wavy" like brain gyri ). Causes excess mucus production with resultant protein loss and parietal cell atrophy with ↓ acid production. Precancerous.

Presents with Weight loss, Anorexia, Vomiting, Epigastric pain, Edema (due to protein loss; pronounce "WAVEE").

---

**Gastric cancer**

Most commonly gastric adenocarcinoma; lymphoma, GI stromal tumor (common mutations include *KIT* or *PDGFRA*), carcinoid (rare). Early aggressive local spread with node/liver metastases. Often presents late, with Weight loss, Early satiety, Abdominal Pain, Obstruction, and in some cases acanthosis Nigricans or Leser-Trélat sign (**WEAPON**).
■ Intestinal—associated with *H pylori*, dietary nitrosamines (smoked foods common in East Asian countries), tobacco smoking, achlorhydria, chronic gastritis. Commonly on lesser curvature; looks like ulcer with raised margins.
■ Diffuse—not associated with *H pylori*; most cases due to E-cadherin mutation; signet ring cells (mucin-filled cells with peripheral nuclei) ; stomach wall grossly thickened and leathery (linitis plastica).

Virchow node—involvement of left supraclavicular node by metastasis from stomach.
Krukenberg tumor—metastasis to ovaries (typically bilateral). Abundant mucin-secreting, signet ring cells.
Sister Mary Joseph nodule—subcutaneous periumbilical metastasis.
Blumer shelf—palpable mass on digital rectal exam suggesting metastasis to rectouterine pouch (pouch of Douglas).

## Peptic ulcer disease

|  | Gastric ulcer | Duodenal ulcer |
|---|---|---|
| PAIN | Can be greater with meals—weight loss | Decreases with meals—weight gain |
| *H PYLORI* INFECTION | ~ 70% | ~ 90% |
| MECHANISM | ↓ mucosal protection against gastric acid | ↓ mucosal protection or ↑ gastric acid secretion |
| OTHER CAUSES | NSAIDs | Zollinger-Ellison syndrome |
| RISK OF CARCINOMA | ↑<br>Biopsy margins to rule out malignancy | Generally benign<br>Not routinely biopsied |

## Ulcer complications

| | |
|---|---|
| Hemorrhage | Gastric, duodenal (posterior > anterior). Most common complication.<br>Ruptured gastric ulcer on the lesser curvature of stomach → bleeding from left gastric artery.<br>An ulcer on the posterior wall of duodenum → bleeding from gastroduodenal artery. |
| Obstruction | Pyloric channel, duodenal. |
| Perforation | Duodenal (anterior > posterior).<br>Anterior duodenal ulcers can perforate into the anterior abdominal cavity, potentially leading to pneumoperitoneum.<br>May see free air under diaphragm (pneumoperitoneum)  with referred pain to the shoulder via irritation of phrenic nerve. |

| Acute gastrointestinal bleeding | Upper GI bleeding—originates **proximal** to ligament of Treitz (suspensory ligament of duodenum). Usually presents with hematemesis and/or melena. Associated with peptic ulcer disease, variceal hemorrhage.<br>Lower GI bleeding—originates **distal** to ligament of Treitz. Usually presents with hematochezia. Associated with IBD, diverticulosis, angiodysplasia, hemorrhoids, anal fissure, cancer. | 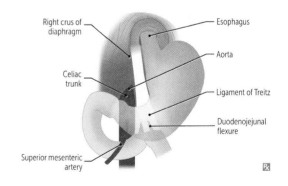 |

| | | |
|---|---|---|
| **Malabsorption syndromes** | Can cause diarrhea, steatorrhea, weight loss, weakness, vitamin and mineral deficiencies. Screen for fecal fat (eg, Sudan stain). | |
| **Celiac disease**  | Also called gluten-sensitive enteropathy, celiac sprue. Autoimmune-mediated intolerance of gliadin (gluten protein found in wheat, barley, rye). Associated with HLA-DQ2, HLA-DQ8, northern European descent. Primarily affects distal duodenum and/or proximal jejunum → malabsorption and steatorrhea. Treatment: gluten-free diet. | Associated with dermatitis herpetiformis, ↓ bone density, iron deficiency anemia, moderately ↑ risk of malignancy (eg, T-cell lymphoma). D-xylose test: abnormal. Serology: ⊕ IgA anti-tissue transglutaminase (IgA tTG), anti-endomysial, and anti-deamidated gliadin peptide antibodies. Histology: Loss of villi, mucosal atrophy, crypt hyperplasia Ⓐ, intraepithelial lymphocytosis. |

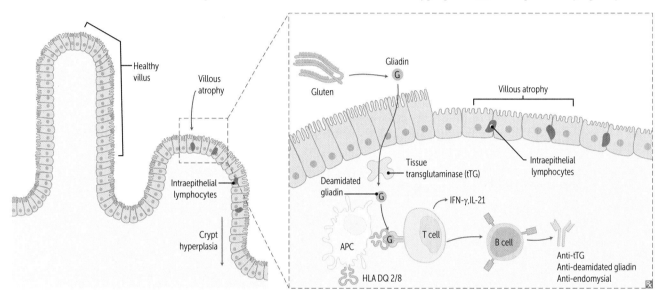

| | | |
|---|---|---|
| **Lactose intolerance** | Lactase deficiency. Normal-appearing villi, except when 2° to injury at tips of villi (eg, viral enteritis). Osmotic diarrhea, ↓ stool pH (colonic bacteria ferment lactose). | Lactose hydrogen breath test: ⊕ for lactose malabsorption if post-lactose breath hydrogen value increases > 20 ppm compared with baseline. |
| **Pancreatic insufficiency** | Due to chronic pancreatitis, cystic fibrosis, obstructing cancer. Causes malabsorption of fat and fat-soluble vitamins (A, D, E, K) as well as vitamin $B_{12}$. | ↓ duodenal bicarbonate (and pH) and fecal elastase. D-xylose test: normal. |
| **Tropical sprue** | Similar findings as celiac sprue (affects small bowel), but responds to antibiotics. Cause is unknown, but seen in residents of or recent visitors to tropics. | ↓ mucosal absorption affecting duodenum and jejunum but can involve ileum with time. Associated with megaloblastic anemia due to folate deficiency and, later, $B_{12}$ deficiency. |
| **Whipple disease**  | Infection with *Tropheryma whipplei* (intracellular gram ⊕); **PAS** ⊕ **foamy** macrophages in intestinal lamina propria Ⓑ. Cardiac symptoms, Arthralgias, and Neurologic symptoms are common. Diarrhea/steatorrhea occur later in disease course. Most common in older males. | **PAS**s the **foamy Whipped** cream in a **CAN**. |

## Inflammatory bowel diseases

| | Crohn disease | Ulcerative colitis |
|---|---|---|
| LOCATION | Any portion of the GI tract, usually the terminal ileum and colon. Skip lesions, rectal sparing. | Colitis = colon inflammation. Continuous colonic lesions, always with rectal involvement. |
| GROSS MORPHOLOGY | Transmural inflammation → fistulas. Cobblestone mucosa, creeping fat, bowel wall thickening ("string sign" on small bowel follow-through ), linear ulcers, fissures. | Mucosal and submucosal inflammation only. Friable mucosa with superficial and/or deep ulcerations (compare normal  with diseased ). Loss of haustra → "lead pipe" appearance on imaging. |
| MICROSCOPIC MORPHOLOGY | Noncaseating granulomas, lymphoid aggregates. | Crypt abscesses/ulcers, bleeding, no granulomas. |
| COMPLICATIONS | Malabsorption/malnutrition, colorectal cancer (↑ risk with pancolitis). | |
| | Fistulas (eg, enterovesical fistulae, which can cause recurrent UTI and pneumaturia), phlegmon/abscess, strictures (causing obstruction), perianal disease. | Fulminant colitis, toxic megacolon, perforation. |
| INTESTINAL MANIFESTATION | Diarrhea that may or may not be bloody. | Bloody diarrhea (usually painful). |
| EXTRAINTESTINAL MANIFESTATIONS | Rash (pyoderma gangrenosum, erythema nodosum), eye inflammation (episcleritis, uveitis), oral ulcerations (aphthous stomatitis), arthritis (peripheral, spondylitis). | |
| | Kidney stones (usually calcium oxalate), gallstones. May be ⊕ for anti-*Saccharomyces cerevisiae* antibodies (ASCA). | 1° sclerosing cholangitis. Associated with MPO-ANCA/p-ANCA. |
| TREATMENT | Glucocorticoids, azathioprine, antibiotics (eg, ciprofloxacin, metronidazole), biologics (eg, infliximab, adalimumab). | 5-aminosalicylic acid preparations (eg, mesalamine), 6-mercaptopurine, infliximab, colectomy. |
| DISEASE ACTIVITY | Fecal calprotectin used to monitor activity and distinguish from noninflammatory diseases (irritable bowel). | |

| | |
|---|---|
| **Microscopic colitis** | Inflammatory disease of colon that causes chronic watery diarrhea. Most common in older females. Colonic mucosa appears normal on endoscopy. Histology shows lymphocytic infiltrate in lamina propria with intraepithelial lymphocytosis or thickened subepithelial collagen band. |

| | |
|---|---|
| **Irritable bowel syndrome** | Recurrent abdominal pain associated with ≥ 2 of the following:<br> ▪ Related to defecation<br> ▪ Change in stool frequency<br> ▪ Change in form (consistency) of stool<br>No structural abnormalities. Most common in middle-aged females. Chronic symptoms may be diarrhea-predominant, constipation-predominant, or mixed. Pathophysiology is multifaceted. May be associated with fibromyalgia and mood disorders (anxiety, depression). First-line treatment is lifestyle modification and dietary changes. |

| | |
|---|---|
| **Appendicitis**<br> | Acute inflammation of the appendix (blue arrow in A), can be due to obstruction by fecalith (in adults) or lymphoid hyperplasia (in children).<br>Proximal appendiceal lumen obstruction → closed-loop obstruction → ↑ intraluminal pressure → stimulation of visceral afferent nerve fibers at T8-T10 → initial diffuse periumbilical pain → inflammation extends to serosa and irritates parietal peritoneum. Pain localized to RLQ/ McBurney point (1/3 the distance from right anterior superior iliac spine to umbilicus). Nausea, fever; may perforate → peritonitis. May elicit psoas, obturator, and Rovsing (severe RLQ pain with palpation of LLQ) signs; guarding and rebound tenderness on exam.<br>Treatment: appendectomy. |

### Diverticula of the GI tract

| | | |
|---|---|---|
| **Diverticulum** | Blind pouch A protruding from the alimentary tract that communicates with the lumen of the gut. Most diverticula (esophagus, stomach, duodenum, colon) are acquired and are termed "false diverticula." | "True" diverticulum—all gut wall layers outpouch (eg, Meckel).<br>"False" diverticulum or pseudodiverticulum—only mucosa and submucosa outpouch. Occur especially where vasa recta perforate muscularis externa. |
| **Diverticulosis** | Many false diverticula of the colon B, commonly sigmoid. Common (in ~ 50% of people > 60 years). Caused by ↑ intraluminal pressure and focal weakness in colonic wall. Associated with obesity and diets low in fiber, high in total fat/red meat. | Often asymptomatic or associated with vague discomfort.<br>Complications include diverticular bleeding (painless hematochezia), diverticulitis. |
| **Diverticulitis** | Inflammation of diverticula with wall thickening (red arrows in C) classically causing LLQ pain, fever, leukocytosis. Treat with supportive care (uncomplicated) or antibiotics (complicated). | Complications: abscess, fistula (colovesical fistula → pneumaturia), obstruction (inflammatory stenosis), perforation (white arrows in C) (→ peritonitis). Hematochezia is rare. |

**Zenker diverticulum**

Pharyngoesophageal **false** diverticulum 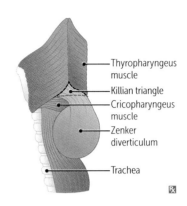. Esophageal dysmotility causes herniation of mucosal tissue at an area of weakness between the thyropharyngeal and cricopharyngeal parts of the inferior pharyngeal constrictor (Killian triangle). Presenting symptoms: dysphagia, obstruction, gurgling, aspiration, foul breath, neck mass. Most common in older males.

- Thyropharyngeus muscle
- Killian triangle
- Cricopharyngeus muscle
- Zenker diverticulum
- Trachea

**Meckel diverticulum**

Umbilicus

Meckel diverticulum

**True** diverticulum. Persistence of the vitelline (omphalomesenteric) duct. May contain ectopic acid–secreting gastric mucosa and/or pancreatic tissue. Most common congenital anomaly of GI tract. Can cause hematochezia/melena (less common), RLQ pain, intussusception, volvulus, or obstruction near terminal ileum.
Diagnosis: $^{99m}$Tc-pertechnetate scan (also called Meckel scan) for uptake by heterotopic gastric mucosa.

The rule of 2's:
2 times as likely in males.
2 inches long.
2 feet from the ileocecal valve.
2% of population.
Commonly presents in first 2 years of life.
May have 2 types of epithelia (gastric/pancreatic).

**Hirschsprung disease**

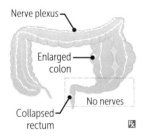

Nerve plexus

Enlarged colon

No nerves

Collapsed rectum

Congenital megacolon characterized by lack of ganglion cells/enteric nervous plexuses (Auerbach and Meissner plexuses) in distal segment of colon. Due to failure of neural crest cell migration. Associated with loss of function mutations in *RET*.
Presents with bilious emesis, abdominal distention, and failure to pass meconium within 48 hours → chronic constipation. Normal portion of the colon proximal to the aganglionic segment is dilated, resulting in a "transition zone."

Risk ↑ with Down syndrome.
Explosive expulsion of feces (squirt sign) → empty rectum on digital exam.
Diagnosed by absence of ganglion cells on rectal suction biopsy.
Treatment: resection.
*RET* mutation in the REcTum.

**Malrotation**

Anomaly of midgut rotation during fetal development → improper positioning of bowel (small bowel clumped on the right side and colon [with contrast] on the left), formation of fibrous bands (Ladd bands).

Can lead to volvulus, duodenal obstruction.

**Intussusception**

Telescoping of a proximal bowel segment into a distal segment, most commonly at ileocecal junction. Typically seen in infants.

Usually idiopathic in children, less frequently due to an identifiable lead point. Idiopathic form is associated with recent viral infections (eg, adenovirus), rotavirus vaccine → Peyer patch hypertrophy may act as a lead point.

Common lead points:
- Children—Meckel diverticulum, small bowel wall hematoma (IgA vasculitis).
- Adults—intraluminal mass/tumor.

Causes small bowel obstruction and vascular compromise → intermittent abdominal pain, vomiting, bloody "currant jelly" stools.

Sausage-shaped mass in right abdomen on exam. Patient may draw their legs to chest to ease pain.

Ultrasound/CT may show "target sign" **A**.

**Volvulus**

Twisting of portion of bowel around its mesentery; can lead to obstruction and infarction. Can occur throughout the GI tract.
- Gastric volvulus more common with abnormalities (paraesophageal hernia) in adults, and presents with severe abdominal pain, dry heaving, and inability to pass nasogastric tube
- Midgut volvulus more common in infants and children (minors)
- Sigmoid volvulus (coffee bean sign on x-ray **A**) more common in older adults (seniors)

**Short bowel syndrome**

Inability to adequately absorb nutrients in the small intestine 2° to significant surgical resection (eg, Crohn disease, malignancy, trauma). Malabsorption of bile salts and fat at the distal ileum → postprandial voluminous diarrhea, dehydration, weight loss, anemia, calcium oxalate kidney stones.

## Other intestinal disorders

| | |
|---|---|
| **Acute mesenteric ischemia** | Critical blockage of intestinal blood flow (often embolic occlusion of SMA) → small bowel necrosis  → abdominal pain out of proportion to physical findings. May see red "currant jelly" stools. Risk factors: atrial fibrillation, peripheral arterial disease, recent MI, CHF. |
| **Angiodysplasia** | Tortuous dilation of vessels → hematochezia. Most often found in the right-sided colon. More common in older patients. Confirmed by angiography. Associated with end-stage renal disease, von Willebrand disease, aortic stenosis. |
| **Chronic mesenteric ischemia** | "Intestinal angina": atherosclerosis of celiac artery, SMA (most commonly affected), or IMA → intestinal hypoperfusion → postprandial epigastric pain → food aversion and weight loss. |
| **Colonic ischemia** | Crampy abdominal pain followed by hematochezia. Commonly occurs at watershed areas (splenic flexure, rectosigmoid junction). Typically affects older adults. Thumbprint sign on imaging due to mucosal edema/hemorrhage. |
| **Ileus** | Intestinal hypomotility without obstruction → constipation and ↓ flatus; distended/tympanic abdomen with ↓ bowel sounds. Associated with abdominal surgeries, opiates, hypokalemia, sepsis. No transition zone on imaging. Treatment: bowel rest, electrolyte correction, cholinergic drugs (stimulate intestinal motility). |
| **Necrotizing enterocolitis** | Seen in premature, formula-fed infants with immature immune system. Necrosis of intestinal mucosa (most commonly terminal ileum and proximal colon), which can lead to pneumatosis intestinalis (arrows in B), pneumoperitoneum, portal venous gas. |
| **Proctitis** | Inflammation of rectal mucosa, usually associated with infection (*N gonorrhea*, *Chlamydia*, *Campylobacter*, *Shigella*, *Salmonella*, HSV, CMV), IBD, and radiation. Patients report tenesmus, rectal bleeding, and rectal pain. Proctoscopy reveals inflamed rectal mucosa (ulcers/vesicles in the case of HSV). Rectal swabs are used to detect other infectious etiologies. |
| **Small bowel obstruction** | Normal flow of intraluminal contents is interrupted → fluid accumulation and intestinal dilation proximal to blockage and intestinal decompression distal to blockage. Presents with abrupt onset of abdominal pain, nausea, vomiting, abdominal distension. Compromised blood flow due to excessive dilation or strangulation may lead to ischemia, necrosis, or perforation. Most commonly caused by intraperitoneal adhesions (fibrous band of scar tissue), tumors, and hernias (in rare cases, meconium plug in newborns → meconium ileus). Upright abdominal x-ray shows air-fluid levels C. Management: gastrointestinal decompression, volume resuscitation, bowel rest. |
| **Small intestinal bacterial overgrowth** | Abnormal bacterial overgrowth in the small intestine (normally low bacterial colony count). Risk factors: altered pH (eg, achlorhydria, PPI use), anatomical (eg, small bowel obstruction, adhesions, fistula, gastric bypass surgery, blind loop), dysmotility (eg, gastroparesis), immune mediated (IgA deficiency, HIV). Presents with bloating, flatulence, abdominal pain, chronic watery diarrhea, malabsorption (vitamin $B_{12}$) in severe cases. Diagnosis: carbohydrate breath test or small bowel culture. |

| Colonic polyps | Growths of tissue within the colon . Grossly characterized as flat, sessile, or pedunculated on the basis of protrusion into colonic lumen. Generally classified by histologic type. |
|---|---|

| HISTOLOGIC TYPE | CHARACTERISTICS |
|---|---|
| **Generally nonneoplastic** | |
| **Hamartomatous polyps** | Solitary lesions do not have significant risk of transformation. Growths of normal colonic tissue with distorted architecture. Associated with Peutz-Jeghers syndrome and juvenile polyposis. |
| **Hyperplastic polyps** | Most common; generally smaller and predominantly located in rectosigmoid region. Occasionally evolves into serrated polyps and more advanced lesions. |
| **Inflammatory pseudopolyps** | Due to mucosal erosion in inflammatory bowel disease. |
| **Mucosal polyps** | Small, usually < 5 mm. Look similar to normal mucosa. Clinically insignificant. |
| **Submucosal polyps** | May include lipomas, leiomyomas, fibromas, and other lesions. |
| **Potentially malignant** | |
| **Adenomatous polyps** | Neoplastic, via chromosomal instability pathway with mutations in *APC* and *KRAS*. Tubular  histology has less malignant potential than villous  ("villous histology is villainous"); tubulovillous has intermediate malignant potential. Usually asymptomatic; may present with occult bleeding. |
| **Serrated polyps** | Neoplastic. Characterized by CpG island methylator phenotype (CIMP; cytosine base followed by guanine, linked by a phosphodiester bond). Defect may silence mismatch repair gene (eg, *MLH1*) expression. Mutations lead to microsatellite instability and mutations in *BRAF*. "Saw-tooth" pattern of crypts on biopsy. Up to 20% of cases of sporadic CRC. |

Sessile  Pedunculated

Stalk

### Polyposis syndromes

| | |
|---|---|
| **Familial adenomatous polyposis** | Autosomal dominant mutation of *APC* tumor suppressor gene on chromosome 5q21-q22. 2-hit hypothesis. Thousands of polyps arise starting after puberty; pancolonic; always involves rectum. Prophylactic colectomy or else 100% progress to CRC. |
| **Gardner syndrome** | FAP + osseous and soft tissue tumors (eg, osteomas of skull or mandible), congenital hypertrophy of retinal pigment epithelium, impacted/supernumerary teeth. |
| **Turcot syndrome** | FAP or Lynch syndrome + malignant CNS tumor (eg, medulloblastoma, glioma). Turcot = Turban. |
| **Peutz-Jeghers syndrome** | Autosomal dominant syndrome featuring numerous hamartomatous polyps throughout GI tract, along with hyperpigmented macules on mouth, lips, hands, genitalia. Associated with ↑ risk of breast and GI cancers (eg, colorectal, stomach, small bowel, pancreatic). |
| **Juvenile polyposis syndrome** | Autosomal dominant syndrome in children (typically < 5 years old) featuring numerous hamartomatous polyps in the colon, stomach, small bowel. Associated with ↑ risk of CRC. |
| ***MUTYH*-associated polyposis syndrome** | Autosomal recessive disorder of the *MUTYH* gene responsible for DNA repair. Associated with significantly ↑ risk of CRC, polyps (adenomatous; may be hyperplastic or serrated), and serrated adenomas. Also associated with duodenal adenomas, ovarian and bladder cancers. |

**Lynch syndrome**

Also called hereditary nonpolyposis colorectal cancer (HNPCC). Autosomal dominant mutation of mismatch repair genes (eg, *MLH1*, *MSH2*) with subsequent microsatellite instability. ~ 80% progress to CRC. Proximal Colon is always involved. Associated with Endometrial, Ovarian, and Skin cancers. Merrill **Lynch** has CEOS.

---

**Colorectal cancer**

| | |
|---|---|
| EPIDEMIOLOGY | Most patients are > 50 years old. ~ 25% have a family history. |
| RISK FACTORS | Adenomatous and serrated polyps, familial cancer syndromes, IBD, tobacco use, diet of processed meat with low fiber. |
| PRESENTATION | Rectosigmoid > ascending > descending. |

Most are asymptomatic. Right side (cecal, ascending) associated with occult bleeding; left side (rectosigmoid) associated with hematochezia and obstruction (narrower lumen → ↓ stool caliber).
Ascending—exophytic mass, iron deficiency anemia, weight loss.
Descending—infiltrating mass, partial obstruction, colicky pain, hematochezia.
Can present with S *bovis* (*gallolyticus*) bacteremia/endocarditis or as an episode of diverticulitis.

DIAGNOSIS

Iron deficiency anemia in males (especially > 50 years old) and postmenopausal females raises suspicion.
Screening:
- Average risk: screen at age 45 with colonoscopy (polyp seen in **A**); alternatives include flexible sigmoidoscopy, fecal occult blood testing (FOBT), fecal immunochemical testing (FIT), FIT-fecal DNA, CT colonography.
- Patients with a first-degree relative who has colon cancer: screen at age 40 with colonoscopy, or 10 years prior to the relative's presentation.
- Patients with IBD: screen 8 years after onset.

"Apple core" lesion seen on barium enema x-ray **B**.
CEA tumor marker: good for monitoring recurrence, should not be used for screening.

---

**Molecular pathogenesis of colorectal cancer**

Chromosomal instability pathway: mutations in APC cause FAP and most sporadic cases of CRC (commonly left-sided) via adenoma-carcinoma sequence.
Microsatellite instability pathway: mutations or methylation of mismatch repair genes (eg, *MLH1*) cause Lynch syndrome and some sporadic CRC via serrated polyp pathway.
Overexpression of COX-2 has been linked to CRC, NSAIDs may be chemopreventive.

Chromosomal instability pathway

Normal colon → Loss of *APC* gene → Colon at risk → *KRAS* mutation → Adenoma → Loss of tumor suppressor gene(s) *(TP53, DCC)* → Carcinoma

↓ Intercellular adhesion
↑ Proliferation

Unregulated intracellular signaling

↑ Tumorigenesis

## Cirrhosis and portal hypertension

Cirrhosis—diffuse bridging fibrosis (via stellate cells) and regenerative nodules disrupt normal architecture of liver A; ↑ risk for hepatocellular carcinoma. Can lead to various systemic changes. Etiologies include alcohol, nonalcoholic steatohepatitis, chronic viral hepatitis, autoimmune hepatitis, biliary disease, genetic/metabolic disorders.

Portal hypertension—↑ pressure in portal venous system. Etiologies include cirrhosis (most common cause in developed countries), vascular obstruction (eg, portal vein thrombosis, Budd-Chiari syndrome), schistosomiasis.

Serum ascites albumin gradient (SAAG)—difference between albumin levels in serum and ascitic fluid.

$$SAAG = albumin_{serum} - albumin_{ascites}$$

Used to evaluate the etiology of ascites.
SAAG ≥ 1.1 = portal hypertension.
SAAG < 1.1 = consider other causes.

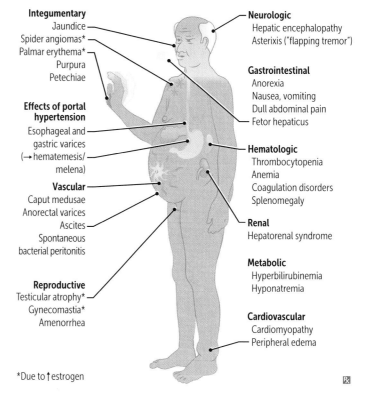

**Integumentary**
Jaundice
Spider angiomas*
Palmar erythema*
Purpura
Petechiae

**Effects of portal hypertension**
Esophageal and gastric varices (→hematemesis/melena)

**Vascular**
Caput medusae
Anorectal varices
Ascites
Spontaneous bacterial peritonitis

**Reproductive**
Testicular atrophy*
Gynecomastia*
Amenorrhea

*Due to ↑ estrogen

**Neurologic**
Hepatic encephalopathy
Asterixis ("flapping tremor")

**Gastrointestinal**
Anorexia
Nausea, vomiting
Dull abdominal pain
Fetor hepaticus

**Hematologic**
Thrombocytopenia
Anemia
Coagulation disorders
Splenomegaly

**Renal**
Hepatorenal syndrome

**Metabolic**
Hyperbilirubinemia
Hyponatremia

**Cardiovascular**
Cardiomyopathy
Peripheral edema

| | |
|---|---|
| **Budd-Chiari syndrome** | Hepatic venous outflow tract obstruction (eg, due to thrombosis, compression) with centrilobular congestion and necrosis → congestive liver disease (hepatomegaly, ascites, varices, abdominal pain, liver failure). Absence of JVD. Associated with hypercoagulable states, polycythemia vera, postpartum state, HCC. May cause nutmeg liver (mottled appearance). 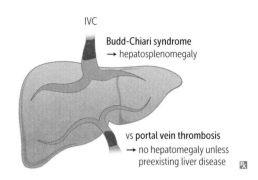 |
| | **Portal vein thrombosis**—thrombosis in portal vein proximal to liver. Usually asymptomatic in the majority of patients, but associated with portal hypertension, abdominal pain, fever. May lead to bowel ischemia if extension to superior mesenteric vein. Etiologies include cirrhosis, malignancy, pancreatitis, and sepsis. |

IVC

Budd-Chiari syndrome
→ hepatosplenomegaly

vs portal vein thrombosis
→ no hepatomegaly unless preexisting liver disease

| | |
|---|---|
| **Spontaneous bacterial peritonitis** | Also called 1° bacterial peritonitis. Common and potentially fatal bacterial infection in patients with cirrhosis and ascites. Often asymptomatic, but can cause fevers, chills, abdominal pain, ileus, or worsening encephalopathy. Commonly caused by gram ⊖ organisms (eg, *E coli*, *Klebsiella*) or less commonly gram ⊕ *Streptococcus*. |
| | Diagnosis: paracentesis with ascitic fluid absolute neutrophil count (ANC) > 250 cells/mm³. Empiric first-line treatment is 3rd generation cephalosporin (eg, ceftriaxone). |

### Serum markers of liver pathology

| ENZYMES RELEASED IN LIVER DAMAGE | |
|---|---|
| **Aspartate aminotransferase and alanine aminotransferase** | ↑ in most liver disease: ALT > AST |
| | ↑ in alcoholic liver disease: AST > ALT (ratio usually > 2:1, AST does not typically exceed 500 U/L in alcoholic hepatitis). Make a toAST with alcohol |
| | AST > ALT in nonalcoholic liver disease suggests progression to advanced fibrosis or cirrhosis |
| | ↑↑↑ aminotransferases (>1000 U/L): differential includes drug-induced liver injury (eg, acetaminophen toxicity), ischemic hepatitis, acute viral hepatitis, autoimmune hepatitis |
| **Alkaline phosphatase** | ↑ in cholestasis (eg, biliary obstruction), infiltrative disorders, bone disease |
| **γ-glutamyl transpeptidase** | ↑ in various liver and biliary diseases (just as ALP can), but not in bone disease (located in canalicular membrane of hepatocytes like ALP); associated with alcohol use |
| FUNCTIONAL LIVER MARKERS | |
| **Bilirubin** | ↑ in various liver diseases (eg, biliary obstruction, alcoholic or viral hepatitis, cirrhosis), hemolysis |
| **Albumin** | ↓ in advanced liver disease (marker of liver's biosynthetic function) |
| **Prothrombin time** | ↑ in advanced liver disease (↓ production of clotting factors, thereby measuring the liver's biosynthetic function) |
| **Platelets** | ↓ in advanced liver disease (↓ thrombopoietin, liver sequestration) and portal hypertension (splenomegaly/splenic sequestration) |

**Reye syndrome**

Rare, often fatal childhood hepatic encephalopathy.

Associated with viral infection (especially VZV and influenza) that has been treated with aspirin. Aspirin metabolites ↓ β-oxidation by reversible inhibition of mitochondrial enzymes.

Findings: mitochondrial abnormalities, fatty liver (microvesicular fatty changes), hyperammonemia, hypoglycemia, vomiting, hepatomegaly, coma.

↑ ICP ↑ morbidity and mortality. Renal and cardiac failure may also occur.

Avoid aspirin (**ASA**) in children, except in Kaw**ASA**ki disease.

Salicylates aren't a ray (**Reye**) of sun**SHINEE** for kids:

**S**teatosis of liver/hepatocytes

**H**ypoglycemia/**H**epatomegaly

**I**nfection (VZV, influenza)

**N**ot awake (coma)

**E**ncephalopathy and diffuse cerebral **E**dema

---

**Alcoholic liver disease**

| | |
|---|---|
| **Hepatic steatosis** | Macrovesicular fatty change **A** that may be reversible with alcohol cessation. |
| **Alcoholic hepatitis** | Requires sustained, long-term consumption. Swollen and necrotic hepatocytes with neutrophilic infiltration. Mallory bodies **B** (intracytoplasmic eosinophilic inclusions of damaged keratin filaments). |
| **Alcoholic cirrhosis** | Final and usually irreversible form. Sclerosis around central vein may be seen in early disease. Regenerative nodules surrounded by fibrous bands (red arrows in **C**) in response to chronic liver injury → portal hypertension and end-stage liver disease. |

---

**Nonalcoholic fatty liver disease**

Associated with metabolic syndrome (obesity, insulin resistance, HTN, hypertriglyceridemia, ↓ HDL); obesity → fatty infiltration of hepatocytes **A** → cellular "ballooning" and eventual necrosis. Steatosis present without evidence of significant inflammation or fibrosis. May persist or even regress over time.

**Nonalcoholic steatohepatitis**—associated with lobular inflammation and hepatocyte ballooning → fibrosis. May progress to cirrhosis and HCC.

| | |
|---|---|
| **Autoimmune hepatitis** | Chronic inflammatory liver disease. More common in females. May be asymptomatic or present with fatigue, nausea, pruritus. Often ⊕ for anti-smooth muscle or anti-liver/kidney microsomal-1 antibodies. Labs: ↑ ALT and AST. Histology: portal and periportal lymphoplasmacytic infiltrate. |

| | |
|---|---|
| **Hepatic encephalopathy** | Cirrhosis → portosystemic shunts → ↓ $NH_3$ metabolism → neuropsychiatric dysfunction (reversible) ranging from disorientation/asterixis to difficult arousal or coma.<br>Triggers:<br>  ▪ ↑ $NH_3$ production and absorption (due to GI bleed, constipation, infection).<br>  ▪ ↓ $NH_3$ removal (due to renal failure, diuretics, bypassed hepatic blood flow post-TIPS).<br>Treatment: lactulose (↑ $NH_4^+$ generation) and rifaximin (↓ $NH_3$-producing gut bacteria). |

## Liver tumors

| | |
|---|---|
| **Hepatic hemangioma** | Also called cavernous hemangioma. Most common benign liver tumor (venous malformation) **A**; typically occurs at age 30–50 years. Biopsy contraindicated because of risk of hemorrhage. |
| **Focal nodular hyperplasia** | Second most common benign liver tumor; occurs predominantly in females aged 35–50 years. Hyperplastic reaction of hepatocytes to an aberrant dystrophic artery. Marked by central stellate scar. Usually asymptomatic and detected incidentally. |
| **Hepatic adenoma** | Rare, benign tumor, often related to oral contraceptive or anabolic steroid use; may regress spontaneously or rupture (abdominal pain and shock). |
| **Hepatocellular carcinoma** | Also called hepatoma. Most common 1° malignant liver tumor in adults **B**. Associated with HBV (+/– cirrhosis) and all other causes of cirrhosis (including HCV, alcoholic and nonalcoholic fatty liver disease, autoimmune disease, hemochromatosis, Wilson disease, $\alpha_1$-antitrypsin deficiency) and specific carcinogens (eg, aflatoxin from *Aspergillus*).<br>Findings: anorexia, jaundice, tender hepatomegaly. May lead to decompensation of previously stable cirrhosis (eg, ascites) and portal vein thrombosis. Spreads hematogenously.<br>Diagnosis: ultrasound (screening) or contrast CT/MRI **C** (confirmation); biopsy if diagnosis is uncertain. |
| **Hepatic angiosarcoma** | Rare, malignant tumor of endothelial origin; associated with exposure to arsenic, vinyl chloride. |
| **Metastases** | Most common malignant liver tumors overall; 1° sources include GI, breast, lung cancers. Metastases are rarely solitary. |

| | | |
|---|---|---|
| **α₁-antitrypsin deficiency**  | Misfolded gene product protein aggregates in hepatocellular ER → cirrhosis with PAS ⊕ globules  in liver. Codominant trait. Often presents in young patients with liver damage and dyspnea without a history of tobacco smoking. | In lungs, ↓ α₁-antitrypsin → uninhibited elastase in alveoli → ↓ elastic tissue → panacinar emphysema. |

| | | |
|---|---|---|
| **Jaundice**  | Abnormal yellowing of the skin and/or sclera (icterus) A due to bilirubin deposition. Hyperbilirubinemia 2° to ↑ production or ↓ clearance (impaired hepatic uptake, conjugation, excretion). | HOT Liver—common causes of ↑ bilirubin level:<br>Hemolysis<br>Obstruction<br>Tumor<br>Liver disease |

| | |
|---|---|
| **Conjugated (direct) hyperbilirubinemia** | Biliary tract obstruction: gallstones, cholangiocarcinoma, pancreatic or liver cancer, liver fluke.<br>Biliary tract disease: 1° sclerosing cholangitis, 1° biliary cholangitis<br>Excretion defect: Dubin-Johnson syndrome, Rotor syndrome. |
| **Unconjugated (indirect) hyperbilirubinemia** | Hemolytic, benign (neonates), Crigler-Najjar, Gilbert syndrome. |
| **Mixed hyperbilirubinemia** | Both direct and indirect hyperbilirubinemia.<br>Hepatitis, cirrhosis. |

| | |
|---|---|
| **Benign neonatal hyperbilirubinemia** | Formerly called physiologic neonatal jaundice. Mild unconjugated hyperbilirubinemia caused by:<br> ▪ ↑ fetal RBC turnover (↑ hematocrit and ↓ fetal RBC lifespan).<br> ▪ Immature newborn liver (↓ UDP-glucuronosyltransferase activity).<br> ▪ Sterile newborn gut (↓ conversion to urobilinogen → ↑ deconjugation by intestinal brush border β-glucuronidase → ↑ enterohepatic circulation).<br>β-glucuronidase—lysosomal enzyme for direct bilirubin deconjugation. Also found in breast milk. May lead to pigment stone formation.<br>Occurs in nearly all newborns after first 24 hours of life and usually resolves without treatment in 1–2 weeks. Exaggerated forms:<br>Breastfeeding failure jaundice—insufficient breast milk intake → ↓ bilirubin elimination in stool → ↑ enterohepatic circulation.<br>Breast milk jaundice—↑ β-glucuronidase in breast milk → ↑ deconjugation → ↑ enterohepatic circulation.<br>Severe cases may lead to kernicterus (deposition of unconjugated, lipid-soluble bilirubin in the brain, particularly basal ganglia).<br>Treatment: phototherapy (non-UV) isomerizes unconjugated bilirubin to water-soluble form. |

| | |
|---|---|
| **Biliary atresia** | Most common reason for pediatric liver transplantation. Fibro-obliterative destruction of bile ducts → cholestasis. Associated with absent/abnormal gallbladder on ultrasonogram. Often presents as a newborn with persistent jaundice after 2 weeks of life, darkening urine, acholic stools, hepatomegaly. Labs: ↑ direct bilirubin and GGT. |

| | |
|---|---|
| **Hereditary hyperbilirubinemias** | All autosomal recessive. |
| ❶ Gilbert syndrome | Mildly ↓ UDP-glucuronosyltransferase conjugation. Asymptomatic or mild jaundice usually with stress, illness, or fasting. ↑ unconjugated bilirubin without overt hemolysis. Relatively common, benign condition. |
| ❷ Crigler-Najjar syndrome, type I | Absent UDP-glucuronosyltransferase. Presents early in life, but some patients may not have neurologic signs until later in life. Findings: jaundice, kernicterus (unconjugated bilirubin deposition in brain), ↑ unconjugated bilirubin. Treatment: plasmapheresis and phototherapy (does not conjugate UCB; but does ↑ polarity and ↑ water solubility to allow excretion). Liver transplant is curative. Type II is less severe and responds to phenobarbital, which ↑ liver enzyme synthesis. |
| ❸ Dubin-Johnson syndrome | Conjugated hyperbilirubinemia due to defective liver excretion. Grossly black (Dark) liver due to impaired excretion of epinephrine metabolites. Benign. |
| ❹ Rotor syndrome | Phenotypically similar to Dubin-Johnson, but milder in presentation without black (Regular) liver. Due to impaired hepatic storage of conjugated bilirubin. |

**Wilson disease**

Also called hepatolenticular degeneration. Autosomal recessive mutations in hepatocyte copper-transporting ATPase (*ATP7B* gene; chromosome 13) → ↓ copper incorporation into apoceruloplasmin and excretion into bile → ↓ serum ceruloplasmin. Copper accumulates, especially in liver, brain (eg, basal ganglia), cornea, kidneys; ↑ urine copper.

Presents before age 40 with liver disease (eg, hepatitis, acute liver failure, cirrhosis), neurologic disease (eg, dysarthria, dystonia, tremor, parkinsonism), psychiatric disease, Kayser-Fleischer rings (deposits in Descemet membrane of cornea) **A**, hemolytic anemia, renal disease (eg, Fanconi syndrome).

Treatment: chelation with penicillamine or trientine, oral zinc. Liver transplant in acute liver failure related to Wilson disease.

**Hemochromatosis**

Autosomal recessive. Mutation in *HFE* gene, located on chromosome 6. Leads to abnormal (low) hepcidin production, ↑ intestinal iron absorption. Iron overload can also be 2° to chronic transfusion therapy (eg, β-thalassemia major). Iron accumulates, especially in liver, pancreas, skin, heart, pituitary, joints. Hemosiderin (iron) can be identified on liver MRI or biopsy with Prussian blue stain **A**.

Presents after age 40 when total body iron > 20 g; iron loss through menstruation slows progression in females. Classic triad of cirrhosis, diabetes mellitus, skin pigmentation ("bronze diabetes"). Also causes restrictive cardiomyopathy (classic) or dilated cardiomyopathy (reversible), hypogonadism, arthropathy (calcium pyrophosphate deposition; especially metacarpophalangeal joints). HCC is common cause of death.

Treatment: repeated phlebotomy, iron (Fe) chelation with deferasirox, deferoxamine, deferiprone.

**Biliary tract disease**

May present with pruritus, jaundice, dark urine, light-colored stool, hepatosplenomegaly. Typically with cholestatic pattern of LFTs (↑ conjugated bilirubin, ↑ cholesterol, ↑ ALP, ↑ GGT).

| | PATHOLOGY | EPIDEMIOLOGY | ADDITIONAL FEATURES |
|---|---|---|---|
| **Primary sclerosing cholangitis** | Unknown cause of concentric "onion skin" bile duct fibrosis → alternating strictures and dilation with "beading" of intra- and extrahepatic bile ducts on ERCP **A**, magnetic resonance cholangiopancreatography (MRCP). | Classically in middle-aged males with ulcerative colitis. | Associated with ulcerative colitis. MPO-ANCA/p-ANCA ⊕. ↑ IgM. Can lead to 2° biliary cirrhosis. ↑ risk of cholangiocarcinoma and gallbladder cancer. |
| **Primary biliary cholangitis** | Autoimmune reaction → lymphocytic infiltrate +/− granulomas → destruction of lobular bile ducts. | Classically in middle-aged females. | Antimitochondrial antibody ⊕, ↑ IgM. Associated with other autoimmune conditions (eg, Hashimoto thyroiditis, rheumatoid arthritis, celiac disease). Treatment: ursodiol. |
| **Secondary biliary cirrhosis** | Extrahepatic biliary obstruction → ↑ pressure in intrahepatic ducts → injury/ fibrosis and bile stasis. | Patients with known obstructive lesions (gallstones, biliary strictures, pancreatic carcinoma). | May be complicated by acute cholangitis. |

## Cholelithiasis and related pathologies

↑ cholesterol and/or bilirubin, ↓ bile salts, and gallbladder stasis all cause sludge or stones.
2 types of stones:

- Cholesterol stones  (radiolucent with 10–20% opaque due to calcifications)—80% of stones. Associated with obesity, Crohn disease, advanced age, estrogen therapy, multiparity, rapid weight loss, medications (eg, fibrates), race (↑ incidence in White and Native American populations).
- Pigment stones (black = radiopaque, Ca²⁺ bilirubinate, hemolysis; brown = radiolucent, infection). Associated with Crohn disease, chronic hemolysis, alcoholic cirrhosis, advanced age, biliary infections, total parenteral nutrition (TPN).

Most common complication is cholecystitis; can also cause acute pancreatitis, acute cholangitis.

Diagnose with ultrasound. Treat with elective cholecystectomy if symptomatic.
Risk factors (7 F's): female, fat, fertile, forty, fair, feeds (TPN), fasting (rapid weight loss).

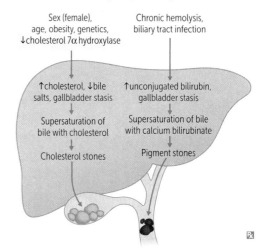

| RELATED PATHOLOGIES | CHARACTERISTICS |
| --- | --- |
| **Biliary colic** | Associated with nausea/vomiting and dull RUQ pain. Neurohormonal activation (eg, by CCK after a fatty meal) triggers contraction of gallbladder, forcing stone into cystic duct. Labs are normal, ultrasound shows cholelithiasis. |
| **Choledocholithiasis** | Presence of gallstone(s) in common bile duct, often leading to elevated ALP, GGT, direct bilirubin, and/or AST/ALT. |
| **Cholecystitis**  | Acute or chronic inflammation of gallbladder.<br>Calculous cholecystitis—most common type; due to gallstone impaction in the cystic duct resulting in inflammation and gallbladder wall thickening (arrows in ); can produce 2° infection.<br>Acalculous cholecystitis—due to gallbladder stasis, hypoperfusion, or infection (CMV); seen in critically ill patients.<br>Murphy sign: inspiratory arrest on RUQ palpation due to pain. Pain may radiate to right shoulder (due to irritation of phrenic nerve). ↑ ALP if bile duct becomes involved (eg, acute cholangitis).<br>Diagnose with ultrasound or cholescintigraphy (HIDA scan). Failure to visualize gallbladder on HIDA scan suggests obstruction.<br>Gallstone ileus—fistula between gallbladder and GI tract → stone enters GI lumen → obstructs at ileocecal valve (narrowest point); can see air in biliary tree (pneumobilia). Rigler triad: radiographic findings of pneumobilia, small bowel obstruction, gallstone (usually in iliac fossa). |
| **Porcelain gallbladder**  | Calcified gallbladder due to chronic cholecystitis; usually found incidentally on imaging .<br>Treatment: prophylactic cholecystectomy generally recommended due to ↑ risk of gallbladder cancer (mostly adenocarcinoma). |
| **Acute cholangitis** | Also called ascending cholangitis. Infection of biliary tree usually due to obstruction that leads to stasis/bacterial overgrowth.<br>Charcot triad of cholangitis includes jaundice, fever, RUQ pain.<br>Reynolds pentad is Charcot triad plus altered mental status and shock (hypotension). |

| | |
|---|---|
| **Cholangiocarcinoma** | Malignant tumor of bile duct epithelium. Most common location is convergence of right and left hepatic ducts. Risk factors include 1° sclerosing cholangitis, liver fluke infections. Usually presents late with fatigue, weight loss, abdominal pain, jaundice. Imaging may show biliary tract obstruction. Histology: infiltrating neoplastic glands associated with desmoplastic stroma. |

| | |
|---|---|
| **Pancreatitis** | Refers to inflammation of the pancreas. Usually sterile. |
| **Acute pancreatitis** | Autodigestion of pancreas by pancreatic enzymes (A shows pancreas [yellow arrows] surrounded by edema [red arrows]).<br><br>Causes: Idiopathic, Gallstones, Ethanol, Trauma, Steroids, Mumps, Autoimmune disease, Scorpion sting, Hypercalcemia/Hypertriglyceridemia (> 1000 mg/dL), ERCP, Drugs (eg, sulfa drugs, NRTIs, protease inhibitors). **I GET SMASHED.**<br><br>Diagnosis by 2 of 3 criteria: acute epigastric pain often radiating to the back, serum amylase or lipase (more specific) to 3× upper limit of normal, or characteristic imaging findings.<br><br>Complications: pancreatic pseudocyst B (lined by granulation tissue, not epithelium), abscess, necrosis, hemorrhage, infection, organ failure (ALI/ARDS, shock, renal failure), hypocalcemia (precipitation of $Ca^{2+}$ soaps). |
| **Chronic pancreatitis** | Chronic inflammation, atrophy, calcification of the pancreas C. Major risk factors include alcohol use disorder and genetic predisposition (eg, cystic fibrosis, *SPINK1* mutations); can be idiopathic. Complications include pancreatic insufficiency and pseudocysts.<br><br>Pancreatic insufficiency (typically when <10% pancreatic function) may manifest with steatorrhea, fat-soluble vitamin deficiency, diabetes mellitus.<br><br>Amylase and lipase may or may not be elevated (almost always elevated in acute pancreatitis). |

**Pancreatic adenocarcinoma**

Very aggressive tumor arising from pancreatic ducts (disorganized glandular structure with cellular infiltration **A**); often metastatic at presentation, with average survival ~ 1 year after diagnosis. Tumors more common in pancreatic head **B** (lead to obstructive jaundice). Associated with CA 19-9 tumor marker (also CEA, less specific).

Risk factors:
- Tobacco smoking (strongest risk factor)
- Chronic pancreatitis (especially > 20 years)
- Diabetes
- Age > 50 years

Often presents with:
- Abdominal pain radiating to back
- Weight loss (due to malabsorption and anorexia)
- Migratory thrombophlebitis—redness and tenderness on palpation of extremities (Trousseau syndrome)
- Obstructive jaundice with palpable, nontender gallbladder (Courvoisier sign)

---

## ▶ GASTROINTESTINAL—PHARMACOLOGY

### Acid suppression therapy

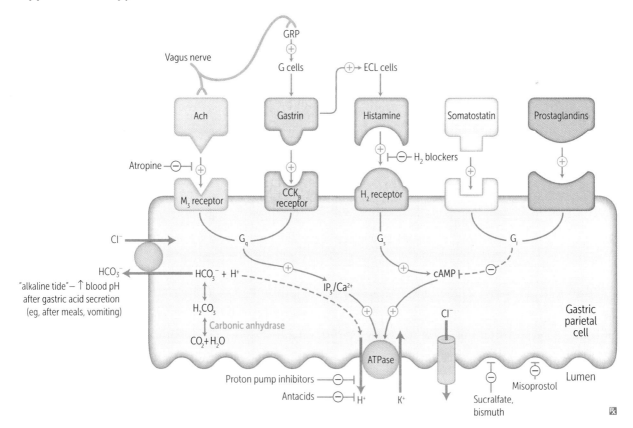

| | |
|---|---|
| **H$_2$-blockers** | Cimetidine, famotidine, nizatidine. |
| | Take H$_2$ blockers before you dine. Think "table for 2" to remember H$_2$. |
| MECHANISM | Reversible block of histamine H$_2$-receptors → ↓ H$^+$ secretion by parietal cells. |
| CLINICAL USE | Peptic ulcer, gastritis, mild esophageal reflux. |
| ADVERSE EFFECTS | Cimetidine is a potent inhibitor of cytochrome P-450 (multiple drug interactions); it also has antiandrogenic effects (prolactin release, gynecomastia, impotence, ↓ libido in males); can cross blood-brain barrier (confusion, dizziness, headaches) and placenta. Cimetidine ↓ renal excretion of creatinine. Other H$_2$ blockers are relatively free of these effects. |

| | |
|---|---|
| **Proton pump inhibitors** | Omeprazole, lansoprazole, esomeprazole, pantoprazole, dexlansoprazole. |
| MECHANISM | Irreversibly inhibit H$^+$/K$^+$-ATPase in stomach parietal cells. |
| CLINICAL USE | Peptic ulcer, gastritis, esophageal reflux, Zollinger-Ellison syndrome, component of therapy for *H pylori*, stress ulcer prophylaxis. |
| ADVERSE EFFECTS | ↑ risk of *C difficile* infection, pneumonia, acute interstitial nephritis. Vitamin B$_{12}$ malabsorption; ↓ serum Mg$^{2+}$/Ca$^{2+}$ absorption (potentially leading to increased fracture risk in older adults). |

| | | |
|---|---|---|
| **Antacids** | Can affect absorption, bioavailability, or urinary excretion of other drugs by altering gastric and urinary pH or by delaying gastric emptying. All can cause hypokalemia. | |
| **Aluminum hydroxide** | Constipation, Hypophosphatemia, Osteodystrophy, Proximal muscle weakness, Seizures | Aluminimum amount of feces CHOPS |
| **Calcium carbonate** | Hypercalcemia (milk-alkali syndrome), rebound acid ↑ | Can chelate and ↓ effectiveness of other drugs (eg, tetracycline) |
| **Magnesium hydroxide** | Diarrhea, hyporeflexia, hypotension, cardiac arrest | Mg$^{2+}$ = Must go 2 the bathroom |

| | |
|---|---|
| **Bismuth, sucralfate** | |
| MECHANISM | Bind to ulcer base, providing physical protection and allowing HCO$_3^-$ secretion to reestablish pH gradient in the mucous layer. Sucralfate requires acidic environment, not given with PPIs/H$_2$ blockers. |
| CLINICAL USE | ↑ ulcer healing, travelers' diarrhea (bismuth). Bismuth also used in quadruple therapy for *H pylori*. |

| | |
|---|---|
| **Misoprostol** | |
| MECHANISM | PGE$_1$ analog. ↑ production and secretion of gastric mucous barrier, ↓ acid production. |
| CLINICAL USE | Prevention of NSAID-induced peptic ulcers (NSAIDs block PGE$_1$ production). Also used off-label for induction of labor (ripens cervix). |
| ADVERSE EFFECTS | Diarrhea. Contraindicated in patients of childbearing potential (abortifacient). |

## Octreotide

| | |
|---|---|
| MECHANISM | Long-acting somatostatin analog; inhibits secretion of various splanchnic vasodilatory hormones. |
| CLINICAL USE | Acute variceal bleeds, acromegaly, VIPoma, carcinoid tumors. |
| ADVERSE EFFECTS | Nausea, cramps, steatorrhea. ↑ risk of cholelithiasis due to CCK inhibition. |

## Sulfasalazine

| | |
|---|---|
| MECHANISM | A combination of sulfapyridine (antibacterial) and 5-aminosalicylic acid (anti-inflammatory). Activated by colonic bacteria. |
| CLINICAL USE | Ulcerative colitis, Crohn disease (colitis component). |
| ADVERSE EFFECTS | Malaise, nausea, sulfonamide toxicity, reversible oligospermia. |

## Loperamide, diphenoxylate

| | |
|---|---|
| MECHANISM | Agonists at μ-opioid receptors → ↓ gut motility. Poor CNS penetration (low addictive potential). |
| CLINICAL USE | Diarrhea. |
| ADVERSE EFFECTS | Constipation, nausea. |

## Antiemetics

All act centrally in chemoreceptor trigger zone of area postrema.

| DRUG | MECHANISM | CLINICAL USE | ADVERSE EFFECTS |
|---|---|---|---|
| Ondansetron, granisetron | 5-HT$_3$-receptor antagonists Also act peripherally (↓ vagal stimulation) | Nausea and vomiting after chemotherapy, radiotherapy, or surgery | Headache, constipation, QT interval prolongation, serotonin syndrome |
| Prochlorperazine, metoclopramide | D$_2$-receptor antagonists Metoclopramide also causes ↑ gastric emptying and ↑ LES tone | Nausea and vomiting Metoclopramide is also used in gastroparesis (eg, diabetic), persistent GERD | Extrapyramidal symptoms, hyperprolactinemia, anxiety, drowsiness, restlessness, depression, GI distress |
| Aprepitant, fosaprepitant | NK$_1$ (neurokinin-1) receptor antagonists NK$_1$ receptor = substance P receptor | Chemotherapy-induced nausea and vomiting | Fatigue, GI distress |

## Orlistat

| | |
|---|---|
| MECHANISM | Inhibits gastric and pancreatic lipase → ↓ breakdown and absorption of dietary fats. Taken with fat-containing meals. |
| CLINICAL USE | Weight loss. |
| ADVERSE EFFECTS | Abdominal pain, flatulence, bowel urgency/frequent bowel movements, steatorrhea; ↓ absorption of fat-soluble vitamins. |

## Anticonstipation drugs

| DRUG | MECHANISM | ADVERSE EFFECTS |
| --- | --- | --- |
| **Bulk-forming laxatives** Methylcellulose, psyllium | Soluble fibers that draw water into gut lumen, forming viscous liquid that promotes peristalsis | Bloating |
| **Osmotic laxatives** Lactulose, magnesium citrate, magnesium hydroxide, polyethylene glycol | Provide osmotic load to draw water into GI lumen Lactulose also treats hepatic encephalopathy: gut microbiota degrades lactulose into metabolites (lactic acid, acetic acid) that promote nitrogen excretion as $NH_4^+$ by trapping it in colon | Diarrhea, dehydration; may be misused by patients with bulimia |
| **Stimulant laxatives** Bisacodyl, senna | Enteric nerve stimulation → colonic contraction | Diarrhea |
| **Emollient laxatives** Docusate | Surfactants that ↓ stool surface tension, promoting water entry into stool | Diarrhea |
| **Lubiprostone** | Chloride channel activator → ↑ intestinal fluid secretion | Diarrhea, nausea |
| **Guanylate cyclase-C agonists** Linaclotide, plecanatide | Activate intracellular cGMP signaling → ↑ fluid and electrolyte secretion in the intestinal lumen | Diarrhea, bloating, abdominal discomfort, flatulence |
| **Serotonergic agonists** Prucalopride | $5HT_4$ agonism → enteric nerve stimulation → ↑ peristalsis, intestinal secretion | Diarrhea, abdominal pain, nausea, headache |
| **NHE₃ inhibitor** Tenapanor | Inhibits $Na^+/H^+$ exchanger → ↓ $Na^+$ absorption → ↑ $H_2O$ secretion in lumen | Diarrhea, abdominal pain, nausea |

# Hematology and Oncology

*"You're always somebody's type! (blood type, that is)"*
—BloodLink

*"The best blood will at some time get into a fool or a mosquito."*
—Austin O'Malley

*"A life touched by cancer is not a life destroyed by cancer."*
—Drew Boswell, *Climbing the Cancer Mountain*

*"Without hair, a queen is still a queen."*
—Prajakta Mhadnak

*"Blood can circulate forever if you keep donating it."*
—Anonymous

When studying hematology, pay close attention to the many cross connections to immunology. Make sure you master the different types of anemias. Be comfortable interpreting blood smears. When reviewing oncologic drugs, focus on mechanisms and adverse effects rather than details of clinical uses, which may be lower yield.

Please note that solid tumors are covered in their respective organ system chapters.

## ▶ HEMATOLOGY AND ONCOLOGY—EMBRYOLOGY

**Fetal erythropoiesis**

Fetal erythropoiesis occurs in:
- Yolk sac (3–8 weeks)
- Liver (6 weeks–birth)
- Spleen (10–28 weeks)
- Bone marrow (18 weeks to adult)

Young liver synthesizes blood.

**Hemoglobin development**

Embryonic globins: $\zeta$ and $\epsilon$.
Fetal hemoglobin (HbF) = $\alpha_2\gamma_2$.
Adult hemoglobin (HbA$_1$) = $\alpha_2\beta_2$.
HbF has higher affinity for $O_2$ due to less avid binding of 2,3-BPG, allowing HbF to extract $O_2$ from maternal hemoglobin (HbA$_1$ and HbA$_2$) across the placenta. HbA$_2$ ($\alpha_2\delta_2$) is a form of adult hemoglobin present in small amounts.

From fetal to adult hemoglobin:
Alpha always; gamma goes, becomes beta.

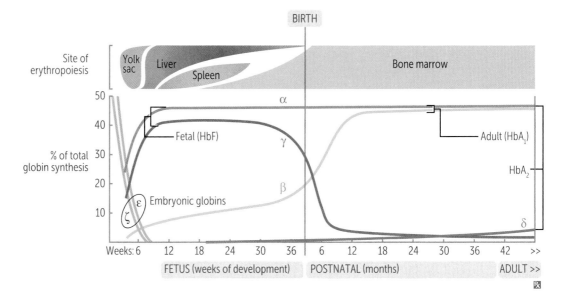

## Blood groups

| | ABO classification | | | | Rh classification | |
|---|---|---|---|---|---|---|
| | **A** | **B** | **AB** | **O** | **Rh⊕** | **Rh⊖** |
| RBC type | | | | | | |
| Group antigens on RBC surface | A | B | A & B | NONE | Rh (D) | NONE |
| Antibodies in plasma | Anti-B | Anti-A | NONE | Anti-A    Anti-B | NONE | Anti-D |
| | IgM | IgM | | IgG, IgM | | IgG |
| **Clinical relevance** | | | | | | |
| Compatible RBC types to receive | A, O | B, O | AB, A, B, O | O | Rh⊕, Rh⊖ | Rh⊖ |
| Compatible RBC types to donate to | A, AB | B, AB | AB | A, B, AB, O | Rh⊕ | Rh⊕, Rh⊖ |

| **Hemolytic disease of the fetus and newborn** | Also called erythroblastosis fetalis. Most commonly involves the antigens of the major blood groups (eg, Rh and ABO), but minor blood group incompatibilities (eg, Kell) can also result in disease, ranging from mild to severe. | |
|---|---|---|
| | **Rh hemolytic disease** | **ABO hemolytic disease** |
| INTERACTION | Rh ⊖ pregnant patient; Rh ⊕ fetus. | Type O pregnant patient; type A or B fetus. |
| MECHANISM | First pregnancy: patient exposed to fetal blood (often during delivery) → formation of maternal anti-D IgG. Subsequent pregnancies: anti-D IgG crosses placenta → attacks fetal and newborn RBCs → hemolysis. | Preexisting pregnant patient anti-A and/or anti-B IgG antibodies cross the placenta → attack fetal and newborn RBCs → hemolysis. |
| PRESENTATION | Hydrops fetalis, jaundice shortly after birth, kernicterus. | Mild jaundice in the neonate within 24 hours of birth. Unlike Rh hemolytic disease, can occur in firstborn babies and is usually less severe. |
| TREATMENT/PREVENTION | Prevent by administration of anti-D IgG to Rh ⊖ pregnant patients during third trimester and early postpartum period (if fetus Rh ⊕). Prevents maternal anti-D IgG production. | Treatment: phototherapy or exchange transfusion. |

### Hematopoiesis

## Neutrophils

Acute inflammatory response cells. Phagocytic. Multilobed nucleus **A**. Specific granules contain leukocyte alkaline phosphatase (LAP), collagenase, lysozyme, and lactoferrin. Azurophilic granules (lysosomes) contain proteinases, acid phosphatase, myeloperoxidase, and β-glucuronidase.

Inflammatory states (eg, bacterial infection) cause neutrophilia and changes in neutrophil morphology, such as left shift, toxic granulation (dark blue, coarse granules), Döhle bodies (light blue, peripheral inclusions, arrow in **B**), and cytoplasmic vacuoles.

Neutrophil chemotactic agents: C5a, IL-8, $LTB_4$, 5-HETE (leukotriene precursor), kallikrein, platelet-activating factor, N-formylmethionine (bacterial proteins).

Hypersegmented neutrophils (nucleus has 5–6+ lobes) are seen in vitamin $B_{12}$/folate deficiency.

Left shift—↑ neutrophil precursors (eg, band cells, metamyelocytes) in peripheral blood. Reflects states of ↑ myeloid proliferation (eg, inflammation, CML).

Leukoerythroblastic reaction—left shift accompanied by immature RBCs. Suggests bone marrow infiltration (eg, myelofibrosis, metastasis).

**Erythrocytes**

Carry $O_2$ to tissues and $CO_2$ to lungs. Anucleate and lack organelles; biconcave **A**, with large surface area-to-volume ratio for rapid gas exchange. Life span of ~120 days in healthy adults; 60–90 days in neonates. Source of energy is glucose (90% used in glycolysis, 10% used in HMP shunt). Membranes contain $Cl^-/HCO_3^-$ antiporter, which allow RBCs to export $HCO_3^-$ and transport $CO_2$ from the periphery to the lungs for elimination.

*Erythro* = red; *cyte* = cell.

Erythrocytosis = polycythemia = ↑ Hct.
Anisocytosis = varying sizes.
Poikilocytosis = varying shapes.

Reticulocyte = immature RBC; reflects erythroid proliferation.
Bluish color (polychromasia) on Wright-Giemsa stain of reticulocytes represents residual ribosomal RNA.

**Thrombocytes (platelets)**

Involved in 1° hemostasis. Anucleate, small cytoplasmic fragments **A** derived from megakaryocytes. Life span of 8–10 days (pl8lets). When activated by endothelial injury, aggregate with other platelets and interact with fibrinogen to form platelet plug. Contain dense granules ($Ca^{2+}$, **A**DP, **S**erotonin, **H**istamine; **CASH**) and α granules (vWF, fibrinogen, fibronectin, platelet factor 4). Approximately 1/3 of platelet pool is stored in the spleen.

Thrombocytopenia or ↓ platelet function results in petechiae.
vWF receptor: GpIb.
Fibrinogen receptor: GpIIb/IIIa.
Thrombopoietin stimulates megakaryocyte proliferation.
Alfa granules contain vWF, fibrinogen, fibronectin, platelet factor four.

**Monocytes**

Found in blood, differentiate into macrophages or dendritic cells. in tissues.
Large, kidney-shaped nucleus **A**. Extensive "frosted glass" cytoplasm.

*Mono* = one (nucleus); *cyte* = cell.

**Macrophages**

A type of antigen-presenting cell. Phagocytose bacteria, cellular debris, and senescent RBCs. Long life in tissues. Differentiate from circulating blood monocytes **A**. Activated by IFN-γ. Can function as antigen-presenting cell via MHC II. Also engage in antibody-dependent cellular cytotoxicity. Important cellular component of granulomas (eg, TB, sarcoidosis), where they may fuse to form giant cells.

*Macro* = large; *phage* = eater.
Macrophage naming varies by specific tissue type (eg, Kupffer cells in liver, histiocytes in connective tissue, osteoclasts in bone, microglial cells in brain).
Lipid A from bacterial LPS binds CD14 on macrophages to initiate septic shock.

**Dendritic cells**

Highly phagocytic antigen-presenting cells (APCs) . Function as link between innate and adaptive immune systems (eg, via T-cell stimulation). Express MHC class II and Fc receptors on surface. Can present exogenous antigens on MHC class I (cross-presentation).

**Eosinophils**

Defend against helminthic infections (major basic protein). Bilobate nucleus. Packed with large eosinophilic granules of uniform size . Highly phagocytic for antigen-antibody complexes.

Produce histaminase, major basic protein (MBP, a helminthotoxin), eosinophil peroxidase, eosinophil cationic protein, and eosinophil-derived neurotoxin.

*Eosin* = pink dye; *philic* = loving.
Causes of eosinophilia (**PACMAN** Eats):
  Parasites
  Asthma
  Chronic adrenal insufficiency
  Myeloproliferative disorders
  Allergic processes
  Neoplasia (eg, Hodgkin lymphoma)
  Eosinophilic granulomatosis with polyangiitis

**Basophils**

Mediate allergic reaction. Densely basophilic granules  contain heparin (anticoagulant) and histamine (vasodilator). Leukotrienes synthesized and released on demand.

**Basophilic**—stains readily with **basic** stains.
Basophilia is uncommon, but can be a sign of myeloproliferative disorders, particularly CML.

**Mast cells**

Mediate local tissue allergic reactions. Contain basophilic granules . Originate from same precursor as basophils but are not the same cell type. Can bind the Fc portion of IgE to membrane. Activated by tissue trauma, C3a and C5a, surface IgE cross-linking by antigen (IgE receptor aggregation) → degranulation → release of histamine, heparin, tryptase, and eosinophil chemotactic factors.

Involved in type I hypersensitivity reactions.
Cromolyn sodium prevents mast cell degranulation (used for asthma prophylaxis).
Vancomycin, opioids, and radiocontrast dye can elicit IgE-independent mast cell degranulation.
Mastocytosis—rare; proliferation of mast cells in skin and/or extracutaneous organs. Associated with c-*KIT* mutations and ↑ serum tryptase.
↑ histamine → flushing, pruritus, hypotension, abdominal pain, diarrhea, peptic ulcer disease.

**Lymphocytes**

Refer to B cells, T cells, and natural killer (NK) cells. B cells and T cells mediate adaptive immunity. NK cells are part of the innate immune response. Round, densely staining nucleus with small amount of pale cytoplasm .

**Natural killer cells**

Important in innate immunity, especially against intracellular pathogens. NK cells are larger than B and T cells, with distinctive cytoplasmic lytic granules (containing perforin and granzymes) that, when released, act on target cells to induce apoptosis. Distinguish between healthy and infected cells by identifying cell surface proteins (induced by stress, malignant transformation, or microbial infections). Induce apoptosis (natural killer) in cells that do not express class I MHC cell surface molecules, eg, virally infected cells in which these molecules are downregulated.

**B cells**

Mediate humoral immune response. Originate from stem cells in bone marrow and matures in marrow. Migrate to peripheral lymphoid tissue (follicles of lymph nodes, white pulp of spleen, unencapsulated lymphoid tissue). When antigen is encountered, B cells differentiate into plasma cells (which produce antibodies) and memory cells. Can function as an APC.

B = bone marrow.

**T cells**

Mediate cellular immune response. Originate from stem cells in the bone marrow, but mature in the thymus. Differentiate into cytotoxic T cells (express CD8, recognize MHC I), helper T cells (express CD4, recognize MHC II), and regulatory T cells. CD28 (costimulatory signal) necessary for T-cell activation. Most circulating lymphocytes are T cells (80%).

T = thymus.
CD4+ helper T cells are the primary target of HIV.

Rule of 8: MHC II × CD4 = 8; MHC I × CD8 = 8.

**Plasma cells**

Produce large amounts of antibody specific to a particular antigen. "Clock-face" chromatin distribution and eccentric nucleus, abundant RER, and well-developed Golgi apparatus (arrows in ). Found in bone marrow and normally do not circulate in peripheral blood.

Multiple myeloma is a plasma cell dyscrasia.

▶ HEMATOLOGY AND ONCOLOGY—PHYSIOLOGY

### Hemoglobin electrophoresis

AA → Normal adult
AF → Normal newborn
AS → Sickle cell trait
SS → Sickle cell disease
AC → Hb C trait
CC → Hb C disease
SC → Hb SC disease

C  S  F  A

⊖ Cathode          ⊕ Anode

A: normal hemoglobin β chain (HbA, adult)
F: normal hemoglobin γ chain (HbF, fetal)
S: sickle cell hemoglobin β chain (HbS)
C: hemoglobin C β chain (HbC)

During gel electrophoresis, hemoglobin migrates from the negatively charged cathode to the positively charged anode. HbA migrates the farthest, followed by HbF, HbS, and HbC. This is because the missense mutations in HbS and HbC replace glutamic acid ⊖ with valine (neutral) and lysine ⊕, respectively, making HbC and HbS more positively charged than HbA.

A Fat Santa Claus can't go far.
HbC is closest to the Cathode. HbA is closest to the Anode.

---

**Antiglobulin test**

Also called Coombs test. Detects the presence of antibodies against circulating RBCs.
Direct antiglobulin test—anti-human globulin (Coombs reagent) added to patient's RBCs. RBCs agglutinate if RBCs are (directly) coated with anti-RBC Abs. Used for AIHA diagnosis.
Indirect (not direct) antiglobulin test—normal RBCs added to patient's serum. If serum has anti-RBC Abs, RBCs agglutinate when Coombs reagent is added. Used for pretransfusion testing.

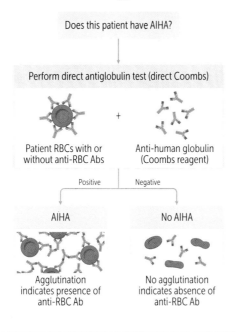

Does this patient have AIHA?

Perform direct antiglobulin test (direct Coombs)

Patient RBCs with or without anti-RBC Abs    +    Anti-human globulin (Coombs reagent)

Positive          Negative

AIHA                No AIHA

Agglutination indicates presence of anti-RBC Ab    No agglutination indicates absence of anti-RBC Ab

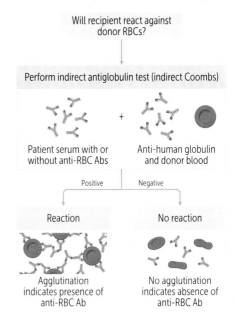

Will recipient react against donor RBCs?

Perform indirect antiglobulin test (indirect Coombs)

Patient serum with or without anti-RBC Abs    +    Anti-human globulin and donor blood

Positive          Negative

Reaction            No reaction

Agglutination indicates presence of anti-RBC Ab    No agglutination indicates absence of anti-RBC Ab

## Platelet plug formation (primary hemostasis)

**❶ INJURY**
Endothelial damage → transient vasoconstriction via neural stimulation reflex and endothelin (released from damaged cell)

**❷ EXPOSURE**
vWF binds to exposed collagen (vWF is from Weibel-Palade bodies of endothelial cells and α-granules of platelets)

**❸ ADHESION**
Platelets bind vWF via Gplb receptor at the site of injury only (specific) → platelets undergo conformational change

Platelets release ADP and $Ca^{2+}$ (necessary for coagulation cascade), $TXA_2$

ADP helps platelets adhere to endothelium

**❹ ACTIVATION**
ADP binding to $P2Y_{12}$ receptor induces GpIIb/IIIa expression at platelet surface → rapid irreversible platelet aggregation

**❺ AGGREGATION**
Fibrinogen binds GpIIb/IIIa receptors and links platelets

Balance between

| Pro-aggregation factors: | Anti-aggregation factors: |
|---|---|
| $TXA_2$ (released by platelets) | $PGI_2$ and NO (released by endothelial cells) |
| ↓ blood flow | ↑ blood flow |
| ↑ platelet aggregation | ↓ platelet aggregation |

Temporary plug stops bleeding; unstable, easily dislodged

Coagulation cascade (secondary hemostasis)

## Thrombogenesis

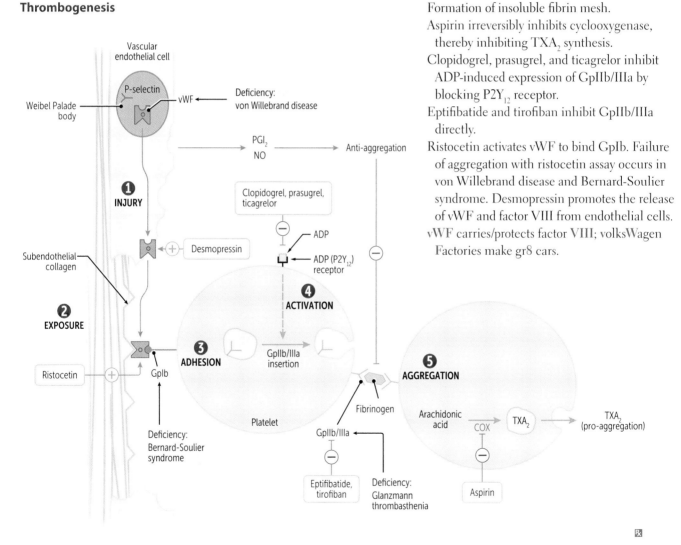

Formation of insoluble fibrin mesh.

Aspirin irreversibly inhibits cyclooxygenase, thereby inhibiting $TXA_2$ synthesis.

Clopidogrel, prasugrel, and ticagrelor inhibit ADP-induced expression of GpIIb/IIIa by blocking $P2Y_{12}$ receptor.

Eptifibatide and tirofiban inhibit GpIIb/IIIa directly.

Ristocetin activates vWF to bind GpIb. Failure of aggregation with ristocetin assay occurs in von Willebrand disease and Bernard-Soulier syndrome. Desmopressin promotes the release of vWF and factor VIII from endothelial cells.

vWF carries/protects factor VIII; volksWagen Factories make gr8 cars.

**Coagulation and kinin pathways**

PT monitors extrinsic and common pathway, reflecting activity of factors I, II, V, VII, and X.
PTT monitors intrinsic and common pathway, reflecting activity of all factors except VII and XIII.

Hemophilia A: deficiency of factor VIII (XR)
Hemophilia B: deficiency of factor IX (XR)
Hemophilia C: deficiency of factor XI (AR)

Note: Kallikrein activates bradykinin
　　　ACE inactivates bradykinin

\# = C1-esterase inhibitor deficiency ⟶ hereditary angioedema
* = require $Ca^{2+}$, phospholipid;
▨ = vitamin K-dependent factors
▨ = cofactor
----- = activates but not part of coagulation cascade
───── = activated by thrombin
LMWH = low-molecular-weight heparin
HMWK = high-molecular-weight kininogen

## Vitamin K–dependent coagulation

### Procoagulation

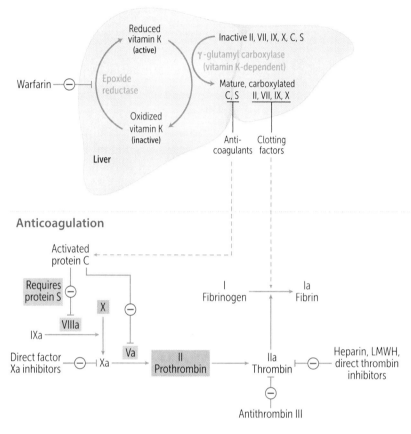

Vitamin K deficiency—↓ synthesis of factors II, VII, IX, X, protein C, protein S.

Warfarin inhibits vitamin K epoxide reductase. Vitamin K administration can potentially reverse inhibitory effect of warfarin on clotting factor synthesis (delayed). FFP or PCC administration reverses action of warfarin immediately and can be given with vitamin K in cases of severe bleeding.

Neonates lack enteric baKteria, which produce vitamin K. Early administration of vitamin K overcomes neonatal deficiency/coagulopathy. Suppression of gut flora by broad spectrum antibiotiKs can also contribute to deficiency.

Factor VII (seven)—shortest half-life.

Factor II (two)—longest (too long) half-life.

Antithrombin inhibits thrombin (factor IIa) and factors VIIa, IXa, Xa, XIa, XIIa.

Heparin enhances the activity of antithrombin.

Principal targets of antithrombin: thrombin and factor Xa.

Factor V Leiden mutation produces a factor V resistant to inhibition by activated protein C.

tPA is used clinically as a thrombolytic.

= vitamin K-dependent factors     − − − = activates but not part of coagulation cascade

= cofactor     LMWH = low-molecular-weight heparin

▶ **HEMATOLOGY AND ONCOLOGY—PATHOLOGY**

### RBC morphology

| TYPE | ASSOCIATED PATHOLOGY | NOTES |
|---|---|---|
| Acanthocytes A ("spur cells") | Liver disease, abetalipoproteinemia, vitamin E deficiency | Projections of varying size at irregular intervals (acanthocytes are asymmetric) |
| Echinocytes B ("burr cells") | Liver disease, ESRD, pyruvate kinase deficiency | Smaller and more uniform projections than acanthocytes (echinocytes are even) |
| Dacrocytes C ("teardrop cells") | Bone marrow infiltration (eg, myelofibrosis) | RBC "sheds a **tear**" because it's mechanically squeezed out of its home in the bone marrow |
| Schistocytes D ("helmet" cells) | Microangiopathic hemolytic anemia (eg, DIC, TTP/HUS, HELLP syndrome), mechanical hemolysis (eg, heart valve prosthesis) | Fragmented RBCs |
| Degmacytes E ("bite cells") | G6PD deficiency | Due to removal of Heinz bodies by splenic macrophages (they "**deg**" them out of/**bite** them off of RBCs) |
| Elliptocytes F | Hereditary elliptocytosis | Caused by mutation in genes encoding RBC membrane proteins (eg, spectrin) |
| Spherocytes G | Hereditary spherocytosis, autoimmune hemolytic anemia | Small, spherical cells without central pallor ↓ surface area-to-volume ratio |
| Macro-ovalocytes H | Megaloblastic anemia (also hypersegmented PMNs) | |
| Target cells I | HbC disease, Asplenia, Liver disease, Thalassemia | "**HALT**," said the hunter to his **target** ↑ surface area-to-volume ratio |
| Sickle cells J | Sickle cell anemia | Sickling occurs with low $O_2$ conditions (eg, high altitude, acidosis), high HbS concentration (ie, dehydration) |

## RBC inclusions

| TYPE | ASSOCIATED PATHOLOGY | NOTES |
|------|---------------------|-------|
| **Bone marrow** | | |
| Iron granules A | Sideroblastic anemias (eg, lead poisoning, myelodysplastic syndromes, chronic alcohol overuse) | Perinuclear mitochondria with excess iron (forming ring in ringed sideroblasts)<br>Require Prussian blue stain to be visualized |
| **Peripheral smear** | | |
| Howell-Jolly bodies B | Functional hyposplenia (eg, sickle cell disease), asplenia | Basophilic nuclear remnants (do not contain iron)<br>Usually removed by splenic macrophages |
| Basophilic stippling C | Sideroblastic anemia, thalassemias | Basophilic ribosomal precipitates (do not contain iron) |
| Pappenheimer bodies | Sideroblastic anemia | Basophilic granules (contain iron)<br>"Pappen-hammer" bodies |
| Heinz bodies D | G6PD deficiency | Denatured and precipitated hemoglobin (contain iron)<br>Phagocytic removal of Heinz bodies → bite cells<br>Requires supravital stain (eg, crystal violet) to be visualized |

## Anemias

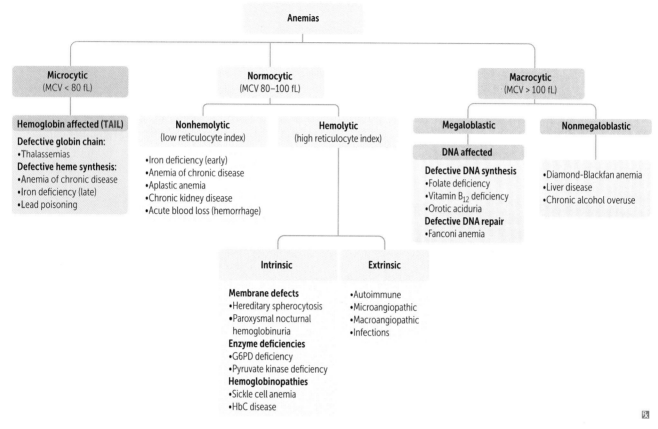

| **Reticulocyte production index** | Also called corrected reticulocyte count. Used to correct falsely elevated reticulocyte count in anemia. Measures appropriate bone marrow response to anemic conditions (effective erythropoiesis). High RPI (> 3) indicates compensatory RBC production; low RPI (< 2) indicates inadequate response to correct anemia. Calculated as: |
|---|---|

$$RPI = \%\ \text{reticulocytes} \times \left( \frac{\text{actual Hct}}{\text{normal Hct}} \right) / \text{maturation time}$$

| **Mentzer index** | Used to differentiate between thalassemia and iron deficiency. An index of < 13 suggests thalassemia. An index of > 13 suggests iron deficiency anemia. |
|---|---|

$$\frac{\text{MCV}}{\text{RBC count}}$$

### Interpretation of iron studies

| | Iron deficiency | Chronic disease | Hemochromatosis | Pregnancy/ OCP use |
|---|---|---|---|---|
| Serum iron | ↓ | ↓ | ↑ | — |
| Transferrin or TIBC | ↑ | ↓[a] | ↓ | ↑ |
| Ferritin | ↓ | ↑ | ↑ | — |
| % transferrin saturation (serum iron/TIBC) | ↓↓ | —/↓ | ↑↑ | ↓ |

↑↓ = 1° disturbance.

Transferrin—**transports** iron in blood.

TIBC—indirectly measures transferrin.

Ferritin—1° iron storage protein of body.

[a]Evolutionary reasoning—pathogens use circulating iron to thrive. The body has adapted a system in which iron is stored within the cells of the body and prevents pathogens from acquiring circulating iron.

| Microcytic, hypochromic anemias | $MCV < 80$ fL. |
|---|---|
| **Iron deficiency** | ↓ iron due to chronic bleeding (eg, GI loss, heavy menstrual bleeding), malnutrition, absorption disorders, GI surgery (eg, gastrectomy), or ↑ demand (eg, pregnancy) → ↓ final step in heme synthesis.<br>Labs: ↓ iron, ↑ TIBC, ↓ ferritin, ↑ free erythrocyte protoporphyrin, ↑ RDW, ↓ RI. Microcytosis and hypochromasia (↑ central pallor) **A**.<br>Symptoms: fatigue, conjunctival pallor **B**, restless leg syndrome, pica (persistent craving and compulsive eating of nonfood substances), spoon nails (koilonychia).<br>May manifest as glossitis, cheilosis, Plummer-Vinson syndrome (triad of iron deficiency anemia, esophageal webs, and dysphagia). |
| **α-thalassemia** | α-globin gene deletions on chromosome 16 → ↓ α-globin synthesis. May have *cis* deletion (deletions occur on same chromosome) or *trans* deletion (deletions occur on separate chromosomes). Normal is αα/αα. Often ↑ RBC count, in contrast to iron deficiency anemia. ↑ prevalence in people of Asian and African descent. Target cells **C** on peripheral smear. |

| # OF α-GLOBIN GENES DELETED<sup>a</sup> | DISEASE | CLINICAL OUTCOME |
|---|---|---|
| 1 | α-thalassemia minima | No anemia (silent carrier) |
| 2 (Cis or Trans) | α-thalassemia minor | Mild microcytic, hypochromic anemia |
| 3 | Hemoglobin H disease (HbH); excess β-globin forms $β_4$ | Moderate to severe microcytic hypochromic anemia |
| 4 | Hemoglobin Barts disease; no α-globin, excess γ-globin forms $γ_4$ | Hydrops fetalis; incompatible with life |

## Microcytic, hypochromic anemias *(continued)*

**β-thalassemia**

Point mutation in splice sites or Kozak consensus sequence (promoter) on chromosome 11 → ↓ β-globin synthesis ($\beta^+$) or absent β-globin synthesis ($\beta^0$). ↑ prevalence in people of Mediterranean descent.

| # OF β-GLOBIN GENES MUTATED[+] | DISEASE | CLINICAL OUTCOME |
|---|---|---|
| 1 <br> β — β | β-thalassemia minor | Mild microcytic anemia. ↑ $HbA_2$. |
| 2 ($\beta^+/\beta^+$ or $\beta^+/\beta^0$) | β-thalassemia intermedia | Variable anemia, ranging from mild/asymptomatic to severe/transfusion-dependent. |
| 2 <br> β — β | β-thalassemia major (Cooley anemia) | Severe microcytic anemia with target cells and ↑ anisopoikilocytosis requiring blood transfusions (↑ risk of 2° hemochromatosis), marrow expansion ("crew cut" on skull x-ray) → skeletal deformities, extramedullary hematopoiesis → HSM. ↑ risk of parvovirus B19-induced aplastic crisis. ↑ HbF and $HbA_2$, becomes symptomatic after 6 months when HbF declines (HbF is protective). Chronic hemolysis → pigmented gallstones. |
| 1 ($\beta^+$/HbS or $\beta^0$/HbS) | Sickle cell β-thalassemia | Mild to moderate sickle cell disease depending on whether there is ↓ ($\beta^+$/HbS) or absent ($\beta^0$/HbS) β-globin synthesis. |

**Lead poisoning**

Lead inhibits ferrochelatase and ALA dehydratase → ↓ heme synthesis and ↑ RBC protoporphyrin. Also inhibits rRNA degradation → RBCs retain aggregates of rRNA (basophilic stippling).
Symptoms of LLEEAAD poisoning:
- **L**ead **L**ines on gingivae (Burton lines) and on metaphyses of long bones **D** on x-ray.
- **E**ncephalopathy and **E**rythrocyte basophilic stippling.
- **A**bdominal colic and sideroblastic **A**nemia.
- **D**rops—wrist and foot drop.
Treatment: chelation with succimer, EDTA, dimercaprol.
Exposure risk ↑ in old houses (built before 1978) with chipped paint (children) and workplace (adults).

**Sideroblastic anemia**

Causes: genetic (eg, X-linked defect in ALA synthase gene), acquired (myelodysplastic syndromes), and reversible (alcohol is most common; also lead poisoning, vitamin $B_6$ deficiency, copper deficiency, drugs [eg, isoniazid, linezolid]).
Lab findings: ↑ iron, normal/↓ TIBC, ↑ ferritin. Ringed sideroblasts (with iron-laden, Prussian blue–stained mitochondria) seen in bone marrow. Peripheral blood smear: basophilic stippling of RBCs. Some acquired variants may be normocytic or macrocytic.
Treatment: pyridoxine ($B_6$, cofactor for ALA synthase).

**Macrocytic anemias**   MCV > 100 fL.

| | DESCRIPTION | FINDINGS |
|---|---|---|
| **Megaloblastic anemia** | Impaired DNA synthesis → maturation of nucleus of precursor cells in bone marrow delayed relative to maturation of cytoplasm. Causes: vitamin $B_{12}$ deficiency, folate deficiency, medications (eg, hydroxyurea, phenytoin, methotrexate, sulfa drugs). | RBC macrocytosis, hypersegmented neutrophils (arrow in A), glossitis. |
| Folate deficiency | Causes: malnutrition (eg, chronic alcohol overuse), malabsorption, drugs (eg, methotrexate, trimethoprim, phenytoin), ↑ requirement (eg, hemolytic anemia, pregnancy). | ↑ homocysteine, normal methylmalonic acid. **No neurologic symptoms** (vs $B_{12}$ deficiency). |
| Vitamin $B_{12}$ (cobalamin) deficiency | Causes: pernicious anemia, malabsorption (eg, Crohn disease), pancreatic insufficiency, gastrectomy, insufficient intake (eg, veganism), *Diphyllobothrium latum* (fish tapeworm). | ↑ homocysteine, ↑ methylmalonic acid. **Neurologic symptoms:** reversible dementia, subacute combined degeneration (due to involvement of $B_{12}$ in fatty acid pathways and myelin synthesis): spinocerebellar tract, lateral corticospinal tract, dorsal column dysfunction. Folate supplementation in vitamin $B_{12}$ deficiency can correct the anemia, but worsens neurologic symptoms. Historically diagnosed with the Schilling test, a test that determines if the cause is dietary insufficiency vs malabsorption. Anemia 2° to insufficient intake may take several years to develop due to liver's ability to store $B_{12}$ (vs folate deficiency, which takes weeks to months). |
| Orotic aciduria | Inability to convert orotic acid to UMP (de novo pyrimidine synthesis pathway) because of defect in UMP synthase. Autosomal recessive. Presents in children as failure to thrive, developmental delay, and megaloblastic anemia refractory to folate and $B_{12}$. No hyperammonemia (vs ornithine transcarbamylase deficiency—↑ orotic acid with hyperammonemia). | Orotic acid in urine. Treatment: uridine monophosphate or uridine triacetate to bypass mutated enzyme. |
| **Nonmegaloblastic anemia** | Macrocytic anemia in which DNA synthesis is normal. Causes: chronic alcohol overuse, liver disease. | RBC macrocytosis without hypersegmented neutrophils. |
| Diamond-Blackfan anemia | A congenital form of pure red cell aplasia (vs Fanconi anemia, which causes pancytopenia). Rapid-onset anemia within 1st year of life due to intrinsic defect in erythroid progenitor cells. | ↑ % HbF (but ↓ total Hb). Short stature, craniofacial abnormalities, and upper extremity malformations (triphalangeal thumbs) in up to 50% of cases. |

| | |
|---|---|
| **Normocytic, normochromic anemias** | Normocytic, normochromic anemias are classified as nonhemolytic or hemolytic. The hemolytic anemias are further classified according to the cause of the hemolysis (intrinsic vs extrinsic to the RBC) and by the location of hemolysis (intravascular vs extravascular). Hemolysis can lead to ↑ in LDH, reticulocytes, unconjugated bilirubin, pigmented gallstones, and urobilinogen in urine. |

Extravascular Hemolysis — Intravascular Hemolysis

| | |
|---|---|
| **Intravascular hemolysis** | Findings: ↓ haptoglobin, ↑ schistocytes on blood smear. Characteristic hemoglobinuria, hemosiderinuria, and urobilinogen in urine. Notable causes are mechanical hemolysis (eg, prosthetic valve), paroxysmal nocturnal hemoglobinuria, microangiopathic hemolytic anemias. |
| **Extravascular hemolysis** | Mechanism: macrophages in spleen clear RBCs. Findings: splenomegaly, spherocytes in peripheral smear (most commonly due to hereditary spherocytosis and autoimmune hemolytic anemia), no hemoglobinuria/hemosiderinuria. Can present with urobilinogen in urine. |

## Nonhemolytic, normocytic anemias

| | DESCRIPTION | FINDINGS |
|---|---|---|
| **Anemia of chronic disease** | Inflammation (eg, ↑ IL-6) → ↑ hepcidin (released by liver, binds ferroportin on intestinal mucosal cells and macrophages, thus inhibiting iron transport) → ↓ release of iron from macrophages and ↓ iron absorption from gut. Associated with conditions such as chronic infections, neoplastic disorders, chronic kidney disease, and autoimmune diseases (eg, SLE, rheumatoid arthritis). | ↓ iron, ↓ TIBC, ↑ ferritin. Normocytic, but can become microcytic. Treatment: address underlying cause of inflammation, judicious use of blood transfusion, consider erythropoiesis-stimulating agents such as EPO (eg, in chronic kidney disease). |
| **Aplastic anemia**  | Failure or destruction of hematopoietic stem cells. Causes (reducing volume from inside diaphysis): <br> ▪ Radiation <br> ▪ Viral agents (eg, EBV, HIV, hepatitis viruses) <br> ▪ Fanconi anemia (autosomal recessive DNA repair defect → bone marrow failure); normocytosis or macrocytosis on CBC. Common associated findings include short stature, café-au-lait spots, thumb/radial defects, predisposition to malignancy. <br> ▪ Idiopathic (immune mediated, 1° stem cell defect); may follow acute hepatitis <br> ▪ Drugs (eg, benzene, chloramphenicol, alkylating agents, antimetabolites) | ↓ reticulocyte count, ↑ EPO. Pancytopenia characterized by anemia, leukopenia, and thrombocytopenia (vs aplastic crisis, which causes anemia only). Normal cell morphology, but hypocellular bone marrow with fatty infiltration A. Symptoms: fatigue, malaise, pallor, purpura, mucosal bleeding, petechiae, infection. Treatment: withdrawal of offending agent, immunosuppressive regimens (eg, antithymocyte globulin, cyclosporine), bone marrow allograft, RBC/platelet transfusion, bone marrow stimulation (eg, GM-CSF). |

## Intrinsic hemolytic anemias

| | DESCRIPTION | FINDINGS |
|---|---|---|
| **Hereditary spherocytosis** | Primarily autosomal dominant. Due to defect in proteins interacting with RBC membrane skeleton and plasma membrane (eg, ankyrin, band 3, protein 4.2, spectrin).<br>Small, round RBCs with no central pallor. ↓ surface area/dehydration → ↑ MCHC → premature removal by spleen (extravascular hemolysis). | Splenomegaly, pigmented gallstones, aplastic crisis (parvovirus B19 infection).<br>Labs: ↓ mean fluorescence of RBCs in eosin 5-maleimide (EMA) binding test, ↑ fragility in osmotic fragility test (RBC hemolysis with exposure to hypotonic solution). Normal to ↓ MCV with abundance of RBCs.<br>Treatment: splenectomy. |
| **Paroxysmal nocturnal hemoglobinuria** | Hematopoietic stem cell mutation → ↑ complement-mediated intravascular hemolysis, especially at night. Acquired *PIGA* mutation → impaired GPI anchor synthesis for decay-accelerating factor (DAF/CD55) and membrane inhibitor of reactive lysis (MIRL/CD59), which protect RBC membrane from complement. | Triad: Coombs ⊖ hemolytic anemia (mainly intravascular), pancytopenia, venous thrombosis (eg, Budd-Chiari syndrome).<br>Pink/red urine in morning. Associated with aplastic anemia, acute leukemias.<br>Labs: CD55/59 ⊖ RBCs on flow cytometry.<br>Treatment: eculizumab (targets terminal complement protein C5). |
| **G6PD deficiency** | X-linked recessive. G6PD defect → ↓ NADPH → ↓ reduced glutathione → ↑ RBC susceptibility to oxidative stress (eg, sulfa drugs, antimalarials, **fava beans**) → hemolysis.<br>Causes extravascular and intravascular hemolysis. | Back pain, hemoglobinuria a few days after oxidant **stress**.<br>Labs: ↓ G6PD activity (may be falsely normal during acute hemolysis), blood smear shows RBCs with **Heinz** bodies and **bite** cells.<br>"**Stress** makes me eat **bites** of **fava beans** with **Heinz** ketchup." |
| **Pyruvate kinase deficiency** | Autosomal recessive. Pyruvate kinase defect → ↓ ATP → rigid RBCs → extravascular hemolysis. Increases levels of 2,3-BPG → ↓ hemoglobin affinity for $O_2$. | Hemolytic anemia in a newborn.<br>Labs: blood smear shows burr cells. |
| **Sickle cell anemia**<br> | Point mutation in β-globin gene → single amino acid substitution (glutamic acid → valine) alters hydrophobic region on β-globin chain → aggregation of hemoglobin. Causes extravascular and intravascular hemolysis.<br>Pathogenesis: low $O_2$, high altitude, or acidosis precipitates sickling (deoxygenated HbS polymerizes) → vaso-occlusive disease.<br>Newborns are initially asymptomatic because of ↑ HbF and ↓ HbS.<br>Heterozygotes (sickle cell trait) have resistance to malaria.<br>Sickle cells are crescent-shaped RBCs Ⓐ.<br>"Crew cut" on skull x-ray due to marrow expansion from ↑ erythropoiesis (also seen in thalassemias). | Complications:<br>▪ Aplastic crisis (transient arrest of erythropoiesis due to parvovirus B19).<br>▪ Autosplenectomy (Howell-Jolly bodies) → ↑ risk of infection by encapsulated organisms (eg, *Salmonella* osteomyelitis).<br>▪ Splenic infarct/sequestration crisis.<br>▪ Painful vaso-occlusive crises: dactylitis (painful swelling of hands/feet), priapism, acute chest syndrome (respiratory distress, new pulmonary infiltrates on CXR, common cause of death), avascular necrosis, stroke.<br>▪ Sickling in renal medulla (↓ $P_{O_2}$) → renal papillary necrosis → hematuria (also seen in sickle cell trait).<br>Hb electrophoresis: ↓↓ HbA, ↑ HbF, ↑↑ HbS.<br>Treatment: hydroxyurea (↑ HbF), hydration. |
| **HbC disease** | Glutamic acid–to-lycine (lysine) mutation in β-globin. Causes extravascular hemolysis. | HbSC (1 of each mutant gene) milder than HbSS.<br>Blood smear in homozygotes: hemoglobin crystals inside RBCs, target cells. |

## Extrinsic hemolytic anemias

| | DESCRIPTION | FINDINGS |
|---|---|---|
| **Autoimmune hemolytic anemia** | A normocytic anemia that is usually idiopathic and Coombs ⊕. Two types:<br>▪ **Warm** AIHA–chronic anemia in which primarily IgG causes extravascular hemolysis. Seen in SLE and CLL and with certain drugs (eg, β-lactams, α-methyldopa). "**Warm** weather is **G**ood."<br>▪ Cold AIHA–acute anemia in which primarily IgM + complement cause RBC agglutination and extravascular hemolysis upon exposure to cold → painful, blue fingers and toes. Seen in CLL, *Mycoplasma pneumoniae* infections, infectious mononucleosis. | Spherocytes and agglutinated RBCs [A] on peripheral blood smear.<br>Warm AIHA treatment: steroids, rituximab, splenectomy (if refractory).<br>Cold AIHA treatment: cold avoidance, rituximab. |
| **Drug-induced hemolytic anemia** | Most commonly due to antibody-mediated immune destruction of RBCs or oxidant injury via free radical damage (may be exacerbated in G6PD deficiency).<br>Common causes include antibiotics (eg, penicillins, cephalosporins), NSAIDs, immunotherapy, chemotherapy. | Spherocytes suggest immune hemolysis.<br>Bite cells suggest oxidative hemolysis.<br>Can cause both extravascular and intravascular hemolysis. |
| **Microangiopathic hemolytic anemia** | RBCs are damaged when passing through obstructed or narrowed vessels. Causes intravascular hemolysis.<br>Seen in DIC, TTP/HUS, SLE, HELLP syndrome, hypertensive emergency. | Schistocytes (eg, "helmet cells") are seen on peripheral blood smear due to mechanical destruction (*schisto* = to split) of RBCs. |
| **Macroangiopathic hemolytic anemia** | Prosthetic heart valves and aortic stenosis may also cause hemolytic anemia 2° to mechanical destruction of RBCs. | Schistocytes on peripheral blood smear. |
| **Hemolytic anemia due to infection** | ↑ destruction of RBCs (eg, malaria, *Babesia*). | |

## Leukopenias

| CELL TYPE | CELL COUNT | CAUSES |
|---|---|---|
| **Neutropenia** | Absolute neutrophil count < 1500 cells/mm³<br>Severe infections typical when < 500 cells/mm³ | Sepsis/postinfection, drugs (including chemotherapy), aplastic anemia, autoimmunity (eg, SLE), radiation, congenital |
| **Lymphopenia** | Absolute lymphocyte count < 1500 cells/mm³<br>(< 3000 cells/mm³ in children) | HIV, DiGeorge syndrome, SCID, SLE, glucocorticoids[a], radiation, sepsis, postoperative |
| **Eosinopenia** | Absolute eosinophil count < 30 cells/mm³ | Cushing syndrome, glucocorticoids[a] |

[a]Glucocorticoids cause neutrophilia, despite causing eosinopenia and lymphopenia. Glucocorticoids ↓ activation of neutrophil adhesion molecules, impairing migration out of the vasculature to sites of inflammation. In contrast, glucocorticoids sequester eosinophils in lymph nodes and cause apoptosis of lymphocytes.

## Heme synthesis, porphyrias, and lead poisoning

The porphyrias are hereditary or acquired conditions of defective heme synthesis that lead to the accumulation of heme precursors. Lead inhibits specific enzymes needed in heme synthesis, leading to a similar condition.

| CONDITION | AFFECTED ENZYME | ACCUMULATED SUBSTRATE | PRESENTING SYMPTOMS |
|---|---|---|---|
| **Lead poisoning**  | Ferrochelatase and ALA dehydratase | Protoporphyrin, ALA (blood) | Microcytic anemia (basophilic stippling in peripheral smear **A**, ringed sideroblasts in bone marrow), GI and kidney disease. Children—exposure to lead paint → mental deterioration. Adults—environmental exposure (eg, batteries, ammunition) → headache, memory loss, demyelination (peripheral neuropathy). |
| **Acute intermittent porphyria** | Porphobilinogen deaminase (autosomal dominant mutation) | Porphobilinogen, ALA | Symptoms (5 P's): <br>▪ Painful abdomen <br>▪ Port wine–colored Pee <br>▪ Polyneuropathy <br>▪ Psychological disturbances <br>▪ Precipitated by factors that ↑ ALA synthase (eg, drugs [CYP450 inducers], alcohol, starvation) <br>Treatment: hemin and glucose. |
| **Porphyria cutanea tarda** | Uroporphyrinogen decarboxylase | Uroporphyrin (tea-colored urine) | Blistering cutaneous photosensitivity and hyperpigmentation **B**. Most common porphyria. Exacerbated with alcohol consumption. Causes: familial, hepatitis C. Treatment: phlebotomy, sun avoidance, antimalarials (eg, hydroxychloroquine). |

## Iron poisoning

|  | Acute | Chronic |
|---|---|---|
| FINDINGS | High mortality rate associated with accidental ingestion by children (adult iron tablets may look like candy). | Seen in patients with 1° (hereditary) or 2° (eg, chronic blood transfusions for thalassemia or sickle cell disease) hemochromatosis. |
| MECHANISM | Cell death due to formation of free radicals and peroxidation of membrane lipids. | |
| SYMPTOMS/SIGNS | Abdominal pain, vomiting, GI bleeding. Radiopaque pill seen on x-ray. May progress to anion gap metabolic acidosis and multiorgan failure. Leads to scarring with GI obstruction. | Arthropathy, cirrhosis, cardiomyopathy, diabetes mellitus and skin pigmentation ("bronze diabetes"), hypogonadism. |
| TREATMENT | Chelation (eg, deferoxamine, deferasirox), gastric lavage. | Phlebotomy (patients without anemia) or chelation. |

## Coagulation disorders

PT—tests function of common and extrinsic pathway (factors I, II, V, VII, and X). Defect → ↑ PT (Play Tennis outside [extrinsic pathway]).

INR (international normalized ratio) = patient PT/control PT. 1 = normal, > 1 = prolonged. Most common test used to follow patients on warfarin, which prolongs INR.

PTT—tests function of common and intrinsic pathway (all factors except VII and XIII). Defect → ↑ PTT (Play Table Tennis inside).

TT—measures the rate of conversion of fibrinogen → fibrin. Prolonged by anticoagulants, hypofibrinogenemia, DIC, liver disease.

Coagulation disorders can be due to clotting factor deficiencies or acquired factor inhibitors (most commonly against factor VIII). Diagnosed with a mixing study, in which normal plasma is added to patient's plasma. Clotting factor deficiencies should correct (the PT or PTT returns to within the appropriate normal range), whereas factor inhibitors will not correct.

| DISORDER | PT | PTT | MECHANISM AND COMMENTS |
|---|---|---|---|
| **Hemophilia A, B, or C** | — | ↑ | Intrinsic pathway coagulation defect (↑ PTT). <ul><li>A: deficiency of factor VIII; X-linked recessive. Pronounce "hemophilia Ate (eight)."</li><li>B: deficiency of factor IX; X-linked recessive.</li><li>C: deficiency of factor XI; autosomal recessive.</li></ul> Hemorrhage in hemophilia—hemarthroses (bleeding into joints, eg, knee A), easy bruising, bleeding after trauma or surgery (eg, dental procedures). Treatment: desmopressin, factor VIII concentrate, emicizumab (A); factor IX concentrate (B); factor XI concentrate (C). |
| **Vitamin K deficiency** | ↑ | ↑ | General coagulation defect. Bleeding time normal. ↓ activity of factors II, VII, IX, X, protein C, protein S. |

**Platelet disorders**    All platelet disorders have ↑ bleeding time (BT), mucous membrane bleeding, and microhemorrhages (eg, petechiae, epistaxis). Platelet count (PC) is usually low, but may be normal in qualitative disorders.

| DISORDER | PC | BT | NOTES |
|---|---|---|---|
| Bernard-Soulier syndrome | –/↓ | ↑ | Autosomal recessive defect in adhesion. ↓ GpIb → ↓ platelet-to-vWF adhesion. Labs: ↓ platelet aggregation, Big platelets. |
| Glanzmann thrombasthenia | – | ↑ | Autosomal recessive defect in aggregation. ↓ GpIIb/IIIa (↓ integrin $\alpha_{IIb}\beta_3$) → ↓ platelet-to-platelet aggregation and defective platelet plug formation. Labs: blood smear shows no platelet clumping. |
| Immune thrombocytopenia | ↓ | ↑ | Destruction of platelets in spleen. Anti-GpIIb/IIIa antibodies → splenic macrophages phagocytose platelets. May be idiopathic or 2° to autoimmune disorders (eg, SLE), viral illness (eg, HIV, HCV), malignancy (eg, CLL), or drug reactions. Labs: ↑ megakaryocytes on bone marrow biopsy, ↓ platelet count. Treatment: glucocorticoids, IVIG, rituximab, TPO receptor agonists (eg, eltrombopag, romiplostim), or splenectomy for refractory ITP. |
| Uremic platelet dysfunction | – | ↑ | In patients with renal failure, uremic toxins accumulate and interfere with platelet adhesion. |

**Thrombotic microangiopathies**    Disorders overlap significantly in symptomatology. May resemble DIC, but do not exhibit lab findings of a consumptive coagulopathy (eg, ↑ PT, ↑ PTT, ↓ fibrinogen), as etiology does not involve widespread clotting factor activation.

| | Thrombotic thrombocytopenic purpura | Hemolytic-uremic syndrome |
|---|---|---|
| EPIDEMIOLOGY | Typically females | Typically children |
| PATHOPHYSIOLOGY | Inhibition or deficiency of ADAMTS13 (a vWF metalloprotease) → ↓ degradation of vWF multimers → ↑ large vWF multimers → ↑ platelet adhesion and aggregation (microthrombi formation) | Predominately caused by Shiga toxin–producing *Escherichia coli* (STEC) infection (serotype O157:H7), which causes profound endothelial dysfunction. |
| PRESENTATION | Triad of thrombocytopenia (↓ platelets), microangiopathic hemolytic anemia (↓ Hb, schistocytes, ↑ LDH), acute kidney injury (↑ Cr) | |
| DIFFERENTIATING SYMPTOMS | Triad + fever + neurologic symptoms | Triad + bloody diarrhea |
| LABS | Normal PT and PTT helps distinguish TTP and HUS (coagulation pathway is not activated) from DIC (coagulation pathway is activated) | |
| TREATMENT | Plasma exchange, glucocorticoids, rituximab | Supportive care |

## Mixed platelet and coagulation disorders

| DISORDER | PC | BT | PT | PTT | NOTES |
|---|---|---|---|---|---|
| von Willebrand disease | — | ↑ | — | —/↑ | Intrinsic pathway coagulation defect: ↓ quantity/function of vWF → ↑ PTT (vWF carries/protects factor VIII). Defect in platelet plug formation: ↓ vWF → defect in platelet-to-vWF adhesion. Most are autosomal dominant. Mild but most common inherited bleeding disorder. Commonly presents with menorrhagia or epistaxis. Treatment: vWF concentrates, desmopressin (releases vWF stored in endothelium). |
| Disseminated intravascular coagulation | ↓ | ↑ | ↑ | ↑ | Widespread clotting factor activation → thromboembolic state with excessive clotting factor consumption → ↑ thromboses, ↑ hemorrhages (eg, blood oozing from puncture sites). May be acute (life-threatening) or chronic (if clotting factor production can compensate for consumption). Causes: heat Stroke, Snake bites, Sepsis (gram ⊖), Trauma, Obstetric complications, acute Pancreatitis, malignancy, nephrotic syndrome, transfusion (SSSTOP making new thrombi). Labs: schistocytes, ↑ fibrin degradation products (D-dimers), ↓ fibrinogen, ↓ factors V and VIII. |

| **Hereditary thrombophilias** | Autosomal dominant disorders resulting in hypercoagulable state (↑ tendency to develop thrombosis). |
|---|---|
| DISEASE | DESCRIPTION |
| Antithrombin deficiency | Has no direct effect on the PT, PTT, or thrombin time but diminishes the increase in PTT following standard heparin dosing. Can also be acquired: renal failure/nephrotic syndrome → antithrombin loss in urine → ↓ inhibition of factors IIa and Xa. |
| Factor V Leiden | Production of mutant factor V (guanine → adenine DNA point mutation → Arg506Gln mutation near the cleavage site) that is resistant to degradation by activated protein C. Complications include DVT, cerebral vein thrombosis, recurrent pregnancy loss. |
| Protein C or S deficiency | ↓ ability to inactivate factors Va and VIIIa. ↑ risk of warfarin-induced skin necrosis. Together, protein C Cancels, and protein S Stops, coagulation. |
| Prothrombin *G20210A* mutation | Point mutation in 3′ untranslated region → ↑ production of prothrombin → ↑ plasma levels and venous clots. |

## Blood transfusion therapy

| COMPONENT | DOSAGE EFFECT | CLINICAL USE |
| --- | --- | --- |
| Packed RBCs | ↑ Hb and $O_2$ binding (carrying) capacity, ↑ hemoglobin ~1 g/dL per unit, ↑ hematocrit ~3% per unit | Acute blood loss, severe anemia |
| Platelets | ↑ platelet count ~30,000/microL per unit (↑ ~5000/mm³/unit) | Stop significant bleeding (thrombocytopenia, qualitative platelet defects) |
| Fresh frozen plasma/ prothrombin complex concentrate | ↑ coagulation factor levels; FFP contains all coagulation factors and plasma proteins; PCC generally contains factors II, VII, IX, and X, as well as protein C and S | Cirrhosis, immediate anticoagulation reversal |
| Cryoprecipitate | Contains fibrinogen, factor VIII, factor XIII, vWF, and fibronectin | Coagulation factor deficiencies involving fibrinogen and factor VIII |
| Albumin | ↑ intravascular volume and oncotic pressure | Post-paracentesis, therapeutic plasmapheresis |

Blood transfusion risks include infection transmission (low), transfusion reactions, transfusion-associated circulatory overload (TACO; volume overload → pulmonary edema, hypertension), transfusion-related acute lung injury (TRALI; hypoxia and inflammation → noncardiogenic pulmonary edema, hypotension), iron overload (may lead to 2° hemochromatosis), hypocalcemia (citrate is a $Ca^{2+}$ chelator), and hyperkalemia (RBCs may lyse in old blood units).

## Leukemia vs lymphoma

| | |
| --- | --- |
| Leukemia | Lymphoid or myeloid neoplasm with widespread involvement of bone marrow. Tumor cells are usually found in peripheral blood. |
| Lymphoma | Discrete tumor mass arising from lymph nodes. Variable clinical presentation (eg, arising in atypical sites, leukemic presentation). |

## Hodgkin vs non-Hodgkin lymphoma

| Hodgkin | Non-Hodgkin |
| --- | --- |
| Both may have constitutional ("B") signs/symptoms: low-grade fever, night sweats, weight loss. | |
| Localized, single group of nodes with contiguous spread (stage is strongest predictor of prognosis). Better prognosis. | Multiple lymph nodes involved; extranodal involvement common; noncontiguous spread. Worse prognosis. |
| Characterized by Reed-Sternberg cells. | Majority involve B cells; rarely of T-cell lineage. |
| Bimodal distribution: young adults, > 55 years. | Can occur in children and adults. |
| Associated with EBV. | May be associated with autoimmune diseases and viral infections (eg, HIV, EBV, HTLV). |

## Hodgkin lymphoma

Contains Reed-Sternberg cells: distinctive tumor giant cells; bilobed nucleus with the 2 halves as mirror images ("owl eyes" A). RS cells are CD15+ and CD30+ B-cell origin. 2 owl eyes × 15 = 30.

| SUBTYPE | NOTES |
| --- | --- |
| Nodular sclerosis | Most common |
| Mixed cellularity | Eosinophilia; seen in immunocompromised patients |
| Lymphocyte rich | Best prognosis (the rich have better bank accounts) |
| Lymphocyte depleted | Worst prognosis (the poor have worse bank accounts); seen in immunocompromised patients |

## Non-Hodgkin lymphoma

| TYPE | OCCURS IN | GENETICS | COMMENTS |
|---|---|---|---|
| **Neoplasms of mature B cells** | | | |
| **Burkitt lymphoma** | Adolescents or young adults "Burkid" lymphoma (more common in kids) | t(8;14)—translocation of c-*myc* (8) and heavy-chain Ig (14) | "Starry sky" appearance (**StarBurst**), sheets of lymphocytes with interspersed "tingible body" macrophages (arrows in ). Associated with EBV. Jaw lesion  in endemic form in Africa; pelvis or abdomen in sporadic form. |
| **Diffuse large B-cell lymphoma** | Usually older adults, but 20% in children | Mutations in *BCL-2*, *BCL-6* | Most common type of non-Hodgkin lymphoma in adults. |
| **Follicular lymphoma** | Adults | t(14;18)—translocation of heavy-chain Ig (14) and *BCL-2* (18) | Indolent course with painless "waxing and waning" lymphadenopathy. Bcl-2 normally inhibits apoptosis. |
| **Mantle cell lymphoma** | Adult males >> adult females | t(11;14)—translocation of cyclin D1 (11) and heavy-chain Ig (14), CD5+ | Very aggressive, patients typically present with late-stage disease. |
| **Marginal zone lymphoma** | Adults | t(11;18) | Associated with chronic inflammation (eg, Sjögren syndrome, chronic gastritis [MALT lymphoma; may regress with *H pylori* eradication]). |
| **Primary central nervous system lymphoma** | Adults | EBV related; associated with HIV/AIDS | Considered an AIDS-defining illness. Variable presentation: confusion, memory loss, seizures. CNS mass (often single, ring-enhancing lesion on MRI) in immunocompromised patients , needs to be distinguished from toxoplasmosis via CSF analysis or other lab tests. |
| **Neoplasms of mature T cells** | | | |
| **Adult T-cell lymphoma** | Adults | Caused by HTLV (associated with IV drug use) | Adults present with cutaneous lesions; common in Japan (T-cell in Tokyo), West Africa, and the Caribbean. Lytic bone lesions, hypercalcemia. |
| **Cutaneous T-cell lymphoma** | Adults | | Heterogenous group of T-cell neoplasms affecting the skin ± blood, lymph nodes, or viscera. Most common subtype is mycosis fungoides  characterized by erythematous patches favoring sun-protected areas that progress to plaques, then eventually tumors. |

| | |
|---|---|
| **Plasma cell dyscrasias**<br> | Group of disorders characterized by proliferation of a single plasma cell clone, typically overproducing a monoclonal immunoglobulin (also called paraprotein). Seen in older adults.<br>Screening with serum protein electrophoresis (**M** spike represents overproduction of **M**onoclonal Ig), serum immunofixation, and serum free light chain assay. Urine protein electrophoresis and immunofixation required to confirm urinary involvement (urine dipstick only detects albumin). Diagnostic confirmation with bone marrow biopsy.<br>Peripheral blood smear may show rouleaux formation **A** (RBCs stacked like poker chips). |
| **Multiple myeloma** | Overproduction of IgG (most common) > IgA > Ig light chains. Clinical features (**CRAB**): hyper**C**alcemia (↑ cytokine secretion [eg, IL-1, TNF-α, RANK-L] by malignant plasma cells → ↑ osteoclast activity), **R**enal insufficiency, **A**nemia, **B**one lytic lesions ("punched out" on x-ray **B** → back pain). Complications: ↑ infection risk, 1° amyloidosis (AL).<br>Urinalysis may show Ig light chains (Bence Jones proteinuria) with ⊖ urine dipstick.<br>Bone marrow biopsy shows >10% monoclonal plasma cells with clock-face chromatin **C** and intracytoplasmic inclusions containing Ig. |
| **Waldenström macroglobulinemia** | Overproduction of IgM (**macro**globulinemia because IgM is the **largest** Ig). Clinical features include anemia, constitutional ("B") signs/symptoms, lymphadenopathy, hepatosplenomegaly, hyperviscosity (eg, headache, bleeding, blurry vision, ataxia), peripheral neuropathy.<br>Funduscopy shows dilated, segmented, and tortuous retinal veins (sausage link appearance).<br>Bone marrow biopsy shows >10% monoclonal B lymphocytes with plasma cell features (lymphoplasmacytic lymphoma) and intranuclear pseudoinclusions containing IgM. |
| **Monoclonal gammopathy of undetermined significance** | Overproduction of any Ig type (M spike <3 g/dL). Asymptomatic (no CRAB findings). 1%–2% risk per year of progressing to multiple myeloma.<br>Bone marrow biopsy shows <10% monoclonal plasma cells. |

| | |
|---|---|
| **Myelodysplastic syndromes**<br> | Stem cell disorders involving ineffective hematopoiesis → defects in cell maturation of nonlymphoid lineages. Bone marrow blasts < 20% (vs > 20% in AML). Caused by de novo mutations or environmental exposure (eg, radiation, benzene, chemotherapy). Risk of transformation to AML. More common in older adults. | Pseudo-Pelger-Huët anomaly—neutrophils with bilobed ("duet") nuclei **A**. Associated with myelodysplastic syndromes or drugs (eg, immunosuppressants). |

| | |
|---|---|
| **Leukemias** | Unregulated growth and differentiation of WBCs in bone marrow → marrow failure → anemia (↓ RBCs), infections (↓ mature WBCs), and hemorrhage (↓ platelets). Usually presents with ↑ circulating WBCs (malignant leukocytes in blood), although some cases present with normal/↓ WBCs.<br>Leukemic cell infiltration of liver, spleen, lymph nodes, and skin (leukemia cutis) possible. |

| TYPE | NOTES |
|---|---|
| **Lymphoid neoplasms** | |
| **Acute lymphoblastic leukemia/lymphoma** | Most frequently occurs in children; less common in adults (worse prognosis). T-cell ALL can present as mediastinal mass (presenting as SVC-like syndrome). Associated with Down syndrome.<br>Peripheral blood and bone marrow have ↑↑↑ lymphoblasts **A**.<br>TdT+ (marker of pre-T and pre-B cells), CD10+ (marker of pre-B cells).<br>Most responsive to therapy.<br>May spread to CNS and testes.<br>t(12;21) → better prognosis; t(9;22) (Philadelphia chromosome) → worse prognosis. |
| **Chronic lymphocytic leukemia/small lymphocytic lymphoma** | Age > 60 years. Most common adult leukemia. CD20+, CD23+, CD5+ B-cell neoplasm. Often asymptomatic, progresses slowly; smudge cells **B** in peripheral blood smear; autoimmune hemolytic anemia. CLL = Crushed Little Lymphocytes (smudge cells).<br>Richter transformation—CLL/SLL transformation into an aggressive lymphoma, most commonly diffuse large B-cell lymphoma (DLBCL). |
| **Hairy cell leukemia** | Adult males. Mature B-cell tumor. Cells have filamentous, hairlike projections (fuzzy appearing on LM **C**). Peripheral lymphadenopathy is uncommon.<br>Causes marrow fibrosis → dry tap on aspiration. Patients usually present with massive splenomegaly and pancytopenia.<br>Stains **TRAP** (Tartrate-Resistant Acid Phosphatase) ⊕ (**TRAP**ped in a **hairy** situation). TRAP stain largely replaced with flow cytometry. Associated with *BRAF* mutations.<br>Treatment: purine analogs (cladribine, pentostatin). |
| **Myeloid neoplasms** | |
| **Acute myelogenous leukemia** | Median onset 65 years. Auer rods **D**; myeloperoxidase ⊕ cytoplasmic inclusions seen mostly in APL (formerly M3 AML); ↑↑↑ circulating myeloblasts on peripheral smear. May present with leukostasis (capillary occlusion by malignant, nondistensible cells → organ damage).<br>Risk factors: prior exposure to alkylating chemotherapy, radiation, benzene, myeloproliferative disorders, Down syndrome (typically acute megakaryoblastic leukemia [formerly M7 AML]).<br>APL: t(15;17), responds to all-*trans* retinoic acid (vitamin A) and arsenic trioxide, which induce differentiation of promyelocytes; DIC is a common presentation. |
| **Chronic myelogenous leukemia** | Peak incidence: 45–85 years; median age: 64 years. Defined by the Philadelphia chromosome (t[9;22], *BCR-ABL*) and myeloid stem cell proliferation. Presents with dysregulated production of mature and maturing granulocytes (eg, neutrophils, metamyelocytes, myelocytes, basophils **E**) and splenomegaly. May accelerate and transform to AML or ALL ("blast crisis").<br>Responds to BCR-ABL tyrosine kinase inhibitors (eg, imatinib). |

| **Myeloproliferative neoplasms** | Malignant hematopoietic neoplasms with varying impacts on WBCs and myeloid cell lines. |
|---|---|
| Polycythemia vera | Primary polycythemia. Disorder of ↑ RBCs, usually due to acquired *JAK2* mutation. May present as intense itching after shower (aquagenic pruritus). Rare but classic symptom is erythromelalgia (severe, burning pain and red-blue coloration) due to episodic blood clots in vessels of the extremities **A**. Associated with hyperviscosity and thrombosis (eg, PE, DVT, Budd-Chiari syndrome). <br> ↓ EPO (vs 2° polycythemia, which presents with endogenous or artificially ↑ EPO). <br> Treatment: phlebotomy, hydroxyurea, ruxolitinib (JAK1/2 inhibitor). |
| Essential thrombocythemia | Characterized by massive proliferation of megakaryocytes and platelets. Symptoms include bleeding and thrombosis. Blood smear shows markedly increased number of platelets, which may be large or otherwise abnormally formed **B**. Erythromelalgia may occur. |
| Myelofibrosis | Atypical megakaryocyte hyperplasia → ↑ TGF-β secretion → ↑ fibroblast activity → obliteration of bone marrow with fibrosis. Associated with massive splenomegaly and "**teardrop**" RBCs **C**. "Bone marrow **cries** because it's fibrosed and is a dry tap." |

|  | RBCs | WBCs | PLATELETS | PHILADELPHIA CHROMOSOME | *JAK2* MUTATIONS |
|---|---|---|---|---|---|
| Polycythemia vera | ↑ | ↑ | ↑ | ⊖ | ⊕ |
| Essential thrombocythemia | – | – | ↑ | ⊖ | ⊕ (30–50%) |
| Myelofibrosis | ↓ | Variable | Variable | ⊖ | ⊕ (30–50%) |
| CML | ↓ | ↑ | ↑ | ⊕ | ⊖ |

### Leukemoid reaction vs chronic myelogenous leukemia

|  | Leukemoid reaction | Chronic myelogenous leukemia |
|---|---|---|
| DEFINITION | Reactive neutrophilia > 50,000 cells/mm³ | Myeloproliferative neoplasm ⊕ for *BCR-ABL* |
| NEUTROPHIL MORPHOLOGY | Toxic granulation, Döhle bodies, cytoplasmic vacuoles | Pseudo-Pelger-Huët anomaly |
| LAP SCORE | ↑ | ↓ (LAP enzyme ↓ in malignant neutrophils) |
| EOSINOPHILS AND BASOPHILS | Normal | ↑ |

## Polycythemia

| | PLASMA VOLUME | RBC MASS | O₂ SATURATION | EPO LEVELS | ASSOCIATIONS |
|---|---|---|---|---|---|
| Relative | ↓ | – | – | – | Dehydration, burns. |
| Appropriate absolute | – | ↑ | ↓ | ↑ | Lung disease, congenital heart disease, high altitude, obstructive sleep apnea. |
| Inappropriate absolute | – | ↑ | – | ↑ | Exogenous EPO (athlete misuse, also called "blood doping"), androgen supplementation. Inappropriate EPO secretion: malignancy (eg, RCC, HCC). |
| Polycythemia vera | ↑ | ↑↑ | – | ↓ | EPO ↓ in PCV due to negative feedback suppressing renal EPO production. |

↑↓ = 1° disturbance

## Chromosomal translocations

| TRANSLOCATION | ASSOCIATED DISORDER | NOTES |
|---|---|---|
| t(8;14) | Burkitt (Burk-8) lymphoma (c-*myc* activation) | The Ig heavy chain genes on chromosome 14 are constitutively expressed. When other genes (eg, c-*myc* and *BCL*-2) are translocated next to this heavy chain gene region, they are overexpressed. |
| t(11;14) | Mantle cell lymphoma (cyclin D1 activation) | |
| t(11;18) | Marginal zone lymphoma | |
| t(14;18) | Follicular lymphoma (*BCL*-2 activation) | |
| t(15;17) | APL (formerly M3 type of AML) | |
| t(9;22) (Philadelphia chromosome) | CML (*BCR-ABL* hybrid), ALL (less common); Philadelphia CreaML cheese | |

## Langerhans cell histiocytosis

Collective group of proliferative disorders of Langerhans cells (antigen-presenting cells normally found in the skin). Presents in a child as lytic bone lesions and skin rash or as recurrent otitis media with a mass involving the mastoid bone. Cells are functionally immature and do not effectively stimulate primary T cells via antigen presentation. Cells express S-100 and CD1a. Birbeck granules ("tennis rackets" or rod shaped on EM) are characteristic .

## Tumor lysis syndrome

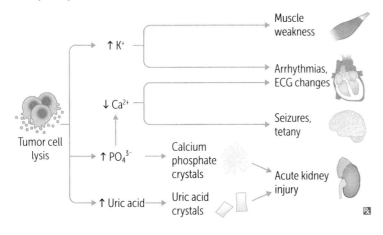

Oncologic emergency triggered by massive tumor cell lysis, seen most often with lymphomas/leukemias. Usually caused by treatment initiation, but can occur spontaneously with fast-growing cancers. Release of $K^+$ → hyperkalemia, release of $PO_4^{3-}$ → hyperphosphatemia, hypocalcemia due to $Ca^{2+}$ sequestration by $PO_4^{3-}$. ↑ nucleic acid breakdown → hyperuricemia → acute kidney injury. Prevention and treatment include aggressive hydration, allopurinol, rasburicase.

---

## ▶ HEMATOLOGY AND ONCOLOGY—PHARMACOLOGY

### Heparin

| | |
|---|---|
| MECHANISM | Activates antithrombin, which ↓ action primarily of factors IIa (thrombin) and Xa. Short half-life. |
| CLINICAL USE | Immediate anticoagulation for pulmonary embolism (PE), acute coronary syndrome, MI, deep venous thrombosis (DVT). Used during pregnancy (does not cross placenta). Monitor PTT. |
| ADVERSE EFFECTS | Bleeding (reverse with protamine sulfate), heparin-induced thrombocytopenia (HIT), osteoporosis (with long-term use), drug-drug interactions, type 4 renal tubular acidosis.<br> ▪ HIT type 1—mild (platelets > 100,000/mm³), transient, nonimmunologic drop in platelet count that typically occurs within the first 2 days of heparin administration. Not clinically significant.<br> ▪ HIT type 2—development of IgG antibodies against heparin-bound platelet factor 4 (PF4) that typically occurs 5–10 days after heparin administration. Antibody-heparin-PF4 complex binds and activates platelets → removal by splenic macrophages and thrombosis → ↓↓ platelet count. Highest risk with unfractionated heparin. Treatment: discontinue heparin, start alternative anticoagulant (eg, argatroban). Fondaparinux safe to use (does not interact with PF4). |
| NOTES | Low-molecular-weight heparins (eg, enoxaparin, dalteparin) act mainly on factor Xa. Fondaparinux acts only on factor Xa. Both are not easily reversible. Unfractionated heparin used in patients with renal insufficiency (low-molecular-weight heparins should be used with caution because they undergo renal clearance). |

## Warfarin

| | |
|---|---|
| MECHANISM | Inhibits vitamin K epoxide reductase by competing with vitamin K → inhibition of vitamin K–dependent γ-carboxylation of clotting factors II, VII, IX, and X and proteins C and S. Metabolism affected by polymorphisms in the gene for vitamin K epoxide reductase complex (*VKORC1*). In laboratory assay, has effect on extrinsic pathway and ↑ PT. Long half-life. "The ex-PresidenT went to war(farin)." |
| CLINICAL USE | Chronic anticoagulation (eg, venous thromboembolism prophylaxis and prevention of stroke in atrial fibrillation). Not used in pregnant patients (because warfarin, unlike heparin, crosses placenta). Monitor PT/INR. |
| ADVERSE EFFECTS | Bleeding, teratogenic effects, skin/tissue necrosis , drug-drug interactions (metabolized by cytochrome P-450 [CYP2C9]). |

Initial risk of hypercoagulation: protein C has shorter half-life than factors II and X. Existing protein C depletes before existing factors II and X deplete, and before warfarin can reduce factors II and X production → hypercoagulation. Skin/tissue necrosis within first few days of large doses believed to be due to small vessel microthrombosis.

Heparin "bridging": heparin frequently used when starting warfarin. Heparin's activation of antithrombin enables anticoagulation during initial, transient hypercoagulable state caused by warfarin. Initial heparin therapy reduces risk of recurrent venous thromboembolism and skin/tissue necrosis.

For reversal of warfarin, give vitamin K. For rapid reversal, give FFP or PCC.

## Heparin vs warfarin

| | Heparin | Warfarin |
|---|---|---|
| ROUTE OF ADMINISTRATION | Parenteral (IV, SC) | Oral |
| SITE OF ACTION | Blood | Liver |
| ONSET OF ACTION | Rapid (seconds) | Slow, limited by half-lives of normal clotting factors |
| DURATION OF ACTION | Hours | Days |
| MONITORING | PTT (intrinsic pathway) | PT/INR (extrinsic pathway) |
| CROSSES PLACENTA | No | Yes (teratogenic) |

## Direct coagulation factor inhibitors

Do not usually require lab monitoring.

| DRUG | MECHANISM | CLINICAL USE | ADVERSE EFFECTS |
|---|---|---|---|
| **Bivalirudin, argatroban, dabigatran** | Directly inhibit thrombin (factor IIa) | Venous thromboembolism, atrial fibrillation. Can be used in HIT, when heparin is BAD for the patient | Bleeding (idarucizumab can be used to inhibit dabigatran) |
| **Apixaban, edoxaban, rivaroxaban** | Directly inhibit (ban) factor Xa | Oral agents. DVT/PE treatment and prophylaxis; stroke prophylaxis in patients with atrial fibrillation | Bleeding (reverse with andexanet alfa) |

## Anticoagulation reversal

| ANTICOAGULANT | REVERSAL AGENT | NOTES |
|---|---|---|
| Heparin | Protamine sulfate | $\oplus$ charged peptide that binds $\ominus$ charged heparin |
| Warfarin | Vitamin K (slow) +/– FFP or PCC (rapid) | |
| Dabigatran | Idarucizumab | Monoclonal antibody Fab fragments |
| Direct factor Xa inhibitors | Andexanet alfa | Recombinant modified factor Xa (inactive) |

## Antiplatelets

All work by ↓ platelet aggregation.

| DRUG | MECHANISM | CLINICAL USE | ADVERSE EFFECTS |
|---|---|---|---|
| Aspirin | Irreversibly blocks COX → ↓ $TXA_2$ release | Acute coronary syndrome; coronary stenting. ↓ incidence or recurrence of thrombotic stroke | Gastric ulcers, tinnitus, allergic reactions, renal injury, Reye syndrome (in children) |
| Clopidogrel, prasugrel, ticagrelor | Block ADP ($P2Y_{12}$) receptor → ↓ ADP-induced expression of GpIIb/IIIa | Same as aspirin; dual antiplatelet therapy | Bleeding |
| Eptifibatide, tirofiban | Block GpIIb/IIIa (fibrinogen receptor) on activated platelets | Unstable angina, percutaneous coronary intervention | Bleeding, thrombocytopenia |
| Cilostazol, dipyridamole | Block phosphodiesterase → ↓ cAMP hydrolysis → ↑ cAMP in platelets | Intermittent claudication, stroke prevention, cardiac stress testing, prevention of coronary stent restenosis | Nausea, headache, facial flushing, hypotension, abdominal pain |

## Thrombolytics

Alteplase (tPA), reteplase (rPA), tenecteplase (TNK-tPA).

| MECHANISM | Directly or indirectly aid conversion of plasminogen to plasmin, which cleaves thrombin and fibrin clots. ↑ PT, ↑ PTT, no change in platelet count. |
|---|---|
| CLINICAL USE | Early MI, early ischemic stroke, direct thrombolysis of high-risk PE. |
| ADVERSE EFFECTS | Bleeding. Contraindicated in patients with active bleeding, history of intracranial bleeding, recent surgery, known bleeding diatheses, or severe hypertension. Nonspecific reversal with antifibrinolytics (eg, aminocaproic acid, tranexamic acid), platelet transfusions, and factor corrections (eg, cryoprecipitate, FFP, PCC). |

## Cancer therapy—cell cycle

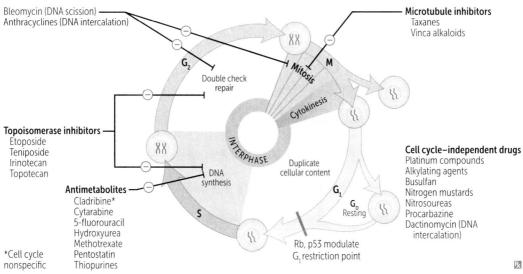

Bleomycin (DNA scission)
Anthracyclines (DNA intercalation)

**Microtubule inhibitors**
Taxanes
Vinca alkaloids

G₂

Double check
repair

Mitosis

M

Cytokinesis

INTERPHASE

**Topoisomerase inhibitors**
Etoposide
Teniposide
Irinotecan
Topotecan

DNA
synthesis

Duplicate
cellular content

**Cell cycle–independent drugs**
Platinum compounds
Alkylating agents
Busulfan
Nitrogen mustards
Nitrosoureas
Procarbazine
Dactinomycin (DNA
intercalation)

**Antimetabolites**
Cladribine*
Cytarabine
5-fluorouracil
Hydroxyurea
Methotrexate
Pentostatin
Thiopurines

S

G₁

G₀
Resting

*Cell cycle
nonspecific

Rb, p53 modulate
G₁ restriction point

## Cancer therapy—targets

Nucleotide synthesis ➡ DNA ➡ RNA ➡ Protein ➡ Cellular division

MTX, 5-FU:
↓ thymidine synthesis

Thiopurines:
↓ de novo purine synthesis

Hydroxyurea:
inhibits ribonucleotide
reductase

Alkylating agents, platinum compounds:
cross-link DNA

Bleomycin:
DNA strand breakage

Anthracyclines, dactinomycin:
DNA intercalators

Etoposide/teniposide:
inhibits topoisomerase II

Irinotecan/topotecan:
inhibits topoisomerase I

Vinca alkaloids:
inhibit microtubule formation

Taxanes:
inhibit microtubule disassembly

## Antibody-drug conjugates

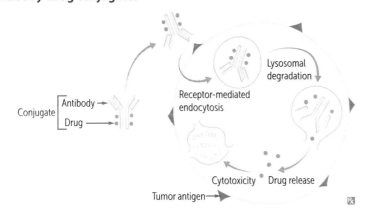

Conjugate
Antibody
Drug

Receptor-mediated
endocytosis

Lysosomal
degradation

Cytotoxicity    Drug release

Tumor antigen ➡

Formed by linking monoclonal antibodies
with cytotoxic chemotherapeutic drugs.
Antibody selectivity against tumor antigens
allows targeted drug delivery to tumor cells
while sparing healthy cells → ↑ efficacy and
↓ toxicity.
Example: ado-trastuzumab emtansine (T-DM1)
for HER2 ⊕ breast cancer.

## Antitumor antibiotics

Dactinomycin is cell cycle nonspecific; bleomycin and anthracycline are $G_2/M$ phase specific.

| DRUG | MECHANISM | CLINICAL USE | ADVERSE EFFECTS |
|---|---|---|---|
| Bleomycin | Induces free radical formation → breaks in DNA strands | Testicular cancer, Hodgkin lymphoma | Pulmonary fibrosis, skin hyperpigmentation |
| Dactinomycin (actinomycin D) | Intercalates into DNA, preventing RNA synthesis | Wilms tumor, Ewing sarcoma, rhabdomyosarcoma | Myelosuppression |
| Anthracyclines Doxorubicin, daunorubicin | Generate free radicals Intercalate in DNA → breaks in DNA → ↓ replication Inhibit topoisomerase II | Solid tumors, leukemias, lymphomas | Dilated cardiomyopathy (often irreversible; prevent with dexrazoxane), myelosuppression |

## Antimetabolites

All are S-phase specific except cladribine, which is cell cycle nonspecific.

| DRUG | MECHANISM | CLINICAL USE | ADVERSE EFFECTS |
|---|---|---|---|
| Thiopurines Azathioprine, 6-mercaptopurine | Purine (thiol) analogs → ↓ de novo purine synthesis AZA is converted to 6-MP, which is then activated by HGPRT | Rheumatoid arthritis, IBD, SLE, ALL; steroid-refractory disease Prevention of organ rejection Weaning from glucocorticoids | Myelosuppression; GI, liver toxicity 6-MP is inactivated by xanthine oxidase (↑ toxicity with allopurinol or febuxostat) |
| Cladribine, pentostatin | Purine analogs → unable to be processed by ADA, interfering with DNA synthesis | Hairy cell leukemia | Myelosuppression |
| Cytarabine (arabinofuranosyl cytidine) | Pyrimidine analog → DNA chain termination Inhibits DNA polymerase | Leukemias (AML), lymphomas | Myelosuppression |
| 5-Fluorouracil | Pyrimidine analog bioactivated to 5-FdUMP → thymidylate synthase inhibition → ↓ dTMP → ↓ DNA synthesis Capecitabine is a prodrug | Colon cancer, pancreatic cancer, actinic keratosis, basal cell carcinoma (topical) Effects enhanced with the addition of leucovorin | Myelosuppression, palmar-plantar erythrodysesthesia (hand-foot syndrome) |
| Hydroxyurea | Inhibits ribonucleotide reductase → ↓ DNA synthesis | Myeloproliferative disorders (eg, CML, polycythemia vera), sickle cell disease (↑ HbF) | Severe myelosuppression, megaloblastic anemia |
| Methotrexate | Folic acid analog that competitively inhibits dihydrofolate reductase → ↓ dTMP → ↓ DNA synthesis | Cancers: leukemias (ALL), lymphomas, choriocarcinoma, sarcomas Nonneoplastic: ectopic pregnancy, medical abortion (with misoprostol), rheumatoid arthritis, psoriasis, IBD, vasculitis | Myelosuppression (reversible with leucovorin "rescue"), hepatotoxicity, mucositis (eg, mouth ulcers), pulmonary fibrosis, folate deficiency (teratogenic), nephrotoxicity |

## Alkylating agents
All are cell cycle nonspecific.

| DRUG | MECHANISM | CLINICAL USE | ADVERSE EFFECTS |
|---|---|---|---|
| **Busulfan** | Cross-links DNA | Used to ablate patient's bone marrow before bone marrow transplantation | Severe myelosuppression (in almost all cases), pulmonary fibrosis, hyperpigmentation |
| **Nitrogen mustards** Cyclophosphamide, ifosfamide | Cross-link DNA Require bioactivation by liver | Solid tumors, leukemia, lymphomas, rheumatic disease (eg, SLE, granulomatosis with polyangiitis) | Myelosuppression, SIADH, Fanconi syndrome (ifosfamide), hemorrhagic cystitis and bladder cancer (prevent with mesna) |
| **Nitrosoureas** Carmustine, lomustine | Cross-link DNA Require bioactivation by liver Cross blood-brain barrier → CNS entry | Brain tumors (including glioblastoma multiforme) Put **nitro** in your **Mustang** and travel the **globe** | CNS toxicity (convulsions, dizziness, ataxia) |
| **Procarbazine** | Mechanism unknown Weak MAO inhibitor | Hodgkin lymphoma, brain tumors | Myelosuppression, pulmonary toxicity, leukemia, disulfiram-like reaction |

## Platinum compounds
Cisplatin, carboplatin, oxaliplatin.

| | |
|---|---|
| MECHANISM | Cross-link DNA. Cell cycle nonspecific. |
| CLINICAL USE | Solid tumors (eg, testicular, bladder, ovarian, GI, lung), lymphomas. |
| ADVERSE EFFECTS | Nephrotoxicity (eg, Fanconi syndrome; prevent with amifostine), peripheral neuropathy, ototoxicity. |

## Microtubule inhibitors
All are M-phase specific.

| DRUG | MECHANISM | CLINICAL USE | ADVERSE EFFECTS |
|---|---|---|---|
| **Taxanes** Docetaxel, paclitaxel | Hyperstabilize polymerized microtubules → prevent mitotic spindle breakdown | Various tumors (eg, ovarian and breast carcinomas) | Myelosuppression, neuropathy, hypersensitivity **Taxes stabilize** society |
| **Vinca alkaloids** Vincristine, vinblastine | Bind β-tubulin and inhibit its polymerization into microtubules → prevent mitotic spindle formation | Solid tumors, leukemias, Hodgkin and non-Hodgkin lymphomas | Vincristine (**crisps** the nerves): neurotoxicity (axonal neuropathy), constipation (including ileus) Vinblastine (**blasts** the marrow): myelosuppression |

## Topoisomerase inhibitors
All cause ↑ DNA degradation resulting in cell cycle arrest in S and $G_2$ phases.

| DRUG | MECHANISM | CLINICAL USE | ADVERSE EFFECTS |
|---|---|---|---|
| **Irinotecan, topotecan** | Inhibit topoisomerase I "-tecone" | Colon, ovarian, small cell lung cancer | Severe myelosuppression, diarrhea |
| **Etoposide, teniposide** | Inhibit topoisomerase II "-bothside" | Testicular, small cell lung cancer, leukemia, lymphoma | Myelosuppression, alopecia |

## Tamoxifen

| | |
|---|---|
| MECHANISM | Selective estrogen receptor modulator with complex mode of action: antagonist in breast tissue, partial agonist in endometrium and bone. Blocks the binding of estrogen to ER in ER ⊕ cells. |
| CLINICAL USE | Prevention and treatment of breast cancer, prevention of gynecomastia in patients undergoing prostate cancer therapy. |
| ADVERSE EFFECTS | Hot flashes, ↑ risk of thromboembolic events (eg, DVT, PE) and endometrial cancer. |

## Anticancer monoclonal antibodies

Work against extracellular targets to neutralize them or to promote immune system recognition (eg, ADCC by NK cells). Eliminated by macrophages (not cleared by kidneys or liver).

| AGENT | TARGET | CLINICAL USE | ADVERSE EFFECTS |
|---|---|---|---|
| Alemtuzumab | CD52 | Chronic lymphocytic leukemia (CLL), multiple sclerosis. | ↑ risk of infections and autoimmunity (eg, ITP) |
| Bevacizumab | VEGF (inhibits blood vessel formation) | Colorectal cancer (CRC), renal cell carcinoma (RCC), non–small cell lung cancer (NSCLC), angioproliferative retinopathy | Hemorrhage, blood clots, impaired wound healing |
| Cetuximab, panitumumab | EGFR | Metastatic CRC (wild-type RAS), head and neck cancer | Rash, elevated LFTs, diarrhea |
| Rituximab | CD20 | Non-Hodgkin lymphoma, CLL, rheumatoid arthritis, ITP, TTP, AIHA, multiple sclerosis | Infusion reaction due to cytokine release following interaction of rituximab with its target on B cells |
| Trastuzumab | Don't **Trast HER**, she will **break your heart** | Breast cancer, gastric cancer | Dilated **cardiomyopathy** (often reversible) |
| Pembrolizumab, nivolumab, cemiplimab | PD-1 | Various tumors (eg, NSCLC, RCC, melanoma, urothelial carcinoma) | ↑ risk of autoimmunity (eg, dermatitis, enterocolitis, hepatitis, pneumonitis, endocrinopathies) |
| Atezolizumab, durvalumab, avelumab | PD-L1 | | |
| Ipilimumab | CTLA-4 | | |

## Anticancer small molecule inhibitors

| AGENT | TARGET | CLINICAL USE | ADVERSE EFFECTS |
|---|---|---|---|
| Alectinib, crizotinib | ALK | Non–small cell lung cancer | Edema, rash, diarrhea |
| Erlotinib, gefitinib, afatinib | EGFR | Non–small cell lung cancer | Rash, diarrhea |
| Imatinib, dasatinib, nilotinib | BCR-ABL (also other tyrosine kinases [eg, c-KIT]) | CML, ALL, GISTs | Myelosuppression, ↑ LFTs, edema, myalgias |
| Ruxolitinib | JAK1/2 | Polycythemia vera | Bruises, ↑ LFTs |
| Bortezomib, ixazomib, carfilzomib | Proteasome (induce arrest at G2-M phase via accumulation of abnormal proteins → apoptosis) | Multiple myeloma, mantle cell lymphoma | Peripheral neuropathy, herpes zoster reactivation (↓ T-cell activation → ↓ cell-mediated immunity) |
| Vemurafenib, encorafenib, dabrafenib | BRAF | Melanoma Often co-administered with MEK inhibitors (eg, trametinib) | Rash, fatigue, nausea, diarrhea |
| Palbociclib | Cyclin-dependent kinase 4/6 (induces arrest at G1-S phase → apoptosis) | Breast cancer | Myelosuppression, pneumonitis |
| Olaparib | Poly(ADP-ribose) polymerase (↓ DNA repair) | Breast, ovarian, pancreatic, and prostate cancers | Myelosuppression, edema, diarrhea |

## Chemotoxicity amelioration

| DRUG | MECHANISM | CLINICAL USE |
|---|---|---|
| Amifostine | Free radical scavenger | Nephrotoxicity from platinum compounds |
| Dexrazoxane | Iron chelator | Cardiotoxicity from anthracyclines |
| Leucovorin (folinic acid) | Tetrahydrofolate precursor | Myelosuppression from methotrexate (leucovorin "rescue"); also enhances the effects of 5-FU |
| Mesna | Sulfhydryl compound that binds acrolein (toxic metabolite of cyclophosphamide/ifosfamide) | Hemorrhagic cystitis from cyclophosphamide/ifosfamide |
| Rasburicase | Recombinant uricase that catalyzes metabolism of uric acid to allantoin | Tumor lysis syndrome |
| Ondansetron, granisetron | 5-HT$_3$ receptor antagonists | Acute nausea and vomiting (usually within 1-2 hr after chemotherapy) |
| Prochlorperazine, metoclopramide | D$_2$ receptor antagonists | |
| Aprepitant, fosaprepitant | NK$_1$ receptor antagonists | Delayed nausea and vomiting (>24 hr after chemotherapy) |
| Filgrastim, sargramostim | Recombinant G(M)-CSF | Neutropenia |
| Epoetin alfa | Recombinant erythropoietin | Anemia |

## Key chemotoxicities

Cisplatin, Carboplatin → ototoxicity

Vincristine → peripheral neuropathy
Bleomycin, Busulfan → pulmonary fibrosis
Doxorubicin, Daunorubicin → cardiotoxicity
Trastuzumab → cardiotoxicity
Cisplatin, Carboplatin → nephrotoxicity

CYclophosphamide → hemorrhagic cystitis

Nonspecific common toxicities of nearly all cytotoxic chemotherapies include myelosuppression (neutropenia, anemia, thrombocytopenia), GI toxicity (nausea, vomiting, mucositis), alopecia.

# Musculoskeletal, Skin, and Connective Tissue

*"Rigid, the skeleton of habit alone upholds the human frame."*
—Virginia Woolf, *Mrs. Dalloway*

*"Beauty may be skin deep, but ugly goes clear to the bone."*
—Redd Foxx

*"The finest clothing made is a person's own skin, but, of course, society demands something more than this."*
—Mark Twain

*"To thrive in life you need three bones. A wishbone. A backbone. And a funny bone."*
—Reba McEntire

This chapter provides information you will need to understand common anatomic dysfunctions, orthopedic conditions, rheumatic diseases, and dermatologic conditions. Be able to interpret 3D anatomy in the context of radiologic imaging. For the rheumatic diseases, create instructional cases that include the most likely presentation and symptoms: risk factors, gender, important markers (eg, autoantibodies), and other epidemiologic factors. Doing so will allow you to answer higher order questions that are likely to be asked on the exam.

▶ MUSCULOSKELETAL, SKIN, AND CONNECTIVE TISSUE—ANATOMY AND PHYSIOLOGY

## Upper extremity nerves

| NERVE | CAUSES OF INJURY | PRESENTATION |
|---|---|---|
| **Axillary (C5-C6)** | Fractured surgical neck of humerus<br>Anterior dislocation of humerus | Flattened deltoid<br>Loss of arm abduction at shoulder (> 15°)<br>Loss of sensation over deltoid and lateral arm |
| **Musculocutaneous (C5-C7)** | Upper trunk compression | ↓ biceps (C5-C6) reflex<br>Loss of forearm flexion and supination<br>Loss of sensation over radial and dorsal forearm |
| **Radial (C5-T1)** | Compression of axilla, eg, due to crutches or sleeping with arm over chair ("Saturday night palsy")<br>Midshaft fracture of humerus<br>Repetitive pronation/supination of forearm, eg, due to screwdriver use ("finger drop") | Injuries above the elbow cause loss of sensation over posterior arm/forearm and dorsal hand, wrist drop (loss of elbow, wrist, and finger extension) with ↓ grip strength (wrist extension necessary for maximal action of flexors)<br>Injuries below the elbow can cause paresthesias of the dorsal forearm (superficial radial nerve) or wrist drop (posterior interosseus nerve)<br>Tricep function and posterior arm sensation spared in midshaft fracture |
| **Median (C5-T1)** | Supracondylar fracture of humerus → proximal lesion of the nerve<br>Carpal tunnel syndrome and wrist laceration → distal lesion of the nerve | "Ape hand" and "Hand of benediction"<br>Loss of wrist flexion and function of the lateral two Lumbricals, Opponens pollicis, Abductor pollicis brevis, Flexor pollicis brevis (**LOAF**)<br>Loss of sensation over thenar eminence and dorsal and palmar aspects of lateral 3 1/2 fingers with proximal lesion |
| **Ulnar (C8-T1)** | Fracture of medial epicondyle of humerus (proximal lesion)<br>Fractured hook of hamate (distal lesion) from fall on outstretched hand<br>Compression of nerve against hamate as the wrist rests on handlebar during cycling | "Ulnar claw" on digit extension<br>Radial deviation of wrist upon flexion (proximal lesion)<br>↓ flexion of ulnar fingers, abduction and adduction of fingers (interossei), thumb adduction, actions of ulnar 2 lumbrical muscles<br>Loss of sensation over ulnar 1 1/2 fingers including hypothenar eminence |
| **Recurrent branch of median nerve (C5-T1)** | Superficial laceration of palm | "Ape hand"<br>Loss of thenar muscle group: opposition, abduction, and flexion of thumb<br>No loss of sensation |

Humerus fractures, proximally to distally, follow the **ARM** (Axillary → Radial → Median) nerves

## Upper extremity nerves *(continued)*

## Rotator cuff muscles

Shoulder muscles that form the rotator cuff:
- Supraspinatus (suprascapular nerve)—abducts arm initially (before the action of the deltoid); most common rotator cuff injury (trauma or degeneration and impingement → tendinopathy or tear [arrow in A]), assessed by "empty/full can" test
- Infraspinatus (suprascapular nerve)—externally rotates arm; pitching injury
- teres minor (axillary nerve)—adducts and externally rotates arm
- Subscapularis (upper and lower subscapular nerves)—internally rotates and adducts arm

Innervated primarily by C5-C6.

SItS (small t is for teres minor).

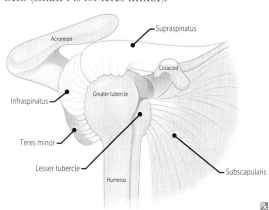

## Arm abduction

| DEGREE | MUSCLE | NERVE |
|---|---|---|
| 0°–15° | Supraspinatus | Suprascapular |
| 15°–90° | Deltoid | Axillary |
| > 90° | Trapezius | Accessory |
| > 90° | Serratus Anterior | Long Thoracic (**SALT**) |

## Brachial plexus lesions

❶ Erb palsy ("waiter's tip")
❷ Klumpke palsy (claw hand)
❸ Wrist drop
❹ Winged scapula
❺ Deltoid paralysis
❻ "Saturday night palsy" (wrist drop)
❼ Difficulty flexing elbow, variable sensory loss
❽ Decreased thumb function, "hand of benediction"
❾ Intrinsic muscles of hand, claw hand

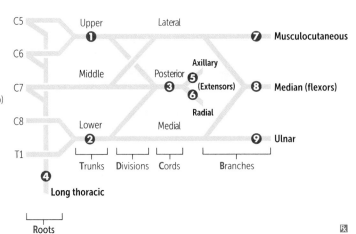

Divisions of brachial plexus:
Remember
To
Drink
Cold
Beer

Trunks of brachial plexus and the subclavian artery pass between anterior and middle scalene muscles. Subclavian vein passes anteromedial to the scalene triangle.

| CONDITION | INJURY | CAUSES | MUSCLE DEFICIT | FUNCTIONAL DEFICIT | PRESENTATION |
|---|---|---|---|---|---|
| **Erb palsy ("waiter's tip")** | Traction or tear of **upper** trunk: C5-C6 roots | Infants—lateral traction on neck during delivery Adults—trauma leading to neck traction (eg, falling on head and shoulder in motorcycle accident) | Deltoid, supraspinatus | Abduction (arm hangs by side) | |
| | | | Infraspinatus, supraspinatus | Lateral rotation (arm medially rotated) | |
| | | | Biceps brachii Herb gets DIBs on **tips** | Flexion, supination (arm extended and pronated) | |
| **Klumpke palsy** | Traction or tear of **lower** trunk: C8-T1 roots | Infants—upward force on arm during delivery Adults—trauma (eg, grabbing a tree branch to break a fall) | Intrinsic hand muscles: lumbricals, interossei, thenar, hypothenar | Claw hand ("Clawmpke" palsy): lumbricals normally flex MCP joints and extend DIP and PIP joints | |
| **Thoracic outlet syndrome** | Compression of **lower** trunk and subclavian vessels, most commonly within the scalene triangle | Cervical/ anomalous first ribs (arrows in Ⓐ), Pancoast tumor | Same as Klumpke palsy | Atrophy of intrinsic hand muscles; ischemia, pain, and edema due to vascular compression | **A** C5 C6 C7 T1 |
| **Winged scapula** | Lesion of long thoracic nerve, roots C5-C7 ("**wings** of heaven") | Axillary node dissection after mastectomy, stab wounds | Serratus anterior | Inability to anchor scapula to thoracic cage → cannot abduct arm above horizontal position **B** | **B** |

**Wrist region**

Scaphoid, lunate, triquetrum, pisiform, hamate, capitate, trapezoid, trapezium **A**. (So long to pinky, here comes the thumb)

Scaphoid (palpable in anatomic snuff box **B**) is the most commonly fractured carpal bone, typically due to a fall on an outstretched hand. Complications of proximal scaphoid fractures include avascular necrosis and nonunion due to retrograde blood supply from a branch of the radial artery. Occult fracture not always seen on initial x-ray.

Dislocation of lunate may impinge median nerve and cause carpal tunnel syndrome.

Fracture of the hook of the hamate can cause ulnar nerve compression—**Guyon canal syndrome**.

**Hand muscles**

Thenar (median)—Opponens pollicis, Abductor pollicis brevis, Flexor pollicis brevis: superficial and deep (by ulnar nerve) heads, adductor pollicis (by ulnar nerve).

Hypothenar (ulnar)—Opponens digiti minimi, Abductor digiti minimi, Flexor digiti minimi brevis.

Dorsal interossei (ulnar)—abduct the fingers.

Palmar interossei (ulnar)—adduct the fingers.

Lumbricals (1st/2nd, median; 3rd/4th, ulnar)— flex at the MCP joint, extend PIP and DIP joints.

Both groups perform the same functions: Oppose, Abduct, and Flex (OAF).

DAB = Dorsals ABduct.
PAD = Palmars ADduct.

---

**Distortions of the hand**

At rest, a balance exists between the extrinsic flexors and extensors of the hand, as well as the intrinsic muscles of the hand—particularly the lumbrical muscles (flexion of MCP, extension of DIP and PIP joints).

"Clawing" A —seen best with **distal** lesions of median or ulnar nerves. Remaining extrinsic flexors of the digits exaggerate the loss of the lumbricals → fingers extend at MCP, flex at DIP and PIP joints.

Deficits less pronounced in **proximal** lesions; deficits present during voluntary flexion of the digits.

| SIGN | "Ulnar claw" | "Hand of benediction" | "Median claw" | "Trouble making a fist" |
|---|---|---|---|---|
| PRESENTATION | | | | |
| CONTEXT | Extending fingers/at rest | Making a fist | Extending fingers/at rest | Closing the hand |
| LOCATION OF LESION | Distal ulnar nerve | Proximal median nerve | Distal median nerve | Proximal ulnar nerve |

Note: Atrophy of the thenar eminence can be seen in median nerve lesions, while atrophy of the hypothenar eminence can be seen in ulnar nerve lesions.

## Actions of hip muscles

| ACTION | MUSCLES |
| --- | --- |
| Abductors | Gluteus medius, gluteus minimus |
| Adductors | Adductor magnus, adductor longus, adductor brevis |
| Extensors | Gluteus maximus, semitendinosus, semimembranosus, long head of biceps femoris |
| Flexors | Iliopsoas (iliacus and psoas), rectus femoris, tensor fascia lata, pectineus, sartorius |
| Internal rotation | Gluteus medius, gluteus minimus, tensor fascia latae |
| External rotation | Iliopsoas, gluteus maximus, piriformis, obturator internus, obturator externus |

| **Knee exam** | Lateral femoral condyle to anterior tibia: ACL.<br>Medial femoral condyle to posterior tibia: PCL.<br>LAMP. | |
| --- | --- | --- |
| TEST | PROCEDURE | |
| Anterior drawer sign | Positive in ACL tear. Tibia glides anteriorly (relative to femur) when knee is at 90° angle. Alternatively, Lachman test done (places knee at 30° angle). | |
| Posterior drawer sign | Bending knee at 90° angle, ↑ posterior gliding of tibia due to PCL injury. | |
| Valgus stress test | Abnormal passive abduction. Knee either extended or at ~ 30° angle, lateral (valgus) force → medial space widening of tibia → MCL injury. | <br>Femur<br>Lateral condyle — Medial condyle<br>ACL — PCL<br>LCL — MCL<br>Lateral meniscus — Medial meniscus<br>Fibula — Tibia |
| Varus stress test | Abnormal passive adduction. Knee either extended or at ~ 30° angle, medial (varus) force → lateral space widening of tibia → LCL injury. | |
| McMurray test | During flexion and extension of knee with rotation of tibia/foot (LIME):<br>▪ Pain, "popping" on internal rotation and varus force → Lateral meniscal tear (Internal rotation stresses lateral meniscus)<br>▪ Pain, "popping" on external rotation and valgus force → Medial meniscal tear (External rotation stresses medial meniscus) | |

## Lower extremity nerves

| NERVE | INNERVATION | CAUSE OF INJURY | PRESENTATION/COMMENTS |
|---|---|---|---|
| **Iliohypogastric (T12-L1)** | Sensory—suprapubic region<br>Motor—transversus abdominis and internal oblique | Abdominal surgery (commonly inguinal hernia repair) | Burning or tingling pain in surgical incision site radiating to inguinal and suprapubic region |
| **Genitofemoral nerve (L1-L2)** | Sensory—scrotum/labia majora, medial thigh<br>Motor—cremaster | Laparoscopic surgery | ↓ upper medial thigh and anterior thigh sensation beneath the inguinal ligament (lateral part of the femoral triangle); absent cremasteric reflex |
| **Lateral femoral cutaneous (L2-L3)** | Sensory—anterior and lateral thigh | Tight clothing, obesity, pregnancy, pelvic procedures | ↓ thigh sensation (anterior and lateral)<br>Meralgia paresthetica—compression of lateral femoral cutaneous nerve → tingling, numbness, burning pain in anterolateral thigh |
| **Obturator (L2-L4)**<br> | Sensory—medial thigh<br>Motor—obturator externus, adductor longus, adductor brevis, gracilis, pectineus, adductor magnus | Pelvic operation | ↓ thigh sensation (medial) and adduction |
| **Femoral (L2-L4)**<br> | Sensory—anterior thigh, medial leg<br>Motor—quadriceps, iliacus, pectineus, sartorius | Pelvic fracture, compression from retroperitoneal hematoma or psoas abscess | ↓ leg extension (↓ patellar reflex) |
| **Sciatic (L4-S3)** | Sensory—posterior thigh, posterior knee, and all below knee (except narrow band on medial lower leg)<br>Motor—semitendinosus, semimembranosus, biceps femoris, adductor magnus | Herniated disc, posterior hip dislocation, piriformis syndrome | Splits into common peroneal and tibial nerves |

## Lower extremity nerves (continued)

| NERVE | INNERVATION | CAUSE OF INJURY | PRESENTATION/COMMENTS |
|---|---|---|---|
| **Common (fibular) peroneal (L4-S2)** | Superficial peroneal nerve:<br>▪ Sensory—dorsum of foot (except webspace between hallux and 2nd digit)<br>▪ Motor—peroneus longus and brevis<br>Deep peroneal nerve:<br>▪ Sensory—webspace between hallux and 2nd digit<br>▪ Motor—tibialis anterior | Trauma or compression of lateral aspect of leg, fibular neck fracture | PED = Peroneal Everts and Dorsiflexes; if injured, foot dropPED<br>Loss of sensation on dorsum of foot<br>Foot drop—inverted and plantarflexed at rest, loss of eversion and dorsiflexion; "steppage gait" |
| **Tibial (L4-S3)** | Sensory—sole of foot<br>Motor—biceps femoris (long head), triceps surae, plantaris, popliteus, flexor muscles of foot | Knee trauma, Baker cyst (proximal lesion); tarsal tunnel syndrome (distal lesion) | TIP = Tibial Inverts and Plantarflexes; if injured, can't stand on TIPtoes<br>Inability to curl toes and loss of sensation on sole; in proximal lesions, foot everted at rest with weakened inversion and plantar flexion |
| **Superior gluteal (L4-S1)** | Motor—gluteus medius, gluteus minimus, tensor fascia latae | Iatrogenic injury during intramuscular injection to superomedial gluteal region (prevent by choosing superolateral quadrant, preferably anterolateral region) | Trendelenburg sign/gait—pelvis tilts because weight-bearing leg cannot maintain alignment of pelvis through hip abduction<br>Lesion is contralateral to the side of the hip that drops, ipsilateral to extremity on which the patient stands |
| **Inferior gluteal (L5-S2)** | Motor—gluteus maximus | Posterior hip dislocation | Difficulty climbing stairs, rising from seated position; loss of hip extension |
| **Pudendal (S2-S4)** | Sensory—perineum<br>Motor—external urethral and anal sphincters | Stretch injury during childbirth, prolonged cycling, horseback riding | ↓ sensation in perineum and genital area; can cause fecal and/or urinary incontinence<br>Can be blocked with local anesthetic during childbirth using ischial spine as a landmark for injection |

Normal    Trendelenburg sign

**Ankle sprains**

Anterior talofibular ligament—most common ankle sprain overall, classified as a low ankle sprain. Due to overinversion/supination of foot. Anterior inferior tibiofibular ligament—most common high ankle sprain. High tide.

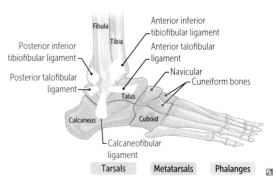

**Signs of lumbosacral radiculopathy**

Paresthesia and weakness related to specific lumbosacral spinal nerves. Intervertebral disc (nucleus pulposus) herniates posterolaterally through annulus fibrosus (outer ring) into spinal canal due to thin posterior longitudinal ligament and thicker anterior longitudinal ligament along midline of vertebral bodies. Nerve affected is usually below the level of herniation. ⊕ straight leg raise, ⊕ contralateral straight leg raise, ⊕ reverse straight leg raise (femoral stretch).

| Disc level herniation | L3-L4 | L4-L5 | L5-S1 |
|---|---|---|---|
| Nerve root affected | L4 | L5 | S1 |
| Dermatome affected | | | |
| Clinical findings | Weakness of knee extension ↓ patellar reflex | Weakness of dorsiflexion Difficulty in heel walking | Weakness of plantar flexion Difficulty in toe walking ↓ Achilles reflex |

**Neurovascular pairing**

Nerves and arteries are frequently named together by the bones/regions with which they are associated. The following are exceptions to this naming convention.

| LOCATION | NERVE | ARTERY |
|---|---|---|
| **Axilla/lateral thorax** | Long thoracic | Lateral thoracic |
| **Surgical neck of humerus** | Axillary | Posterior circumflex |
| **Midshaft of humerus** | Radial | Deep brachial |
| **Distal humerus/cubital fossa** | Median | Brachial |
| **Popliteal fossa** | Tibial | Popliteal |
| **Posterior to medial malleolus** | Tibial | Posterior tibial |

**Motor neuron action potential to muscle contraction**

T-tubules are extensions of plasma membrane in contact with the sarcoplasmic reticulum, allowing for coordinated contraction of striated muscles.

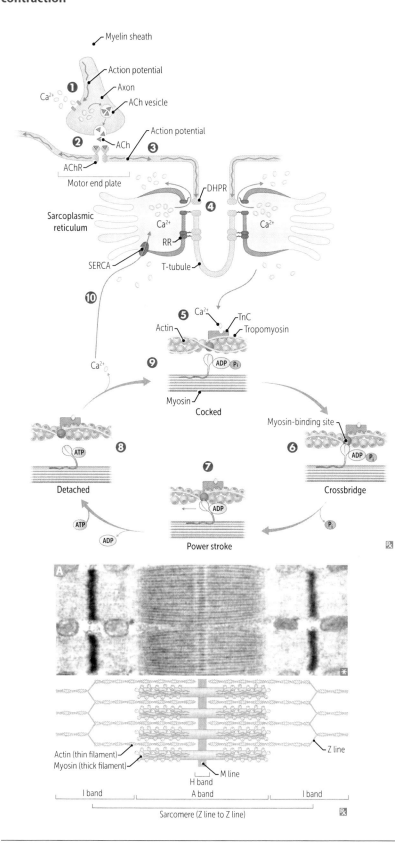

❶ Action potential opens presynaptic voltage-gated $Ca^{2+}$ channels, inducing acetylcholine (ACh) release.

❷ Postsynaptic ACh binding leads to muscle cell depolarization at the motor end plate.

❸ Depolarization travels over the entire muscle cell and deep into the muscle via the T-tubules.

❹ Membrane depolarization induces conformational changes in the voltage-sensitive dihydropyridine receptor (DHPR) and its mechanically coupled ryanodine receptor (RR) → $Ca^{2+}$ release from the sarcoplasmic reticulum (buffered by calsequestrin) into the cytoplasm.

❺ Tropomyosin is blocking myosin-binding sites on the actin filament. Released $Ca^{2+}$ binds to troponin C (TnC), shifting tropomyosin to expose the myosin-binding sites.

❻ Myosin head binds strongly to actin (crossbridge). $P_i$ released, initiating power stroke.

❼ During the power stroke, force is produced as myosin pulls on the thin filament Ⓐ. Muscle shortening occurs, with shortening of **H** and **I** bands and between **Z** lines (**HI**, I'm wearing short**Z**). The A band remains the same length (**A** band is **A**lways the same length). ADP is released at the end of the power stroke.

❽ Binding of new ATP molecule causes detachment of myosin head from actin filament. $Ca^{2+}$ is resequestered.

❾ ATP hydrolysis into ADP and $P_i$ results in myosin head returning to high-energy position (cocked). The myosin head can bind to a new site on actin to form a crossbridge if $Ca^{2+}$ remains available.

❿ Reuptake of calcium by sarco(endo)plasmic reticulum $Ca^{2+}$ ATPase (SERCA) → muscle relaxation.

### Types of skeletal muscle fibers

Two types, normally distributed randomly within muscle. Muscle fiber type grouping commonly occurs due to reinnervation of denervated muscle fibers in peripheral nerve damage.

|  | Type I | Type II |
|---|---|---|
| CONTRACTION VELOCITY | Slow | Fast |
| FIBER COLOR | Red | White |
| PREDOMINANT METABOLISM | Oxidative phosphorylation → sustained contraction | Anaerobic glycolysis |
| MITOCHONDRIA, MYOGLOBIN | ↑ | ↓ |
| TYPE OF TRAINING | Endurance training | Weight/resistance training, sprinting |
| NOTES | Think "1 slow red ox" | Think "2 fast white antelopes" |

### Skeletal muscle adaptations

|  | Atrophy | Hypertrophy |
|---|---|---|
| MYOFIBRILS | ↓ (removal via ubiquitin-proteasome system) | ↑ (addition of sarcomeres in parallel) |
| MYONUCLEI | ↓ (selective apoptosis) | ↑ (fusion of satellite cells, which repair damaged myofibrils; absent in cardiac muscles) |

### Vascular smooth muscle contraction and relaxation

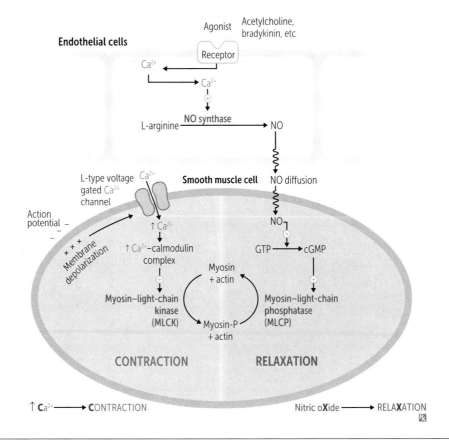

| **Muscle proprioceptors** | Specialized sensory receptors that relay information about muscle dynamics. | |
|---|---|---|
| | **Muscle stretch receptors** | **Golgi tendon organ** |
| PATHWAY | ❶ ↑ length and speed of stretch → ❷ via dorsal root ganglion (DRG) → ❸ activation of inhibitory interneuron and α motor neuron → ❹ simultaneous inhibition of antagonist muscle (prevents overstretching) and activation of agonist muscle (contraction). | ❶ ↑ tension → ❷ via DRG → ❸ activation of inhibitory interneuron → ❹ inhibition of agonist muscle (reduced tension within muscle and tendon) |
| LOCATION/INNERVATION | Body of muscle/type Ia and II sensory axons | Tendons/type Ib sensory axons |
| ACTIVATION BY | ↑ muscle stretch. Responsible for deep tendon reflexes | ↑ muscle tension |

 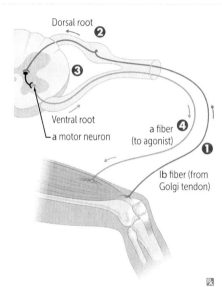

**Bone formation**

| Endochondral ossification | Bones of axial skeleton, appendicular skeleton, and base of skull. Cartilaginous model of bone is first made by chondrocytes. Osteoclasts and osteoblasts later replace with woven bone and then remodel to lamellar bone. In adults, woven bone occurs after fractures and in Paget disease. Defective in achondroplasia. |
|---|---|
| Membranous ossification | Bones of calvarium, facial bones, and clavicle. Woven bone formed directly without cartilage. Later remodeled to lamellar bone. |

## Cell biology of bone

| | |
|---|---|
| Osteoblast | Builds bone by secreting collagen and catalyzing mineralization in alkaline environment via ALP. Differentiates from mesenchymal stem cells in periosteum. Osteoblastic activity measured by bone ALP, osteocalcin, propeptides of type I procollagen. |
| Osteoclast | Dissolves ("crushes") bone by secreting $H^+$ and collagenases. Differentiates from a fusion of monocyte/macrophage lineage precursors. RANK receptors on osteoclasts are stimulated by RANKL (RANK ligand, expressed on osteoblasts). OPG (osteoprotegerin, a RANKL decoy receptor) binds RANKL to prevent RANK-RANKL interaction → ↓ osteoclast activity. |
| Parathyroid hormone | At low, intermittent levels, exerts anabolic effects (building bone) on osteoblasts and osteoclasts (indirect). Chronically ↑ PTH levels (1° hyperparathyroidism) cause catabolic effects (osteitis fibrosa cystica). |
| Estrogen | Inhibits apoptosis in bone-forming osteoblasts and induces apoptosis in bone-resorbing osteoclasts. Causes closure of epiphyseal plate during puberty. Estrogen deficiency (surgical or postmenopausal) → ↑ cycles of remodeling and bone resorption → ↑ risk of osteoporosis. |

## ▶ MUSCULOSKELETAL, SKIN, AND CONNECTIVE TISSUE—PATHOLOGY

## Overuse injuries of the elbow

| | |
|---|---|
| Medial (golfer's) elbow tendinopathy | Repetitive wrist flexion or idiopathic → pain near medial epicondyle. |
| Lateral (tennis) elbow tendinopathy | Repetitive wrist extension (backhand shots) or idiopathic → pain near lateral epicondyle. |

**Clavicle fractures**

Common in children and as birth trauma. Usually caused by a fall on outstretched hand or by direct trauma to shoulder. Weakest point at the junction of middle and lateral thirds **A**; fractures at the middle third segment are most common. Presents as shoulder drop, shortened clavicle (lateral fragment is depressed due to arm weight and medially rotated by arm adductors [eg, pectoralis major]).

## Wrist and hand injuries

| | | |
|---|---|---|
| **Guyon canal syndrome** | Compression of ulnar nerve at wrist. Classically seen in cyclists due to pressure from handlebars. | May also be seen with fracture/dislocation of the hook of hamate. |
| **Carpal tunnel syndrome** | Entrapment of median nerve in carpal tunnel (between transverse carpal ligament and carpal bones) → nerve compression → paresthesia, pain, and numbness in distribution of median nerve. Thenar eminence atrophies but sensation spared, because palmar cutaneous branch enters hand external to carpal tunnel. | Suggested by ⊕ Tinel sign (percussion of wrist causes tingling) and Phalen maneuver (90° flexion of wrist causes tingling). Associated with pregnancy (due to edema), rheumatoid arthritis, hypothyroidism, diabetes, acromegaly, dialysis-related amyloidosis; may be associated with repetitive use. |
| **Metacarpal neck fracture**  | Also called boxer's fracture. Common fracture caused by direct blow with a closed fist (eg, from punching a wall). Most commonly seen in the 5th metacarpal **A**. | |

**Psoas abscess**

Collection of pus in iliopsoas compartment. May spread from blood (hematogenous) or from adjacent structures (eg, vertebral osteomyelitis, tuberculous spondylitis [also called Pott disease], pyelonephritis). Associated with Crohn disease, diabetes, and immunocompromised states.

*Staphylococcus aureus* most commonly isolated, but may also occur 2° to tuberculosis.

Findings: flank pain, fever, inguinal mass, ⊕ psoas sign (hip extension exacerbates lower abdominal pain).

Labs: leukocytosis. Imaging (CT/MRI) will show focal hypodense lesion within the muscle plane (red arrow in **A**).

Treatment: abscess drainage, antibiotics.

## Common knee conditions

| | | |
|---|---|---|
| "Unhappy triad" | Common injury in contact sports due to lateral force impacting the knee when foot is planted on the ground. Consists of damage to the ACL 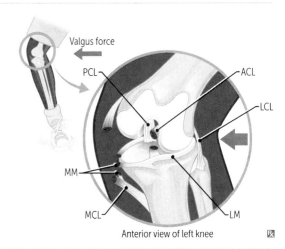, MCL, and medial meniscus (attached to MCL). However, lateral meniscus involvement is more common than medial meniscus involvement in conjunction with ACL and MCL injury. Presents with acute pain and signs of joint instability. | Anterior view of left knee |
| Prepatellar bursitis | Inflammation of the prepatellar bursa in front of the kneecap (red arrow in **B**). Can be caused by repeated trauma or pressure from excessive kneeling (also called "housemaid's knee"). |  |
| Popliteal cyst | Also called Baker cyst. Popliteal fluid collection (red arrow in **C**) in gastrocnemius-semimembranosus bursa commonly communicating with synovial space and related to chronic joint disease (eg, osteoarthritis, rheumatoid arthritis). |  |

## Common musculoskeletal conditions

| | |
|---|---|
| **Costochondritis** | Inflammation of costochondral or costosternal junctions. Presents with focal tenderness to palpation and sharp, positional chest pain that may worsen with deep inspiration. More common in younger female patients. May mimic cardiac (eg, MI) or pulmonary (eg, pulmonary embolism) diseases. |
| **De Quervain tenosynovitis** | Noninflammatory thickening of abductor pollicis longus and extensor pollicis brevis tendons → pain or tenderness at radial styloid. ⊕ Finkelstein test (pain at radial styloid with active or passive stretch of thumb tendons). ↑ risk in new mothers (lifting baby), golfers, racquet sport players, "thumb" texters. |
| **Dupuytren contracture** | Caused by fibroblastic proliferation and thickening of superficial palmar fascia. Typically involves the fascia at the base of the ring and little fingers. Unknown etiology; most frequently seen in males > 50 years old of Northern European descent. |
| **Ganglion cyst** | Fluid-filled swelling overlying joint or tendon sheath, most commonly at dorsal side of wrist. Transilluminates with shining light (tumors lack transillumination). Usually resolves spontaneously. |
| **Iliotibial band syndrome** | Overuse injury of lateral knee that occurs primarily in runners. Pain develops 2° to friction of iliotibial band against lateral femoral epicondyle. |
| **Limb compartment syndrome** | ↑ pressure within fascial compartment of a limb → venous outflow obstruction and arteriolar collapse → anoxia, necrosis, rhabdomyolysis → acute tubular necrosis. Causes include significant long bone fractures (eg, tibia), reperfusion injury, animal venoms. Presents with severe pain and tense, swollen compartments with passive stretch of muscles in the affected compartment. Increased serum creatine kinase and motor deficits are late signs of irreversible muscle and nerve damage. 5 P's: pain, pallor, paresthesia, pulselessness, paralysis. |
| **Medial tibial stress syndrome** | Also called shin splints. Common cause of shin pain and diffuse tenderness in runners and military recruits. Caused by bone resorption that outpaces bone formation in tibial cortex. |
| **Plantar fasciitis** | Inflammation of plantar aponeurosis characterized by heel pain (worse with first steps in the morning or after period of inactivity) and tenderness. Associated with obesity, prolonged standing or jumping (eg, dancers, runners), and flat feet. Heel spurs often coexist. |
| **Temporomandibular disorders** | Group of disorders that involve the temporomandibular joint (TMJ) and muscles of mastication. Multifactorial etiology; associated with TMJ trauma, poor head and neck posture, abnormal trigeminal nerve pain processing, psychological factors. Present with dull, constant unilateral facial pain that worsens with jaw movement, otalgia, headache, TMJ dysfunction (eg, limited range of motion). |

## Childhood musculoskeletal conditions

| | |
|---|---|
| **Radial head subluxation**  | Also called nursemaid's elbow. Common elbow injury in children < 5 years. Caused by a sudden pull on the arm → immature annular ligament slips over head of radius. Injured arm held in slightly flexed and pronated position. |
| **Osgood-Schlatter disease**  | Also called traction apophysitis. Overuse injury caused by repetitive strain and chronic avulsion of the secondary ossification center of the tibial tuberosity. Occurs in adolescents after growth spurt. Common in athletes who run and jump. Presents with progressive anterior knee pain. |
| **Patellofemoral syndrome**  | Overuse injury that commonly presents in young, female athletes as anterior knee pain. Exacerbated by prolonged sitting or weight-bearing on a flexed knee. |
| **Developmental dysplasia of the hip** | Abnormal acetabulum development in newborns. Risk factor is breech presentation. Results in hip instability/dislocation. Commonly tested with Ortolani and Barlow maneuvers (manipulation of newborn hip reveals a "clunk"). Confirmed via ultrasound (x-ray not used until ~4–6 months because cartilage is not ossified). |
| **Legg-Calvé-Perthes disease** | Idiopathic avascular necrosis of femoral head. Commonly presents between 5–7 years with insidious onset of hip pain that may cause child to limp. More common in males (4:1 ratio). Initial x-ray often normal. |
| **Slipped capital femoral epiphysis**  | Classically presents in an obese young adolescent with hip/knee pain and altered gait. Increased axial force on femoral head → epiphysis displaces relative to femoral neck (like a scoop of ice cream slipping off a cone). Diagnosed via x-ray A. |

## Common pediatric fractures

| | | |
|---|---|---|
| **Greenstick fracture** | Incomplete fracture extending partway through width of bone  following bending stress; bone fails on tension side; compression side intact (compare to torus fracture). Bone is bent like a green twig. |  |
| **Torus (buckle) fracture** | Axial force applied to immature bone → cortex buckles on compression (concave) side and fractures . Tension (convex) side remains solid (intact). | |

Normal    Complete fracture    Greenstick fracture    Torus fracture

---

**Achondroplasia**

Failure of longitudinal bone growth (endochondral ossification) → short limbs. Membranous ossification is not affected → large head relative to limbs. Constitutive activation of fibroblast growth factor receptor (FGFR3) actually inhibits chondrocyte proliferation. > 85% of mutations occur sporadically; autosomal dominant with full penetrance (homozygosity is lethal). Associated with ↑ paternal age. Most common cause of short-limbed dwarfism.

---

**Osteoporosis**

Trabecular (spongy) and cortical bone lose mass despite normal bone mineralization and lab values (serum $Ca^{2+}$ and $PO_4^{3-}$).

Most commonly due to ↑ bone resorption (↑ osteoclast number and activity) related to ↓ estrogen levels, old age, and cigarette smoking. Can be 2° to drugs (eg, steroids, alcohol, anticonvulsants, anticoagulants, thyroid replacement therapy) or other conditions (eg, hyperparathyroidism, hyperthyroidism, multiple myeloma, malabsorption syndromes, anorexia), low BMI (or weight), and prolonged microgravity exposure (eg, space travel).

Diagnosed by bone mineral density measurement by DEXA (dual-energy x-ray absorptiometry) at the lumbar spine, total hip, and femoral neck, with a T-score of ≤ −2.5 or by a fragility fracture (eg, fall from standing height, minimal trauma) at hip or vertebra. One-time screening recommended in females ≥ 65 years old.

Prophylaxis: regular weight-bearing exercise and adequate $Ca^{2+}$ and vitamin D intake throughout adulthood.

Treatment: bisphosphonates, teriparatide, SERMs, denosumab (monoclonal antibody against RANKL), romosozumab (sclerostin inhibitor).

Can lead to vertebral compression fractures —acute back pain, loss of height, kyphosis. Also can present with fractures of femoral neck, distal radius (Colles fracture).

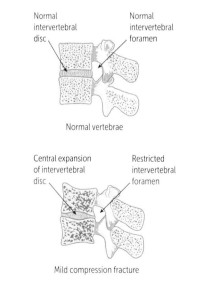

Normal intervertebral disc    Normal intervertebral foramen

Normal vertebrae

Central expansion of intervertebral disc    Restricted intervertebral foramen

Mild compression fracture

**Osteopetrosis**

Failure of normal bone resorption due to defective osteoclasts → thickened, dense bones that are prone to fracture. Mutations (eg, carbonic anhydrase II) impair ability of osteoclast to generate acidic environment necessary for bone resorption. Overgrowth of cortical bone fills marrow space → pancytopenia, extramedullary hematopoiesis. Can result in cranial nerve impingement and palsies due to narrowed foramina.

X-rays show diffuse symmetric sclerosis (bone-in-bone, "stone bone" A). Bone marrow transplant is potentially curative as osteoclasts are derived from monocytes.

**Osteomalacia/rickets**

Defective mineralization of osteoid (osteomalacia) or cartilaginous growth plates (rickets, only in children). Most commonly due to vitamin D deficiency.

X-rays show osteopenia and pseudofractures in osteomalacia, epiphyseal widening and metaphyseal cupping/fraying in rickets. Children with rickets have pathologic bow legs (genu varum A), beadlike costochondral junctions (rachitic rosary B), craniotabes (soft skull).

↓ vitamin D → ↓ serum $Ca^{2+}$ → ↑ PTH secretion → ↓ serum $PO_4^{3-}$.

Hyperactivity of osteoblasts → ↑ ALP.

**Osteitis deformans**

Also called Paget disease of bone. Common, localized disorder of bone remodeling caused by ↑ osteoclastic activity followed by ↑ osteoblastic activity that forms poor-quality bone. Serum $Ca^{2+}$, phosphorus, and PTH levels are normal. ↑ ALP. Mosaic pattern of woven and lamellar bone (osteocytes within lacunae in chaotic juxtapositions); long bone chalk-stick fractures. ↑ blood flow from ↑ arteriovenous shunts may cause high-output heart failure. ↑ risk of osteosarcoma.

Hat size can be increased due to skull thickening A; hearing loss is common due to skull deformity.

Stages of Paget disease:
- Early destructive (lytic): osteoclasts
- Intermediate (mixed): osteoclasts + osteoblasts
- Late (sclerotic/blastic): osteoblasts

May enter quiescent phase.

Treatment: bisphosphonates.

**Avascular necrosis of bone**

Infarction of bone and marrow, usually very painful. Most common site is femoral head (watershed area) A (due to insufficiency of medial circumflex femoral artery). Causes include glucoCorticoids, chronic Alcohol overuse, Sickle cell disease, Trauma, SLE, "the Bends" (caisson/decompression disease), LEgg-Calvé-Perthes disease (idiopathic), Gaucher disease, Slipped capital femoral epiphysis—CASTS Bend LEGS.

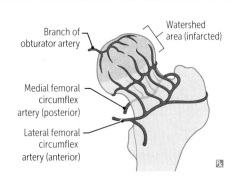

Branch of obturator artery

Watershed area (infarcted)

Medial femoral circumflex artery (posterior)

Lateral femoral circumflex artery (anterior)

## Lab values in bone disorders

| DISORDER | SERUM $Ca^{2+}$ | $PO_4^{3-}$ | ALP | PTH | COMMENTS |
|---|---|---|---|---|---|
| **Osteoporosis** | — | — | — | — | ↓ bone mass; if concurrent ↓ vitamin D → ↑ PTH with normal $Ca^{2+}$ |
| **Osteopetrosis** | —/↓ | — | — | — | Dense, brittle bones. $Ca^{2+}$ ↓ in severe, malignant disease |
| **Paget disease of bone** | — | — | ↑ | — | Abnormal "mosaic" bone architecture |
| **Osteitis fibrosa cystica** | | | | | |
| Primary hyperparathyroidism | ↑ | ↓ | ↑ | ↑ | "Brown tumors" due to fibrous replacement of bone, subperiosteal thinning<br>Idiopathic or parathyroid hyperplasia, adenoma, carcinoma |
| Secondary hyperparathyroidism | ↓ | ↑ | ↑ | ↑ | Often as compensation for CKD (↓ $PO_4^{3-}$ excretion and production of activated vitamin D) |
| **Osteomalacia/rickets** | ↓ | ↓ | ↑ | ↑ | Soft bones; vitamin D deficiency also causes 2° hyperparathyroidism |
| **Hypervitaminosis D** | ↑ | ↑ | — | ↓ | Caused by oversupplementation or granulomatous disease (eg, sarcoidosis) |

↑↓ = 1° change.

**Primary bone tumors**    Metastatic disease is more common than 1° bone tumors. Benign bone tumors that start with c and
o are more common in boys.

| TUMOR TYPE | EPIDEMIOLOGY | LOCATION | CHARACTERISTICS |
|---|---|---|---|
| **Benign tumors** | | | |
| **Osteochondroma (exostosis)** | Most common benign bone tumor<br>Males < 25 years old | Metaphysis of long bones (most common around knee—distal femur) | Lateral bony projection of growth plate (continuous with marrow space) covered by cartilaginous cap A; points away from joint<br>*EXT1* or *EXT2* gene mutation—hereditary multiple exostoses<br>Rarely transforms to chondrosarcoma |
| **Osteoma** | Middle age | Surface of facial bones | Associated with Gardner syndrome |
| **Osteoid osteoma** | Adults < 25 years old<br>Males > females | Cortex of long bones | Classically presents as bone pain (worse at night) caused by prostaglandins; thus relieved by NSAIDs (vs osteoblastoma)<br>Bony mass (< 1.5 cm) with radiolucent osteoid core B |
| **Osteoblastoma** | Males > females | Vertebrae | Similar histology to osteoid osteoma<br>Larger size (> 2 cm); pain unresponsive to NSAIDs<br>X-ray similar to aneurysmal bone cyst |
| **Giant cell tumor** | 20–40 years old<br>Females > males | Epiphysis of long bones after skeletal maturation (often in knee region), radiographic epicenter is metaphysis | Locally aggressive benign tumor neoplastic mononuclear cells that express RANKL and reactive multinucleated giant (osteoclastlike) cells; "osteoclastoma"<br>"Soap bubble" appearance on x-ray C |
| **Chondroblastoma** | Adolescents<br>Males > females | Epiphysis of long bones before skeletal maturation (often in knee region) | May complain of joint pain<br>Cross physis on x-ray |

**Primary bone tumors** *(continued)*

| TUMOR TYPE | EPIDEMIOLOGY | LOCATION | CHARACTERISTICS |
|---|---|---|---|
| **Malignant tumors** | | | |
| **Osteosarcoma (osteogenic sarcoma)** | Accounts for 20% of 1° bone cancers. Peak incidence of 1° tumor in males < 20 years. Less common in older adults; usually 2° to predisposing factors, such as Paget disease of bone, bone infarcts, radiation, familial retinoblastoma, Li-Fraumeni syndrome. | Metaphysis of long bones (often in knee region). | Pleomorphic osteoid-producing cells (malignant osteoblasts). Presents as painful enlarging mass or pathologic fractures. Codman triangle  (from elevation of periosteum) or sunburst pattern on x-ray (think of an osteocod [bone fish] swimming in the sun). Aggressive. 1° usually responsive to treatment (surgery, chemotherapy), poor prognosis for 2°. |
| **Chondrosarcoma** | Most common in adults > 50 years old. | Medulla of pelvis, proximal femur and humerus. | Tumor of malignant chondrocytes. Lytic (> 50%) cases with intralesional calcifications, endosteal erosion, cortex breach. |
| **Ewing sarcoma** | Most common in White patients, generally males < 15 years old. | Diaphysis of long bones (especially femur), pelvic flat bones. | Anaplastic small blue cells of neuroectodermal (mesenchymal) origin (resemble lymphocytes). Differentiate from conditions with similar morphology (eg, lymphoma, chronic osteomyelitis) by testing for t(11;22) (fusion protein EWS-FLI1). "Onion skin" periosteal reaction. Aggressive with early metastases, but responsive to chemotherapy. 11 + 22 = 33 (Patrick Ewing's jersey number). |

## Osteoarthritis vs rheumatoid arthritis

| | Osteoarthritis A | Rheumatoid arthritis B |
|---|---|---|
| PATHOGENESIS | Mechanical—wear and tear destroys articular cartilage (degenerative joint disorder) → inflammation with inadequate repair (mediated by chondrocytes). | Autoimmune—inflammation C induces formation of pannus (proliferative granulation tissue), which erodes articular cartilage and bone. |
| PREDISPOSING FACTORS | Age, female, obesity, joint trauma. | Female, HLA-DR4 (4-walled "rheum"), HLA-DRB1, tobacco smoking. ⊕ rheumatoid factor (IgM antibody that targets IgG Fc region; in 80%), anti-cyclic citrullinated peptide antibody (more specific). |
| PRESENTATION | Pain in weight-bearing joints after use (eg, at the end of the day), improving with rest. Asymmetric joint involvement. Knee cartilage loss begins medially ("bowlegged"). No systemic symptoms. | Pain, swelling, and morning stiffness lasting > 1 hour, improving with use. Symmetric joint involvement. Systemic symptoms (fever, fatigue, weight loss). Extraarticular manifestations common.* |
| JOINT FINDINGS | Osteophytes (bone spurs), joint space narrowing (asymmetric), subchondral sclerosis and cysts, loose bodies. Synovial fluid noninflammatory (WBC < 2000/mm³). Development of Heberden nodes D (at DIP) and Bouchard nodes E (at PIP), and 1st CMC; not MCP. | Erosions, juxta-articular osteopenia, soft tissue swelling, subchondral cysts, joint space narrowing (symmetric). Deformities: cervical subluxation, ulnar finger deviation, swan neck F, boutonniere G. Involves MCP, PIP, wrist; not DIP or 1st CMC. |
| TREATMENT | Activity modification, acetaminophen, NSAIDs, intra-articular glucocorticoids. | NSAIDs, glucocorticoids, disease-modifying agents (eg, methotrexate, sulfasalazine), biologic agents (eg, TNF-α inhibitors). |

*Extraarticular manifestations include cervical subluxation, rheumatoid nodules (fibrinoid necrosis with palisading histiocytes) in subcutaneous tissue and lung (+ pneumoconiosis = Caplan syndrome), interstitial lung disease, pleuritis, pericarditis, anemia of chronic disease, neutropenia + splenomegaly (Felty syndrome: **SANTA**—**S**plenomegaly, **A**nemia, **N**eutropenia, **T**hrombocytopenia, **A**rthritis [Rheumatoid]), AA amyloidosis, Sjögren syndrome, scleritis, carpal tunnel syndrome.

## Gout

**FINDINGS**

Acute inflammatory monoarthritis caused by precipitation of monosodium urate crystals in joints. Risk factors: male sex, hypertension, obesity, diabetes, dyslipidemia, alcohol use. Strongest risk factor is hyperuricemia, which can be caused by:

- Underexcretion of uric acid (90% of patients)—largely idiopathic, potentiated by renal failure; can be exacerbated by certain medications (eg, thiazide diuretics).
- Overproduction of uric acid (10% of patients)—Lesch-Nyhan syndrome, PRPP excess, ↑ cell turnover (eg, tumor lysis syndrome).
- Combined mechanism—alcohol use and von Gierke disease.

Crystals are needle shaped and ⊖ birefringent under polarized light (yellow under parallel light, blue under perpendicular light ). Serum uric acid levels may be normal during an acute attack.

**SYMPTOMS**

Asymmetric joint distribution. Joint is swollen, red, and painful. Classic manifestation is painful MTP joint of big toe (podagra). Tophus formation **B** (often on external ear, olecranon bursa, or Achilles tendon). Acute attack tends to occur after a large meal with foods rich in purines (eg, red meat, seafood), trauma, surgery, dehydration, diuresis, or alcohol consumption (↑ blood lactate from metabolism → ↑ resorption of uric acid → hyperuricemia).

**TREATMENT**

Acute: NSAIDs (eg, indomethacin), glucocorticoids, colchicine.
Chronic (preventive): xanthine oxidase inhibitors (eg, allopurinol, febuxostat).

---

**Calcium pyrophosphate deposition disease**

Formerly called pseudogout. Deposition of calcium pyrophosphate crystals within the joint space. Occurs in patients > 50 years old; both sexes affected equally. Usually idiopathic, sometimes associated with hemochromatosis, hyperparathyroidism, joint trauma.
Pain and swelling with acute inflammation (pseudogout) and/or chronic degeneration (pseudo-osteoarthritis). Most commonly affected joint is the knee.

Chondrocalcinosis (cartilage calcification) on x-ray.
Crystals are rhomboid and weakly ⊕ birefringent under polarized light (blue when parallel to light) **A**.
Acute treatment: NSAIDs, colchicine, glucocorticoids.
Prophylaxis: colchicine.
The blue P's of CPPD—blue (when parallel), positive birefringence, calcium pyrophosphate, pseudogout.

**Systemic juvenile idiopathic arthritis**

Systemic arthritis seen in < 16 years of age. Usually presents with daily spiking fevers, salmon-pink macular rash, arthritis (commonly 2+ joints). Associated with anterior uveitis. Frequently presents with leukocytosis, thrombocytosis, anemia, ↑ ESR, ↑ CRP.

**Sjögren syndrome**

Autoimmune disorder characterized by destruction of exocrine glands (especially lacrimal and salivary) by lymphocytic infiltrates. Predominantly affects females 40–60 years old.

Findings:

- Inflammatory joint pain
- Keratoconjunctivitis sicca (decreased tear production and subsequent corneal damage) → gritty or sandy feeling in eyes
- Xerostomia (↓ saliva production) → mucosal atrophy, fissuring of the tongue
- Presence of antinuclear antibodies, rheumatoid factor (can be positive in the absence of rheumatoid arthritis), antiribonucleoprotein antibodies: SS-A (anti-Ro) and/or SS-B (anti-La)
- Bilateral parotid enlargement

Anti-SSA and anti-SSB may also be seen in SLE.

A common 1° disorder or a 2° syndrome associated with other autoimmune disorders (eg, rheumatoid arthritis, SLE, systemic sclerosis).

Complications: dental caries; mucosa-associated lymphoid tissue (MALT) lymphoma (may present as parotid enlargement); ↑ risk of giving birth to baby with neonatal lupus.

Focal lymphocytic sialadenitis on labial salivary gland biopsy can confirm diagnosis.

**Septic arthritis**

*S aureus*, *Streptococcus*, and *Neisseria gonorrhoeae* are common causes. Usually monoarticular. Affected joint is often swollen A, red, and painful. Synovial fluid purulent (WBC > 50,000/mm³). Complications: osteomyelitis, chronic pain, irreversible joint damage, sepsis. Treatment: antibiotics, aspiration, and drainage (+/− debridement) to prevent irreversible joint damage.

Disseminated gonococcal infection—STI that presents as either purulent arthritis (eg, knee) or triad of polyarthralgia, tenosynovitis (eg, hand), dermatitis (eg, pustules).

**Osteomyelitis**

Chronic or acute infection of the bone; *S aureus* most common (overall), *S epidermidis* (prosthetics), *Salmonella* (sickle cell anemia), *P aeruginosa* (plantar puncture wounds). Spread is commonly hematogenous (usually in children, affecting the metaphysis of the long bones) or exogenous (usually in adults, post-traumatic, iatrogenic, or spread from nearby tissues). Pain, redness, swelling, fever, limping are common.

Diagnosis: x-ray (bone destruction and periosteal elevation if chronic), MRI, bone biopsy with cultures and blood cultures.

Treatment: antibiotics (+/− surgery).

| | | |
|---|---|---|
| **Seronegative spondyloarthritis** | Arthritis without rheumatoid factor (no anti-IgG antibody). Strong association with HLA-B27 (MHC class I serotype). Subtypes (**PAIR**) share variable occurrence of inflammatory back pain (associated with morning stiffness, improves with exercise), peripheral arthritis, enthesitis (inflamed insertion sites of tendons, eg, Achilles), dactylitis ("sausage fingers"), uveitis. | |
| **Psoriatic arthritis** | Associated with skin psoriasis and nail lesions. Asymmetric and patchy involvement **A**. Dactylitis and "pencil-in-cup" deformity of DIP on x-ray **B**. | Seen in fewer than 1/3 of patients with psoriasis. |
| **Ankylosing spondylitis** | Symmetric involvement of spine and sacroiliac joints → ankylosis (joint fusion), uveitis, aortic regurgitation. | Bamboo spine (vertebral fusion) **C**. Costovertebral and costosternal ankylosis may cause restrictive lung disease. More common in males, with age of onset usually 20–40 years. |
| **Inflammatory bowel disease** | Crohn disease and ulcerative colitis are often associated with spondyloarthritis. | |
| **Reactive arthritis** | Classic triad:<br>▪ Conjunctivitis<br>▪ Urethritis<br>▪ Arthritis<br>Commonly associated with hyperkeratotic skin lesions in the palms and soles (keratoderma blennorrhagica). | "Can't see, can't pee, can't bend my knee." Associated with infections by *Shigella*, *Campylobacter*, *E coli*, *Salmonella*, *Chlamydia*, *Yersinia*. "She Caught Every Student Cheating Yesterday and overreacted." |

**Systemic lupus erythematosus**

Systemic, remitting, and relapsing autoimmune disease. Organ damage primarily due to a type III hypersensitivity reaction and, to a lesser degree, a type II hypersensitivity reaction. Associated with deficiency of early complement proteins (eg, C1q, C4, C2) → ↓ clearance of immune complexes. Classic presentation: facial rash (spares nasolabial folds), joint pain, and fever in a female of reproductive age. ↑ prevalence in Black, Caribbean, Asian, and Hispanic populations in the US.

Libman-Sacks Endocarditis (**LSE** in **SLE**).

Lupus nephritis (glomerular deposition of DNA-anti-DNA immune complexes) can be nephritic or nephrotic (causing hematuria or proteinuria). Most common and severe type is diffuse proliferative.

Common causes of death in SLE: renal disease (most common), infections, cardiovascular disease (accelerated CAD). Lupus patients die with redness in their cheeks.

In an anti-SSA ⊕ pregnant patient, ↑ risk of newborn developing neonatal lupus → congenital heart block, periorbital/diffuse rash, transaminitis, and cytopenias at birth.

**RASH OR PAIN**:

Rash (malar  or discoid **B**)

Arthritis (nonerosive)

Serositis (eg, pleuritis, pericarditis)

Hematologic disorders (eg, cytopenias)

Oral/nasopharyngeal ulcers (usually painless)

Renal disease

Photosensitivity

Antinuclear antibodies

Immunologic disorder (anti-dsDNA, anti-Sm, antiphospholipid)

Neurologic disorders (eg, seizures, psychosis)

**Mixed connective tissue disease**

Features of SLE, systemic sclerosis, and/or polymyositis. Associated with anti-U1 RNP antibodies (speckled ANA).

**Antiphospholipid syndrome**

1° or 2° autoimmune disorder (most commonly in SLE).

Diagnosed based on clinical criteria including history of thrombosis (arterial or venous) or recurrent abortion along with laboratory findings of lupus anticoagulant, anticardiolipin, anti-$\beta_2$ glycoprotein I antibodies.

Treatment: systemic anticoagulation.

Anticardiolipin antibodies can cause false-positive VDRL/RPR.

Lupus anticoagulant can cause prolonged PTT that is not corrected by the addition of normal platelet-free plasma.

## Polymyalgia rheumatica

| | |
|---|---|
| SYMPTOMS | Pain and stiffness in proximal muscles (eg, shoulders, hips), often with fever, malaise, weight loss. Does not cause muscular weakness. More common in females > 50 years old; associated with giant cell (temporal) arteritis. |
| FINDINGS | ↑ ESR, ↑ CRP, normal CK. |
| TREATMENT | Rapid response to low-dose glucocorticoids. |

## Fibromyalgia

Most common in females 20–50 years old. Chronic, widespread musculoskeletal pain associated with "tender points," stiffness, paresthesias, poor sleep, fatigue, cognitive disturbance ("fibro fog"). Normal inflammatory markers like ESR. Treatment: regular exercise, antidepressants (TCAs, SNRIs), neuropathic pain agents (eg, gabapentinoids).

## Polymyositis/ dermatomyositis

Nonspecific: ⊕ ANA, ↑ CK. Specific: ⊕ anti-Jo-1 (histidyl-tRNA synthetase), ⊕ anti-SRP (signal recognition particle), ⊕ anti-Mi-2 (helicase).

### Polymyositis

Progressive symmetric proximal muscle weakness, characterized by endomysial inflammation with CD8+ T cells. Most often involves shoulders.

### Dermatomyositis

Clinically similar to polymyositis, but also involves Gottron papules , photodistributed facial erythema (eg, heliotrope [violaceous] edema of the eyelids ), "shawl and face" rash , mechanic's hands (thickening, cracking, irregular "dirty"-appearing marks due to hyperkeratosis of digital skin . ↑ risk of occult malignancy. Perimysial inflammation and atrophy with CD4+ T cells.

## Myositis ossificans

Heterotopic ossification involving skeletal muscle (eg, quadriceps). Associated with blunt muscle trauma. Presents as painful soft tissue mass. Imaging: eggshell calcification. Histology: metaplastic bone surrounding area of fibroblastic proliferation. Benign, but may be mistaken for sarcoma.

## IgG4-related disease

Immune-mediated spectrum of conditions, characterized by fibrosis and lymphoplasmacytic infiltrate, that can affect multiple organs. Patients usually have elevated serum IgG4 levels. Most common IgG4-related conditions are:

- Sialadenitis and dacryoadenitis
- Riedel thyroiditis
- Autoimmune pancreatitis
- Autoimmune aortitis (may lead to TAA, AAA)
- Retroperitoneal fibrosis (may affect the ureters and present with signs of acute kidney injury/ CKD and/or hydronephrosis)

## Vasculitides

| | EPIDEMIOLOGY/PRESENTATION | NOTES |
|---|---|---|
| **Large-vessel vasculitis** | | |
| **Giant cell (temporal) arteritis** | Females > 50 years old. Unilateral headache, possible temporal artery tenderness, jaw claudication. May lead to irreversible blindness due to anterior ischemic optic neuropathy. Associated with polymyalgia rheumatica. Most commonly affects carotid artery branches. | May also cause aortitis or vertebral artery infarct. Focal granulomatous inflammation ▣. ↑↑ ESR. IL-6 levels correlate with disease activity. Treat with high-dose glucocorticoids prior to temporal artery biopsy to prevent blindness. |
| **Takayasu arteritis** | Usually Asian females < 40 years old. "Pulseless disease" (weak upper extremity pulses), fever, night sweats, arthritis, myalgias, skin nodules, ocular disturbances. | Granulomatous thickening and narrowing of aortic arch and proximal great vessels ▣. ↑ ESR. Treatment: glucocorticoids. |
| **Medium-vessel vasculitis** | | |
| **Buerger disease (thromboangiitis obliterans)** | Heavy tobacco smoking history, males < 40 years old. Intermittent claudication. May lead to gangrene ▣, autoamputation of digits, superficial nodular phlebitis. | Raynaud phenomenon is often present. Segmental thrombosing vasculitis with vein and nerve involvement. Treatment: smoking cessation. |
| **Kawasaki disease** | Usually Asian children < 4 years old. Bilateral nonexudative bulbar Conjunctivitis, Rash (polymorphous → desquamating), Adenopathy (cervical), Strawberry tongue (oral mucositis) ▣, Hand-foot changes (edema, erythema), fever (≥ 5 days). | Formerly called mucocutaneous lymph node syndrome. **CRASH** and **burn** on a **Kawasaki**. May develop coronary artery aneurysms ▣; thrombosis or rupture can cause death. Treatment: IV immunoglobulin and aspirin. |
| **Polyarteritis nodosa** | Usually middle-aged males. Hepatitis B seropositivity in 30% of patients. Fever, weight loss, malaise, headache. GI: abdominal pain, melena. Hypertension, neurologic dysfunction, cutaneous eruptions, renal damage. Typically involves renal and visceral vessels, spares pulmonary arteries. | Different stages of transmural inflammation with fibrinoid necrosis. Innumerable renal microaneurysms ▣ and spasms on arteriogram (string of pearls appearance). Treatment: glucocorticoids, cyclophosphamide. PAN usually affects the **SKIN**: Skin, Kidneys, Intestines (GI), Nerves. |
| **Small-vessel vasculitis** | | |
| **Behçet syndrome** | ↑ incidence in people of Turkish and eastern Mediterranean descent. Recurrent aphthous ulcers, genital ulcerations, uveitis, erythema nodosum. Can be precipitated by HSV or parvovirus. Flares last 1–4 weeks. | Immune complex vasculitis. Associated with HLA-B51. |
| **Cutaneous small-vessel vasculitis** | Occurs 7–10 days after certain medications (penicillins, cephalosporins, sulfonamides, phenytoin, allopurinol) or infections (eg, HCV, HIV). Palpable purpura, no visceral involvement. | Immune complex–mediated leukocytoclastic vasculitis; late involvement indicates systemic vasculitis. |

## Vasculitides *(continued)*

| | EPIDEMIOLOGY/PRESENTATION | NOTES |
|---|---|---|
| **Small-vessel vasculitis** *(continued)* | | |
| **Eosinophilic granulomatosis with polyangiitis** | Asthma, sinusitis, skin nodules or purpura, peripheral neuropathy (eg, wrist/foot drop). Can also involve heart, GI, kidneys (pauci-immune glomerulonephritis). | Formerly called Churg-Strauss syndrome. Granulomatous, necrotizing vasculitis with eosinophilia **G**. MPO-ANCA/p-ANCA, ↑ IgE level. |
| **Granulomatosis with polyangiitis** | Upper respiratory tract: perforation of nasal septum, chronic sinusitis, otitis media, mastoiditis. Lower respiratory tract: hemoptysis, cough, dyspnea. Renal: pauci-immune rapidly progressive glomerulonephritis (hematuria, red cell casts). Skin: purpura, typically on lower extremities. | Triad: <ul><li>Focal necrotizing vasculitis</li><li>Necrotizing granulomas in lung and upper airway</li><li>Necrotizing glomerulonephritis</li></ul> PR3-ANCA/c-ANCA **H** (anti-proteinase 3). CXR: large nodular densities. Treatment: glucocorticoids in combination with rituximab or cyclophosphamide. |
| **Immunoglobulin A vasculitis** | Most common childhood systemic vasculitis. Often follows URI. Classic triad: <ul><li>Hinge pain (arthralgias)</li><li>Stomach pain (abdominal pain associated with intussusception)</li><li>Palpable purpura on buttocks/legs **I**</li></ul> | Formerly called Henoch-Schönlein purpura. Vasculitis 2° to IgA immune complex deposition. Associated with IgA nephropathy (Berger disease). Treatment: supportive care, possibly glucocorticoids. |
| **Microscopic polyangiitis** | Necrotizing vasculitis commonly involving lung, kidneys, and skin with pauci-immune glomerulonephritis **J** and palpable purpura. Presentation similar to granulomatosis with polyangiitis but without nasopharyngeal involvement. | No granulomas. MPO-ANCA/p-ANCA (anti-myeloperoxidase). Treatment: cyclophosphamide, glucocorticoids. |
| **Mixed cryoglobulinemia** | Often due to viral infections, especially HCV. Triad of palpable purpura, weakness, arthralgias. May also have peripheral neuropathy and renal disease (eg, glomerulonephritis). | Cryoglobulins are immunoglobulins that precipitate in the Cold. Vasculitis due to mixed IgG and IgM immune complex deposition. |

## Neuromuscular junction diseases

| | Myasthenia gravis | Lambert-Eaton myasthenic syndrome |
|---|---|---|
| FREQUENCY | Most common NMJ disorder | Uncommon |
| PATHOPHYSIOLOGY | Autoantibodies to postsynaptic ACh receptor | Autoantibodies to presynaptic $Ca^{2+}$ channel → ↓ ACh release; L comes before M |
| CLINICAL | Fatigable muscle weakness—ptosis; diplopia; proximal weakness; respiratory muscle involvement → dyspnea; bulbar muscle involvement → dysphagia, difficulty chewing | Proximal muscle weakness, autonomic symptoms (dry mouth, constipation, impotence) |
| | Spared reflexes | Hyporeflexia |
| | Worsens with muscle use | Improves with muscle use |
| ASSOCIATED WITH | Thymoma, thymic hyperplasia | Small cell lung cancer |
| AChE INHIBITOR ADMINISTRATION | Reverses symptoms (pyridostigmine for treatment) | Minimal effect |

Myasthenia gravis

Lambert-Eaton myasthenic syndrome

| **Raynaud phenomenon** | ↓ blood flow to skin due to arteriolar (small vessel) vasospasm in response to cold or stress: color change from white (ischemia) to blue (hypoxia) to red (reperfusion). Most often in the fingers A and toes. Called Raynaud disease when 1° (idiopathic), Raynaud syndrome when 2° to a disease process such as mixed connective tissue disease, SLE, or CREST syndrome (limited form of systemic sclerosis). Digital ulceration (critical ischemia) seen in 2° Raynaud syndrome. Treat with calcium channel blockers. |
|---|---|

**Scleroderma**

Systemic sclerosis. Triad of autoimmunity, noninflammatory vasculopathy, and collagen deposition with fibrosis. Commonly sclerosis of skin, manifesting as puffy, taut skin **A** without wrinkles, fingertip pitting **B**. Can involve other systems, eg, renal (scleroderma renal crisis; treat with ACE inhibitors), pulmonary (interstitial fibrosis, pulmonary HTN), GI (↓ peristalsis and LES tone → dysphagia, heartburn), cardiovascular. 75% female. 2 major types:

- **Diffuse scleroderma**—widespread skin involvement, rapid progression, early visceral involvement. Associated with anti-Scl-70 antibody (anti-DNA topoisomerase-I antibody) and anti-RNA polymerase III.

- **Limited scleroderma**—limited skin involvement confined to fingers and face. Also with CREST syndrome: Calcinosis cutis **C**, anti-Centromere antibody, Raynaud phenomenon, Esophageal dysmotility, Sclerodactyly, and Telangiectasia. More benign clinical course.

---

### ▶ MUSCULOSKELETAL, SKIN, AND CONNECTIVE TISSUE—DERMATOLOGY

**Skin layers**

Skin has 3 layers: epidermis, dermis, subcutaneous fat (hypodermis, subcutis).
Epidermal layers: come, let's get sunburned.

## Epithelial cell junctions

Apical

Tight junction — Claudin/occludin

Adherens junction — Cadherins

Desmosome — Intermediate filaments

Gap junction — Connexon

Basal

Hemidesmosome — Integrin / Fibronectin/laminin / ECM/collagen

Tight junctions (zonula occludens) **A**—prevents paracellular movement of solutes; composed of claudins and occludins.

Adherens junction (belt desmosome, zonula adherens) **B**—forms "belt" connecting actin cytoskeletons of adjacent cells with **cad**herins (Ca$^{2+}$-dependent **ad**hesion proteins). Loss of E-cadherin promotes metastasis.

Desmosome (spot desmosome, macula adherens) **C**—structural support via intermediate filament interactions. Autoantibodies to desmoglein 3 +/– desmoglein 1 → pemphigus vulgaris.

Gap junction **D**—channel proteins called connexons permit electrical and chemical communication between cells.

Hemidesmosome **E**—connects keratin in basal cells to underlying basement membrane. Autoantibodies → **bullous** pemphigoid. (Hemidesmosomes are down "**bullow**.")

**Integrins**—membrane proteins that maintain **integrity** of basolateral membrane by binding to collagen, laminin, and fibronectin in basement membrane.

## Exocrine glands

Glands that produce substances other than hormones (vs endocrine glands, which secrete hormones) that are released through ducts to the exterior of the body. Can be merocrine (eg, salivary and sweat glands), apocrine (eg, mammary glands), or holocrine (eg, sebaceous glands).

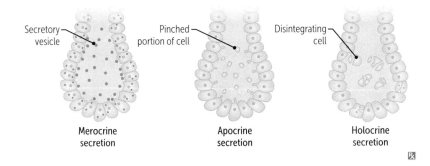

Secretory vesicle — Merocrine secretion

Pinched portion of cell — Apocrine secretion

Disintegrating cell — Holocrine secretion

## Dermatologic macroscopic terms

| LESION | CHARACTERISTICS | EXAMPLES |
| --- | --- | --- |
| Macule | Flat lesion with well-circumscribed change in skin color < 1 cm | Freckle (ephelis), labial macule **A** |
| Patch | Macule > 1 cm | Vitiligo **B** |
| Papule | Elevated solid skin lesion < 1 cm | Neurofibroma **C**, acne |
| Plaque | Papule > 1 cm | Psoriasis **D** |
| Vesicle | Small fluid-containing blister < 1 cm | Chickenpox (varicella), shingles (zoster) **E** |
| Bulla | Large fluid-containing blister > 1 cm | Bullous pemphigoid **F** |
| Pustule | Vesicle containing pus | Pustular psoriasis **G** |
| Wheal | Transient smooth papule or plaque | Hives (urticaria) **H** |
| Scale | Flaking off of stratum corneum | Eczema, psoriasis, SCC **I** |
| Crust | Dry exudate | Impetigo **J** |

## Dermatologic microscopic terms

| LESION | CHARACTERISTICS | EXAMPLES |
| --- | --- | --- |
| Dyskeratosis | Abnormal premature keratinization | Squamous cell carcinoma |
| Hyperkeratosis | ↑ thickness of stratum corneum | Psoriasis, calluses |
| Parakeratosis | Retention of nuclei in stratum corneum | Psoriasis, actinic keratosis |
| Hypergranulosis | ↑ thickness of stratum granulosum | Lichen planus |
| Spongiosis | Epidermal accumulation of edematous fluid in intercellular spaces | Eczematous dermatitis |
| Acantholysis | Separation of epidermal cells | Pemphigus vulgaris |
| Acanthosis | Epidermal hyperplasia (↑ spinosum) | Acanthosis nigricans, psoriasis |

## Pigmented skin disorders

| | |
|---|---|
| Albinism | Normal melanocyte number with ↓ melanin production  due to ↓ tyrosinase activity or defective tyrosine transport. ↑ risk of skin cancer. |
| Melasma (chloasma) | Acquired hyperpigmentation associated with pregnancy ("mask of pregnancy" B) or OCP use. More common in patients with darker skin tones. |
| Vitiligo | Irregular patches of complete depigmentation C. Caused by destruction of melanocytes (believed to be autoimmune). Associated with other autoimmune disorders. |
| Waardenburg syndrome | Patchy depigmentation of skin, hair, and irises that can be associated with deafness. Caused by defects in the differentiation of neural crest cells into melanocytes. |

**Seborrheic dermatitis**

Erythematous, well-demarcated plaques A with greasy yellow scales in areas rich in sebaceous glands, such as scalp, face, and periocular region. Common in both infants (cradle cap) and adults. Extensive disease may be associated with HIV infection and Parkinson disease. Sebaceous glands are not inflamed, but play a role in disease development. Possibly associated with *Malassezia* spp. Treatment: topical antifungals and glucocorticoids.

## Common skin disorders

| | |
|---|---|
| Acne | Multifactorial etiology—↑ sebum/androgen production, abnormal keratinocyte desquamation, *Cutibacterium acnes* colonization of the pilosebaceous unit (comedones), and inflammation (papules/pustules **A**, nodules, cysts). Treatment: retinoids, benzoyl peroxide, and antibiotics. |
| Atopic dermatitis (eczema) | Pruritic eruption associated with ichthyosis vulgaris and other atopic diseases (asthma, allergic rhinitis, food allergies); ↑ serum IgE. Often appears on face in infancy **B** and then on flexural surfaces **C** in children and adults. |
| Allergic contact dermatitis | Type IV hypersensitivity reaction secondary to contact allergen (eg, nickel **D**, poison ivy **E**, neomycin). |
| Keratosis pilaris | Follicular-based papules from keratin plugging, most often on extensor surfaces of arms and thighs. |
| Melanocytic nevus | Common mole. Benign, but melanoma can arise in congenital or atypical moles. Intradermal nevi are papular **F**. Junctional nevi are flat macules **G**. |
| Pseudofolliculitis barbae | Inflammatory reaction to hair penetrating the skin characterized by firm papules and pustules that are painful and pruritic. Commonly occurs near jawline as a result of shaving ("razor bumps"), more common with naturally curly hair. |
| Psoriasis | Papules and plaques with silvery scaling **H**, especially on knees and elbows. Acanthosis with parakeratotic scaling (nuclei still in stratum corneum), Munro microabscesses. ↑ stratum spinosum, ↓ stratum granulosum. Auspitz sign (**I**)—pinpoint bleeding spots from exposure of dermal papillae when scales are scraped off. Associated with nail pitting and psoriatic arthritis. |
| Rosacea | Inflammatory facial skin disorder characterized by erythematous papules and pustules **J**, but no comedones. May be associated with facial flushing in response to external stimuli (eg, alcohol, heat). Complications include ocular involvement, rhinophyma (bulbous deformation of nose). |
| Seborrheic keratosis | Well-demarcated, verrucous, benign squamous epithelial proliferation of immature keratinocytes with keratin-filled cysts (horn cysts) **K**. Looks "stuck on." Leser-Trélat sign **L**—rapid onset of multiple seborrheic keratoses, indicates possible malignancy (eg, GI adenocarcinoma). |
| Verrucae | Warts; caused by low-risk HPV strains. Soft, tan-colored, cauliflowerlike papules **M**. Epidermal hyperplasia, hyperkeratosis, koilocytosis. Condyloma acuminatum on anus or genitals **N**. |
| Urticaria | Hives. Pruritic wheals that form after mast cell degranulation **O**. Characterized by superficial dermal edema and lymphatic channel dilation. |

## Vascular tumors of skin

| | |
|---|---|
| **Angiosarcoma** | Rare blood vessel malignancy typically occurring in the head, neck, and breast areas. Usually in older adults, on sun-exposed areas. Associated with radiation therapy and chronic postmastectomy lymphedema. Stewart-Treves syndrome—cutaneous angiosarcoma developing after chronic lymphedema. Hepatic angiosarcoma associated with vinyl chloride and arsenic exposures. Very aggressive and difficult to resect due to delay in diagnosis. |
| **Bacillary angiomatosis** | Benign capillary skin papules  found in patients with AIDS. Caused by *Bartonella* infections. Frequently mistaken for Kaposi sarcoma, but has neutrophilic infiltrate. |
| **Cherry angioma** | Benign capillary hemangioma  commonly appearing in middle-aged adults. Does not regress. Frequency ↑ with age. |
| **Glomus tumor** | Benign, painful, red-blue tumor, commonly under fingernails . Arises from modified smooth muscle cells of the thermoregulatory glomus body. |
| **Kaposi sarcoma** | Endothelial malignancy most commonly affecting the skin, mouth, GI tract, respiratory tract. Classically seen in older Eastern European males, patients with AIDS, and organ transplant patients. Associated with HHV-8 and HIV. Lymphocytic infiltrate, unlike bacillary angiomatosis. |
| **Pyogenic granuloma** | Polypoid lobulated capillary hemangioma  that can ulcerate and bleed. Associated with trauma and pregnancy. |
| **Infantile hemangioma** | Benign capillary hemangioma of infancy . Appears in first few weeks of life (1/200 births); initially grows rapidly, then involutes starting at age 1. Infantile hemangiomas spontaneously involute; cherry angiomas cannot. |

## Skin infections

### Bacterial infections

| | |
|---|---|
| Impetigo | Skin infection involving superficial epidermis. Usually from S aureus or S pyogenes. Highly contagious. Honey-colored crusting **A**.<br>Bullous impetigo **B** has bullae and is usually caused by S aureus. |
| Erysipelas | Infection involving upper dermis and superficial lymphatics, usually from S pyogenes. Presents with well-defined, raised demarcation between infected and normal skin **C**. |
| Cellulitis | Acute, painful, spreading infection of deeper dermis and subcutaneous tissues. Usually from S pyogenes or S aureus. Often starts with a break in skin from trauma or another infection **D**. |
| Abscess | Collection of pus from a walled-off infection within deeper layers of skin **E**. Offending organism is almost always S aureus. |
| Necrotizing fasciitis | Deeper tissue injury, usually from anaerobic bacteria or S pyogenes. Pain may be out of proportion to exam findings. Results in crepitus from methane and $CO_2$ production. "Flesh-eating bacteria." Causes bullae and skin necrosis → violaceous color of bullae, surrounding skin **F**. Surgical emergency. |
| Staphylococcal scalded skin syndrome | Exotoxin destroys keratinocyte attachments in stratum granulosum only (vs toxic epidermal necrolysis, which destroys epidermal-dermal junction). No mucosal involvement. Characterized by fever and generalized erythematous rash with sloughing of the upper layers of the epidermis **G** that heals completely. ⊕ Nikolsky sign (separation of epidermis upon manual stroking of skin). Commonly seen in newborns and children/adults with renal insufficiency. |

### Viral infections

| | |
|---|---|
| Herpes | Herpes virus infections (HSV-1 and HSV-2) of skin can occur anywhere from mucosal surfaces to normal skin. These include herpes labialis, herpes genitalis, herpetic whitlow **H** (finger). |
| Molluscum contagiosum | Umbilicated papules **I** caused by a poxvirus. While frequently seen in children, it may be sexually transmitted in adults. |
| Varicella zoster | Causes varicella (chickenpox) and zoster (shingles). Varicella presents with multiple crops of lesions in various stages from vesicles to crusts. Zoster is a reactivation of the virus in dermatomal distribution (unless it is disseminated). |
| Hairy leukoplakia | Irregular, white, painless plaques on lateral tongue that cannot be scraped off **J**. EBV mediated. Occurs in patients living with HIV, organ transplant recipients. Contrast with thrush (scrapable) and leukoplakia (precancerous). |

## Cutaneous mycoses

| | |
|---|---|
| **Tinea (dermatophytes)** | Clinical name for dermatophyte (cutaneous fungal) infections. Dermatophytes include *Microsporum, Trichophyton,* and *Epidermophyton.* Branching septate hyphae visible on KOH preparation with blue fungal stain **A**. Associated with pruritus. |
| Tinea capitis | Occurs on head, scalp. Associated with lymphadenopathy, alopecia, scaling **B**. |
| Tinea corporis | Occurs on body (usually torso). Characterized by enlarging erythematous, scaly rings ("ringworm") with central clearing **C**. Can be acquired from contact with infected pets or farm animals. |
| Tinea cruris | Occurs in inguinal area ("jock itch") **D**. Often does not show the central clearing seen in tinea corporis. |
| Tinea pedis | Three varieties ("athlete's foot"):<br>▪ Interdigital **E**; most common<br>▪ Moccasin distribution **F**<br>▪ Vesicular type |
| Tinea unguium | Onychomycosis; occurs on nails. |
| **Tinea (pityriasis) versicolor** | Caused by *Malassezia* spp. (*Pityrosporum* spp.), a yeastlike fungus (not a dermatophyte despite being called tinea). Degradation of lipids produces acids that inhibit tyrosinase (involved in melanin synthesis) → hypopigmentation **G**; hyperpigmentation and/or pink patches can also occur due to inflammatory response. Less pruritic than dermatophytes.<br>Can occur any time of year, but more common in summer (hot, humid weather). "Spaghetti and meatballs" appearance on microscopy **H**.<br>Treatment: selenium sulfide, topical and/or oral antifungal medications. |

**Autoimmune blistering skin disorders**

| | Pemphigus vulgaris | Bullous pemphigoid |
|---|---|---|
| PATHOPHYSIOLOGY | Potentially fatal. Most commonly seen in older adults. Type II hypersensitivity reaction. IgG antibodies against desmoglein 3 +/– desmoglein 1 (component of desmosomes, which connect keratinocytes in the stratum spinosum). | Less severe than pemphigus vulgaris. Most commonly seen in older adults. Type II hypersensitivity reaction. IgG antibodies against hemidesmosomes (epidermal basement membrane; antibodies are "bullow" the epidermis). |
| GROSS MORPHOLOGY | Flaccid intraepidermal bullae A caused by acantholysis (separation of keratinocytes, "row of tombstones" on H&E stain); oral mucosa is involved. Nikolsky sign ⊕. | Tense blisters C containing eosinophils; oral mucosa spared. Nikolsky sign ⊖. |
| IMMUNOFLUORESCENCE | Reticular pattern around epidermal cells B. | Linear pattern at epidermal-dermal junction D. |

## Other blistering skin disorders

| | |
|---|---|
| Dermatitis herpetiformis | Pruritic papules, vesicles, and bullae (often found on elbows, knees, buttocks) . Deposits of IgA at tips of dermal papillae. Associated with celiac disease. Treatment: dapsone, gluten-free diet. |
| Erythema multiforme | Associated with infections (eg, *Mycoplasma pneumoniae*, HSV), drugs (eg, sulfa drugs, β-lactams, phenytoin). Presents with multiple types of lesions—macules, papules, vesicles, target lesions (look like targets with multiple rings and dusky center showing epithelial disruption) . |
| Stevens-Johnson syndrome | Characterized by fever, bullae formation and necrosis, sloughing of skin at dermal-epidermal junction (⊕ Nikolsky), high mortality rate. Typically mucous membranes are involved . Targetoid skin lesions may appear, as seen in erythema multiforme. Usually associated with adverse drug reaction. Toxic epidermal necrolysis (TEN)   is more severe form of SJS involving > 30% body surface area. 10–30% involvement denotes SJS-TEN. |

## Cutaneous ulcers

| | Venous ulcer | Arterial ulcer | Neuropathic ulcer | Pressure injury |
|---|---|---|---|---|
| ETIOLOGY | Chronic venous insufficiency; most common ulcer type | Peripheral artery disease (eg, atherosclerotic stenosis) | Peripheral neuropathy (eg, diabetic foot) | Prolonged unrelieved pressure (eg, immobility) |
| LOCATION | Gaiter area (ankle to midcalf), typically over malleoli | Distal toes, anterior shin, pressure points | Bony prominences (eg, metatarsal heads, heel) | Weightbearing points (eg, sacrum, ischium, calcaneus) |
| APPEARANCE | Irregular border, shallow, exudative  | Symmetric with well-defined punched-out appearance  | Hyperkeratotic edge with undermined borders  | Varies based on stage from non-blanchable erythema to full-thickness skin loss  |
| PAIN | Mild to moderate | Severe | Absent | Present |
| ASSOCIATED SIGNS | Telangiectasias, varicose veins, edema, stasis dermatitis (erythematous eczematous patches) | Arterial insufficiency, cold and pale atrophic skin, hair loss, absent pulses | Claw toes, Charcot joints, absent reflexes | Soft tissue infection and osteomyelitis are frequent complications |

## Miscellaneous skin disorders

| | |
|---|---|
| **Acanthosis nigricans** | Epidermal hyperplasia causing symmetric, hyperpigmented thickening of skin, especially in axilla or on neck A. Associated with insulin resistance (eg, diabetes, obesity, Cushing syndrome, PCOS), visceral malignancy (eg, gastric adenocarcinoma). |
| **Erythema nodosum** | Painful, raised inflammatory lesions of subcutaneous fat (panniculitis), usually on anterior shins. Often idiopathic, but can be associated with sarcoidosis, coccidioidomycosis, histoplasmosis, TB, streptococcal infections B, leprosy C, inflammatory bowel disease. |
| **Ichthyosis vulgaris** | Disorder of defective keratinocyte desquamation due to filaggrin gene mutations resulting in diffuse scaling of the skin D most commonly on the extensor side of extremities and the trunk. Manifests in infancy or early childhood. Strong association with atopic dermatitis. |
| **Lichen Planus** | Pruritic, purple, polygonal planar papules and plaques are the **6 P's** of lichen **P**lanus E F. Mucosal involvement manifests as Wickham striae (reticular white lines) and hypergranulosis. Sawtooth infiltrate of lymphocytes at dermal-epidermal junction. Associated with hepatitis C. |
| **Pityriasis rosea** | "Herald patch" G followed days later by other scaly erythematous plaques, often in a "Christmas tree" distribution on trunk H. Multiple pink plaques with collarette scale. Self-resolving in 6–8 weeks. |
| **Sunburn** | Acute cutaneous inflammatory reaction due to excessive UV irradiation. Causes DNA mutations, inducing apoptosis of keratinocytes. UVB is dominant in sun**B**urn, UVA in t**A**nning and photo**A**ging. Exposure to UVA and UVB ↑ risk of skin cancer. |

**Estimation of body surface area**

Approximated by the rule of 9's. Used to assess the extent of burn injuries.

Inhalation injury—complication of inhalation of noxious stimuli (eg, smoke). Heat, particulates (< 1 μm diameter), or irritants (eg, $NH_3$) → chemical tracheobronchitis, edema, pneumonia, acute respiratory distress syndrome. Singed nasal hairs or soot in oropharynx common on exam. Bronchoscopy shows severe edema, congestion of bronchus, and soot deposition ( A , 18 hours after inhalation injury; B , resolution at 11 days after injury).

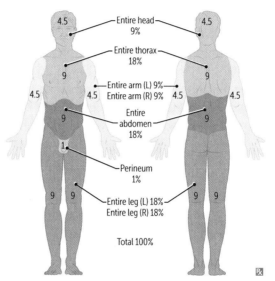

Entire head 9%
Entire thorax 18%
Entire arm (L) 9%
Entire arm (R) 9%
Entire abdomen 18%
Perineum 1%
Entire leg (L) 18%
Entire leg (R) 18%

Total 100%

## Burn classification

| DEPTH | INVOLVEMENT | APPEARANCE | SENSATION |
|---|---|---|---|
| **Superficial burn** | Epidermis only | Similar to sunburn; histamine release causes localized, dry, blanching redness without blisters | Painful |
| **Superficial partial-thickness burn** | Epidermis and papillary dermis | Blisters, blanches with pressure, swollen, warm | Painful to temperature and air |
| **Deep partial-thickness burn** | Epidermis and reticular dermis | Blisters (easily unroofed), does not blanch with pressure | Painless; perception of pressure only |
| **Full-thickness burn** | Epidermis and full-thickness dermis | White, waxy, dry, inelastic, leathery, does not blanch with pressure | Painless; perception of deep pressure only |
| **Deeper injury burn** | Epidermis, dermis, and involvement of underlying tissue (eg, fascia, muscle) | White, dry, inelastic, does not blanch with pressure | Painless; some perception of deep pressure |

| | |
|---|---|
| **Skin cancer** | Basal cell carcinoma (BCC) more common above **upper lip**.<br>Squamous cell carcinoma (SCC) more common below **lower lip**.<br>Sun exposure strongly predisposes to skin cancer.  |
| **Basal cell carcinoma** | Most common skin cancer. Found in sun-exposed areas of body (eg, face). Locally invasive, but rarely metastasizes. Waxy, pink, pearly nodules, commonly with telangiectasias, rolled borders **A**, central crusting or ulceration. BCCs also appear as a scaling plaque (superficial BCC) **B**. |
| **Squamous cell carcinoma** | Second most common skin cancer. Associated with immunosuppression, chronic nonhealing wounds, and occasionally arsenic exposure. Marjolin ulcer—SCC arising in chronic wounds or scars; usually develops > 20 years after insult. Commonly appears on face **C**, lower lip **D**, ears, hands. Locally invasive, may spread to lymph nodes, and will rarely metastasize. Ulcerative red lesions. Histopathology: keratin "pearls" **E**.<br>Actinic keratosis—Premalignant lesions caused by sun exposure. Small, rough, erythematous or brownish papules or plaques **F**. Risk of squamous cell carcinoma is proportional to degree of epithelial dysplasia. |
| **Melanoma** | Common tumor with significant risk of metastasis. S-100 tumor marker. Associated with dysplastic nevi; people with lighter skin tones are at ↑ risk. Depth of tumor (Breslow thickness) correlates with risk of metastasis. Look for the ABCDEs: Asymmetry, Border irregularity, Color variation, Diameter > 6 mm, and Evolution over time. At least 4 different types of melanoma, including superficial spreading **G**, nodular **H**, lentigo maligna **I**, and acral lentiginous (highest prevalence in people with darker skin tones) **J**. Often driven by activating mutation in BRAF kinase. Primary treatment is excision with appropriately wide margins. Advanced melanoma also treated with immunotherapy (eg, ipilimumab) and/or BRAF inhibitors (eg, vemurafenib). |

## ▶ MUSCULOSKELETAL, SKIN, AND CONNECTIVE TISSUE—PHARMACOLOGY

### Arachidonic acid pathways

$LTB_4$ is a neutrophil chemotactic agent.
$PGI_2$ is a vasodilator and platelet aggregation inhibitor.

Neutrophils arrive "B4" others.
Platelet-Gathering Inhibitor.

### Acetaminophen

| | |
|---|---|
| MECHANISM | Reversibly inhibits cyclooxygenase, mostly in CNS. Inactivated peripherally. |
| CLINICAL USE | Antipyretic, analgesic, but not anti-inflammatory. Used instead of aspirin to avoid Reye syndrome in children with viral infection. |
| ADVERSE EFFECTS | Overdose produces hepatic necrosis; acetaminophen metabolite (NAPQI) depletes glutathione and forms toxic tissue byproducts in liver. N-acetylcysteine is antidote—regenerates glutathione. |

## Aspirin

| | |
|---|---|
| MECHANISM | NSAID that irreversibly (aspirin) inhibits cyclooxygenase (both COX-1 and COX-2) by covalent acetylation → ↓ synthesis of $TXA_2$ and prostaglandins. ↑ bleeding time. No effect on PT, PTT. Effect lasts until new platelets are produced. |
| CLINICAL USE | Low dose (< 300 mg/day): ↓ platelet aggregation. Intermediate dose (300–2400 mg/day): antipyretic and analgesic. High dose (2400–4000 mg/day): anti-inflammatory. |
| ADVERSE EFFECTS | Gastric ulceration, tinnitus (CN VIII), allergic reactions (especially in patients with asthma or nasal polyps). Chronic use can lead to acute kidney injury, interstitial nephritis, GI bleeding. Risk of Reye syndrome in children treated for viral infection. Toxic doses cause respiratory alkalosis early, but transitions to mixed metabolic acidosis-respiratory alkalosis. Overdose treatment: $NaHCO_3$. |

## Celecoxib

| | |
|---|---|
| MECHANISM | Reversibly and selectively inhibits the cyclooxygenase (**COX**) isoform 2 ("**Selecoxib**"), which is found in inflammatory cells and vascular endothelium and mediates inflammation and pain; spares COX-1, which helps maintain gastric mucosa. Thus, does not have the corrosive effects of other NSAIDs on the GI lining. Spares platelet function as $TXA_2$ production is dependent on COX-1. |
| CLINICAL USE | Rheumatoid arthritis, osteoarthritis. |
| ADVERSE EFFECTS | ↑ risk of thrombosis, sulfa allergy. |

## Nonsteroidal anti-inflammatory drugs

Ibuprofen, naproxen, indomethacin, ketorolac, diclofenac, meloxicam, piroxicam.

| | |
|---|---|
| MECHANISM | Reversibly inhibit cyclooxygenase (both COX-1 and COX-2). Block prostaglandin synthesis. |
| CLINICAL USE | Antipyretic, analgesic, anti-inflammatory. Indomethacin is used to close a PDA. |
| ADVERSE EFFECTS | Interstitial nephritis, gastric ulcer (prostaglandins protect gastric mucosa), renal ischemia (prostaglandins vasodilate afferent arteriole), aplastic anemia. |

## Leflunomide

| | |
|---|---|
| MECHANISM | Reversibly inhibits dihydroorotate dehydrogenase, preventing pyrimidine synthesis. Suppresses T-cell proliferation. |
| CLINICAL USE | Rheumatoid arthritis, psoriatic arthritis. |
| ADVERSE EFFECTS | Diarrhea, hypertension, hepatotoxicity, teratogenicity. |

## Bisphosphonates

Alendronate, ibandronate, risedronate, zoledronate.

| | |
|---|---|
| MECHANISM | Pyrophosphate analogs; bind hydroxyapatite in bone, inhibiting osteoclast activity and promoting osteoclast apoptosis. |
| CLINICAL USE | Osteoporosis, hypercalcemia, Paget disease of bone, metastatic bone disease, osteogenesis imperfecta. |
| ADVERSE EFFECTS | Esophagitis, osteonecrosis of jaw, atypical femoral stress fractures. |

## Teriparatide

| | |
|---|---|
| MECHANISM | Recombinant PTH analog. ↑ osteoblastic activity when administered in pulsatile fashion. |
| CLINICAL USE | Osteoporosis. Causes ↑ bone growth compared to antiresorptive therapies (eg, bisphosphonates). |
| ADVERSE EFFECTS | Dizziness, tachycardia, transient hypercalcemia, muscle spasms. |

## Gout drugs

### Chronic gout drugs (preventive)

| | | |
|---|---|---|
| Allopurinol | Competitive inhibitor of xanthine oxidase → ↓ conversion of hypoxanthine and xanthine to urate. Also used in lymphoma and leukemia to prevent tumor lysis–associated urate nephropathy. ↑ concentrations of xanthine oxidase active metabolites, azathioprine, and 6-MP. | All painful flares are preventable. |
| Pegloticase | Recombinant uricase catalyzing uric acid to allantoin (a more water-soluble product). | |
| Febuxostat | Inhibits xanthine oxidase. Think, "febu-xo-stat makes Xanthine Oxidase static." | |
| Probenecid | Inhibits reabsorption of uric acid in proximal convoluted tubule (also inhibits secretion of penicillin). Can precipitate uric acid calculi or lead to sulfa allergy. | |

### Acute gout drugs

| | |
|---|---|
| NSAIDs | Any NSAID. Use salicylates with caution (may decrease uric acid excretion, particularly at low doses). |
| Glucocorticoids | Oral, intra-articular, or parenteral. |
| Colchicine | Binds and stabilizes tubulin to inhibit microtubule polymerization, impairing neutrophil chemotaxis and degranulation. Acute and prophylactic value. GI, neuromyopathic adverse effects. Can also cause myelosuppression, nephrotoxicity. |

## TNF-α inhibitors

| DRUG | MECHANISM | CLINICAL USE | ADVERSE EFFECTS |
|------|-----------|--------------|-----------------|
| Etanercept | Fusion protein (decoy receptor for TNF-α + IgG1 Fc), produced by recombinant DNA. Etanercept intercepts TNF. | Rheumatoid arthritis, psoriasis, ankylosing spondylitis. | Predisposition to infection, including reactivation of latent TB, since TNF is important in granuloma formation and stabilization. Can also lead to drug-induced lupus. |
| Adalimumab, infliximab | Anti-TNF-α monoclonal antibody. | Inflammatory bowel disease, rheumatoid arthritis, ankylosing spondylitis, psoriasis. | |

## Psoriasis biologics

| DRUG | TARGET |
|------|--------|
| Ustekinumab | IL-12/IL-23 |
| Ixekizumab Secukinumab | IL-17 |
| Brodalumab | IL-17 receptor |
| Guselkumab Risankizumab Tildrakizumab | IL-23 |

## Imiquimod

| | |
|---|---|
| MECHANISM | Binds toll-like receptor 7 (TLR-7) of macrophages, monocytes, and dendritic cells to activate them → topical antitumor immune response modifier. |
| CLINICAL USE | Anogenital warts, actinic keratosis. |
| ADVERSE EFFECTS | Itching, burning pain at site of application, rashes. |

# Neurology and Special Senses

"We are all now connected by the Internet, like neurons in a giant brain."
—Stephen Hawking

"Exactly how [the brain] operates remains one of the biggest unsolved mysteries, and it seems the more we probe its secrets, the more surprises we find."
—Neil deGrasse Tyson

"It's not enough to be nice in life. You've got to have nerve."
—Georgia O'Keeffe

"I not only use all the brains that I have, but all that I can borrow."
—Woodrow Wilson

"The chief function of the body is to carry the brain around."
—Thomas Edison

"I opened two gifts this morning. They were my eyes."
—Zig Ziglar

Understand the difference between the findings and underlying anatomy of upper motor neuron and lower motor neuron lesions. Know the major motor, sensory, cerebellar, and visual pathways and their respective locations in the CNS. Connect key neurological associations with certain pathologies (eg, cerebellar lesions, stroke manifestations, Brown-Séquard syndrome). Recognize common findings on MRI/CT (eg, ischemic and hemorrhagic stroke) and on neuropathology (eg, neurofibrillary tangles and Lewy bodies). High-yield medications include those used to treat epilepsy, Parkinson disease, migraine, and pain (eg, opioids).

## ▶ NEUROLOGY—EMBRYOLOGY

**Neural development**

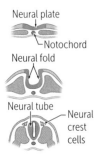

Notochord induces overlying ectoderm to differentiate into neuroectoderm and form neural plate. Notochord becomes nucleus pulposus of intervertebral disc in adults.

Neural plate gives rise to neural tube and neural crest cells.

Lateral walls of neural tube are divided into alar and basal plates.

Alar plate (dorsal): sensory; induced by bone morphogenetic proteins (BMPs)

Basal plate (ventral): motor; induced by sonic hedgehog (SHH)

⎱ Same orientation as spinal cord

---

**Regionalization of neural tube**

Telencephalon is the 1st part. Diencephalon is the 2nd part. The rest are arranged alphabetically: mesencephalon, metencephalon, myelencephalon.

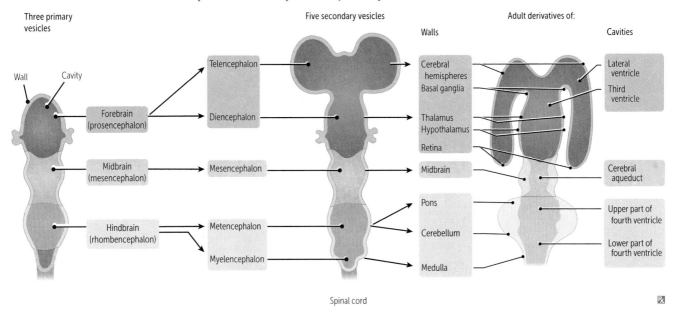

---

**Central and peripheral nervous systems origins**

Neuroepithelia in neural tube—CNS neurons, CNS glial cells (astrocytes, oligodendrocytes, ependymal cells).

Neural crest—PNS neurons (dorsal root ganglia, autonomic ganglia [sympathetic, parasympathetic, enteric]), PNS glial cells (Schwann cells, satellite cells), adrenal medulla.

Mesoderm—microglia (like macrophages).

| **Neural tube defects** | Failure of neural tube to close completely by week 4 of development. Associated with maternal folate deficiency during pregnancy. Diagnosis: ultrasound, maternal serum AFP (↑ in open NTDs). |
|---|---|

### Spinal dysraphism

| **Spina bifida occulta** | Closed NTD. Failure of caudal neural tube to close, but no herniation. Dura is intact. Usually seen at lower vertebral levels. Associated with tuft of hair or skin dimple at level of bony defect. |
|---|---|
| **Meningocele** | Open NTD. Meninges (but no neural tissue) herniate through bony defect. |
| **Myelomeningocele** | Open NTD. Meninges and neural tissue (eg, cauda equina) herniate through bony defect. |
| **Myeloschisis** | Open NTD. Exposed, unfused neural tissue without skin/meningeal covering. |

### Cranial dysraphism

| Anencephaly | Open NTD. Failure of rostral neuropore to close → no forebrain, open calvarium. Often presents with polyhydramnios (↓ fetal swallowing due to lack of neural control). |
|---|---|

| **Brain malformations** | Often incompatible with postnatal life. Survivors may be profoundly disabled. |
|---|---|

| Holoprosencephaly | Failure of forebrain (prosencephalon) to divide into 2 cerebral hemispheres; developmental field defect usually occurring at weeks 3–4 of development. Associated with *SHH* mutations. May be seen in Patau syndrome (trisomy 13), fetal alcohol syndrome.<br>Presents with midline defects: monoventricle **A**, fused basal ganglia, cleft lip/palate, hypotelorism, cyclopia, proboscis. ↑ risk for pituitary dysfunction (eg, diabetes insipidus). | <br> |
|---|---|---|
| Lissencephaly | Failure of neuronal migration → smooth brain surface that lacks sulci and gyri **B**.<br>Presents with dysphagia, seizures, microcephaly, facial anomalies. | |

## Posterior fossa malformations

| | |
|---|---|
| Chiari I malformation | Downward displacement of cerebellar **tonsils** through foramen magnum (1 structure) . Usually asymptomatic in childhood, manifests in adulthood with headaches and cerebellar symptoms. Associated with spinal cord cavitations (eg, syringomyelia). |
| Chiari II malformation | Downward displacement of **cerebellum** (vermis and tonsils) and **medulla** (2 structures) through foramen magnum → noncommunicating hydrocephalus. More severe than Chiari I, usually presents early in life with dysphagia, stridor, apnea, limb weakness. Associated with myelomeningocele (usually lumbosacral). |
| Dandy-Walker malformation | Agenesis of cerebellar vermis → cystic enlargement of 4th ventricle (arrow in B) that fills the enlarged posterior fossa. Associated with noncommunicating hydrocephalus, spina bifida. |

Chiari I malformation

Syrinx

## Syringomyelia

Fluid-filled, gliosis-lined cavity within spinal cord (yellow arrows in A). Fibers crossing in anterior white commissure (spinothalamic tract) are typically damaged first → "cape-like" loss of pain and temperature sensation in bilateral upper extremities. As lesion expands it may damage anterior horns → LMN deficits.

*Syrinx* (Greek) = tube, as in "syringe." Most lesions occur between C2 and T9. Usually associated with Chiari I malformation (red arrow in A). Less commonly associated with other malformations, infections, tumors, trauma.

Dorsal root ganglion

Expanding syrinx
*can affect multiple dermatomes*

Afferent
Lateral spinothalamic tract
*pain, temperature*

Anterior white commissure
compressed by syrinx

Loss of pain and temperature sensation at affected dermatomes
*C5-T4 shown here*

## ▶ NEUROLOGY—ANATOMY AND PHYSIOLOGY

| | | |
|---|---|---|
| **Cells of the nervous system** | Neurons and nonneuronal (glial) cells. Neurons—permanent, signal-transmitting cells of the nervous system composed of dendrites (receive input), cell bodies, and axons (send output). Dendrites and cell bodies can be seen on Nissl staining (stains RER; not present in axons). Markers: neurofilament protein, synaptophysin. | CNS glial cells—neuroectoderm (except microglia, which derive from mesoderm). PNS glial cells—neural crest ectoderm. Myelin is a multilayer wrapping of electrical insulation formed around axons → ↑ conduction velocity of transmitted signals via saltatory conduction of action potentials at nodes of Ranvier (↑↑ $Na^+$ channel density). |

### CNS glial cells

| | | |
|---|---|---|
| **Astrocytes** | Physical support, repair, removal of excess neurotransmitters, component of blood-brain barrier, glycogen fuel reserve buffer. GFAP ⊕. | Largest and most abundant glial cell in CNS. Reactive gliosis in response to neural injury. |
| **Oligodendrocytes** | Myelinate axons in CNS (including CN II). "Fried egg" appearance histologically ("oleggodendrocytes"). | Each myelinates many axons (~ 30). Predominant type of glial cell in white matter. Injured in multiple sclerosis, leukodystrophies, progressive multifocal leukoencephalopathy. |
| **Ependymal cells** | Ciliated simple columnar glial cells lining ventricles and central canal of spinal cord. Apical surfaces are covered with cilia (which circulate CSF) and microvilli (which help with CSF absorption). | Specialized ependymal cells (choroid plexus) produce CSF. |
| **Microglia** | Activation in response to tissue damage → release of inflammatory mediators (eg, nitric oxide, glutamate). Not readily discernible by Nissl stain. | Phagocytic scavenger cells of CNS. HIV-infected microglia fuse to form multinucleated giant cells in CNS in HIV-associated dementia. |

### PNS glial cells

| | | |
|---|---|---|
| **Satellite cells** | Surround neuronal cell bodies in ganglia. | Similar supportive role to astrocytes. |
| **Schwann cells** | Myelinate axons in PNS (including CN III-XII). S100 ⊕. | Each myelinates a **single** axon ("Schwone"). Injured in Guillain-Barré syndrome. |

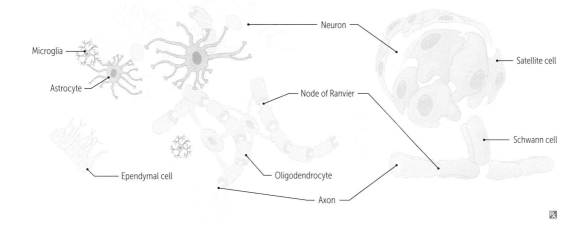

Central nervous system      Peripheral nervous system

Microglia · Astrocyte · Neuron · Satellite cell · Node of Ranvier · Schwann cell · Ependymal cell · Oligodendrocyte · Axon

## Neuron action potential

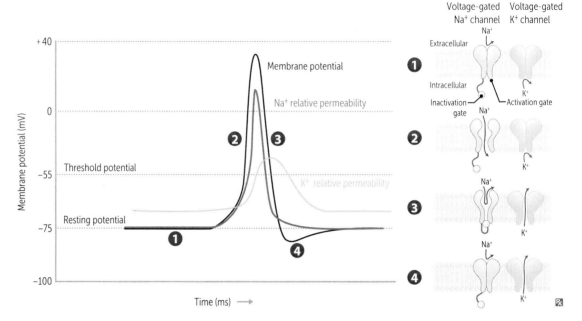

❶ Resting membrane potential: membrane is more permeable to K⁺ than Na⁺ at rest. Voltage-gated Na⁺ and K⁺ channels are closed.

❷ Membrane depolarization: Na⁺ activation gate opens → Na⁺ flows inward.

❸ Membrane repolarization: Na⁺ inactivation gate closes at peak potential, thus stopping Na⁺ inflow. K⁺ activation gate opens → K⁺ flows outward.

❹ Membrane hyperpolarization: K⁺ activation gates are slow to close → excess K⁺ efflux and brief period of hyperpolarization. Voltage-gated Na⁺ channels switch back to resting state. Na⁺/K⁺ pump restores ions concentration.

## Sensory receptors

| RECEPTOR TYPE | SENSORY NEURON FIBER TYPE | LOCATION | SENSES |
|---|---|---|---|
| **Free nerve endings** | Aδ—fast, myelinated fibers C—slow, unmyelinated A Delta plane is fast, but a taxC is slow | All tissues except cartilage and eye lens; numerous in skin | Pain, temperature |
| **Meissner corpuscles** | Large, myelinated fibers; adapt quickly | Glabrous (hairless) skin | Dynamic, fine/light touch, low-frequency vibration, skin indentation |
| **Pacinian corpuscles** | Large, myelinated fibers; adapt quickly | Deep skin layers, ligaments, joints | High-frequency vibration, pressure |
| **Merkel discs** | Large, myelinated fibers; adapt slowly | Finger tips, superficial skin | Pressure, deep static touch (eg, shapes, edges) |
| **Ruffini corpuscles** | Large, myelinated fiber intertwined among collagen fiber bundles; adapt slowly | Finger tips, joints | Stretch, joint angle change |

**Peripheral nerve**

Endoneurium—thin, supportive connective tissue that ensheathes and supports individual myelinated nerve fibers. May be affected in Guillain-Barré syndrome.

Perineurium (blood-nerve permeability barrier)—surrounds a fascicle of nerve fibers.

Epineurium—dense connective tissue that surrounds entire nerve (fascicles and blood vessels).

*Endo* = inner
*Peri* = around
*Epi* = outer

**Neuronal response to axonal injury**

Chromatolysis—dispersion of Nissl substance throughout cytoplasm (not visible on stain). Neuronal cell body reaction reflecting ↑ protein synthesis in effort to repair damaged axon. Accompanied by round cellular swelling and displacement of nucleus to periphery.

Axonal retraction—proximal axon segment retracts and sprouts new protrusions that grow toward other neurons for potential reinnervation. In PNS, Schwann cells create a tract that guides axonal regeneration.

Wallerian degeneration—distal axon segment and associated myelin sheath disintegrates with macrophages removing debris. In CNS, persistence of myelin debris and reactive gliosis prevent axonal regeneration.

**Injured neuron**

## Neurotransmitter changes with disease

| | LOCATION OF SYNTHESIS | ANXIETY | DEPRESSION | SCHIZOPHRENIA | ALZHEIMER DISEASE | HUNTINGTON DISEASE | PARKINSON DISEASE |
|---|---|---|---|---|---|---|---|
| **Acetylcholine** | Basal nucleus of Meynert (forebrain) | | | | ↓ | ↓ | ↑ |
| **Dopamine** | Ventral tegmentum, SNc (midbrain) | | ↓ | ↑ | | ↑ | ↓ |
| **GABA** | Nucleus accumbens (basal ganglia) | ↓ | | | | ↓ | |
| **Norepinephrine** | Locus ceruleus (pons) | ↑ | ↓ | | | | |
| **Serotonin** | Raphe nuclei (brainstem) | ↓ | ↓ | | | | ↓ |

## Meninges

Three membranes that surround and protect the brain and spinal cord. Derived from both neural crest and mesoderm:

- Dura mater—thick outer layer closest to skull.
- Arachnoid mater—middle layer, contains weblike connections.
- Pia mater—thin, fibrous inner layer that firmly adheres to brain and spinal cord.

CSF flows in the subarachnoid space, located between arachnoid and pia mater.

Epidural space—potential space between dura mater and skull/vertebral column containing fat and blood vessels. Site of blood collection associated with middle meningeal artery injury.

## Blood-brain barrier

Prevents circulating blood substances (eg, bacteria, drugs) from reaching the CSF/CNS. Formed by 4 structures:

- Tight junctions between nonfenestrated capillary endothelial cells
- Basement membrane
- Pericytes
- Astrocyte foot processes

Glucose and amino acids cross slowly by carrier-mediated transport mechanisms.

Nonpolar/lipid-soluble substances cross rapidly via diffusion.

Circumventricular organs with fenestrated capillaries and no blood-brain barrier allow molecules in blood to affect brain function (eg, area postrema—vomiting after chemotherapy; OVLT [organum vasculosum lamina terminalis]—osmoreceptors) or neurosecretory products to enter circulation (eg, neurohypophysis—ADH release).

BBB disruption (eg, stroke) → vasogenic edema.

Hyperosmolar agents (eg, mannitol) can disrupt the BBB → ↑ permeability of medications.

## Vomiting center

Coordinated by NTS in the medulla, which receives information from the chemoreceptor trigger zone (CTZ, located within area postrema (pronounce "puke"-strema) in 4th ventricle), GI tract (via vagus nerve), vestibular system, and CNS.

CTZ and adjacent vomiting center nuclei receive input through 5 major receptors: histamine ($H_1$), muscarinic ($M_1$), neurokinin (NK-1), dopamine ($D_2$), and serotonin (5-$HT_3$).

- 5-$HT_3$, $D_2$, and NK-1 antagonists treat chemotherapy-induced vomiting.
- $H_1$ and $M_1$ antagonists treat motion sickness; $H_1$ antagonists treat hyperemesis gravidarum.

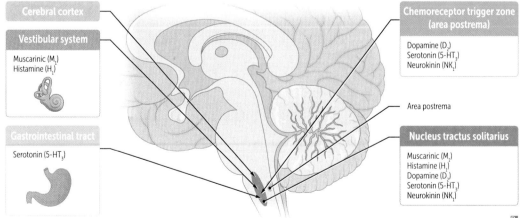

| Sleep physiology | Sleep occurs in 4-6 cycles per night, each lasting ~90 mins and consisting of 2 main stages: | Sleep-wake cycle is regulated by circadian rhythm, which is driven by suprachiasmatic nucleus (SCN) of hypothalamus. Low light conditions → ↓ SCN activity → ↑ norepinephrine from superior cervical ganglion → ↑ melatonin from pineal gland. |
|---|---|---|
|  | ▪ Non-rapid eye movement (non-REM) sleep<br>▪ Rapid-eye movement (REM) sleep; duration of REM sleep ↑ through the night |  |

| SLEEP STAGE (% OF TOTAL SLEEP) | DESCRIPTION | EEG WAVEFORM |
|---|---|---|
| Awake | Alert, active mental concentration.<br>Eyes open—beta waves (highest frequency, lowest amplitude).<br>Eyes closed—alpha waves. | Beta      Alpha |
| **Non-REM sleep** | | |
| Stage N1 (5%) | Light sleep; theta waves. | Theta |
| Stage N2 (45%) | Deeper sleep; sleep spindles and K complexes. When bruxism occurs ("twoth" grinding in N2). | Sleep spindle    K-complex |
| Stage N3 (25%) | Deepest non-REM sleep (slow-wave sleep); delta waves (lowest frequency, highest amplitude). When bedwetting, sleepwalking, and night terrors occur (wee and flee in N3). | Delta |
| REM sleep (25%) | Loss of motor tone, ↑ brain $O_2$ use, variable pulse/BP. Extraocular movements due to activity of PPRF (paramedian pontine reticular formation/conjugate gaze center). May serve memory processing function. When dreaming, nightmares, and penile/clitoral tumescence occur (remember dreams in REM). | Beta |

| Factors affecting sleep architecture | Alcohol, benzodiazepines, barbiturates: ↓ N3 and REM sleep (benzodiazepines are useful for sleepwalking and night terrors).<br>Aging: ↓ N3 and REM sleep, ↑ sleep-onset latency, early morning awakening.<br>Depression: ↓ N3 sleep, ↑ REM sleep, ↓ REM latency, repeated nighttime awakenings, early morning awakening (terminal insomnia).<br>Narcolepsy: ↓ REM latency. |
|---|---|

| | | |
|---|---|---|
| **Hypothalamus** | Maintains homeostasis by regulating Thirst and water balance, controlling Adenohypophysis (anterior pituitary) and Neurohypophysis (posterior pituitary) release of hormones produced in the hypothalamus, and regulating Hunger, Autonomic nervous system, Temperature, and Sexual urges (TAN HATS). Inputs (areas not protected by blood-brain barrier): OVLT (senses change in osmolarity), area postrema (found in dorsal medulla, responds to emetics). | |
| **Lateral nucleus** | Hunger. Stimulated by ghrelin, inhibited by leptin. | Lateral injury makes you lean. Destruction → anorexia, failure to thrive (infants). |
| **Ventromedial nucleus** | Satiety. Stimulated by leptin. | Ventromedial injury makes you very massive. Destruction (eg, craniopharyngioma) → hyperphagia. |
| **Anterior nucleus** | Cooling, parasympathetic. | A/C = Anterior Cooling. |
| **Posterior nucleus** | Heating, sympathetic. | Heating controlled by posterior nucleus ("hot pot"). |
| **Suprachiasmatic nucleus** | Circadian rhythm. | SCN is a Sun-Censing Nucleus. |
| **Supraoptic and paraventricular nuclei** | Synthesize ADH and oxytocin. | SAD POX: Supraoptic = ADH, Paraventricular = OXytocin. ADH and oxytocin are carried by neurophysins down axons to posterior pituitary, where these hormones are stored and released. |
| **Preoptic nucleus** | Thermoregulation, sexual behavior. Releases GnRH. | Failure of GnRH-producing neurons to migrate from olfactory pit → Kallmann syndrome. |

| | | |
|---|---|---|
| **Thalamus** | Major relay for all ascending sensory information except olfaction. | |

| NUCLEI | INPUT | SENSES | DESTINATION | MNEMONIC |
|---|---|---|---|---|
| **Ventral posterolateral nucleus** | Spinothalamic and dorsal columns/medial lemniscus | Vibration, pain, pressure, proprioception (conscious), light touch, temperature | 1° somatosensory cortex (parietal lobe) | |
| **Ventral postero-medial nucleus** | Trigeminal and gustatory pathway | Face sensation, taste | 1° somatosensory cortex (parietal lobe) | Very pretty makeup goes on the face |
| **Lateral geniculate nucleus** | CN II, optic chiasm, optic tract | Vision | 1° visual cortex (occipital lobe) | Lateral = light (vision) |
| **Medial geniculate nucleus** | Superior olive and inferior colliculus of tectum | Hearing | 1° auditory cortex (temporal lobe) | Medial = music (hearing) |
| **Ventral anterior and ventral lateral nuclei** | Basal ganglia, cerebellum | Motor | Motor cortices (frontal lobe) | Venus astronauts vow to love moving |

**Limbic system**

Collection of neural structures involved in emotion, long-term memory, olfaction, behavior modulation, ANS function.
Consists of hippocampus (red arrows in A), amygdalae, mammillary bodies, anterior thalamic nuclei, cingulate gyrus (yellow arrows in A), entorhinal cortex. Responsible for feeding, fleeing, fighting, feeling, and sex.

The famous 5 F's.

---

**Dopaminergic pathways**

Commonly altered by drugs (eg, antipsychotics) and movement disorders (eg, Parkinson disease). The mesocortical and mesolimbic pathways are involved in addiction behaviors.

| PATHWAY | PROJECTION | FUNCTION | SYMPTOMS OF ALTERED ACTIVITY | NOTES |
|---|---|---|---|---|
| **Mesocortical** | Ventral tegmental area → prefrontal cortex | Motivation and reward | ↓ activity → negative symptoms | Antipsychotics have limited effect |
| **Mesolimbic** | Ventral tegmental area → nucleus accumbens | | ↑ activity → positive symptoms | 1° therapeutic target of antipsychotics |
| **Nigrostriatal** | Substantia nigra → dorsal striatum | **Motor** control (pronounce "nigrostrideatal") | ↓ activity → extrapyramidal symptoms | Significantly affected by antipsychotics and in Parkinson disease |
| **Tuberoinfundibular** | Hypothalamus → pituitary | Regulation of prolactin secretion | ↓ activity → ↑ prolactin | Significantly affected by antipsychotics |

Prefrontal cortex

Dorsal striatum

Substantia nigra

Hypothalamus

Nucleus accumbens

Pituitary gland

Ventral tegmental area

- Mesocortical pathway
- Mesolimbic pathway
- Nigrostriatal pathway
- Tuberoinfundibular pathway

## Cerebellum

Modulates movement; aids in coordination and balance .

- Ipsilateral (unconscious) proprioceptive information via inferior cerebellar peduncle from spinal cord
- Deep nuclei (lateral → medial)—dentate, emboliform, globose, fastigial (**d**on't **e**at **g**reasy **f**oods)

**Medial** cerebellum (eg, vermis) controls axial and proximal limb musculature bilaterally (**medial** structures).

**Lateral** cerebellum (ie, hemisphere) controls distal limb musculature ipsilaterally (**lateral** structures).

Tests: rapid alternating movements (pronation/supination), finger-to-nose, heel-to-shin, gait, look for intention tremor.

## Basal ganglia

Important in voluntary movements and adjusting posture **A**.
Receives cortical input, provides negative feedback to cortex to modulate movement.
Striatum = putamen (motor) + Caudate nucleus (cognitive).
Lentiform nucleus = putamen + globus pallidus.

$D_1$ Receptor = DIRect pathway.
Indirect ($D_2$) = Inhibitory.

Direct (excitatory) pathway—cortical input (via glutamate) stimulates GABA release from the striatum, which inhibits GABA release from GPi, disinhibiting (activating) the Thalamus → ↑ motion.

Indirect (inhibitory) pathway—cortical input (via glutamate) stimulates GABA release from the striatum, which inhibits GABA release from GPe, disinhibiting (activating) the STN. STN input (via glutamate) stimulates GABA release from GPi, inhibiting the Thalamus → ↓ motion.

Dopamine from SNc (nigrostriatal pathway) stimulates the direct pathway (by binding to $D_1$ receptor) and inhibits the indirect pathway (by binding to $D_2$ receptor) → ↑ motion.

## Cerebral cortex regions

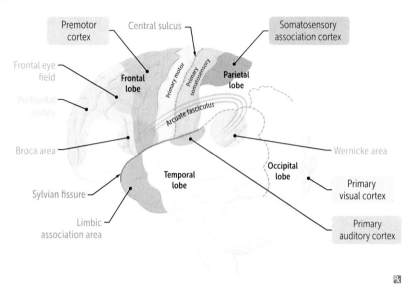

## Cerebral perfusion

Relies on tight autoregulation. Primarily driven by $P_{CO_2}$ ($P_{O_2}$ also modulates perfusion in severe hypoxia).

Also relies on a pressure gradient between mean arterial pressure (MAP) and intracranial pressure (ICP). ↓ blood pressure or ↑ ICP → ↓ cerebral perfusion pressure (CPP).

Cushing reflex—triad of hypertension, bradycardia, and respiratory depression in response to ↑ ICP.

Therapeutic hyperventilation → ↓ $P_{CO_2}$ → vasoconstriction → ↓ cerebral blood flow → ↓ ICP. May be used to treat acute cerebral edema (eg, 2° to stroke) unresponsive to other interventions.

CPP = MAP – ICP. If CPP = 0, there is no cerebral perfusion → brain death (coma, absent brainstem reflexes, apnea).

Hypoxemia increases CPP only if $P_{O_2}$ < 50 mm Hg.

CPP is directly proportional to $P_{CO_2}$ until $P_{CO_2}$ > 90 mm Hg.

**Homunculus**   Topographic representation of motor and sensory areas in the cerebral cortex. Distorted appearance is due to certain body regions being more richly innervated and thus having ↑ cortical representation.

**Cerebral arteries—cortical distribution**

☐ Anterior cerebral artery (supplies anteromedial surface)
☐ Middle cerebral artery (supplies lateral surface)
☐ Posterior cerebral artery (supplies posterior and inferior surfaces)

**Watershed zones**

Cortical border zones occur between anterior and middle cerebral arteries and posterior and middle cerebral arteries (blue areas in **A**). Internal border zones occur between the superficial and deep vascular territories of the middle cerebral artery (red areas in **A**).

Common locations for brain metastases. Infarct due to severe hypoperfusion:
- ACA-MCA watershed infarct—proximal upper and lower extremity weakness ("man-in-a-barrel syndrome").
- PCA-MCA watershed infarct—higher-order visual dysfunction.

**Circle of Willis**   System of anastomoses between anterior and posterior blood supplies to brain.

ACom | Anterior communicating
Optic chiasm
A2
ACA | Anterior cerebral
A1
**Internal carotid | ICA**
CIRCLE
MCA | Middle cerebral
Lenticulo-striate
M1
OF
PCom | Posterior communicating
WILLIS
Anterior choroidal
P2   P1
PCA | Posterior cerebral
SCA | Superior cerebellar
Pontine
AICA | Anterior inferior cerebellar
**Basilar | BA**
PICA | Posterior inferior cerebellar
**Vertebral | VA**
Anterior spinal | ASA

Anterior circulation
☐ ACA
☐ ICA
☐ MCA
Posterior circulation

*INFERIOR VIEW*

ACA
MCA
PCA
BA
PCom
ECA
CCA
ICA
Brachio-cephalic
VA
Sub-clavian
Aorta

*OBLIQUE-LATERAL VIEW*

---

**Dural venous sinuses**   Large venous channels 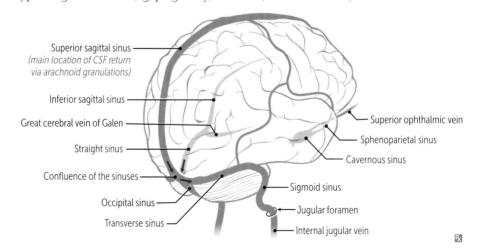 **A** that run through the periosteal and meningeal layers of the dura mater. Drain blood from cerebral veins (arrow) and receive CSF from arachnoid granulations. Empty into internal jugular vein.

**Venous sinus thrombosis**—presents with signs/symptoms of ↑ ICP (eg, headache, seizures, papilledema, focal neurologic deficits). May lead to venous hemorrhage. Associated with hypercoagulable states (eg, pregnancy, OCP use, factor V Leiden).

Superior sagittal sinus *(main location of CSF return via arachnoid granulations)*
Inferior sagittal sinus
Great cerebral vein of Galen
Straight sinus
Confluence of the sinuses
Occipital sinus
Transverse sinus
Superior ophthalmic vein
Sphenoparietal sinus
Cavernous sinus
Sigmoid sinus
Jugular foramen
Internal jugular vein

## Ventricular system

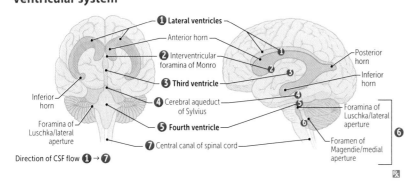

Lateral ventricles → 3rd ventricle via right and left interventricular foramina of Monro.

3rd ventricle → 4th ventricle via cerebral aqueduct of Sylvius.

4th ventricle → subarachnoid space via:
- Foramina of Luschka = lateral.
- Foramen of Magendie = medial.

CSF made by choroid plexuses located in the lateral, third, and fourth ventricles. Travels to subarachnoid space via foramina of Luschka and Magendie, is reabsorbed by arachnoid granulations, and then drains into dural venous sinuses.

## Brainstem—ventral view

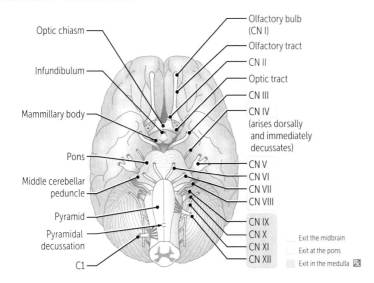

4 CN are above pons (I, II, III, IV).
4 CN exit the pons (V, VI, VII, VIII).
4 CN are in medulla (IX, X, XI, XII).
4 CN nuclei are medial (III, IV, VI, XII).
"Factors of 12, except 1 and 2."

## Brainstem—dorsal view (cerebellum removed)

Pineal gland—melatonin secretion, circadian rhythm.

Superior colliculi—direct eye movements to stimuli (noise/movements) or objects of interest.

Inferior colliculi—auditory.

Your eyes are **above** your ears, and the superior colliculus (visual) is **above** the inferior colliculus (auditory).

**Cranial nerve nuclei**    Located in tegmentum portion of brainstem (between dorsal and ventral portions):
- Midbrain—nuclei of CN III, IV
- Pons—nuclei of CN V, VI, VII, VIII
- Medulla—nuclei of CN IX, X, XII
- Spinal cord—nucleus of CN XI

Lateral nuclei = sensory (alar plate).
—Sulcus limitans—
Medial nuclei = motor (basal plate).

## Vagal nuclei

| NUCLEUS | FUNCTION | CRANIAL NERVES |
|---|---|---|
| Nucleus tractus solitarius | Visceral sensory information (eg, taste, baroreceptors, gut distention) <br> May play a role in vomiting | VII, IX, X |
| Nucleus ambiguus | Motor innervation of pharynx, larynx, upper esophagus (eg, swallowing, palate elevation) | IX, X |
| Dorsal motor nucleus | Sends autonomic (parasympathetic) fibers to heart, lungs, upper GI | X |

## Brainstem cross sections

### Midbrain

Superior colliculus
Cerebral aqueduct
CN III nucleus
CN III fibers
Medial lemniscus
Red nucleus
Substantia nigra
Cerebral peduncle

**Brainstem cross sections** *(continued)*

Pons

Fourth ventricle

Medial longitudinal fasciculus

Middle cerebellar peduncle

CN V

Corticospinal and corticobulbar tracts

Superior cerebellar peduncle

Locus ceruleus

Medial lemniscus

Medulla

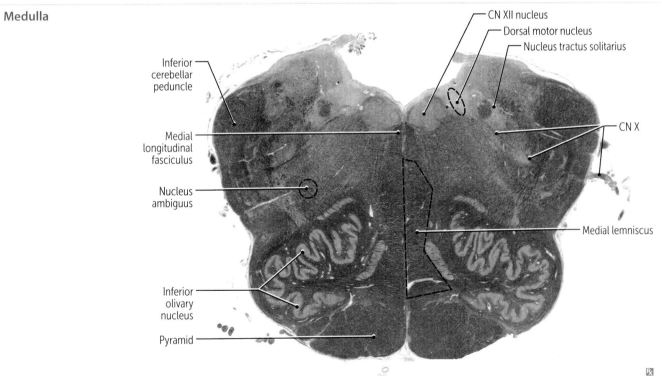

Inferior cerebellar peduncle

Medial longitudinal fasciculus

Nucleus ambiguus

Inferior olivary nucleus

Pyramid

CN XII nucleus

Dorsal motor nucleus

Nucleus tractus solitarius

CN X

Medial lemniscus

## Cranial nerves and vessel pathways

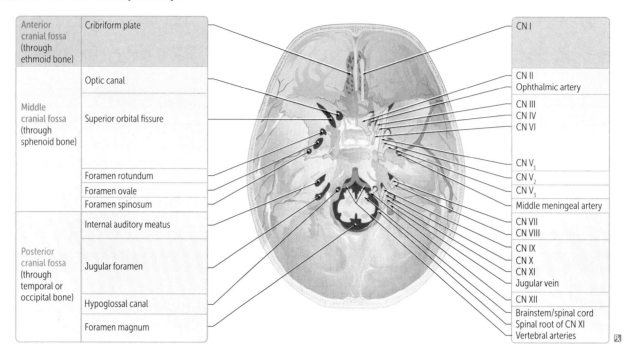

| | Cribriform plate | CN I |
|---|---|---|
| Anterior cranial fossa (through ethmoid bone) | | |
| Middle cranial fossa (through sphenoid bone) | Optic canal | CN II / Ophthalmic artery |
| | Superior orbital fissure | CN III / CN IV / CN VI / CN V₁ |
| | Foramen rotundum | CN V₂ |
| | Foramen ovale | CN V₃ |
| | Foramen spinosum | Middle meningeal artery |
| Posterior cranial fossa (through temporal or occipital bone) | Internal auditory meatus | CN VII / CN VIII |
| | Jugular foramen | CN IX / CN X / CN XI / Jugular vein |
| | Hypoglossal canal | CN XII |
| | Foramen magnum | Brainstem/spinal cord / Spinal root of CN XI / Vertebral arteries |

## Cranial nerves and arteries

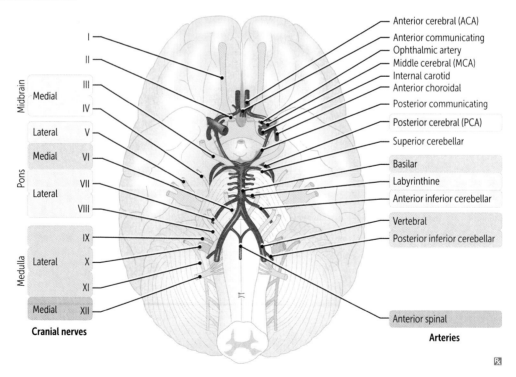

Midbrain — Medial: III, IV
Pons — Lateral: V; Medial: VI; Lateral: VII, VIII
Medulla — Lateral: IX, X, XI; Medial: XII

Cranial nerves: I, II

**Cranial nerves**

Anterior cerebral (ACA)
Anterior communicating
Ophthalmic artery
Middle cerebral (MCA)
Internal carotid
Anterior choroidal
Posterior communicating
Posterior cerebral (PCA)
Superior cerebellar
Basilar
Labyrinthine
Anterior inferior cerebellar
Vertebral
Posterior inferior cerebellar
Anterior spinal

**Arteries**

## Cranial nerves

| NERVE | CN | FUNCTION | TYPE | MNEMONIC |
|---|---|---|---|---|
| Olfactory | I | Smell (only CN without thalamic relay to cortex) | Sensory | Some |
| Optic | II | Sight | Sensory | Say |
| Oculomotor | III | Eye movement (SR, IR, MR, IO), pupillary constriction (sphincter pupillae), accommodation (ciliary muscle), eyelid opening (levator palpebrae) | Motor | Marry |
| Trochlear | IV | Eye movement (SO) | Motor | Money |
| Trigeminal | V | Mastication, facial sensation (ophthalmic, maxillary, mandibular divisions), somatosensation from anterior 2/3 of tongue, dampening of loud noises (tensor tympani) | Both | But |
| Abducens | VI | Eye movement (LR) | Motor | My |
| Facial | VII | Facial movement, eye closing (orbicularis oculi), auditory volume modulation (stapedius), taste from anterior 2/3 of tongue (chorda tympani), lacrimation, salivation (submandibular and sublingual glands are innervated by CN seven) | Both | Brother |
| Vestibulocochlear | VIII | Hearing, balance | Sensory | Says |
| Glossopharyngeal | IX | Taste and sensation from posterior 1/3 of tongue, swallowing, salivation (parotid gland), monitoring carotid body and sinus chemo- and baroreceptors, and elevation of pharynx/larynx (stylopharyngeus) | Both | Big |
| Vagus | X | Taste from supraglottic region, swallowing, soft palate elevation, midline uvula, talking, cough reflex, parasympathetics to thoracoabdominal viscera, monitoring aortic arch chemo- and baroreceptors | Both | Brains |
| Accessory | XI | Head turning, shoulder shrugging (SCM, trapezius) | Motor | Matter |
| Hypoglossal | XII | Tongue movement | Motor | Most |

## Cranial nerve reflexes

| REFLEX | AFFERENT | EFFERENT |
|---|---|---|
| Accommodation | II | III |
| Corneal | $V_1$ ophthalmic (nasociliary branch) | Bilateral VII (temporal and zygomatic branches—orbicularis oculi) |
| Cough | X | X (also phrenic and spinal nerves) |
| Gag | IX | X |
| Jaw jerk | $V_3$ (sensory—muscle spindle from masseter) | $V_3$ (motor—masseter) |
| Lacrimation | $V_1$ (loss of reflex does not preclude emotional tears) | VII |
| Pupillary | II | III |

| | | |
|---|---|---|
| **Mastication muscles** | 3 muscles close jaw: masseter, temporalis, medial pterygoid (**M**'s munch). Lateral pterygoid protrudes jaw. All are innervated by mandibular branch of trigeminal nerve (CN V₃). | 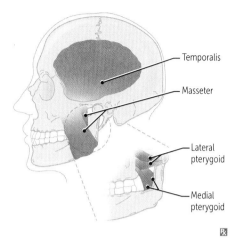 |

Temporalis

Masseter

Lateral pterygoid

Medial pterygoid

---

**Spinal nerves**

There are 31 pairs of spinal nerves: 8 cervical, 12 thoracic, 5 lumbar, 5 sacral, 1 coccygeal.
Nerves C1–C7 exit above the corresponding vertebrae (eg, C3 exits above the 3rd cervical vertebra).
C8 spinal nerve exits below C7 and above T1. All other nerves exit below (eg, L2 exits below the 2nd lumbar vertebra).

---

**Spinal cord—lower extent**

In adults, spinal cord ends at lower border of L1–L2 vertebrae. Subarachnoid space (which contains the CSF) extends to lower border of S2 vertebra. Lumbar puncture is usually performed between L3–L4 or L4–L5 (level of cauda equina) to obtain sample of CSF while avoiding spinal cord. To keep the cord **alive**, keep the spinal needle between **L3** and **L5**.
Needle passes through:
❶ Skin
❷ Fascia and fat
❸ Supraspinous ligament
❹ Interspinous ligament
❺ Ligamentum flavum
❻ Epidural space (epidural anesthesia needle stops here)
❼ Dura mater
❽ Arachnoid mater
❾ Subarachnoid space (CSF collection occurs here)

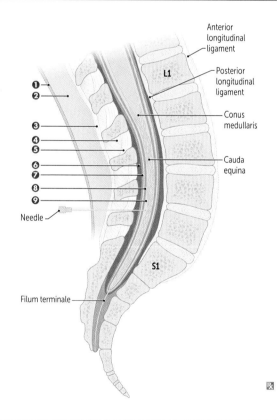

Anterior longitudinal ligament

Posterior longitudinal ligament

Conus medullaris

Cauda equina

L1

S1

Needle

Filum terminale

---

**Conus medullaris and cauda equina syndrome**

Rare neurosurgical emergencies caused by compression (eg, disc herniation, tumors, trauma) of terminal end of spinal cord (conus medullaris) or lumbosacral spinal nerve roots (cauda equina).
Present with radicular low back pain, saddle/perianal anesthesia, bladder and bowel dysfunction, lower limb weakness → symmetric with UMN signs (eg, spastic) in conus medullaris syndrome, asymmetric with LMN signs (eg, flaccid) in cauda equina syndrome.

**Spinal cord levels and associated tracts**

Legs (lumbosacral) are lateral in lateral corticospinal, spinothalamic tracts.
Dorsal columns are organized as you are, with hands at sides. "Arms outside, legs inside."

Cervical
— Two dorsal columns
— White matter
— Gray matter

Thoracic
— Two dorsal columns
— Lateral horn

Lumbosacral
— One dorsal column
— Ventral horn

## Spinal tract anatomy and functions

Spinothalamic tract and dorsal column (ascending tracts) synapse and then cross.
Corticospinal tract (descending tract) crosses and then synapses.

| | Spinothalamic tract | Dorsal column | Corticospinal tract |
|---|---|---|---|
| FUNCTION | Pain, temperature | Pressure, vibration, fine touch, proprioception (conscious) | Voluntary movement |
| 1ST-ORDER NEURON | Sensory nerve ending (Aδ and C fibers) of pseudounipolar neuron in dorsal root ganglion → enters spinal cord | Sensory nerve ending of pseudounipolar neuron in dorsal root ganglion → enters spinal cord → ascends ipsilaterally in dorsal columns | UMN: 1° motor cortex → descends ipsilaterally (through posterior limb of internal capsule and cerebral peduncle), decussates at caudal medulla (pyramidal decussation) → descends contralaterally |
| 1ST SYNAPSE | Posterior horn (spinal cord) | Nucleus gracilis, nucleus cuneatus (ipsilateral medulla) | Anterior horn (spinal cord) |
| 2ND-ORDER NEURON | Decussates in spinal cord as the anterior white commissure → ascends contralaterally | Decussates in medulla → ascends contralaterally as the medial lemniscus | LMN: leaves spinal cord |
| 2ND SYNAPSE | VPL (thalamus) | VPL (thalamus) | NMJ (skeletal muscle) |
| 3RD-ORDER NEURON | Projects to 1° somatosensory cortex | Projects to 1° somatosensory cortex | |

## Clinical reflexes

Reflexes count up in order (main nerve root in **bold**):

- Achilles reflex = **S1**, S2 ("buckle my shoe")
- Patellar reflex = L2-**L4** ("kick the door")
- Biceps and brachioradialis reflexes = **C5**, C6 ("pick up sticks")
- Triceps reflex = C6, **C7**, C8 ("lay them straight")

Additional reflexes:

- Cremasteric reflex = L1, L2 ("testicles move")
- Anal wink reflex = S3, S4 ("winks galore")

Reflex grading:

- 0: absent
- 1+: hypoactive
- 2+: normal
- 3+: hyperactive
- 4+: clonus

## Primitive reflexes

CNS reflexes that are present in a healthy infant, but are absent in a neurologically intact adult. Normally disappear within 1st year of life. These primitive reflexes are inhibited by a mature/developing frontal lobe. They may reemerge in adults following frontal lobe lesions → loss of inhibition of these reflexes.

| | |
|---|---|
| Moro reflex | "Hang on for life" reflex—abduct/extend arms when startled, and then draw together. |
| Rooting reflex | Movement of head toward one side if cheek or mouth is stroked (nipple seeking). |
| Sucking reflex | Sucking response when roof of mouth is touched. |
| Palmar reflex | Curling of fingers if palm is stroked. |
| Plantar reflex | Dorsiflexion of large toe and fanning of other toes with plantar stimulation. Babinski sign—presence of this reflex in an adult, which may signify a UMN lesion. |
| Galant reflex | Stroking along one side of the spine while newborn is in ventral suspension (face down) causes lateral flexion of lower body toward stimulated side. |

## Landmark dermatomes

| DERMATOME | CHARACTERISTICS |
|---|---|
| C2 | Posterior half of skull |
| C3 | High turtleneck shirt<br>Diaphragm and gallbladder pain referred to the right shoulder via phrenic nerve<br>C3, 4, 5 keeps the diaphragm **alive** |
| C4 | Low-collar shirt |
| C6 | Includes thumbs<br>**Thumbs up** sign on left hand looks like a 6 |
| T4 | At the **nipple**<br>T4 at the teat **pore** |
| T7 | At the xiphoid process<br>7 letters in xiphoid |
| T10 | At the umbilicus (belly butten)<br>Point of referred pain in early appendicitis |
| L1 | At the Inguinal Ligament |
| L4 | Includes the kneecaps<br>Down on **ALL** 4's |
| S2, S3, S4 | Sensation of penile and anal zones<br>S2, 3, 4 keep the penis off the **floor** |

▶ **NEUROLOGY—PATHOLOGY**

## Common brain lesions

| AREA OF LESION | COMPLICATIONS |
|---|---|
| **Prefrontal cortex** | Frontal lobe syndrome—disinhibition, hyperphagia, impulsivity, loss of empathy, impaired executive function, akinetic mutism. Seen in frontotemporal dementia. |
| **Frontal eye fields** | Eyes look toward brain lesion (ie, away from side of hemiplegia). Seen in MCA stroke. |
| **Paramedian pontine reticular formation** | Eyes look away from brain lesion (ie, toward side of hemiplegia). |
| **Dominant parietal cortex** | Gerstmann syndrome—agraphia, acalculia, finger agnosia, left-right disorientation. |
| **Nondominant parietal cortex** | Hemispatial neglect syndrome—agnosia of the contralateral side of the world. |
| **Basal ganglia** | Tremor at rest, chorea, athetosis. Seen in Parkinson disease, Huntington disease. |
| **Subthalamic nucleus** | Contralateral hemiballismus. |
| **Mammillary bodies** | Bilateral lesions → Wernicke-Korsakoff syndrome (due to thiamine deficiency). |
| **Amygdala** | Bilateral lesions → Klüver-Bucy syndrome—disinhibition (eg, hyperphagia, hypersexuality, hyperorality). Seen in HSV-1 encephalitis. |
| **Hippocampus** | Bilateral lesions → anterograde amnesia (no new memory formation). Seen in Alzheimer disease. |
| **Dorsal midbrain** | Parinaud syndrome (often due to pineal gland tumors). |
| **Reticular activating system** | Reduced levels of arousal and wakefulness, coma. |
| **Medial longitudinal fasciculus** | Internuclear ophthalmoplegia (impaired adduction of ipsilateral eye; nystagmus of contralateral eye with abduction). Seen in multiple sclerosis. |
| **Cerebellar hemisphere** | Intention tremor, limb ataxia, loss of balance; damage to cerebellum → ipsilateral deficits; fall toward side of lesion. Cerebellar hemispheres are **laterally** located—affect **lateral** limbs. |
| **Cerebellar vermis** | Truncal ataxia (wide-based, "drunken sailor" gait), nystagmus, dysarthria. Degeneration associated with chronic alcohol overuse. Vermis is **centrally** located—affects **central** body. |

## Abnormal motor posturing

| | Decorticate (flexor) posturing | Decerebrate (extensor) posturing |
|---|---|---|
| SITE OF LESION | Above red nucleus (often cerebral cortex) | Between red and vestibular nuclei (brainstem) |
| OVERACTIVE TRACTS | Rubrospinal and vestibulospinal tracts | Vestibulospinal tract |
| PRESENTATION | Upper limb flexion, lower limb extension | Upper and lower limb extension |
| NOTES | "Your hands are near the **cor** (heart)" | Worse prognosis |

**Ischemic brain disease/stroke**

Irreversible neuronal injury begins after 5 minutes of hypoxia. Most vulnerable: hippocampus (CA1 region), neocortex, cerebellum (**Purkinje** cells), watershed areas ("**vulnerable hippos need pure water**").

Stroke imaging: noncontrast CT to exclude hemorrhage (before tPA can be given). CT detects ischemic changes in 6–24 hr. Diffusion-weighted MRI can detect ischemia within 3–30 min.

| TIME SINCE ISCHEMIC EVENT | 12–24 HOURS | 24–72 HOURS | 3–5 DAYS | 1–2 WEEKS | > 2 WEEKS |
|---|---|---|---|---|---|
| Histologic features | Eosinophilic cytoplasm + pyknotic nuclei (red neurons) | Necrosis + neutrophils | Macrophages (microglia) | Reactive gliosis (astrocytes) + vascular proliferation | Glial scar |

**Ischemic stroke**

Ischemia → infarction → liquefactive necrosis.

3 types:
- Thrombotic—due to a clot forming directly at site of infarction (commonly the MCA ), usually over a ruptured atherosclerotic plaque.
- Embolic—due to an embolus from another part of the body. Can affect multiple vascular territories. Examples: atrial fibrillation, carotid artery stenosis, DVT with patent foramen ovale (paradoxical embolism), infective endocarditis.
- Hypoxic—due to systemic hypoperfusion or hypoxemia. Common during cardiovascular surgeries, tends to affect watershed areas.

Treatment: tPA (if within 3–4.5 hr of onset and no hemorrhage/risk of hemorrhage) and/or thrombectomy (if large artery occlusion). Reduce risk with medical therapy (eg, aspirin, clopidogrel); optimum control of blood pressure, blood sugars, lipids; smoking cessation; and treat conditions that ↑ risk (eg, atrial fibrillation, carotid artery stenosis).

**Transient ischemic attack**

Brief, reversible episode of focal neurologic dysfunction without acute infarction (⊖ MRI), with the majority resolving in < 15 minutes; ischemia (eg, embolus, small vessel stenosis). May present with amaurosis fugax (transient visual loss) due to retinal artery emboli from carotid artery disease.

**Cerebral edema**

Fluid accumulation in brain parenchyma → ↑ ICP. Types:
- Cytotoxic edema—intracellular fluid accumulation due to osmotic shift (eg, Na⁺/K⁺-ATPase dysfunction → ↑ intracellular Na⁺). Caused by ischemia (early), hyperammonemia, SIADH.
- Vasogenic edema—extracellular fluid accumulation due to disruption of BBB (↑ permeability). Caused by ischemia (late), trauma, hemorrhage, inflammation, tumors (arrows in  show surrounding vasogenic edema).

### Effects of strokes

| ARTERY | AREA OF LESION | SYMPTOMS | NOTES |
|---|---|---|---|
| **Anterior circulation** | | | |
| **Anterior cerebral artery** | Motor and sensory cortices—lower limb. | Contralateral paralysis and sensory loss—lower limb, urinary incontinence. | |
| **Middle cerebral artery** | Motor and sensory cortices A—upper limb and face. Temporal lobe (Wernicke area); frontal lobe (Broca area). | Contralateral paralysis and sensory loss—lower face and upper limb. Aphasia if in dominant (usually left) hemisphere. Hemineglect if lesion affects nondominant (usually right) hemisphere. | Wernicke aphasia is associated with right superior quadrant visual field defect due to temporal lobe involvement. |
| **Lenticulo-striate artery** | Striatum, internal capsule. | Contralateral paralysis. Absence of cortical signs (eg, neglect, aphasia, visual field loss). | Pure motor stroke (most common). Common location of lacunar infarcts B, due to microatheroma and hyaline arteriosclerosis (lipohyalinosis) 2° to unmanaged hypertension. |
| **Posterior circulation** | | | |
| **Posterior cerebral artery** | Occipital lobe C. | Contralateral hemianopia with macular sparing; alexia without agraphia (dominant hemisphere, extending to splenium of corpus callosum); prosopagnosia (nondominant hemisphere). | Weber syndrome—midbrain stroke due to occlusion of paramedian branches of PCA → ipsilateral CN III palsy and contralateral hemiplegia (damage to ipsilateral cerebral peduncle). |
| **Basilar artery** | Pons, medulla, lower midbrain. | If RAS spared, consciousness is preserved. | Locked-in syndrome (locked in the basement). |
| | Corticospinal and corticobulbar tracts. | Quadriplegia; loss of voluntary facial (except blinking), mouth, and tongue movements. | |
| | Ocular cranial nerve nuclei, paramedian pontine reticular formation. | Loss of horizontal, but not vertical, eye movements. | |
| **Anterior inferior cerebellar artery** | Facial nerve nuclei. | Paralysis of face (LMN lesion vs UMN lesion in cortical stroke), ↓ lacrimation, ↓ salivation, ↓ taste from anterior 2/3 of tongue. | Lateral pontine syndrome. Facial nerve nuclei effects are specific to AICA lesions. |
| | Vestibular nuclei. Spinothalamic tract, spinal trigeminal nucleus. | Vomiting, vertigo, nystagmus ↓ pain and temperature sensation from contralateral body, ipsilateral face. | |
| | Sympathetic fibers. Middle and inferior cerebellar peduncles. | Ipsilateral Horner syndrome. Ipsilateral ataxia, dysmetria. | |
| | Inner ear. | Ipsilateral sensorineural deafness, vertigo. | Supplied by labyrinthine artery, a branch of AICA. |

## Effects of strokes *(continued)*

| ARTERY | AREA OF LESION | SYMPTOMS | NOTES |
|---|---|---|---|
| Posterior inferior cerebellar artery | Nucleus ambiguus (CN IX, X). | Dysphagia, hoarseness, ↓ gag reflex, hiccups. | Lateral medullary (Wallenberg) syndrome. |
| | Vestibular nuclei. | Vomiting, vertigo, nystagmus | Nucleus ambiguus effects are specific to PICA lesions . |
| | Lateral spinothalamic tract, spinal trigeminal nucleus. | ↓ pain and temperature sensation from contralateral body, ipsilateral face. | "Don't pick a (PICA) lame (lateral medullary syndrome) horse (hoarseness) that can't |
| | Sympathetic fibers. | Ipsilateral Horner syndrome. | eat (dysphagia)." |
| | Inferior cerebellar peduncle. | Ipsilateral ataxia, dysmetria. | |
| Anterior spinal artery | Corticospinal tract. | Contralateral paralysis—upper and lower limbs. | Medial Medullary syndrome— caused by infarct of |
| | Medial lemniscus. | ↓ contralateral proprioception. | paramedian branches of ASA and/or vertebral arteries. Ants |
| | Caudal medulla—hypoglossal nerve. | Ipsilateral hypoglossal dysfunction (tongue deviates ipsilaterally). | love **M&M's**. |

| | |
|---|---|
| **Neonatal intraventricular hemorrhage** | Bleeding into ventricles (arrows in  show blood in intraventricular spaces on ultrasound). Increased risk in premature and low-birth-weight infants. Originates in germinal matrix, a highly vascularized layer within the subventricular zone. Due to reduced glial fiber support and impaired autoregulation of BP in premature infants. Can present with altered level of consciousness, bulging fontanelle, hypotension, seizures, coma. |

## Intracranial hemorrhage

| | | |
|---|---|---|
| Epidural hematoma | Rupture of middle meningeal artery (branch of maxillary artery), often 2° to skull fracture (circle in **A**) involving the pterion (thinnest area of the lateral skull). Might present with transient loss of consciousness → recovery ("lucid interval") → rapid deterioration due to hematoma expansion.<br><br>Scalp hematoma (arrows in **A**) and rapid intracranial expansion (arrows in **B**) under systemic arterial pressure → transtentorial herniation, CN III palsy.<br><br>CT shows biconvex (lentiform), hyperdense blood collection **B** **not crossing suture lines**. |  |
| Subdural hematoma | Rupture of bridging veins. Can be acute (traumatic, high-energy impact → hyperdense on CT) or chronic (associated with mild trauma, cerebral atrophy, ↑ age, chronic alcohol overuse → hypodense on CT). Also seen in shaken babies.<br><br>Crescent-shaped hemorrhage (red arrows in **C** and **D**) that **crosses suture lines**. Can cause midline shift, findings of "acute on chronic" hemorrhage (blue arrows in **D**). |  |
| Subarachnoid hemorrhage | Bleeding **E** **F** due to trauma, or rupture of an aneurysm (such as a saccular aneurysm) or arteriovenous malformation. Rapid time course. Patients complain of "worst headache of my life." Bloody or yellow (xanthochromic) lumbar puncture.<br><br>Vasospasm can occur due to blood breakdown or rebleed 3–10 days after hemorrhage → ischemic infarct; nimodipine used to prevent/reduce vasospasm. ↑ risk of developing communicating and/or obstructive hydrocephalus. |  |
| Intraparenchymal hemorrhage | Most commonly caused by systemic hypertension. Also seen with amyloid angiopathy (recurrent lobar hemorrhagic stroke in older adults), arteriovenous malformations, vasculitis, neoplasm. May be 2° to reperfusion injury in ischemic stroke.<br><br>Hypertensive hemorrhages (Charcot-Bouchard microaneurysm) most often occur in putamen/globus pallidus of basal ganglia (lenticulostriate vessels **G**), followed by internal capsule, thalamus, pons, and cerebellum **H**. |  |

| | |
|---|---|
| **Central poststroke pain** | Neuropathic pain due to thalamic lesions. Initial paresthesias followed in weeks to months by allodynia (ordinarily painless stimuli cause pain) and dysesthesia (altered sensation) on the contralateral side. Occurs in 10% of stroke patients. |
| **Phantom limb pain** | Sensation of pain in a limb that is no longer present. Common after amputation. Associated with reorganization of 1° somatosensory cortex. Characterized by burning, aching, or electric shock–like pain. |
| **Diffuse axonal injury**  | Traumatic shearing of white matter tracts during rapid acceleration and/or deceleration of the brain (eg, motor vehicle accident). Usually results in devastating neurologic injury, often causing coma or persistent vegetative state. MRI shows multiple lesions (punctate hemorrhages) involving white matter tracts A. |
| **Aphasia** | Aphasia—higher-order language deficit (inability to understand/produce/use language appropriately); caused by pathology in dominant cerebral hemisphere (usually left). Dysarthria—motor inability to produce speech (movement deficit). |

| TYPE | COMMENTS |
|---|---|
| Broca (expressive) | Broca area in inferior frontal gyrus of frontal lobe. Associated with defective language production. Patients appear frustrated, insight intact. Broca = broken boca (*boca* = mouth in Spanish). |
| Wernicke (receptive) | Wernicke area in superior temporal gyrus of temporal lobe. Associated with impaired language comprehension. Patients do not have insight. Wernicke is a word salad and makes no sense. |
| Conduction | Can be caused by damage to arcuate fasciculus. |
| Global | Broca and Wernicke areas affected. |

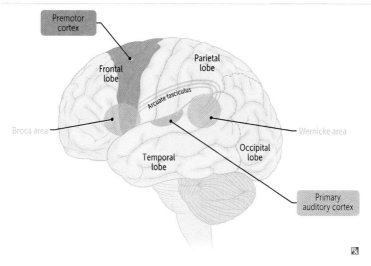

| Aneurysms | Abnormal dilation of an artery due to weakening of vessel wall. |
|---|---|
| Saccular aneurysm  | Also called berry aneurysm **A**. Occurs at bifurcations in the circle of Willis. Most common site is junction of ACom and ACA. Associated with ADPKD, Ehlers-Danlos syndrome. Other risk factors: advanced age, hypertension, tobacco smoking. <br> Usually clinically silent until rupture (most common complication) → subarachnoid hemorrhage ("worst headache of my life" or "thunderclap headache") → focal neurologic deficits. Can also cause symptoms via direct compression of surrounding structures by growing aneurysm. <br> ▪ ACom—compression → bitemporal hemianopia (compression of optic chiasm); visual acuity deficits; rupture → ischemia in ACA distribution → contralateral lower extremity hemiparesis, sensory deficits. <br> ▪ MCA—rupture → ischemia in MCA distribution → contralateral upper extremity and lower facial hemiparesis, sensory deficits. <br> ▪ PCom—compression → ipsilateral CN III palsy → mydriasis ("blown pupil"); may also see ptosis, "down and out" eye. |
| Charcot-Bouchard microaneurysm | Common, associated with chronic hypertension; affects small vessels (eg, lenticulostriate arteries in basal ganglia, thalamus) and can cause hemorrhagic intraparenchymal strokes. Not visible on angiography. |

### Fever vs heat stroke

| | Fever | Heat stroke |
|---|---|---|
| PATHOPHYSIOLOGY | Cytokine activation during inflammation (eg, infection) | Inability of body to dissipate heat (eg, exertion) |
| TEMPERATURE | Usually < 40°C (104°F) | Usually > 40°C (104°F) |
| COMPLICATIONS | Febrile seizure (benign, usually self-limiting) | CNS dysfunction (eg, confusion), rhabdomyolysis, acute kidney injury, ARDS, DIC |
| MANAGEMENT | Acetaminophen or ibuprofen for comfort (does not prevent future febrile seizures), antibiotic therapy if indicated | Rapid external cooling, rehydration and electrolyte correction |

| | | |
|---|---|---|
| **Seizures** | Characterized by synchronized, high-frequency neuronal firing. Consist of 3 phases: | |
| | ▪ Aura—early part of a seizure, may include odd smells or tastes. | |
| | ▪ Ictal—time from first symptom to end of seizure activity. | |
| | ▪ Postictal—period of gradual recovery back to preseizure baseline level of function/awareness. | |

| | | |
|---|---|---|
| **Focal seizures** | Affect single area of the brain. Most commonly originate in medial temporal lobe. Types:<br>▪ Focal aware (formerly called simple partial)—consciousness intact; motor, sensory, autonomic, psychic symptoms<br>▪ Focal impaired awareness (formerly called complex partial)—impaired consciousness, automatisms | Epilepsy—disorder of recurrent, unprovoked seizures (febrile seizures are not epilepsy).<br>Status epilepticus—continuous (≥ 5 min) or recurring seizures without interictal return to baseline consciousness that may result in brain injury.<br>Causes of seizures by age:<br>▪ Children < 18—genetic, infection (febrile), trauma, congenital, metabolic<br>▪ Adults 18–65—tumor, trauma, stroke, infection<br>▪ Adults > 65—stroke, tumor, trauma, metabolic, infection |
| **Generalized seizures** | Diffuse. Types:<br>▪ Absence (petit mal)—3 Hz spike-and-wave discharges, short (usually 10 seconds) and frequent episodes of blank stare, no postictal confusion. Can be triggered by hyperventilation<br>▪ Myoclonic—quick, repetitive jerks; no loss of consciousness<br>▪ Tonic-clonic (grand mal)—alternating stiffening and movement, postictal confusion, urinary incontinence, tongue biting<br>▪ Tonic—stiffening<br>▪ Atonic—"drop" seizures (falls to floor); commonly mistaken for fainting | |

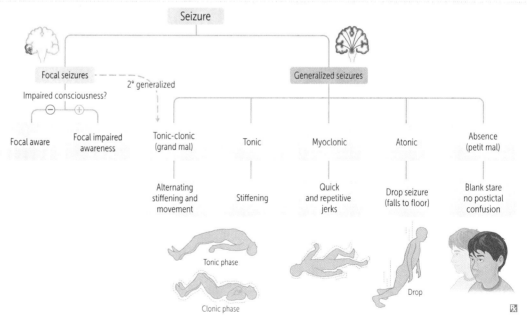

## Headaches

Pain due to irritation of intra- or extracranial structures (eg, meninges, blood vessels). Primary headaches include tension-type, migraine, and cluster. Secondary headaches include medication overuse, meningitis, subarachnoid hemorrhage, hydrocephalus, neoplasia, giant cell arteritis.

| CLASSIFICATION | LOCALIZATION | DURATION | DESCRIPTION | TREATMENT |
|---|---|---|---|---|
| **Tension-type** | Bilateral | > 30 min (typically 4–6 hr); constant | Steady, "bandlike" pain. No nausea or vomiting. No more than one of photophobia or phonophobia. No aura. Most common primary headache; more common in females. | Acute: analgesics, NSAIDs, acetaminophen. Prophylaxis: TCAs (eg, amitriptyline), behavioral therapy. |
| **Migraine** | Unilateral | 4–72 hr | Pulsating pain with nausea, photophobia, and/or phonophobia. May have "aura." Due to irritation of CN V, meninges, or blood vessels (release of vasoactive neuropeptides [eg, substance P, calcitonin gene-related peptide]). More common in females. POUND–Pulsatile, One-day duration, Unilateral, Nausea, Disabling. | Acute: NSAIDs, triptans, dihydroergotamine, antiemetics (eg, prochlorperazine, metoclopramide). Prophylaxis: lifestyle changes (eg, sleep, exercise, diet), β-blockers, amitriptyline, topiramate, valproate, botulinum toxin, anti-CGRP monoclonal antibodies. |
| **Cluster** | Unilateral | 15 min–3 hr; repetitive | Excruciating periorbital pain with autonomic symptoms (eg, lacrimation, rhinorrhea, conjunctival injection). May present with Horner syndrome. More common in males. | Acute: sumatriptan, 100% $O_2$. Prophylaxis: verapamil. |

## Trigeminal neuralgia

Recurrent brief episodes of intense unilateral pain in CN V distribution (usually $V_2$ and/or $V_3$). Most cases are due to compression of CN V root by an aberrant vascular loop. Pain is described as electric shock–like or stabbing and usually lasts seconds. Typically triggered by light facial touch or facial movements (eg, chewing, talking). Treatment: carbamazepine, oxcarbazepine.

▨ $V_1$
▢ $V_2$
▨ $V_3$

**Dyskinesias**

| DISORDER | PRESENTATION | NOTES |
|---|---|---|
| Akathisia | Restlessness and intense urge to move | Can be seen with neuroleptic use or as an adverse effect of Parkinson disease treatment |
| Asterixis | "Flapping" motion upon extension of wrists | Associated with hepatic encephalopathy, Wilson disease, and other metabolic derangements |
| Athetosis | Slow, snakelike, writhing movements; especially seen in the fingers | Caused by lesion to basal ganglia <br> Seen in Huntington disease |
| Chorea | Sudden, jerky, purposeless movements | *Chorea* (Greek) = dancing <br> Caused by lesion to basal ganglia <br> Seen in Huntington disease and acute rheumatic fever (Sydenham chorea). |
| Dystonia | Sustained, involuntary muscle contractions | Writers cramp, blepharospasm, torticollis <br> Treatment: botulinum toxin injection |
| Essential tremor | High-frequency tremor with sustained posture (eg, outstretched arms); worsened with movement or anxiety | Often familial <br> Patients often self-medicate with alcohol, which ↓ tremor amplitude <br> Treatment: nonselective β-blockers (eg, propranolol), barbiturates (primidone) |
| Intention tremor | Slow, zigzag motion when pointing/extending toward a target | Caused by cerebellar dysfunction |
| Resting tremor | Uncontrolled movement of distal appendages (most noticeable in hands); tremor alleviated by intentional movement | Caused by lesion to substantia nigra <br> Occurs at **rest**; "pill-rolling tremor" of **Parkinson** disease; when you **park** your car, it is at **rest** |
| Hemiballismus | Sudden, wild flailing of one side of the body | Caused by lesion to contralateral subthalamic nucleus (eg, due to lacunar stroke) <br> In hemiballismus, **half**-of-body is going **ballistic** |
| Myoclonus | Sudden, brief, uncontrolled muscle contraction | Jerks; hiccups; common in metabolic abnormalities (eg, renal and liver failure), Creutzfeldt-Jakob disease |

| | |
|---|---|
| **Restless legs syndrome** | Uncomfortable sensations in legs causing irresistible urge to move them. Emerge during periods of inactivity; most prominent in the evening or at night. Transiently relieved by movement (eg, walking). Usually idiopathic (often with genetic predisposition), but may be associated with iron deficiency, CKD, diabetes mellitus (especially with neuropathy). Treatment: gabapentinoids, dopamine agonists. |

## Neurodegenerative movement disorders

| | | |
|---|---|---|
| **Parkinson disease**  | Loss of dopaminergic neurons in substantia nigra pars compacta (depigmentation in A). Symptoms typically manifest after age 60 ("body TRAP"): <br> ▪ Tremor (pill-rolling tremor at rest) <br> ▪ Rigidity (cogwheel or leadpipe) <br> ▪ Akinesia/bradykinesia → shuffling gait, small handwriting (micrographia) <br> ▪ Postural instability (tendency to fall) <br> Dementia is usually a late finding. | Affected neurons contain Lewy bodies: intracellular eosinophilic inclusions composed of α-synuclein B. Think "Parkinsynuclein."   |
| **Huntington disease**  | Loss of GABAergic neurons in striatum. Autosomal dominant trinucleotide $(CAG)_n$ repeat expansion in **huntingtin** (*HTT*) gene on chromosome 4 (**4 letters**) → toxic gain of function. <br> Symptoms typically manifest between age 30 and 50: chorea, athetosis, aggression, depression, dementia (sometimes initially mistaken for substance use). | Atrophy of caudate and putamen with ex vacuo ventriculomegaly. <br> ↑ dopamine, ↓ GABA, ↓ ACh in brain. Neuronal death via NMDA receptor binding and glutamate excitotoxicity. <br> Anticipation results from expansion of **CAG** repeats. Caudate loses ACh and GABA. |

| | |
|---|---|
| **Dementia** | Decline in cognitive ability (eg, memory, executive function) with intact consciousness. Reversible causes of dementia include depression (pseudodementia), hypothyroidism, vitamin $B_{12}$ deficiency, neurosyphilis, normal pressure hydrocephalus. |

### Neurodegenerative

| | | |
|---|---|---|
| **Alzheimer disease**  | Most common cause of dementia in older adults. Advanced age is the strongest risk factor. Down syndrome patients have ↑ risk of developing early-onset Alzheimer disease, as amyloid precursor protein (APP) is located on chromosome 21. ↓ ACh in brain. <br> Associated with the following altered proteins: <br> ▪ ApoE-2: ↓ risk of sporadic form <br> ▪ ApoE-4: ↑ risk of sporadic form <br> ▪ APP, presenilin-1, presenilin-2: familial forms (10%) with earlier onset <br> ApoE-2 is "protwoctive," ApoE-4 is "four" Alzheimer disease. | Widespread cortical atrophy, especially hippocampus. Narrowing of gyri and widening of sulci. <br> Senile plaques A in gray matter: extracellular β-amyloid core; may cause amyloid angiopathy → intraparenchymal hemorrhage; Aβ (amyloid-β) is derived from cleavage of APP. <br> Neurofibrillary tangles B: intracellular, hyperphosphorylated tau protein = insoluble cytoskeletal elements; number of tangles correlates with degree of dementia. <br> Hirano bodies: intracellular eosinophilic proteinaceous rods in hippocampus. |
| **Frontotemporal dementia** | Formerly called Pick disease. Early changes in personality and behavior (behavioral variant), or aphasia (primary progressive aphasia). May have associated movement disorders. | Frontal and/or temporal lobe atrophy. Inclusions of hyperphosphorylated tau (round Pick bodies C) or ubiquitinated TDP-43. |
| **Lewy body dementia** | Visual hallucinations ("haLewycinations"), dementia with fluctuating cognition/alertness, REM sleep behavior disorder, and parkinsonism. | Intracellular Lewy bodies primarily in cortex. Called Lewy body dementia if cognitive and motor symptom onset < 1 year apart, otherwise considered dementia 2° to Parkinson disease. |

**Dementia** *(continued)*

| Vascular | | |
|---|---|---|
| **Vascular dementia** | 2nd most common cause of dementia in older adults. Result of multiple arterial infarcts and/or chronic ischemia.<br>Step-wise decline in cognitive ability with late-onset memory impairment. | MRI or CT shows multiple cortical and/or subcortical infarcts **D**. |

| Infective | | |
|---|---|---|
| **Creutzfeldt-Jakob disease** | Rapidly progressive (weeks to months) dementia with myoclonus ("startle myoclonus") and ataxia. Fatal. Caused by prions: $PrP^c \rightarrow PrP^{sc}$ (β-pleated sheet resistant to proteases).<br>Typically sporadic, but may be transmitted by contaminated materials (eg, corneal transplant, neurosurgical equipment). | Spongiform cortex **E** (vacuolation without inflammation).<br>Associated with periodic sharp waves on EEG and ↑ 14-3-3 protein in CSF. |
| **HIV-associated dementia** | Subcortical dysfunction associated with advanced HIV infection. Characterized by cognitive deficits, gait disturbance, irritability, depressed mood. | Diffuse gray matter and subcortical atrophy. Microglial nodules with multinucleated giant cells. |

| | |
|---|---|
| **Idiopathic intracranial hypertension** | Also called pseudotumor cerebri. ↑ ICP with no obvious findings on imaging. Risk factors include female sex, Tetracyclines, Obesity, vitamin A excess, Danazol (female TOAD). Associated with dural venous sinus stenosis. Findings: headache, tinnitus, diplopia (usually from CN VI palsy), no change in mental status. Impaired optic nerve axoplasmic flow → papilledema. Visual field testing shows enlarged blind spot and peripheral constriction. Lumbar puncture reveals ↑ opening pressure and provides temporary headache relief.<br><br>Treatment: weight loss, acetazolamide, invasive procedures for refractory cases (eg, CSF shunt placement, optic nerve sheath fenestration surgery for visual loss). |

| | |
|---|---|
| **Hydrocephalus** | ↑ CSF volume → ventricular dilation +/− ↑ ICP. |

### Communicating

| | |
|---|---|
| **Communicating hydrocephalus** | ↓ CSF absorption by arachnoid granulations (eg, arachnoid scarring post-meningitis) → ↑ ICP, papilledema, herniation. All ventricles are dilated. |
| **Normal pressure hydrocephalus** | Affects older adults; idiopathic; CSF pressure elevated only episodically; does not result in increased subarachnoid space volume. Expansion of ventricles  distorts the fibers of the corona radiata → triad of gait apraxia (magnetic gait), cognitive dysfunction, and urinary incontinence. "Wobbly, wacky, and wet." Treatment: CSF drainage via lumbar puncture or shunt placement. |

### Noncommunicating (obstructive)

| | |
|---|---|
| **Noncommunicating hydrocephalus** | Caused by structural blockage of CSF circulation within ventricular system (eg, stenosis of aqueduct of Sylvius, colloid cyst blocking foramen of Monro, tumor ). Ventricles "upstream" of the obstruction are dilated. |

### Hydrocephalus mimics

| | |
|---|---|
| **Ex vacuo ventriculomegaly** | Appearance of ↑ CSF on imaging , but is actually due to ↓ brain tissue and neuronal atrophy (eg, Alzheimer disease, advanced HIV, frontotemporal dementia, Huntington disease). ICP is normal; NPH triad is not seen. |

| | |
|---|---|
| **Multiple sclerosis** | Autoimmune inflammation and demyelination of CNS (brain and spinal cord) with subsequent axonal damage. Most often affects females aged 20–40; more common in individuals who grew up farther from equator and with low serum vitamin D levels. Can present with <br> ▪ Optic neuritis (acute painful monocular visual loss, associated with relative afferent pupillary defect) <br> ▪ Brainstem/cerebellar syndromes (eg, diplopia, ataxia, vertigo, scanning speech, dysarthria, intention tremor, nystagmus/INO [bilateral > unilateral]) <br> ▪ Pyramidal tract demyelination (eg, weakness, spasticity) <br> ▪ Spinal cord syndromes (eg, electric shock–like sensation along cervical spine on neck flexion, neurogenic bladder, paraparesis, sensory manifestations affecting the trunk or one or more extremities) <br> Symptoms may exacerbate with increased body temperature (eg, hot bath, exercise). Relapsing and remitting is most common clinical course. |
| FINDINGS | ↑ IgG level and myelin basic protein in CSF. Oligoclonal bands aid in diagnosis. MRI is gold standard. Periventricular plaques  (areas of oligodendrocyte loss and reactive gliosis). Multiple white matter lesions disseminated in space and time. |
| TREATMENT | Stop relapses and halt/slow progression with disease-modifying therapies (eg, β-interferon, glatiramer, natalizumab). Treat acute flares with IV steroids. Symptomatic treatment for neurogenic bladder (muscarinic antagonists, botulinum toxin injection), spasticity (baclofen, $GABA_B$ receptor agonists), pain (TCAs, anticonvulsants). |

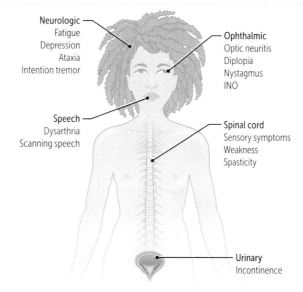

**Neurologic**
Fatigue
Depression
Ataxia
Intention tremor

**Ophthalmic**
Optic neuritis
Diplopia
Nystagmus
INO

**Speech**
Dysarthria
Scanning speech

**Spinal cord**
Sensory symptoms
Weakness
Spasticity

**Urinary**
Incontinence

## Other demyelinating and dysmyelinating disorders

| | |
|---|---|
| **Osmotic demyelination syndrome**<br> | Also called central pontine myelinolysis. Massive axonal demyelination in pontine white matter  2° to rapid osmotic changes, most commonly iatrogenic correction of hyponatremia but also rapid shifts of other osmolytes (eg, glucose). Acute paralysis, dysarthria, dysphagia, diplopia, loss of consciousness. Can cause "locked-in syndrome."<br>Correcting serum Na⁺ too fast:<br>　▪ "From low to high, your pons will die" (osmotic demyelination syndrome)<br>　▪ "From high to low, your brains will blow" (cerebral edema/herniation) |
| **Acute inflammatory demyelinating polyneuropathy** | Most common subtype of **Guillain-Barré syndrome**.<br>Autoimmune condition that destroys Schwann cells via inflammation and demyelination of motor fibers, sensory fibers, peripheral nerves (including CN III-XII). Likely facilitated by molecular mimicry and triggered by inoculations or stress. Despite association with infections (eg, *Campylobacter jejuni*, viruses [eg, Zika]), no definitive causal link to any pathogen.<br>Results in symmetric ascending muscle weakness/paralysis and depressed/absent DTRs beginning in lower extremities. Facial paralysis (usually bilateral) and respiratory failure are common. May see autonomic dysregulation (eg, cardiac irregularities, hypertension, hypotension) or sensory abnormalities. Most patients survive with good functional recovery.<br>↑ CSF protein with normal cell count (albuminocytologic dissociation).<br>Respiratory support is critical until recovery. Disease-modifying treatment: plasma exchange or IV immunoglobulins. No role for steroids. |
| **Acute disseminated (postinfectious) encephalomyelitis** | Multifocal inflammation and demyelination after infection or vaccination. Presents with rapidly progressive multifocal neurologic symptoms, altered mental status. |
| **Charcot-Marie-Tooth disease** | Also called hereditary motor and sensory neuropathy. Group of progressive hereditary nerve disorders related to the defective production of proteins involved in the structure and function of peripheral nerves or the myelin sheath. Typically autosomal dominant and associated with foot deformities (eg, pes cavus, hammer toe), lower extremity weakness (eg, foot drop), and sensory deficits (Can't Move Toes). Most common type, CMT1A, is caused by *PMP22* gene duplication. |
| **Progressive multifocal leukoencephalopathy**<br> | Demyelination of CNS  due to destruction of oligodendrocytes (2° to reactivation of latent JC virus infection). Associated with severe immunosuppression (eg, lymphomas and leukemias, AIDS, organ transplantation). Rapidly progressive, usually fatal. Predominantly involves parietal and occipital areas; visual symptoms are common. ↑ risk associated with natalizumab. |
| **Other disorders** | Krabbe disease, metachromatic leukodystrophy, adrenoleukodystrophy. |

## Neurocutaneous disorders

| DISORDER | GENETICS | PRESENTATION | NOTES |
|---|---|---|---|
| **Sturge-Weber syndrome** | Congenital nonhereditary anomaly of neural crest derivatives. Somatic mosaicism of an activating mutation in one copy of the GNAQ gene. | Capillary vascular malformation → port-wine stain A (nevus flammeus or non-neoplastic birthmark) in CN $V_1/V_2$ distribution; ipsilateral leptomeningeal angioma with calcifications B → seizures/epilepsy; intellectual disability; episcleral hemangioma → ↑ IOP → early-onset glaucoma. | Also called encephalotrigeminal angiomatosis. |
| **Tuberous sclerosis complex** | AD, variable expression. Mutation in tumor suppressor genes TSC1 on chromosome 9 (hamartin), TSC2 on chromosome 16 (tuberin; pronounce "twoberin"). | Hamartomas in CNS and skin, angiofibromas C, mitral regurgitation, ash-leaf spots D, cardiac rhabdomyoma, intellectual disability, renal angiomyolipoma E, seizures, shagreen patches. | ↑ incidence of subependymal giant cell astrocytomas and ungual fibromas. |
| **Neurofibromatosis type I** | AD, 100% penetrance. Mutation in NF1 tumor suppressor gene on chromosome 17 (encodes neurofibromin, a negative RAS regulator). | Café-au-lait spots F, Intellectual disability, Cutaneous neurofibromas G, Lisch nodules (pigmented iris hamartomas H), Optic gliomas, Pheochromocytomas, Seizures/focal neurologic Signs (often from meningioma), bone lesions (eg, sphenoid dysplasia). | Also called von Recklinghausen disease. 17 letters in "von Recklinghausen." CICLOPSS. |
| **Neurofibromatosis type II** | AD. Mutation in NF2 tumor suppressor gene (merlin) on chromosome 22. | Bilateral vestibular schwannomas, juvenile cataracts, meningiomas, ependymomas. | NF2 affects 2 ears, 2 eyes. |
| **von Hippel-Lindau disease** | AD. Deletion of VHL gene on chromosome 3p. pVHL ubiquitinates hypoxia-inducible factor 1a. | Hemangioblastomas (high vascularity with hyperchromatic nuclei I) in retina, brainstem, cerebellum, spine J; Angiomatosis; bilateral Renal cell carcinomas; Pheochromocytomas. | Numerous tumors, benign and malignant. HARP. VHL = 3 letters = chromosome 3; associated with RCC (also 3 letters). |

## Adult primary brain tumors

| TUMOR | DESCRIPTION | HISTOLOGY |
|---|---|---|
| Glioblastoma | Common, highly malignant 1° brain tumor with ~ 1-year median survival. Found in cerebral hemispheres. Can cross corpus callosum ("butterfly glioma" A). Associated with *EGFR* amplification. | Astrocyte origin, GFAP ⊕. "Pseudopalisading" pleomorphic tumor cells B border central areas of necrosis, hemorrhage, and/or microvascular proliferation. |
| Oligodendroglioma | Relatively rare, slow growing. Most often in frontal lobes C. Often calcified. | Oligodendrocyte origin. "Fried egg" cells—round nuclei with clear cytoplasm D. "Chicken-wire" capillary pattern. |
| Meningioma | Common, typically benign. Females > males. Occurs along surface of brain or spinal cord. Extra-axial (external to brain parenchyma) and may have a dural attachment ("tail" E). Often asymptomatic; may present with seizures or focal neurologic signs. Resection and/or radiosurgery. | Arachnoid cell origin. Spindle cells concentrically arranged in a whorled pattern; psammoma bodies (laminated calcifications, arrow in F). |
| Hemangioblastoma | Most often cerebellar G. Associated with von Hippel-Lindau syndrome when found with retinal angiomas. Can produce erythropoietin → 2° polycythemia. | Blood vessel origin. Closely arranged, thin-walled capillaries with minimal intervening parenchyma H. |
| Pituitary adenoma | May be nonfunctioning (silent) or hyperfunctioning (hormone-producing). Nonfunctional tumors present with mass effect (eg, bitemporal hemianopia [due to pressure on optic chiasm I]). Pituitary apoplexy → hypopituitarism. Prolactinoma classically presents as galactorrhea, amenorrhea, ↓ bone density due to suppression of estrogen in females and as ↓ libido, infertility in males. Treatment: dopamine agonists (eg, bromocriptine, cabergoline), transsphenoidal resection. | Hyperplasia of only one type of endocrine cells found in pituitary. Most commonly from lactotrophs (prolactin) J → hyperprolactinemia. Less commonly, from somatotrophs (GH) → acromegaly, gigantism; corticotrophs (ACTH) → Cushing disease. Rarely, from thyrotrophs (TSH), gonadotrophs (FSH, LH). |
| Schwannoma | Classically at the cerebellopontine angle K, benign, involving CNs V, VII, and VIII, but can be along any peripheral nerve. Often localized to CN VIII in internal acoustic meatus → vestibular schwannoma (can present as hearing loss and tinnitus). Bilateral vestibular schwannomas found in NF-2. Resection or stereotactic radiosurgery. | Schwann cell origin, S-100 ⊕. Biphasic, dense, hypercellular areas containing spindle cells alternating with hypocellular, myxoid areas L. |

## Adult primary brain tumors *(continued)*

## Childhood primary brain tumors

| TUMOR | DESCRIPTION | HISTOLOGY |
|---|---|---|
| Pilocytic astrocytoma | Most common 1° brain tumor in childhood. Usually well circumscribed. In children, most often found in posterior fossa (eg, cerebellum). May be supratentorial. Cystic appearance with mural nodule A. Benign; good prognosis. | Astrocyte origin, GFAP ⊕. Bipolar neoplastic cells with hairlike projections. Associated with microcysts and Rosenthal fibers (eosinophilic, corkscrew fibers B). |
| Medulloblastoma | Most common malignant brain tumor in childhood. Commonly involves cerebellum C. Can compress 4th ventricle, causing noncommunicating hydrocephalus → headaches, papilledema. Can involve the cerebellar vermis → truncal ataxia. Can send "drop metastases" to spinal cord. | Form of primitive neuroectodermal tumor (PNET). Homer-Wright rosettes (small blue cells surrounding central area of neuropil D). Synaptophysin ⊕. |
| Ependymoma | Most commonly found in 4th ventricle E. Can cause hydrocephalus. Poor prognosis. | Ependymal cell origin. Characteristic perivascular pseudorosettes F. Rod-shaped blepharoplasts (basal ciliary bodies) found near the nucleus. |
| Craniopharyngioma | Most common childhood supratentorial tumor. Calcification is common G. May be confused with pituitary adenoma (both cause bitemporal hemianopia). Associated with a high recurrence rate. | Derived from remnants of Rathke pouch (ectoderm) H. Cholesterol crystals found in "motor oil"-like fluid within tumor. |
| Pineal gland tumors | Most commonly extragonadal germ cell tumors. ↑ incidence in males. Present with obstructive hydrocephalus (compression of cerebral aqueduct), Parinaud syndrome (compression of dorsal midbrain)—triad of upward gaze palsy, convergence-retraction nystagmus, and light-near dissociation. | Similar to testicular seminomas. |

## Herniation syndromes

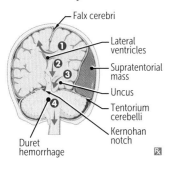

Falx cerebri
Lateral ventricles
Supratentorial mass
Uncus
Tentorium cerebelli
Kernohan notch
Duret hemorrhage

| | |
|---|---|
| ❶ Cingulate (subfalcine) herniation under falx cerebri | Can compress anterior cerebral artery. |
| ❷ Central/downward transtentorial herniation | Caudal displacement of brainstem → rupture of paramedian basilar artery branches → Duret hemorrhages. Usually fatal. |
| ❸ Uncal transtentorial herniation | Uncus = medial temporal lobe. Early herniation → ipsilateral blown pupil (unilateral CN III compression), contralateral hemiparesis. Late herniation → coma, Kernohan phenomenon (misleading contralateral blown pupil and ipsilateral hemiparesis due to contralateral compression against Kernohan notch). |
| ❹ Cerebellar tonsillar herniation into the foramen magnum | Coma and death result when these herniations compress the brainstem. |

## Motor neuron signs

| SIGN | UMN LESION | LMN LESION | COMMENTS |
|---|---|---|---|
| Weakness | + | + | Lower motor neuron (LMN) = everything lowered (less muscle mass, ↓ muscle tone, ↓ reflexes, downgoing toes) |
| Atrophy | – | + | |
| Fasciculations | – | + | |
| Reflexes | ↑ | ↓ | Upper motor neuron (UMN) = everything up (tone, DTRs, toes) |
| Tone | ↑ | ↓ | |
| Babinski | + | – | Fasciculations = muscle twitching |
| Spastic paresis | + | – | Positive Babinski is normal in infants |
| Flaccid paralysis | – | + | |
| Clasp knife spasticity | + | – | |

## Spinal cord lesions

| | |
|---|---|
| **Poliomyelitis**  | Destruction of anterior horns by poliovirus. Fecal-oral transmission → replication in lymphoid tissue of oropharynx and small intestine → spread to CNS via bloodstream. Acute LMN signs (**asymmetric** weakness) and symptoms of viral meningitis (eg, fever, headache, neck stiffness). Respiratory muscle involvement leads to respiratory failure. CSF shows ↑ WBCs (lymphocytic pleocytosis) and slight ↑ of protein (with no change in CSF glucose). Poliovirus can be isolated from stool or throat secretions. |
| **Spinal muscular atrophy**  | Congenital degeneration of anterior horns. Autosomal recessive *SMN1* mutation (encodes survival motor neuron protein) → defective snRNP assembly → LMN apoptosis. Spinal muscular atrophy type 1 (most common) is also called Werdnig-Hoffmann disease. LMN signs only (**symmetric** weakness). "Floppy baby" with marked hypotonia (flaccid paralysis) and tongue fasciculations. |
| **Amyotrophic lateral sclerosis**  | Combined UMN (corticospinal/corticobulbar) and LMN (brainstem/spinal cord) degeneration. Usually idiopathic. Familial form (less common) may be linked to *SOD1* mutations (encodes superoxide dismutase 1). ALS is also called Lou Gehrig disease. LMN signs: flaccid limb weakness, fasciculations, atrophy, bulbar palsy (dysarthria, dysphagia, tongue atrophy). UMN signs: spastic limb weakness, hyperreflexia, clonus, pseudobulbar palsy (dysarthria, dysphagia, emotional lability). No sensory or bowel/bladder deficits. Fatal (most often from respiratory failure). Treatment: riluzole ("ri**Lou**zole"). |
| **Tabes dorsalis**  | Degeneration/demyelination of dorsal columns and roots by *T pallidum* (3° syphilis). Causes progressive sensory ataxia (impaired proprioception → poor coordination). ⊕ Romberg sign and absent DTRs. Associated with shooting pain, Argyll Robertson pupils, Charcot joints. |
| **Subacute combined degeneration**  | Demyelination of Spinocerebellar tracts, lateral Corticospinal tracts, and Dorsal columns (SCD) due to vitamin $B_{12}$ deficiency. Ataxic gait, paresthesias, impaired position/vibration sense (⊕ Romberg sign), UMN signs. |
| **Anterior spinal artery occlusion**  Posterior spinal arteries<br>Anterior spinal artery | Spinal cord infarction sparing dorsal horns and dorsal columns. Watershed area is mid-thoracic ASA territory, as the artery of Adamkiewicz supplies ASA below T8. Can be caused by aortic aneurysm repair. Presents with UMN signs below the lesion (corticospinal tract), LMN signs at the level of the lesion (anterior horn), and loss of pain and temperature sensation below the lesion (spinothalamic tract). |

## Brown-Séquard syndrome

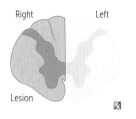

Hemisection of spinal cord. Findings:
1. Ipsilateral loss of all sensation **at** level of lesion
2. Ipsilateral LMN signs (eg, flaccid paralysis) **at** level of lesion
3. Ipsilateral UMN signs **below** level of lesion (due to corticospinal tract damage)
4. Ipsilateral loss of proprioception, vibration, and fine (2-point discrimination) touch **below** level of lesion (due to dorsal column damage)
5. Contralateral loss of pain, temperature, and crude (non-discriminative) touch **below** level of lesion (due to spinothalamic tract damage)

If lesion occurs above T1, patient may present with ipsilateral Horner syndrome due to damage of oculosympathetic pathway.

## Friedreich ataxia

Autosomal recessive trinucleotide repeat disorder $(GAA)_n$ on chromosome 9 in gene that encodes frataxin (iron-binding protein). Leads to impairment in mitochondrial functioning. Degeneration of lateral corticospinal tract (spastic paralysis), spinocerebellar tract (ataxia), dorsal columns (↓ vibratory sense, proprioception), and dorsal root ganglia (loss of DTRs). **Staggering** gait, frequent **falling**, nystagmus, dysarthria, pes cavus, hammer toes, diabetes mellitus, **hypertrophic cardiomyopathy** (cause of death). Presents in childhood with kyphoscoliosis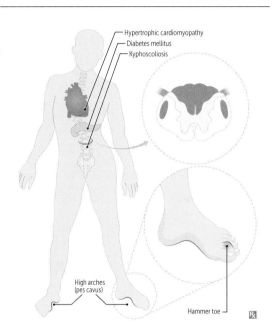

Friedreich is fratastic (**frataxin**): he's your favorite **frat** brother, always **staggering** and **falling** but has a sweet, big heart. Ataxic GAAit.

## Cerebral palsy

Permanent motor dysfunction resulting from nonprogressive injury to developing fetal/infant brain. Most common movement disorder in children.

Multifactorial etiology; prematurity and low birth weight are the strongest risk factors. Associated with development of periventricular leukomalacia (focal necrosis of white matter tracts).

Presents with UMN signs (eg, spasticity, hyperreflexia) affecting ≥ 1 limbs, persistence of primitive reflexes, abnormal posture, developmental delay in motor skills, neurobehavioral abnormalities (excessive docility, irritability).

Treatment: muscle relaxants (eg, baclofen), botulinum toxin injections, selective dorsal rhizotomy.

Prevention: prenatal magnesium sulfate for high-risk pregnancies ↓ incidence and severity.

### Common cranial nerve lesions

| | |
|---|---|
| **CN V motor lesion** | Jaw deviates **toward** side of lesion due to unopposed force from the opposite pterygoid muscle. |
| **CN X lesion** | Uvula deviates **away** from side of lesion. Weak side collapses and uvula points away. |
| **CN XI lesion** | Weakness turning head **away** from side of lesion (SCM). Shoulder droop on side of lesion (trapezius). |
| **CN XII lesion** | LMN lesion. Tongue deviates **toward** side of lesion ("lick your wounds") due to weakened tongue muscles on affected side. |

### Facial nerve lesions

**Bell palsy** is the most common cause of peripheral facial palsy **A**. Usually develops after HSV reactivation. Treatment: glucocorticoids +/– acyclovir. Most patients gradually recover function, but aberrant regeneration can occur. Other causes of peripheral facial palsy include Lyme disease, herpes zoster (Ramsay Hunt syndrome), sarcoidosis, tumors (eg, parotid gland), diabetes mellitus.

| | Upper motor neuron lesion | Lower motor neuron lesion |
|---|---|---|
| LESION LOCATION | Motor cortex, connection from motor cortex to facial nucleus in pons | Facial nucleus, anywhere along CN VII |
| AFFECTED SIDE | Contralateral | Ipsilateral |
| MUSCLES INVOLVED | Lower muscles of facial expression | Upper and lower muscles of facial expression |
| FOREHEAD INVOLVEMENT | Spared, due to bilateral UMN innervation | Affected |
| OTHER SYMPTOMS | Variable; depends on size of lesion | Incomplete eye closure (dry eyes, corneal ulceration), hyperacusis, loss of taste sensation to anterior tongue |

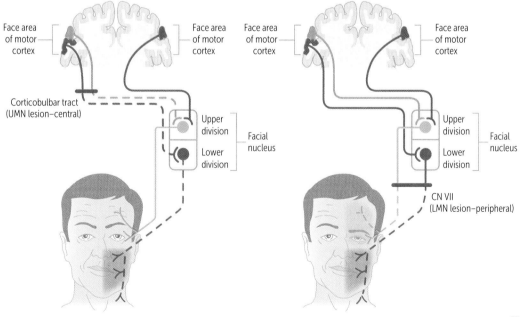

## ▶ NEUROLOGY—OTOLOGY

**Auditory anatomy and physiology**

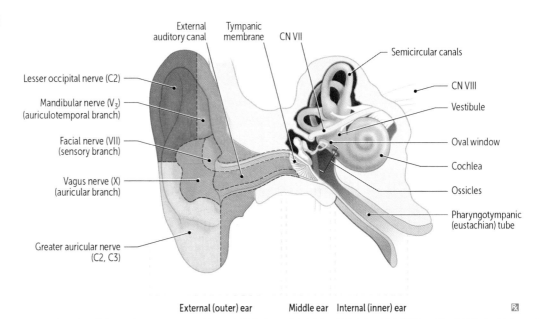

Lesser occipital nerve (C2)
Mandibular nerve (V₃) (auriculotemporal branch)
Facial nerve (VII) (sensory branch)
Vagus nerve (X) (auricular branch)
Greater auricular nerve (C2, C3)

External auditory canal — Tympanic membrane — CN VII
Semicircular canals
CN VIII
Vestibule
Oval window
Cochlea
Ossicles
Pharyngotympanic (eustachian) tube

External (outer) ear     Middle ear    Internal (inner) ear

| | |
|---|---|
| **Outer ear** | Visible portion of ear (pinna), includes auditory canal and tympanic membrane. Transfers sound waves via vibration of tympanic membrane. |
| **Middle ear** | Air-filled space with three bones called the ossicles (malleus, incus, stapes). Ossicles conduct and amplify sound from tympanic membrane to inner ear. |
| **Inner ear** | Snail-shaped, fluid-filled cochlea. Contains basilar membrane that vibrates 2° to sound waves. Vibration transduced via specialized hair cells → auditory nerve signaling → brainstem. Each frequency leads to vibration at specific location on basilar membrane (tonotopy): ▪ Low frequency heard at apex near helicotrema (wide and flexible). ▪ High frequency heard best at base of cochlea (thin and rigid). |

**Otitis externa**

Inflammation of external auditory canal. Most commonly due to *Pseudomonas*. Associated with water exposure (swimmer's ear), ear canal trauma/occlusion (eg, hearing aids).
Presents with otalgia that worsens with ear manipulation, pruritus, hearing loss, discharge A.
Malignant (necrotizing) otitis externa—invasive infection causing osteomyelitis. Complication of otitis externa mostly seen in older patients with diabetes. Presents with severe otalgia and otorrhea. May lead to cranial nerve palsies. Physical exam shows granulation tissue in ear canal.

**Otitis media**

Inflammation of middle ear. Most commonly due to nontypeable *Haemophilus influenzae*, *Streptococcus pneumoniae*, *Moraxella catarrhalis*. Associated with eustachian tube dysfunction, which promotes overgrowth of bacterial colonizers of upper respiratory tract.
Usually seen in children < 2 years old. Presents with fever, otalgia, hearing loss. Physical exam shows bulging, erythematous tympanic membrane A that may rupture.
Mastoiditis—infection of mastoid process of temporal bone. Complication of acute otitis media due to continuity of middle ear cavity with mastoid air cells. Presents with postauricular pain, erythema, swelling. May lead to brain abscess.

## Common causes of hearing loss

| | |
|---|---|
| Noise-induced hearing loss | Damage to stereociliated cells in organ of Corti. Loss of high-frequency hearing first. Sudden extremely loud noises can produce hearing loss due to tympanic membrane rupture. |
| Presbycusis | Aging-related progressive bilateral/symmetric sensorineural hearing loss (often of higher frequencies) due to destruction of hair cells at the cochlear base (preserved low-frequency hearing at apex). |

## Diagnosing hearing loss

| | Normal | Conductive | Sensorineural |
|---|---|---|---|
| **Weber test** Tuning fork on vertex of skull | No localization | Localizes to affected ear ↓ transmission of background noise | Localizes to unaffected ear ↓ transmission of all sound |
| **Rinne test** Tuning fork in front of ear (air conduction, AC), Tuning fork on mastoid process (bone conduction, BC) | AC > BC | BC > AC | AC > BC |

## Cholesteatoma

Abnormal growth of keratinized squamous epithelium in middle ear 🅐 ("skin in wrong place"). Usually acquired, but can be congenital. 1° acquired results from tympanic membrane retraction pockets that form due to eustachian tube dysfunction. 2° acquired results from tympanic membrane perforation (eg, due to otitis media) that permits migration of squamous epithelium to middle ear. Classically presents with painless otorrhea. May erode ossicles → conductive hearing loss.

## Vertigo

Sensation of spinning while actually stationary. Subtype of "dizziness," but distinct from "lightheadedness." Peripheral vertigo is more common than central vertigo.

| | |
|---|---|
| Peripheral vertigo | Due to inner ear pathologies such as semicircular canal debris (benign paroxysmal positional vertigo), vestibular neuritis, **Mén**ière disease—endolymphatic hydrops (↑ endolymph in inner ear) → triad of vertigo, sensorineural hearing loss, tinnitus ("**men** wear **vests**"). Findings: mixed horizontal-torsional nystagmus (never purely torsional or vertical) that does not change direction and is suppressible with visual fixation. |
| Central vertigo | Due to brainstem or cerebellar lesions (eg, stroke affecting vestibular nuclei, demyelinating disease, or posterior fossa tumor). Findings: nystagmus of any direction that is not suppressible with visual fixation, neurologic findings (eg, diplopia, ataxia, dysmetria). |

▶ NEUROLOGY—OPHTHALMOLOGY

### Normal eye anatomy

---

### Conjunctivitis

Inflammation of the conjunctiva → red eye .

Allergic—itchy eyes, bilateral.

Bacterial—pus; treat with antibiotics.

Viral—most common, often adenovirus; sparse mucous discharge, swollen preauricular node, ↑ lacrimation; self-resolving.

---

| Refractive errors | Common cause of impaired vision, correctable with glasses. |
|---|---|
| Hyperopia | Also called "farsightedness." Eye too short for refractive power of cornea and lens → light focused behind retina. Correct with convex (converging) lenses. |
| Myopia | Also called "nearsightedness." Eye too long for refractive power of cornea and lens → light focused in front of retina. Correct with concave (diverging) lens. |
| Astigmatism | Abnormal curvature of cornea → different refractive power at different axes. Correct with cylindrical lens. |

## Lens disorders

| | |
|---|---|
| Presbyopia | Aging-related impaired accommodation (focusing on near objects), primarily due to ↓ lens elasticity. Patients often need reading glasses or magnifiers. |
| Cataract  | Painless, often bilateral, opacification of lens A. Can result in glare and ↓ vision, especially at night, and loss of the red reflex. <br> Acquired risk factors: ↑ age, tobacco smoking, alcohol overuse, excessive sunlight, prolonged glucocorticoid use, diabetes mellitus, trauma, infection. <br> Congenital risk factors: classic galactosemia, galactokinase deficiency, trisomies (13, 18, 21), TORCH infections (eg, rubella), Marfan syndrome, Alport syndrome, myotonic dystrophy, NF-2. <br> Treatment: surgical removal of lens and replacement with an artificial lens. |
| Lens dislocation | Also called ectopia lentis. Displacement or malposition of lens. Usually due to trauma, but may occur in association with systemic diseases (eg, Marfan syndrome, homocystinuria). |

## Aqueous humor pathway

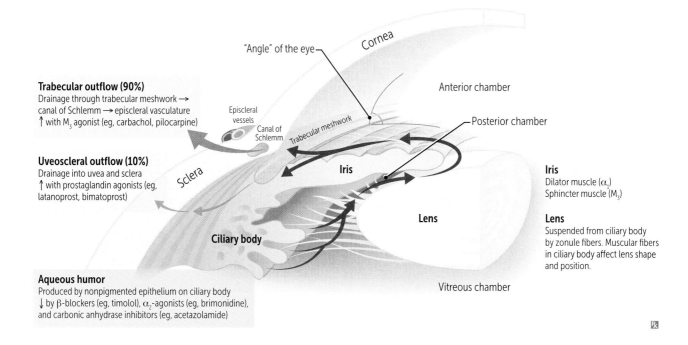

**Trabecular outflow (90%)**
Drainage through trabecular meshwork → canal of Schlemm → episcleral vasculature
↑ with $M_3$ agonist (eg, carbachol, pilocarpine)

**Uveoscleral outflow (10%)**
Drainage into uvea and sclera
↑ with prostaglandin agonists (eg, latanoprost, bimatoprost)

**Aqueous humor**
Produced by nonpigmented epithelium on ciliary body
↓ by β-blockers (eg, timolol), $\alpha_2$-agonists (eg, brimonidine), and carbonic anhydrase inhibitors (eg, acetazolamide)

"Angle" of the eye
Cornea
Anterior chamber
Episcleral vessels
Canal of Schlemm
Trabecular meshwork
Posterior chamber
Iris
Sclera
Ciliary body
Lens
Vitreous chamber

**Iris**
Dilator muscle ($\alpha_1$)
Sphincter muscle ($M_3$)

**Lens**
Suspended from ciliary body by zonule fibers. Muscular fibers in ciliary body affect lens shape and position.

| | |
|---|---|
| **Glaucoma** | Optic neuropathy causing progressive vision loss (peripheral → central). Usually, but not always, accompanied by ↑ intraocular pressure (IOP). Etiology is most often 1°, but can be 2° to an identifiable cause (eg, uveitis, glucocorticoids). Funduscopy: optic disc cupping (normal **A** vs thinning of outer rim of optic disc **B**). Treatment: pharmacologic or surgical lowering of IOP. |
| **Open-angle glaucoma** | Anterior chamber angle is open (normal). Most common type in US. Associated with ↑ resistance to aqueous humor drainage through trabecular meshwork. Risk factors: ↑ age, race (↑ incidence in Black population), family history, diabetes mellitus. Typically asymptomatic and discovered incidentally. |
| **Angle-closure glaucoma** | Anterior chamber angle is narrowed or closed. Associated with anatomic abnormalities (eg, anteriorly displaced lens resting against central iris) → ↓ aqueous flow through pupil (pupillary block) → pressure buildup in posterior chamber → peripheral iris pushed against cornea → obstruction of drainage pathways by the iris. Usually chronic and asymptomatic, but may develop acutely. |
| | Acute angle-closure glaucoma—complete pupillary block causing abrupt angle closure and rapid ↑ IOP. Presents with severe eye pain, conjunctival erythema **C**, sudden vision loss, halos around lights, headache, fixed and mid-dilated pupil, nausea and vomiting. Hurts in a hurry with halos, a headache, and a "half-dilated" pupil. True ophthalmic emergency that requires immediate management to prevent blindness. Mydriatic agents are contraindicated. |

Open-angle glaucoma

Angle-closure glaucoma

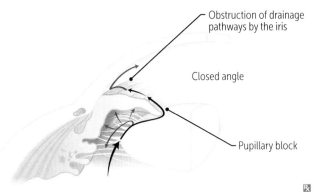

## Retinal disorders

| | |
|---|---|
| Age-related macular degeneration | Degeneration of macula (central area of retina) → loss of central vision (scotomas). Two types:<br>▪ Dry (most common)—gradual ↓ in vision with subretinal deposits (drusen, arrow in **A**).<br>▪ Wet—rapid ↓ in vision due to bleeding 2° to choroidal neovascularization. Distortion of straight lines (metamorphopsia) is an early symptom. |
| Diabetic retinopathy | Chronic hyperglycemia → ↑ permeability and occlusion of retinal vessels. Two types:<br>▪ Nonproliferative (most common)—microaneurysms, hemorrhages (arrows in **B**), cotton-wool spots, hard exudates. Vision loss mainly due to macular edema.<br>▪ Proliferative—retinal neovascularization due to chronic hypoxia. Abnormal new vessels may cause vitreous hemorrhage and tractional retinal detachment. |
| Hypertensive retinopathy | Chronic hypertension → spasm, sclerosis, and fibrinoid necrosis of retinal vessels. Funduscopy: arteriovenous nicking, microaneurysms, hemorrhages, cotton-wool spots (blue arrow in **C**), hard exudates (may form macular "star," red arrow in **C**). Presence of papilledema is indicative of hypertensive emergency and warrants immediate lowering of blood pressure. |
| Retinal artery occlusion | Blockage of central or branch retinal artery usually due to embolism (carotid artery atherosclerosis > cardiogenic); less commonly due to giant cell arteritis. Presents with acute, painless monocular vision loss. Funduscopy: cloudy retina with "cherry-red" spot at fovea **D**, identifiable retinal emboli (eg, cholesterol crystals appear as small, yellow, refractile deposits in arterioles). |
| Retinal vein occlusion | Central retinal vein occlusion is due to 1° thrombosis; branch retinal vein occlusion is due to 2° thrombosis at arteriovenous crossings (sclerotic arteriole compresses adjacent venule causing turbulent blood flow). Funduscopy: retinal hemorrhage and venous engorgement ("blood and thunder" appearance; arrows in **E**), retinal edema in affected areas. |
| Retinal detachment | Separation of neurosensory retina from underlying retinal pigment epithelium → loss of choroidal blood supply → hypoxia and degeneration of photoreceptors. Two types:<br>▪ Rhegmatogenous (most common)—due to retinal tears; often associated with posterior vitreous detachment (↑ risk with advanced age, high myopia), less frequently traumatic.<br>▪ Nonrhegmatogenous—tractional or exudative (fluid accumulation).<br>Commonly presents with symptoms of posterior vitreous detachment (eg, floaters, light flashes) followed by painless monocular vision loss ("dark curtain"). Funduscopy: opacification and wrinkling of detached retina **F**, change in vessel direction. Surgical emergency. |
| Retinitis pigmentosa | Group of inherited dystrophies causing progressive degeneration of photoreceptors and retinal pigment epithelium. May be associated with abetalipoproteinemia. Early symptoms: night blindness (nyctalopia) and peripheral vision loss. Funduscopy: triad of optic disc pallor, retinal vessel attenuation, and retinal pigmentation with bone spicule-shaped deposits **G**. |
| Retinopathy of prematurity | Preterm birth → loss of normal hypoxic environment in utero → relative hyperoxia (↑ with supplemental $O_2$ for NRDS) → ↓ VEGF → arrest of normal retinal vascularization. As the eyes grow → hypoxia of avascular retina → ↑ VEGF → retinal neovascularization (may cause tractional retinal detachment). Common cause of childhood blindness. |
| Papilledema | Optic disc swelling (usually bilateral) due to ↑ ICP (eg, 2° to mass effect). Results from impaired axoplasmic flow in optic nerve. Funduscopy: elevated optic disc with blurred margins **H**. |

## Retinal disorders *(continued)*

| | |
|---|---|
| **Retinoblastoma**  | Most common intraocular malignancy in children. Arises from immature retinal cells . Caused by mutations to both *RB1* tumor suppressor genes on chromosome 13, which normally impede $G_1 \rightarrow S$ phase progression. Can be sporadic or familial (loss of heterozygosity). Presents with leukocoria, strabismus, nystagmus, eye redness. |
| **Leukocoria**  | Loss (whitening) of the red reflex. Important causes in children include retinoblastoma A, congenital cataract. |
| **Uveitis**  | Inflammation of uvea; specific name based on location within affected eye. Anterior uveitis: iritis; posterior uveitis: choroiditis and/or retinitis. May have hypopyon (accumulation of pus in anterior chamber A) or conjunctival redness. Associated with systemic inflammatory disorders (eg, sarcoidosis, Behçet syndrome, juvenile idiopathic arthritis, HLA-B27–associated conditions). |

## Pupillary control

| | |
|---|---|
| **Miosis** | Constriction, parasympathetic:<br>▪ 1st neuron: Edinger-Westphal nucleus to ciliary ganglion via CN III<br>▪ 2nd neuron: short ciliary nerves to sphincter pupillae muscles<br>Short ciliary nerves shorten the pupil diameter. |
| **Pupillary light reflex** | Light in either retina sends a signal via CN II to pretectal nuclei (dashed lines in image) in midbrain that activates bilateral Edinger-Westphal nuclei; pupils constrict bilaterally (direct and consensual reflex).<br>Result: illumination of 1 eye results in bilateral pupillary constriction. 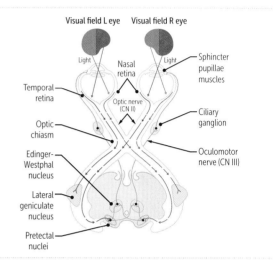 |
| **Mydriasis** | Dilation, sympathetic:<br>▪ 1st neuron: hypothalamus to ciliospinal center of Budge (C8–T2)<br>▪ 2nd neuron: exit at T1 to superior cervical ganglion (travels along cervical sympathetic chain near lung apex, subclavian vessels)<br>▪ 3rd neuron: plexus along internal carotid, through cavernous sinus; enters orbit as long ciliary nerve to pupillary dilator muscles. Sympathetic fibers also innervate smooth muscle of eyelids (minor retractors) and sweat glands of forehead and face.<br>Long ciliary nerves make the pupil diameter longer. |

| | |
|---|---|
| **Relative afferent pupillary defect** | Also called Marcus Gunn pupil. Extent of pupillary constriction differs when light is shone in one eye at a time due to unilateral or asymmetric lesions of afferent limb of pupillary reflex (eg, retina, optic nerve). When light shines into a normal eye, constriction of the ipsilateral eye (direct reflex) and contralateral eye (consensual reflex) is observed. When light is swung from a normal eye to an affected eye, both pupils dilate instead of constricting. |

## Horner syndrome

Sympathetic denervation of face:
- Ptosis (slight drooping of eyelid: superior tarsal muscle)
- Miosis (pupil constriction)
- Anhidrosis (absence of sweating) and absence of flushing of affected side of face

Associated with lesions along the sympathetic chain:
- 1st neuron: pontine hemorrhage, lateral medullary syndrome, spinal cord lesion above T1 (eg, Brown-Séquard syndrome, late-stage syringomyelia)
- 2nd neuron: stellate ganglion compression by Pancoast tumor
- 3rd neuron: carotid dissection (painful); anhidrosis is usually absent

## Ocular motility

CN **VI** innervates the **L**ateral **R**ectus.
CN **IV** innervates the **S**uperior **O**blique.
CN **III** innervates the **R**est.
The "chemical formula" $LR_6SO_4R_3$.

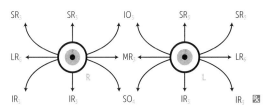

**O**bliques go **O**pposite (left SO and IO tested with patient looking right)
**IOU: IO** tested looking **U**p

**Blowout fracture**—orbital floor fracture; usually caused by direct trauma to eyeball or infraorbital rim. ↑ risk of IR muscle A and/or orbital fat entrapment. May lead to infraorbital nerve injury

## Strabismus

Eye misalignment ("crossed eyes"). Deviation of eye toward the nose (esotropia) is the most common type of strabismus in children. Complications include amblyopia, diplopia, adverse psychosocial impact.

**Amblyopia** ("lazy eye")—↓ visual acuity due to maldevelopment of visual cortex. Caused by abnormal visual experience early in life (eg, due to strabismus). Typically unilateral.

## Cranial nerve III, IV, VI palsies

| | | |
|---|---|---|
| **CN III damage** | CN III has both motor (central) and parasympathetic (peripheral) components. Common causes include: | Motor = **m**iddle (central) Parasympathetic = **p**eripheral |

- Ischemia → pupil sparing (motor fibers affected more than parasympathetic fibers)
- Uncal herniation → coma
- PCom aneurysm → sudden-onset headache
- Cavernous sinus thrombosis → proptosis, involvement of CNs IV, $V_1/V_2$, VI
- Midbrain stroke → contralateral hemiplegia

CN III

**M**otor output to extraocular muscles—affected primarily by vascular disease (eg, diabetes mellitus: glucose → sorbitol) due to ↓ diffusion of oxygen and nutrients to the interior (**m**iddle) fibers from compromised vasculature that resides on outside of nerve. Signs: ptosis, "down-and-out" gaze.

**P**arasympathetic output—fibers on the **p**eriphery are first affected by compression (eg, PCom aneurysm, uncal herniation). Signs: diminished or absent pupillary light reflex, "blown pupil" often with "down-and-out" gaze A.

| | |
|---|---|
| **CN IV damage** | Pupil is higher in the affected eye B. Characteristic head tilt to contralateral/ unaffected side to compensate for lack of intorsion in affected eye. Can't see the **floor** with CN **IV** damage (eg, difficulty going down stairs, reading). |

| | |
|---|---|
| **CN VI damage** | Affected eye unable to abduct C and is displaced medially in primary position of gaze. |

**Visual field defects**

Ventral optic radiation (Meyer loop)—lower retina; travels through temporal lobe; loops around inferior horn of lateral ventricle.

Dorsal optic radiation—superior retina; travels through parietal lobe.

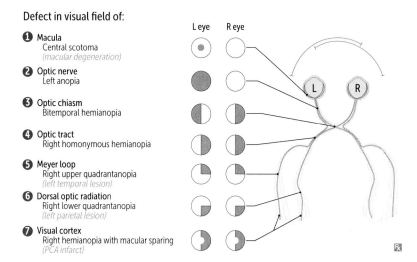

Defect in visual field of:

❶ Macula
Central scotoma
*(macular degeneration)*

❷ Optic nerve
Left anopia

❸ Optic chiasm
Bitemporal hemianopia

❹ Optic tract
Right homonymous hemianopia

❺ Meyer loop
Right upper quadrantanopia
*(left temporal lesion)*

❻ Dorsal optic radiation
Right lower quadrantanopia
*(left parietal lesion)*

❼ Visual cortex
Right hemianopia with macular sparing
*(PCA infarct)*

Note: When an image hits 1° visual cortex, it is upside down and left-right reversed.

**Cavernous sinus**

Collection of venous sinuses on either side of pituitary. Blood from eye and superficial cortex → cavernous sinus → internal jugular vein.

CNs III, IV, $V_1$, $V_2$, and VI plus postganglionic sympathetic pupillary fibers en route to orbit all pass through cavernous sinus. Cavernous portion of internal carotid artery is also here.

Cavernous sinus syndrome—presents with variable ophthalmoplegia (eg, CN III and CN VI), ↓ corneal sensation, Horner syndrome and occasional decreased maxillary sensation. 2° to pituitary tumor mass effect, carotid-cavernous fistula, or cavernous sinus thrombosis related to infection (spread due to lack of valves in dural venous sinuses).

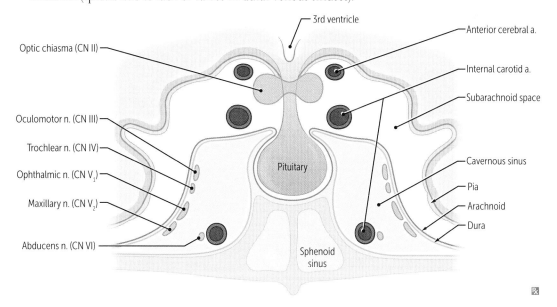

- 3rd ventricle
- Anterior cerebral a.
- Optic chiasma (CN II)
- Internal carotid a.
- Subarachnoid space
- Oculomotor n. (CN III)
- Trochlear n. (CN IV)
- Ophthalmic n. (CN $V_1$)
- Pituitary
- Cavernous sinus
- Maxillary n. (CN $V_2$)
- Pia
- Arachnoid
- Dura
- Abducens n. (CN VI)
- Sphenoid sinus

**Internuclear ophthalmoplegia**

Medial longitudinal fasciculus (MLF): pair of tracts that interconnect CN VI and CN III nuclei. Coordinates both eyes to move in same horizontal direction. Highly myelinated (must communicate quickly so eyes move at same time). Lesions may be unilateral or bilateral (latter classically seen in multiple sclerosis, stroke).

Lesion in MLF = internuclear ophthalmoplegia (INO), a conjugate horizontal gaze palsy. Lack of communication such that when CN VI nucleus activates ipsilateral lateral rectus, contralateral CN III nucleus does not stimulate medial rectus to contract. Abducting eye displays nystagmus (CN VI overfires to stimulate CN III). Convergence normal.

MLF in MS.

When looking left, the left nucleus of CN VI fires, which contracts the left lateral rectus and stimulates the contralateral (right) nucleus of CN III via the right MLF to contract the right medial rectus.

Directional term (eg, right INO, left INO) refers to the eye that is unable to adduct.

INO = **I**psilateral adduction failure, **N**ystagmus **O**pposite.

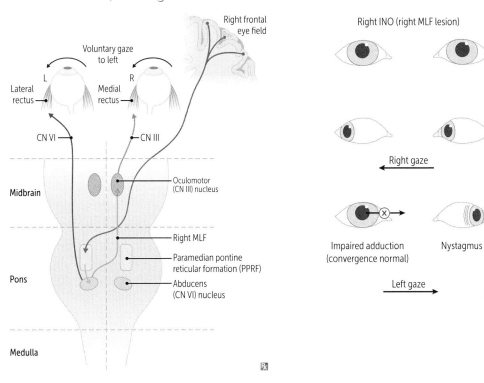

▸ NEUROLOGY—PHARMACOLOGY

**Anticonvulsants**

| | MECHANISM | COMMON ADVERSE EFFECTS | RARE BUT SERIOUS ADVERSE EFFECTS |
|---|---|---|---|
| **Narrow spectrum (focal seizures)** | | | |
| **Phenytoin** | Block Na$^+$ channel | Sedation, dizziness, diplopia, gingival hypertrophy, rash, hirsutism, drug interactions (CYP450 induction) | SJS, DRESS, hepatotoxicity, neuropathy, osteoporosis, folate depletion, teratogenicity |
| **Carbamazepine** | | Sedation, dizziness, diplopia, vomiting, diarrhea, SIADH, rash, drug interactions (CYP450 induction) | SJS, DRESS, hepatotoxicity, agranulocytosis, aplastic anemia, folate depletion, teratogenicity |
| **Gabapentinoids** Gabapentin, pregabalin | Block Ca$^{2+}$ channel | Sedation, dizziness, ataxia, weight gain | |
| **Narrow spectrum (absence seizures only)** | | | |
| **Ethosuximide** | Blocks Ca$^{2+}$ channel | Sedation, dizziness, vomiting | |
| **Broad spectrum (focal and generalized seizures)** | | | |
| **Valproate** | Blocks Na$^+$ channel Blocks Ca$^{2+}$ channel Blocks GABA transaminase | Sedation, dizziness, vomiting, weight gain, hair loss, easy bruising, drug interactions (CYP450 inhibition) | Hepatotoxicity, pancreatitis, teratogenicity |
| **Lamotrigine** | Blocks Na$^+$ channel | Sedation, dizziness, rash | SJS, DRESS |
| **Levetiracetam** | Blocks Synaptic Vesicle protein 2A (SV2A) | Sedation, dizziness, fatigue | Neuropsychiatric (eg, psychosis) |
| **Topiramate** | Blocks Na$^+$ channel Potentiates GABA$_A$ receptor | Sedation, dizziness, mood disturbance (eg, depression), weight loss, paresthesia | Kidney stones, angle-closure glaucoma |

## Anticonvulsants *(continued)*

| **Barbiturates** | Phenobarbital, pentobarbital. |
|---|---|
| MECHANISM | Facilitate $GABA_A$ action by ↑ **duration** of $Cl^-$ channel opening, thus ↓ neuron firing (barbidurates ↑ duration). |
| CLINICAL USE | Sedative for anxiety, seizures, insomnia. |
| ADVERSE EFFECTS | Respiratory and cardiovascular depression (can be fatal); CNS depression (can be exacerbated by alcohol use); dependence; drug interactions (induces cytochrome P-450). Overdose treatment is supportive (assist respiration and maintain BP). Contraindicated in porphyria. |

| **Benzodiazepines** | Diazepam, lorazepam, triazolam, temazepam, oxazepam, midazolam, chlordiazepoxide, alprazolam. |
|---|---|
| MECHANISM | Facilitate $GABA_A$ action by ↑ **frequency** of $Cl^-$ channel opening ("frenzodiazepines" ↑ frequency). ↓ REM sleep. Most have long half-lives and active metabolites (exceptions [**ATOM**]: Alprazolam, Triazolam, Oxazepam, and Midazolam are short acting → higher addictive potential). |
| CLINICAL USE | Anxiety, panic disorder, spasticity, status epilepticus (lorazepam, diazepam, midazolam), eclampsia, medically supervised withdrawal (eg, alcohol/DTs; long-acting chlordiazepoxide and diazepam are preferred), night terrors, sleepwalking, general anesthetic (amnesia, muscle relaxation), hypnotic (insomnia). Lorazepam, Oxazepam, and Temazepam can be used for those with liver disease who drink a LOT due to minimal first-pass metabolism. |
| ADVERSE EFFECTS | Dependence, additive CNS depression effects with alcohol and barbiturates (all bind the $GABA_A$ receptor). Less risk of respiratory depression and coma than with barbiturates. Treat overdose with flumazenil (competitive antagonist at GABA benzodiazepine receptor). Can precipitate seizures by causing acute benzodiazepine withdrawal. |

## Insomnia therapy

| AGENT | MECHANISM | ADVERSE EFFECTS | NOTES |
|---|---|---|---|
| Nonbenzodiazepine hypnotics | Examples: Zolpidem, Zaleplon, esZopiclone Act via the $BZ_1$ subtype of GABA receptor | Ataxia, headaches, confusion Cause only modest day-after psychomotor depression and few amnestic effects (vs older sedative-hypnotics) | These **ZZZ**s put you to sleep Short duration due to rapid metabolism by liver enzymes; effects reversed by flumazenil ↓ dependency risk and ↓ sleep cycle disturbance (vs benzodiazepine hypnotics) |
| Suvorexant | Orexin (hypocretin) receptor antagonist | CNS depression (somnolence), headache, abnormal sleep-related activities | Contraindications: narcolepsy, combination with strong CYP3A4 inhibitors Not recommended in patients with liver disease Limited risk of dependency |
| Ramelteon | Melatonin receptor agonist: binds MT1 and MT2 in suprachiasmatic nucleus | Dizziness, nausea, fatigue, headache | No known risk of dependency |

## Triptans

| Triptans | Sumatriptan |
|---|---|
| MECHANISM | $5\text{-HT}_{1B/1D}$ agonists. Inhibit trigeminal nerve activation, prevent vasoactive peptide release, induce vasoconstriction. |
| CLINICAL USE | Acute migraine, cluster headache attacks. A **sumo** wrestler **trips** and falls on their **head**. |
| ADVERSE EFFECTS | Coronary vasospasm (contraindicated in patients with CAD or vasospastic angina), mild paresthesia, serotonin syndrome (in combination with other 5-HT agonists). |

| | |
|---|---|
| **Parkinson disease therapy** | The most effective treatments are non-ergot dopamine agonists which are usually started in younger patients, and levodopa (with carbidopa) which is usually started in older patients. Deep brain stimulation of the STN or GPi may be helpful in advanced disease. |

| STRATEGY | AGENTS |
|---|---|
| **Dopamine agonists** | Non-ergot (preferred)—pramipexole, ropinirole; toxicity includes nausea, impulse control disorder (eg, gambling), postural hypotension, hallucinations, confusion, sleepiness, edema. Ergot—bromocriptine; rarely used due to toxicity. |
| **↑ dopamine availability** | Amantadine (↑ dopamine release and ↓ dopamine reuptake); mainly used to reduce levodopa-induced dyskinesias; toxicity = peripheral edema, livedo reticularis, ataxia. |
| **↑ L-DOPA availability** | Agents prevent peripheral (pre-BBB) L-DOPA degradation → ↑ L-DOPA entering CNS → ↑ central L-DOPA available for conversion to dopamine.<br>▪ Levodopa (L-DOPA)/carbidopa—carbidopa blocks peripheral conversion of L-DOPA to dopamine by inhibiting DOPA decarboxylase. Also reduces adverse effects of peripheral L-DOPA conversion into dopamine (eg, nausea, vomiting).<br>▪ Entacapone and tolcapone prevent peripheral L-DOPA degradation to 3-O-methyldopa (3-OMD) by inhibiting COMT. Used in conjunction with levodopa. |
| **Prevent dopamine breakdown** | Agents act centrally (post-BBB) to inhibit breakdown of dopamine.<br>▪ Selegiline, rasagiline—block conversion of dopamine into DOPAC by selectively inhibiting MAO-B, which is more commonly found in the Brain than in the periphery.<br>▪ Tolcapone—crosses BBB and blocks conversion of dopamine to 3-methoxytyramine (3-MT) in the brain by inhibiting central COMT. |
| **Curb excess cholinergic activity** | Benztropine, trihexyphenidyl (Antimuscarinic; improves tremor and rigidity but has little effect on bradykinesia in Parkinson disease). **Tri Parking my Mercedes-Benz.** |

## Carbidopa/levodopa

| | |
|---|---|
| MECHANISM | ↑ dopamine in brain. Unlike dopamine, L-DOPA can cross BBB and is converted by DOPA decarboxylase in the CNS to dopamine. Carbidopa, a peripheral DOPA decarboxylase inhibitor that cannot cross BBB, is given with L-DOPA to ↑ bioavailability of L-DOPA in the brain and to limit peripheral adverse effects. |
| CLINICAL USE | Parkinson disease. |
| ADVERSE EFFECTS | Nausea, hallucinations, postural hypotension. With progressive disease, L-DOPA can lead to "on-off" phenomenon with improved mobility during "on" periods, then impaired motor function during "off" periods when patient responds poorly to L-DOPA or medication wears off. |

## Neurodegenerative disease therapy

| DISEASE | AGENT | MECHANISM | NOTES |
|---|---|---|---|
| **Alzheimer disease** | Donepezil, rivastigmine, galantamine | AChE inhibitor | 1st-line treatment<br>Adverse effects: nausea, dizziness, insomnia; contraindicated in patients with cardiac conduction abnormalities<br>**Dona Riva** dances at the gala |
| | Memantine | NMDA receptor antagonist; helps prevent excitotoxicity (mediated by $Ca^{2+}$) | Used for moderate to advanced dementia<br>Adverse effects: dizziness, confusion, hallucinations |
| **Amyotrophic lateral sclerosis** | Riluzole | ↓ neuron glutamate excitotoxicity | ↑ survival<br>Treat **Lou** Gehrig disease with ri**Lou**zole |
| **Huntington disease** | Deutetrabenazine, tetrabenazine | Inhibit vesicular monoamine transporter (VMAT) → ↓ dopamine vesicle packaging and release | May be used for Huntington chorea and tardive dyskinesia |

| | |
|---|---|
| **Local anesthetics** | Esters—benzocaine, chloroprocaine, cocaine, tetracaine. <br> Amides—bupivacaine, lidocaine, mepivacaine, prilocaine, ropivacaine (amides have 2 i's in name). |

| | |
|---|---|
| MECHANISM | Block neurotransmission via binding to voltage-gated $Na^+$ channels on inner portion of the channel along nerve fibers. Most effective in rapidly firing neurons. 3° amine local anesthetics penetrate membrane in uncharged form, then bind to ion channels as charged form. <br> Can be given with vasoconstrictors (usually epinephrine) to enhance block duration of action by ↓ systemic absorption. <br> In infected (acidic) tissue, alkaline anesthetics are charged and cannot penetrate membrane effectively → need more anesthetic. <br> Order of loss: (1) pain, (2) temperature, (3) touch, (4) pressure. |
| CLINICAL USE | Minor surgical procedures, spinal anesthesia. If allergic to esters, give amides. |
| ADVERSE EFFECTS | CNS excitation, severe cardiovascular toxicity (bupivacaine), hypertension, hypotension, arrhythmias (cocaine), methemoglobinemia (benzocaine, prilocaine). |

| | |
|---|---|
| **General anesthetics** | CNS drugs must be lipid soluble (cross the BBB) or be actively transported. <br> Drugs with ↓ solubility in blood (eg, nitrous oxide [$N_2O$]) = rapid induction and recovery times. <br> Drugs with ↑ solubility in lipids (eg, isoflurane) = ↑ potency. <br> MAC = Minimum Alveolar Concentration (of inhaled anesthetic) required to prevent 50% of subjects from moving in response to noxious stimulus (eg, skin incision). Potency = 1/MAC. |

| | MECHANISM | ADVERSE EFFECTS/NOTES |
|---|---|---|
| **Inhaled anesthetics** | | |
| **Sevoflurane** | | Respiratory depression, ↓ cough reflex |
| **Desflurane** | | Myocardial depression, ↓ BP |
| **Isoflurane** | Mechanism unknown | ↑ cerebral blood flow (↑ ICP), ↓ metabolic rate <br> ↓ skeletal and smooth muscle tone <br> Postoperative nausea and vomiting <br> Malignant hyperthermia |
| $N_2O$ | | Diffusion into and expansion ($N_2O$) of gas-filled cavities (eg, pneumothorax); very low potency |
| **Intravenous anesthetics** | | |
| **Propofol** | Potentiates $GABA_A$ receptor <br> Inhibits NMDA receptor | Respiratory depression, ↓ BP; most commonly used IV agent for induction of anesthesia |
| **Etomidate** | Potentiates $GABA_A$ receptor | Acute adrenal insufficiency, postoperative nausea and vomiting; hemodynamically neutral |
| **Ketamine** | Inhibits NMDA receptor | Sympathomimetic: ↑ BP, ↑ HR, ↑ cerebral blood flow (↑ ICP), bronchodilation <br> Psychotomimetic: hallucinations, vivid dreams |

| | |
|---|---|
| **Neuromuscular blocking drugs** | Muscle paralysis in surgery or mechanical ventilation. Selective for $N_m$ nicotinic receptors at neuromuscular junction but not autonomic $N_n$ receptors. |
| Depolarizing neuromuscular blocking drugs | Succinylcholine—strong $N_m$ nicotinic receptor agonist; produces sustained depolarization and prevents muscle contraction. Reversal of blockade: <br> • Phase I (prolonged depolarization)—no antidote. Block potentiated by cholinesterase inhibitors. <br> • Phase II (repolarized but blocked; $N_m$ nicotinic receptors are available, but desensitized)—may be reversed with cholinesterase inhibitors. <br> Complications include hypercalcemia, hyperkalemia, malignant hyperthermia. ↑ risk of prolonged muscle paralysis in patients with pseudocholinesterase deficiency. |
| Nondepolarizing neuromuscular blocking drugs | Atracurium, cisatracurium, pancuronium, rocuronium, vecuronium—competitive $N_m$ nicotinic receptor antagonist. Reversal of blockade—sugammadex or cholinesterase inhibitors (eg, neostigmine). Anticholinergics (eg, atropine, glycopyrrolate) are given with cholinesterase inhibitors to prevent muscarinic effects (eg, bradycardia). |
| **Malignant hyperthermia** | Rare, life-threatening, hypermetabolic condition caused by the administration of potent inhaled anesthetics (sevoflurane, desflurane, isoflurane) or succinylcholine in susceptible individuals. Susceptibility to malignant hyperthermia is caused by de novo or inherited (autosomal dominant) mutations to ryanodine (*RYR1*) or dihydropyridine receptors (*DHPR*). ↑↑ $Ca^{2+}$ release from sarcoplasmic reticulum → sustained muscle contraction → hypercapnia, tachycardia, masseter/generalized muscle rigidity, rhabdomyolysis, hyperthermia. Treatment: dantrolene (ryanodine receptor antagonist). |

## Skeletal muscle relaxants

| DRUG | MECHANISM | CLINICAL USE | NOTES |
|---|---|---|---|
| **Baclofen** | GABA$_B$ receptor agonist in spinal cord | Muscle spasticity, dystonia, multiple sclerosis | Acts on the back (spinal cord) May cause sedation |
| **Cyclobenzaprine** | Acts within CNS, mainly at the brainstem | Muscle spasms | Centrally acting Structurally related to TCAs May cause anticholinergic adverse effects, sedation |
| **Dantrolene** | Prevents release of Ca$^{2+}$ from sarcoplasmic reticulum of skeletal muscle by inhibiting the ryanodine receptor | Malignant hyperthermia (toxicity of inhaled anesthetics and succinylcholine) and neuroleptic malignant syndrome (toxicity of antipsychotics) | Acts directly on muscle |
| **Tizanidine** | $\alpha_2$ agonist, acts centrally | Muscle spasticity, multiple sclerosis, ALS, cerebral palsy | |

## Opioid analgesics

| | |
|---|---|
| MECHANISM | Act as agonists at opioid receptors ($\mu$ = $\beta$-endorphin, $\delta$ = enkephalin, $\kappa$ = dynorphin) to modulate synaptic transmission—close presynaptic Ca$^{2+}$ channels, open postsynaptic K$^+$ channels → ↓ synaptic transmission. Inhibit release of ACh, norepinephrine, 5-HT, glutamate, substance P. |
| EFFICACY | Full agonist: morphine, meperidine (long acting), methadone, codeine (prodrug; activated by CYP2D6), fentanyl. Partial agonist: buprenorphine. Mixed agonist/antagonist: butorphanol, nalbuphine. Antagonist: naloxone, naltrexone, methylnaltrexone. |
| CLINICAL USE | Moderate to severe or refractory pain, diarrhea (loperamide, diphenoxylate), acute pulmonary edema, maintenance programs for opiate use disorder (methadone, buprenorphine + naloxone), neonatal abstinence syndrome (methadone, morphine). |
| ADVERSE EFFECTS | Nausea, vomiting, pruritus (histamine release), opiate use disorder, respiratory depression, constipation, sphincter of Oddi spasm, miosis (except meperidine → mydriasis), additive CNS depression with other drugs. Tolerance does not develop to miosis and constipation. Treat toxicity with naloxone and prevent relapse with naltrexone once detoxified. |

## Tramadol

| | |
|---|---|
| MECHANISM | Very weak opioid agonist; also inhibits the reuptake of norepinephrine and serotonin. |
| CLINICAL USE | Chronic pain. |
| ADVERSE EFFECTS | Similar to opioids; decreases seizure threshold; serotonin syndrome. |

## Butorphanol, nalbuphine

| | |
|---|---|
| MECHANISM | μ-opioid receptor partial agonists and κ-opioid receptor full agonists. |
| CLINICAL USE | Analgesia for severe pain (eg, labor). |
| NOTES | Mixed opioid agonists/antagonists cause less respiratory depression than full opioid agonists. Can cause opioid withdrawal symptoms if patient is also taking full opioid agonist (due to competition for opioid receptors). Not easily reversed with naloxone. |

## Capsaicin

Naturally found in hot peppers.

| | |
|---|---|
| MECHANISM | Excessive stimulation and desensitization of nociceptive fibers → ↓ substance P release → ↓ pain. |
| CLINICAL USE | Musculoskeletal and neuropathic pain. |

## Glaucoma therapy

↓ IOP via ↓ amount of aqueous humor (inhibit synthesis/secretion or ↑ drainage).
"βαD humor may not be politically correct."

| DRUG CLASS | EXAMPLES | MECHANISM | ADVERSE EFFECTS |
|---|---|---|---|
| β-blockers | Timolol, betaxolol, carteolol | ↓ aqueous humor synthesis | No pupillary or vision changes |
| α-agonists | Epinephrine ($\alpha_1$), apraclonidine, brimonidine ($\alpha_2$) | ↓ aqueous humor synthesis via vasoconstriction (epinephrine) <br> ↓ aqueous humor synthesis (apraclonidine, brimonidine) <br> ↑ outflow of aqueous humor via uveoscleral pathway | Mydriasis ($\alpha_1$); do not use in closed-angle glaucoma <br> Blurry vision, ocular hyperemia, foreign body sensation, ocular allergic reactions, ocular pruritus |
| Diuretics | Acetazolamide | ↓ aqueous humor synthesis via inhibition of carbonic anhydrase | No pupillary or vision changes |
| Prostaglandins | Bimatoprost, latanoprost ($PGF_{2\alpha}$) | ↑ outflow of aqueous humor via ↓ resistance of flow through uveoscleral pathway | Darkens color of iris (browning), eyelash growth |
| Cholinomimetics ($M_3$) | Direct: pilocarpine, carbachol <br> Indirect: physostigmine, echothiophate | ↑ outflow of aqueous humor via contraction of ciliary muscle and opening of trabecular meshwork <br> Use pilocarpine in acute angle closure glaucoma—very effective at opening meshwork into canal of Schlemm | Miosis (contraction of pupillary sphincter muscles) and cyclospasm (contraction of ciliary muscle) |

# Psychiatry

*"Words of comfort, skillfully administered, are the oldest therapy known to man."*

—Louis Nizer

*"Psychiatry at its best is what all medicine needs more of—humanity, art, listening, and sympathy."*

—Susannah Cahalan

*"It's time to tell everyone who's dealing with a mental health issue that they're not alone, and that getting support and treatment isn't a sign of weakness, it's a sign of strength."*

—Michelle Obama

*"I have schizophrenia. I am not schizophrenia. I am not my mental illness. My illness is a part of me."*

—Jonathan Harnisch

This chapter encompasses overlapping areas in psychiatry, psychology, sociology, and psychopharmacology. High-yield topics include schizophrenia, mood disorders, eating disorders, personality disorders, somatic symptom disorders, substance use disorders, and antipsychotics. Know the DSM-5 criteria for diagnosing common psychiatric disorders.

▶ **PSYCHIATRY—PSYCHOLOGY**

| | | |
|---|---|---|
| **Classical conditioning** | Learning in which a natural response (salivation) is elicited by a conditioned, or learned, stimulus (bell) that previously was presented in conjunction with an unconditioned stimulus (food). | Usually elicits **involuntary** responses. Pavlov's classical experiments with dogs— ringing the bell provoked salivation. |

| | | |
|---|---|---|
| **Operant conditioning** | Learning in which a particular action is elicited because it produces a punishment or reward. Usually elicits **voluntary** responses. | |
| Reinforcement | Target behavior (response) is followed by desired reward (positive reinforcement) or removal of aversive stimulus (negative reinforcement). | Skinner operant conditioning quadrants: |
| Punishment | Repeated application of aversive stimulus (positive punishment) or removal of desired reward (negative punishment) to extinguish unwanted behavior. | |
| Extinction | Discontinuation of reinforcement (positive or negative) eventually eliminates behavior. Can occur in operant or classical conditioning. | |

Skinner operant conditioning quadrants:

| | Increase behavior | Decrease behavior |
|---|---|---|
| **Add a stimulus** | Positive reinforcement | Positive punishment |
| **Remove a stimulus** | Negative reinforcement | Negative punishment |

**Transference and countertransference**

| | |
|---|---|
| Transference | Patient projects feelings about formative or other important persons onto physician (eg, psychiatrist is seen as parent). |
| Countertransference | Physician projects feelings about formative or other important persons onto patient (eg, patient reminds physician of younger sibling). |

**Ego defenses** Thoughts and behaviors (voluntary or involuntary) used to resolve conflict and prevent undesirable feelings (eg, anxiety, depression).

| IMMATURE DEFENSES | DESCRIPTION | EXAMPLE |
|---|---|---|
| **Acting out** | Subconsciously coping with stressors or emotional conflict using actions rather than reflections or feelings. | A patient skips therapy appointments after deep discomfort from dealing with his past. |
| **Denial** | Avoiding the awareness of some painful reality. | A patient with cancer plans a full-time work schedule despite being warned of significant fatigue during chemotherapy. |
| **Displacement** | Redirection of emotions or impulses to a neutral person or object (vs projection). | After being reprimanded by her principal, a frustrated teacher returns home and criticizes her wife's cooking instead of confronting the principal directly. |
| **Dissociation** | Temporary, drastic change in personality, memory, consciousness, or motor behavior to avoid emotional stress. Patient has incomplete or no memory of traumatic event. | A survivor of sexual abuse sees the abuser and suddenly becomes numb and detached. |

## Ego defenses (continued)

| IMMATURE DEFENSES | DESCRIPTION | EXAMPLE |
|---|---|---|
| Fixation | Partially remaining at a more childish level of development (vs regression). | A college student continues to suck her thumb when studying for stressful exams. |
| Idealization | Expressing extremely positive thoughts of self and others while ignoring negative thoughts. | A patient boasts about his physician and his accomplishments while ignoring any flaws. |
| Identification | Largely unconscious assumption of the characteristics, qualities, or traits of another person or group. | A resident starts putting her stethoscope in her pocket like her favorite attending, instead of wearing it around her neck like before. |
| Intellectualization | Using facts and logic to emotionally distance oneself from a stressful situation. | A patient diagnosed with cancer discusses the pathophysiology of the disease. |
| Isolation (of affect) | Separating feelings from ideas and events. | Describing murder in graphic detail with no emotional response. |
| Passive aggression | Demonstrating hostile feelings in a nonconfrontational manner; showing indirect opposition. | A disgruntled employee is repeatedly late to work, but won't admit it is a way to get back at the manager. |
| Projection | Attributing an unacceptable internal impulse to an external source (vs displacement). | A man who wants to cheat on his wife accuses his wife of being unfaithful. |
| Rationalization | Asserting plausible explanations for events that actually occurred for other reasons, usually to avoid self-blame. | An employee who was recently fired claims that the job was not important anyway. |
| Reaction formation | Replacing a warded-off idea or feeling with an emphasis on its opposite (vs sublimation). | A stepfather treats a child he resents with excessive nurturing and overprotection. |
| Regression | Involuntarily turning back the maturational clock to behaviors previously demonstrated under stress (vs fixation). | A previously toilet-trained child begins bedwetting again following the birth of a sibling. |
| Repression | Involuntarily withholding an idea or feeling from conscious awareness (vs suppression). | A 20-year-old does not remember going to counseling during his parents' divorce 10 years earlier. |
| Splitting | Believing that people are either all good or all bad at different times due to intolerance of ambiguity. Common in **borderline** personality disorder. **Borders split** countries. | A patient says that all the nurses are cold and insensitive, but the physicians are warm and friendly. |
| MATURE DEFENSES | | |
| Sublimation | Replacing an unacceptable wish with a course of action that is similar to the wish but socially acceptable (vs reaction formation). | A teenager's aggression toward her parents because of their high expectations is channeled into excelling in sports. |
| Altruism | Alleviating negative feelings via unsolicited generosity, which provides gratification (vs reaction formation). | A mafia boss makes a large donation to charity. |
| Suppression | Intentionally withholding an idea or feeling from conscious awareness (vs repression); temporary. | An athlete focuses on other tasks to prevent worrying about an important upcoming match. |
| Humor | Lightheartedly expressing uncomfortable feelings to shift the internal focus away from the distress. | A nervous medical student jokes about the boards. |
| | Mature adults wear a **SASH**. | |

**Grief**

Natural feeling that occurs in response to the death of a loved one. Symptoms and trajectory vary for each individual, are specific to each loss, and do not follow a fixed series of stages. In addition to guilt, sadness, and yearning, patients may experience somatic symptoms, hallucinations of the deceased, and/or transient episodes of wishing they had died with or instead of their loved one. Typical acute grief is time limited (adaptations within 6 months) and is not a disorder.

Prolonged grief disorder—diagnosed if grief remains intense, persistent, and prolonged (at least 6–12 months), significantly impair functioning, is inconsistent with patient's cultural or religious norms, and do not meet criteria for another disorder (eg, major depressive disorder [MDD]).

---

**Normal infant and child development**

Milestone dates are ranges that have been approximated and vary by source. Children not meeting milestones may need assessment for potential developmental delay.

| AGE | MOTOR | SOCIAL | VERBAL/COGNITIVE |
|---|---|---|---|
| **Infant** | **Parents** | **Start** | **Observing,** |
| 0–12 mo | Primitive reflexes disappear—Moro, rooting, palmar, Babinski (**Mr. Peanut Butter**) <br> Posture—lifts head up prone (by 1 mo), rolls and sits (by 6 mo), crawls (by 8 mo), stands (by 10 mo), walks (by 12–18 mo) <br> Picks—passes toys hand to hand (by 6 mo), Pincer grasp (by 10 mo) <br> Points to objects (by 12 mo) | Social smile (by 2 mo) <br> Stranger anxiety (by 6 mo) <br> Separation anxiety (by 9 mo) | Orients—first to voice (by 4 mo), then to name and gestures (by 9 mo) <br> Object permanence (by 9 mo) <br> Oratory—says "mama" and "dada" (by 10 mo) |
| **Toddler** | **Child** | **Rearing** | **Working,** |
| 12–36 mo | Cruises, takes first steps (by 12 mo) <br> Climbs stairs (by 18 mo) <br> Cubes stacked (number) = age (yr) × 3 <br> Cutlery—feeds self with fork and spoon (by 20 mo) <br> Kicks ball (by 24 mo) | Recreation—parallel play (by 24–36 mo) <br> Rapprochement—moves away from and returns to parent (by 24 mo) <br> Realization—core gender identity formed (by 36 mo) | Words—uses 50-200 words (by 2 yr), uses 300+ words (by 3 yr) |
| **Preschool** | **Don't** | **Forget, they're still** | **Learning!** |
| 3–5 yr | Drive—tricycle (3 wheels at 3 yr) <br> Drawings—copies line or circle, stick figure (by 4 yr) <br> Dexterity—hops on one foot by 4 yr ("4 on one foot"), uses buttons or zippers, grooms self (by 5 yr) | Freedom—comfortably spends part of day away from parent (by 3 yr) <br> Friends—cooperative play, has imaginary friends (by 4 yr) | Language—understands 1000 (**3 zeros**) words (by 3 yr), uses complete sentences and prepositions (by 4 yr) <br> Legends—can tell detailed stories (by 4 yr) |

▶ **PSYCHIATRY—PATHOLOGY**

**Child abuse**  All cases of suspected child abuse must be reported to local child protective services.

| | SIGNS | EPIDEMIOLOGY |
|---|---|---|
| **Neglect** | Poor hygiene, malnutrition, withdrawn affect, impaired social/emotional development, failure to thrive due to failure to provide a child with adequate food, shelter, supervision, education, and/or affection. | Most common form of child maltreatment. |
| **Physical abuse** | Nonaccidental trauma (eg, fractures, bruises, burns). Injuries often in different stages of healing or in patterns resembling possible implements of injury. Includes abusive head trauma (shaken baby syndrome), characterized by subdural hematomas or retinal hemorrhages.<br>Caregivers may delay seeking medical attention for the child or provide explanations inconsistent with the child's developmental stage or pattern of injury. | 40% of deaths related to child abuse or neglect occur in children < 1 year old. |
| **Sexual abuse** | STIs, UTIs, and genital, anal, or oral trauma. Most often, there are no physical signs; sexual abuse should not be excluded from a differential diagnosis in the absence of physical trauma.<br>Children often exhibit sexual knowledge or behavior incongruent with their age. | Peak incidence 9–12 years old. |
| **Emotional abuse** | Babies or young children may lack a bond with the caregiver but are overly affectionate with less familiar adults. They may be aggressive towards children and animals or unusually anxious.<br>Older children are often emotionally labile and prone to angry outbursts. They may distance themselves from caregivers and other children. They can experience vague somatic symptoms for which a medical cause cannot be found. | ~ 80% of young adult victims of child emotional abuse meet the criteria for ≥ 1 psychiatric illness by age 21. |

**Vulnerable child syndrome**  Parents perceive the child as especially susceptible to illness or injury (vs factitious disorder imposed on another). Usually follows a serious illness or life-threatening event. Can result in missed school or overuse of medical services.

## Childhood and early-onset disorders

| | |
|---|---|
| **Attention-deficit hyperactivity disorder** | Onset before age 12, but diagnosis can only be established after age 4. Characterized by hyperactivity, impulsivity, and/or inattention in ≥ 2 settings (eg, school, home, places of worship). Normal intelligence, but commonly coexists with difficulties in school. Often persists into adulthood. Commonly coexists with other behavioral, cognitive, or developmental disorders. Treatment: stimulants (eg, methylphenidate) +/– behavioral therapy; alternatives include atomoxetine and $\alpha_2$-agonists (eg, clonidine, guanfacine). |
| **Autism spectrum disorder** | Onset in early childhood. Social and communication deficits, repetitive/ritualized behaviors, restricted interests. May be accompanied by intellectual disability and/or above average abilities in specific skills (eg, music). More common in males. Associated with ↑ head and/or brain size. |
| **Conduct disorder** | Repetitive, pervasive behavior violating societal norms or the basic rights of others (eg, aggression toward people and animals, destruction of property, theft). After age 18, often reclassified as antisocial personality disorder. Conduct = children, antisocial = adults. Treatment: psychotherapy (eg, cognitive behavioral therapy [CBT]). |
| **Disruptive mood dysregulation disorder** | Onset before age 10. Severe, recurrent temper outbursts out of proportion to situation. Child is constantly angry and irritable between outbursts. Treatment: CBT, stimulants, antipsychotics. |
| **Intellectual disability** | Global cognitive deficits (vs specific learning disorder) that affect reasoning, memory, abstract thinking, judgment, language, learning. Adaptive functioning is impaired, leading to major difficulties with education, employment, communication, socialization, independence. Treatment: psychotherapy, occupational therapy, special education. |
| **Intermittent explosive disorder** | Onset after age 6. Recurrent verbal or physical outbursts representing a failure to control aggressive impulses. Outbursts last < 30 minutes and are out of proportion to provocation and may lead to legal, financial, or social consequences. Episodes are not premeditated and may provide an immediate sense of relief, followed by remorse. Treatment: psychotherapy, SSRIs. |
| **Oppositional defiant disorder** | Pattern of anger and irritability with argumentative, vindictive, and defiant behavior toward authority figures lasting ≥ 6 months. Treatment: psychotherapy (eg, CBT). |
| **Selective mutism** | Onset before age 5. Anxiety disorder lasting ≥ 1 month involving refraining from speech in certain situations despite speaking in other, usually more comfortable situations. Development (eg, speech and language) not typically impaired. Interferes with social, academic, and occupational tasks. Commonly coexists with social anxiety disorder. Treatment: behavioral, family, and play therapy; SSRIs. |
| **Separation anxiety disorder** | Overwhelming fear of separation from home or attachment figure lasting ≥ 4 weeks. Can be normal behavior up to age 3–4. May lead to factitious physical complaints to avoid school. Treatment: CBT, play therapy, family therapy. |
| **Specific learning disorder** | Onset during school-age years. Inability to acquire or use information from a specific subject (eg, math, reading, writing) near age-expected proficiency for ≥ 6 months despite focused intervention. General functioning and intelligence are normal (vs intellectual disability). Treatment: academic support, counseling, extracurricular activities. |
| **Tourette syndrome** | Onset before age 18. Sudden, recurrent, nonrhythmic, stereotyped motor (eg, grimacing, shrugging) and vocal (eg, grunting, throat clearing) tics that persist for > 1 year. Coprolalia (involuntary obscene speech) found in some patients. Associated with OCD and ADHD. Treatment: psychoeducation, behavioral therapy. For intractable and distressing tics: tetrabenazine, antipsychotics, $\alpha_2$-agonists. |

| | |
|---|---|
| **Orientation** | Patients' ability to know the date and time, where they are, and who they are (order of loss: time → place → person). Common causes of loss of orientation: alcohol, drugs, fluid/electrolyte imbalance, head trauma, hypoglycemia, infection, nutritional deficiencies, hypoxia. |

### Amnesias

| | |
|---|---|
| Retrograde amnesia | Inability to remember things that occurred before a CNS insult. |
| Anterograde amnesia | Inability to remember things that occurred after a CNS insult (↓ acquisition of new memory). |
| Korsakoff syndrome | Amnesia (anterograde > retrograde) and disorientation caused by vitamin $B_1$ deficiency. Associated with disruption and destruction of the limbic system, especially mammillary bodies and anterior thalamus. Seen in chronic alcohol use as a late neuropsychiatric manifestation of Wernicke encephalopathy. Confabulations are characteristic. |

### Dissociative disorders

| | |
|---|---|
| Depersonalization/ derealization disorder | Persistent feelings of detachment or estrangement from one's own body, thoughts, perceptions, and actions (depersonalization) or one's environment (derealization). Intact reality testing (vs psychosis). |
| Dissociative amnesia | Inability to recall important personal information, usually following severe trauma or stress. May be accompanied by dissociative fugue (abrupt, unexpected travelling away from home). |
| Dissociative identity disorder | Formerly called multiple personality disorder. Presence of ≥ 2 distinct identities or personality states, typically with distinct memories and patterns of behavior. More common in females. Associated with history of sexual abuse, PTSD, depression, substance use, borderline personality disorder, somatic symptom disorders. |

| | | |
|---|---|---|
| **Delirium** | "Waxing and waning" level of consciousness with acute onset, ↓ attention span, ↓ level of arousal. Characterized by disorganized thinking, hallucinations (often visual), misperceptions (eg, illusions), disturbance in sleep-wake cycle, cognitive dysfunction, agitation. Reversible. Usually 2° to other identifiable illness (eg, CNS disease, infection, trauma, substance use/ withdrawal, metabolic/electrolyte disturbances, hemorrhage, urinary/fecal retention), or medications (eg, anticholinergics), especially in older adults. Most common presentation of altered mental status in inpatient setting, especially in the ICU or during prolonged hospital stays. | Delirium = changes in sensorium. EEG may show diffuse background rhythm slowing. Treatment: identification and management of underlying condition. Orientation protocols (eg, keeping a clock or calendar nearby), ↓ sleep disturbances, and ↑ cognitive stimulation to manage symptoms. Antipsychotics (eg, haloperidol) as needed. Avoid unnecessary restraints and drugs that may worsen delirium (eg, anticholinergics, benzodiazepines, opioids). |

| | |
|---|---|
| **Psychosis** | Distorted perception of reality characterized by delusions, hallucinations, and/or disorganized thought/speech. Can occur in patients with psychiatric illness or another medical condition, or secondary to substance or medication use. |
| Delusions | False, fixed, idiosyncratic beliefs that persist despite evidence to the contrary and are not typical of a patient's culture or religion (eg, a patient who believes that others are reading his thoughts). Types include erotomanic, grandiose, jealous, persecutory, somatic, mixed, and unspecified. |
| Disorganized thought | Speech may be incoherent ("word salad"), tangential, or derailed ("loose associations"). |
| Hallucinations | Perceptions in the absence of external stimuli (eg, seeing a light that is not actually present). Contrast with misperceptions (eg, illusions) of real external stimuli. Types include:<br>▪ Auditory—more commonly due to psychiatric illness (eg, schizophrenia) than neurologic disease.<br>▪ Visual—more commonly due to neurologic disease (eg, dementia), delirium, or drug intoxication than psychiatric illness.<br>▪ Tactile—common in alcohol withdrawal and stimulant use (eg, "cocaine crawlies," a type of delusional parasitosis).<br>▪ Olfactory—often occur as an aura of temporal lobe epilepsy (eg, burning rubber) and in brain tumors.<br>▪ Gustatory—rare, but seen in epilepsy.<br>▪ Hypnagogic—occurs while going to sleep. Sometimes seen in narcolepsy.<br>▪ Hypnopompic—occurs while waking from sleep ("get pomped up in the morning"). Sometimes seen in narcolepsy.<br>Contrast with illusions, which are misperceptions of real external stimuli (eg, mistaking a shadow for a black cat). |

| | |
|---|---|
| **Mood disorder** | Characterized by an abnormal range of moods or internal emotional states and loss of control over them. Severity of moods causes distress and impairment in social and occupational functioning. Includes major depressive, bipolar, dysthymic, and cyclothymic disorders. Episodic superimposed psychotic features (delusions, hallucinations, disorganized speech/behavior) may be present at any time during mood episodes (other than hypomania). |

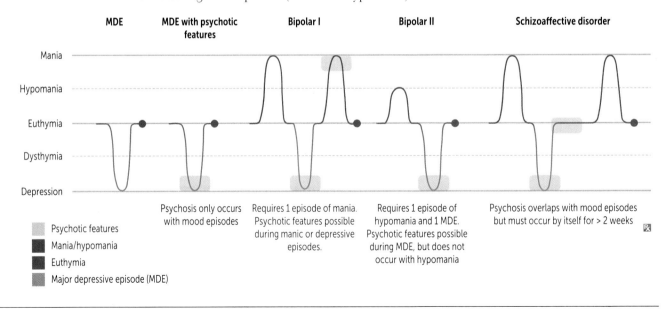

MDE | MDE with psychotic features | Bipolar I | Bipolar II | Schizoaffective disorder

Mania — Hypomania — Euthymia — Dysthymia — Depression

Psychosis only occurs with mood episodes

Requires 1 episode of mania. Psychotic features possible during manic or depressive episodes.

Requires 1 episode of hypomania and 1 MDE. Psychotic features possible during MDE, but does not occur with hypomania

Psychosis overlaps with mood episodes but must occur by itself for > 2 weeks

■ Psychotic features
■ Mania/hypomania
■ Euthymia
■ Major depressive episode (MDE)

## Schizophrenia spectrum disorders

| | | |
|---|---|---|
| **Schizophrenia** | Chronic illness causing profound functional impairment. Symptom categories include:<br>▪ Positive—excessive or distorted functioning (eg, hallucinations, delusions, unusual thought processes, disorganized speech, bizarre behavior)<br>▪ Negative—diminished functioning (eg, flat or blunted affect, apathy, anhedonia, alogia, social withdrawal)<br>▪ Cognitive—reduced ability to understand or make plans, diminished working memory, inattention<br>Diagnosis requires ≥ 2 of the following active symptoms, including ≥ 1 from symptoms #1–3:<br>1. Delusions<br>2. Hallucinations, often auditory<br>3. Disorganized speech<br>4. Disorganized or catatonic behavior<br>5. Negative symptoms<br>Symptom onset ≥ 6 months prior to diagnosis; requires ≥ 1 month of active symptoms over the past 6 months. | Associated with altered dopaminergic activity, ↑ serotonergic activity, and ↓ dendritic branching. Ventriculomegaly on brain imaging. Lifetime prevalence—1.5% (males > females). Presents earlier in males (late teens to early 20s) than in females (late 20s to early 30s). ↑ suicide risk.<br>Heavy cannabis use in adolescence is associated with ↑ incidence and worsened course of psychotic, mood, and anxiety disorders.<br>Treatment: atypical antipsychotics (eg, risperidone) are first line.<br>Negative symptoms often persist after treatment, despite resolution of positive symptoms. |
| | **Brief psychotic disorder**—≥ 1 positive symptom(s) lasting between 1 day and 1 month, usually stress-related. | |
| | **Schizophreniform disorder**—≥ 2 symptoms lasting 1–6 months. | |
| **Schizoaffective disorder** | Shares symptoms with both schizophrenia and mood disorders (MDD or bipolar disorder). To differentiate from a mood disorder with psychotic features, patient must have ≥ 2 weeks of psychotic symptoms without a manic or depressive episode. | |
| **Delusional disorder** | ≥ 1 delusion(s) lasting > 1 month, but without a mood disorder or other psychotic symptoms. Daily functioning, including socialization, may be impacted by the pathological, fixed belief but is otherwise unaffected. Can be shared by individuals in close relationships (folie à deux). | |
| **Schizotypal personality disorder** | Cluster A personality disorder that also falls on the schizophrenia spectrum. May include brief psychotic episodes (eg, delusions) that are less frequent and severe than in schizophrenia. | |

| | | |
|---|---|---|
| **Manic episode** | Distinct period of abnormally and persistently elevated, expansive, or irritable mood and ↑ activity or energy. Diagnosis requires marked functional impairment with ≥ 3 of the following for ≥ 1 week, or any duration if hospitalization is required (people with mania **DIG FAST**):<br>▪ Distractibility<br>▪ Impulsivity/Indiscretion—seeks pleasure without regard to consequences (hedonistic)<br>▪ Grandiosity—inflated self-esteem | ▪ Flight of ideas—racing thoughts<br>▪ ↑ goal-directed Activity/psychomotor Agitation<br>▪ ↓ need for Sleep<br>▪ Talkativeness or pressured speech |

| | |
|---|---|
| **Hypomanic episode** | Similar to a manic episode except mood disturbance is not severe enough to cause marked impairment in social and/or occupational functioning or to necessitate hospitalization. Abnormally ↑ activity or energy usually present. No psychotic features. Lasts ≥ 4 consecutive days. |

| | |
|---|---|
| **Bipolar disorder** | Bipolar I (requires 1 type of episode)—≥ 1 manic episode +/– a hypomanic or depressive episode (may be separated by any length of time). <br> Bipolar II (requires 2 types of episodes)—a hypomanic and a depressive episode (no history of manic episodes). <br> Patient's mood and functioning usually normalize between episodes. Use of antidepressants can destabilize mood. High suicide risk. Treatment: atypical antipsychotics, mood stabilizers (eg, lithium, lamotrigine, valproate, carbamazepine). A little less variable character. <br><br> **Cyclothymic disorder**—milder form of bipolar disorder fluctuating between mild depressive and hypomanic symptoms. Must last ≥ 2 years with symptoms present at least half of the time, with any remission lasting ≤ 2 months. |

| | |
|---|---|
| **Major depressive disorder** | Recurrent episodes lasting ≥ 2 weeks characterized by ≥ 5 of 9 diagnostic symptoms including depressed mood or anhedonia (or irritability in children). SIG: E CAPS: <br> ▪ Sleep disturbances <br> ▪ ↓ Interest in pleasurable activities (anhedonia) <br> ▪ Guilt or feelings of worthlessness <br> ▪ ↓ Energy <br> ▪ ↓ Concentration <br> ▪ Appetite/weight changes <br> ▪ Psychomotor retardation or agitation <br> ▪ Suicidal ideation <br> Screen for previous manic or hypomanic episodes to rule out bipolar disorder. <br> Treatment: CBT and SSRIs are first line; alternatives include SNRIs, mirtazapine, bupropion, electroconvulsive therapy (ECT), ketamine. <br> Responses to a significant loss (eg, bereavement, natural disaster, disability) may resemble a depressive episode. Diagnosis of MDD is made if criteria are met. |
| **MDD with psychotic features** | MDD + hallucinations or delusions. Psychotic features are typically mood congruent (eg, depressive themes of inadequacy, guilt, punishment, nihilism, disease, or death) and occur only in the context of major depressive episode (vs schizoaffective disorder). Treatment: antidepressant with atypical antipsychotic, ECT. |
| **Persistent depressive disorder** | Also called dysthymia. Often milder than MDD; ≥ 2 depressive symptoms lasting ≥ 2 years (≥ 1 year in children), with any remission lasting ≤ 2 months. |
| **MDD with seasonal pattern** | Formerly called seasonal affective disorder. Major depressive episodes occurring only during a particular season (usually winter) in ≥ 2 consecutive years and in most years across a lifetime. Atypical symptoms common. Treatment: standard MDD therapies + light therapy. |

| | |
|---|---|
| **Depression with atypical features** | Characterized by mood reactivity (transient improvement in response to a positive event), hypersomnia, hyperphagia, leaden paralysis (heavy feeling in arms and legs), long-standing interpersonal rejection sensitivity. Most common subtype of depression. Treatment: CBT and SSRIs are first line. MAO inhibitors are effective but not first line because of their risk profile. |

| **Peripartum mood disturbances** | Onset during pregnancy or within 4 weeks of delivery. ↑ risk with history of mood disorders. | |
| --- | --- | --- |
| Postpartum blues | 50–85% incidence rate. Characterized by depressed affect, tearfulness, and fatigue starting 2–3 days after delivery. Usually resolves within 2 weeks. Treatment: supportive. Follow up to assess for possible MDD with peripartum onset. | |
| MDD with peripartum onset | 10–15% incidence rate. Formerly called postpartum depression. Meets MDD criteria with onset either during pregnancy or within 4 weeks after delivery. Treatment: CBT and SSRIs are first line. | |
| Postpartum psychosis | 0.1–0.2% incidence rate. Characterized by mood-congruent delusions, hallucinations, and thoughts of harming the baby or self. Risk factors include first pregnancy, family history, bipolar disorder, psychotic disorder, recent medication change. Treatment: hospitalization and initiation of atypical antipsychotic; if insufficient, ECT may be used. | |

| **Electroconvulsive therapy** | Rapid-acting method to treat refractory depression, depression with psychotic symptoms, catatonia, and acute suicidality. Induces tonic-clonic seizure under anesthesia and neuromuscular blockade. Adverse effects include disorientation, headache, partial anterograde/retrograde amnesia usually resolving in 6 months. No absolute contraindications. Safe in pregnant individuals and older adults. |
| --- | --- |

| **Risk factors for suicide death** | Sex (male)<br>Age (young adult or older adult)<br>Depression<br>Previous attempt (highest risk factor)<br>Ethanol or drug use<br>Rational thinking loss (psychosis)<br>Sickness (medical illness)<br>Organized plan<br>No spouse or other social support<br>Stated future intent | SAD PERSONS are more likely to die from suicide.<br>Most common method in US is firearms; access to guns ↑ risk of suicide death.<br>Women try more often; men die more often.<br>Other risk factors include recent psychiatric hospitalization and family history of suicide death.<br>Protective factors include effective care for comorbidities; medical, familial, or community connectedness; cultural/religious beliefs encouraging self-preservation; and strong problem-solving skills. |
| --- | --- | --- |

| **Anxiety disorders** | Inappropriate experiences of fear/worry and their physical manifestations incongruent with the magnitude of the stressors. Symptoms are not attributable to another medical condition (eg, psychiatric disorder, hyperthyroidism) or substance use. Includes panic disorder, phobias, generalized anxiety disorder, and selective mutism. |
| --- | --- |

**Panic disorder**

Recurrent panic attacks involving intense fear and discomfort +/– a known trigger. Attacks typically peak in 10 minutes with ≥ 4 of the following: palpitations, paresthesias, depersonalization or derealization, abdominal distress or nausea, intense fear of dying, intense fear of losing control, lightheadedness, chest pain, chills, choking, sweating, shaking, shortness of breath. Strong genetic component. ↑ risk of suicide.

Diagnosis requires attack followed by ≥ 1 month of ≥ 1 of the following:
- Persistent concern of additional attacks
- Worrying about consequences of attack
- Behavioral change related to attacks

Symptoms are systemic manifestations of fear. Treatment: CBT, SSRIs, and venlafaxine are first line. Benzodiazepines occasionally used in acute setting.

**Phobias**

Severe, persistent (≥ 6 months) fear or anxiety due to presence or anticipation of a specific object or situation. Person often recognizes fear is excessive. Treatment: CBT with exposure therapy.

**Social anxiety disorder**—exaggerated fear of embarrassment in social situations (eg, public speaking, using public restrooms). Treatment: CBT, SSRIs, SNRIs. For performance type (eg, anxiety restricted to public speaking), use β-blockers or benzodiazepines as needed.

**Agoraphobia**—irrational fear, anxiety, and/or avoidance while facing or anticipating ≥ 2 specific situations (eg, public transportation, open/closed spaces, lines/crowds, being outside of home alone). Symptoms stem from the concern that help or escape may be unavailable. Associated with panic disorder. Treatment: CBT, SSRIs.

**Generalized anxiety disorder**

Excessive anxiety and worry about different aspects of daily life (eg, work, school, children) for most days of ≥ 6 months. Associated with ≥ 3 of the following for adults (≥ 1 for kids): difficulty **C**oncentrating, **R**estlessness, **I**rritability, **M**uscle tension, fatigue (low **E**nergy), **S**leep disturbance (anxiety over **CRIMES**). Treatment: CBT, SSRIs, SNRIs are first line. Buspirone, TCAs, benzodiazepines are second line.

**Obsessive-compulsive disorders**

Obsessions (recurring intrusive thoughts or sensations that can cause severe distress), and/or compulsions (repetitive, often time-consuming actions that may relieve distress). Associated with tic disorders. Poor insight into beliefs/actions linked to worse outcomes. Treatment: CBT and SSRIs; clomipramine and venlafaxine are second line.

**Body dysmorphic disorder**—preoccupation with minor or imagined defects in appearance. Causes significant emotional distress and repetitive appearance-related behaviors (eg, mirror checking, excessive grooming). Common in eating disorders. Treatment: CBT.

**Trichotillomania**—compulsively pulling out one's hair. Causes significant distress and persists despite attempts to stop. Presents with areas of thinning hair or baldness on any area of the body, most commonly the scalp . Remaining hair shafts are of different lengths (vs alopecia). Incidence highest in childhood but spans all ages. Treatment: CBT and SSRIs.

## Trauma and stress-related disorders

| Adjustment disorder | Emotional or behavioral symptoms (eg, anxiety, outbursts) that occur within 3 months of an identifiable psychosocial stressor (eg, divorce, illness) lasting < 6 months once the stressor has ended. Symptoms do not meet criteria for another psychiatric illness. If symptoms persist > 6 months after stressor ends, reevaluate for other explanations (eg, MDD, GAD). Treatment: CBT is first line; antidepressants and anxiolytics may be considered. |
|---|---|
| Post-traumatic stress disorder | Experiencing, witnessing, or discovering that a loved one has experienced a life-threatening situation (eg, serious injury, sexual assault) → persistent **H**yperarousal, **A**voidance of associated stimuli, intrusive **R**e-experiencing of the event (eg, nightmares, flashbacks), changes in cognition or mood (eg, fear, horror, **D**istress) (having PTSD is **HARD**). Disturbance lasts > 1 month with significant distress or impaired functioning. Treatment: CBT, SSRIs, and venlafaxine are first line. Prazosin can reduce nightmares. |
| | Acute stress disorder—lasts between 3 days and 1 month. Treatment: CBT; pharmacotherapy is usually not indicated. |

## Diagnostic criteria by symptom duration

| | |
|---|---|
| **Personality disorders** | Inflexible, maladaptive, and rigidly pervasive patterns of behavior causing subjective distress and/ or impaired functioning; person is usually not aware of problem (egosyntonic). Usually present by early adulthood. Contrast with **personality traits**—nonpathologic enduring patterns of perception and behavior. <br> Three clusters: <br> ▪ Cluster A (remember as "weird")—odd or eccentric; inability to develop meaningful social relationships. No psychosis; genetic association with schizophrenia. <br> ▪ Cluster B (remember as "wild")—dramatic, emotional, or erratic; genetic association with mood disorders and substance use. <br> ▪ Cluster C (remember as "worried")—anxious or fearful; genetic association with anxiety disorders. |

### Cluster A

| | |
|---|---|
| **Paranoid** | Pervasive distrust (accusatory), suspiciousness, hypervigilance, and a profoundly cynical view of the world. |
| **Schizoid** | Prefers social withdrawal and solitary activities (vs avoidant), limited emotional expression, indifferent to others' opinions (aloof). |
| **Schizotypal** | Eccentric appearance, odd beliefs or magical thinking, interpersonal awkwardness. Included on the schizophrenia spectrum. Pronounce "schizo-type-al" for odd-type thoughts. |

### Cluster B

| | |
|---|---|
| **Antisocial** | Disregard for the rights of others with lack of remorse (bad). Involves criminality, impulsivity, hostility, and manipulation (sociopath). Males > females. Must be ≥ 18 years old with evidence of conduct disorder onset before age 15. If patient is < 18, diagnosis is conduct disorder. |
| **Borderline** | Unstable mood and interpersonal relationships, fear of abandonment, impulsivity, self-mutilation, suicidality, sense of emotional emptiness (borderline). Females > males. Splitting is a major defense mechanism. Treatment: dialectical behavior therapy. |
| **Histrionic** | Attention-seeking, dramatic speech and emotional expression, shallow and labile emotions, sexually provocative. May use physical appearance to draw attention (flamboyant). |
| **Narcissistic** | Grandiosity, sense of entitlement; lacks empathy and requires excessive admiration; often demands the "best" and reacts to criticism with rage and/or defensiveness (must be the best). Fragile self-esteem. Often envious of others. |

### Cluster C

| | |
|---|---|
| **Avoidant** | Hypersensitive to rejection and criticism, socially inhibited, timid (cowardly), feelings of inadequacy, desires relationships with others (vs schizoid). |
| **Obsessive-compulsive** | Preoccupation with order, perfectionism, and control (obsessive-compulsive); egosyntonic: behavior consistent with one's own beliefs and attitudes (vs OCD). |
| **Dependent** | Excessive need for support (clingy), submissive, low self-confidence. Patients often get stuck in abusive relationships. |

| **Malingering** | Symptoms are intentional, motivation is intentional. Patient consciously fakes, profoundly exaggerates, or claims to have a disorder in order to attain a specific 2° (external) gain (eg, avoiding work, obtaining compensation). Poor compliance with treatment or follow-up of diagnostic tests. Complaints cease after gain (vs factitious disorder). |

| **Factitious disorders** | Symptoms are intentional, motivation is unconscious. Patient consciously creates physical and/or psychological symptoms in order to assume "sick role" and to get medical attention and sympathy (1° [internal] gain). |
| --- | --- |
| Factitious disorder imposed on self | Formerly called Munchausen syndrome. Chronic factitious disorder with predominantly physical signs and symptoms. Characterized by a history of multiple hospital admissions and willingness to undergo invasive procedures. More common in females and healthcare workers. |
| Factitious disorder imposed on another | Formerly called Munchausen syndrome by proxy. Illness in an individual being cared for (most often a child, also seen in disabled or older adults) is directly caused (eg, physically harming a child) or fabricated (eg, lying about a child's symptoms) by the caregiver. Form of child/elder abuse. |

| **Somatic symptom and related disorders** | Symptoms are unconscious, motivation is unconscious. Category of disorders characterized by physical symptoms causing significant distress and impairment. Symptoms not intentionally produced or feigned. |
| --- | --- |
| Somatic symptom disorder | ≥ 1 bodily complaints (eg, abdominal pain, fatigue) lasting months to years. Associated with excessive, persistent thoughts and anxiety about symptoms. May co-occur with medical illness. Treatment: regular office visits with the same physician with the goals of addressing active symptoms, reassuring the patient, and avoiding unnecessary tests or medications. |
| Conversion disorder | Also called functional neurologic symptom disorder. Unexplained loss of sensory or motor function (eg, paralysis, blindness, mutism), often following an acute stressor; patient may be aware of but indifferent toward symptoms ("la belle indifférence"); more common in females, adolescents, and young adults. |
| Illness anxiety disorder | Preoccupation with acquiring or having a serious illness, often despite medical evaluation and reassurance; minimal to no somatic symptoms. |

**Malingering vs factitious disorder vs somatic symptom disorders**

|  | Malingering | Factitious disorder | Somatic symptom disorders |
| --- | --- | --- | --- |
| SYMPTOMS | Intentional | Intentional | Unconscious |
| MOTIVATION | Intentional | Unconscious | Unconscious |

| | |
|---|---|
| **Eating disorders** | Most common in young women. |
| Anorexia nervosa | Intense fear of weight gain, overvaluation of thinness, and body image distortion leading to calorie restriction and severe weight loss resulting in inappropriately low body weight (BMI < 18.5 kg/m² for adults). Physiological disturbances may present as bradycardia, hypotension, hypothermia, hypothyroidism, osteoporosis, lanugo, amenorrhea (low calorie intake → ↓ leptin → ↓ GnRH → ↓ LH, FSH → ↓ estrogen → amenorrhea).<br><br>Binge-eating/purging type—recurring purging behaviors (eg, laxative or diuretic abuse, self-induced vomiting) or binge eating over the last 3 months. Associated with hypokalemia.<br><br>Restricting type—primary disordered behaviors include dieting, fasting, and/or over-exercising. No recurring purging behaviors or binge eating over the last 3 months.<br><br>Refeeding syndrome—often occurs in significantly malnourished patients with sudden ↑ calorie intake → ↑ insulin → ↓ $PO_4^{3-}$, ↓ $K^+$, ↓ $Mg^{2+}$ → cardiac complications, rhabdomyolysis, seizures.<br><br>Treatment: nutritional rehabilitation, psychotherapy, olanzapine. |
| Bulimia nervosa | Recurring episodes of binge eating with compensatory purging behaviors at least weekly over the last 3 months. BMI often normal or slightly overweight (vs anorexia). Associated with parotid gland hypertrophy (may see ↑ serum amylase), enamel erosion, Mallory-Weiss syndrome, electrolyte disturbances (eg, ↓ $K^+$, ↓ $Cl^-$), metabolic alkalosis, dorsal hand calluses from induced vomiting (Russell sign).<br><br>Treatment: psychotherapy, nutritional rehabilitation, antidepressants (eg, SSRIs). Bupropion is contraindicated due to seizure risk. |
| Binge-eating disorder | Recurring episodes of binge eating without purging behaviors at least weekly over the last 3 months. ↑ diabetes risk. Most common eating disorder in adults.<br><br>Treatment: psychotherapy (first line); SSRIs; lisdexamfetamine. |
| Pica | Recurring episodes of eating non-food substances (eg, ice, dirt, hair, paint chips) over ≥ 1 month that are not culturally or developmentally recognized as normal. May provide temporary emotional relief. Common in children and during pregnancy. Associated with malnutrition, iron deficiency anemia, developmental disabilities, emotional trauma.<br><br>Treatment: psychotherapy and nutritional rehabilitation (first line); SSRIs (second line). |

| | |
|---|---|
| **Gender dysphoria** | Significant incongruence between one's gender identity and one's gender assigned at birth, lasting > 6 months and leading to persistent distress. Individuals experience marked discomfort with their assigned gender, which interferes with social, academic, and other areas of function. Individuals may pursue multiple domains of gender affirmation, including social, legal, and medical.<br><br>Transgender—any individual who transiently or persistently experiences incongruence between their gender identity and their gender assigned at birth. Some individuals who are transgender will experience gender dysphoria. Nonconformity to one's assigned gender itself is not a mental disorder. |

| | |
|---|---|
| **Sexual dysfunction** | Includes sexual desire disorders (hypoactive sexual desire or sexual aversion), sexual arousal disorders (erectile dysfunction), orgasmic disorders (anorgasmia, premature ejaculation), sexual pain disorders (genito-pelvic pain/penetration disorder).<br><br>Differential diagnosis includes (**PENIS**):<br>▪ Psychological (if nighttime erections still occur)<br>▪ Endocrine (eg, diabetes, low testosterone)<br>▪ Neurogenic (eg, postoperative, spinal cord injury)<br>▪ Insufficient blood flow (eg, atherosclerosis)<br>▪ Substances (eg, antihypertensives, antidepressants, ethanol) |

**Sleep terror disorder**

Periods of inconsolable terror with screaming in the middle of the night. Most common in children. Occurs during slow-wave/deep (stage N3) non-REM sleep with no memory of the arousal episode, as opposed to nightmares that occur during **REM** sleep (remembering a scary dream). Triggers include emotional stress, fever, and lack of sleep. Usually self limited.

**Enuresis**

Nighttime urinary incontinence ≥ 2 times/week for ≥ 3 months in person > 5 years old. First-line treatment: behavioral modification (eg, scheduled voids, nighttime fluid restriction) and positive reinforcement. For refractory cases: bedwetting alarm, oral desmopressin (ADH analog; preferred over imipramine due to fewer adverse effects).

**Narcolepsy**

Excessive daytime sleepiness (despite awakening well-rested) with recurrent episodes of rapid-onset, overwhelming sleepiness ≥ 3 times/week for the last 3 months. Due to ↓ orexin (hypocretin) production in lateral hypothalamus and dysregulated sleep-wake cycles. Associated with:
- Hypnagogic (just before going to sleep) or hypnopompic (just before awakening; get pomped up in the morning) hallucinations.
- Nocturnal and narcoleptic sleep episodes that start with REM sleep (sleep paralysis).
- Cataplexy (loss of all muscle tone following strong emotional stimulus, such as laughter).

Treatment: good sleep hygiene (scheduled naps, regular sleep schedule), daytime stimulants (eg, amphetamines, modafinil) and/or nighttime sodium oxybate (GHB).

**Substance use disorder**

Maladaptive pattern of substance use involving ≥ 2 of the following in the past year:
- Tolerance
- Withdrawal
- Intense, distracting cravings
- Using more, or longer, than intended
- Persistent desire but inability to cut down
- Time-consuming substance acquisition, use, or recovery
- Impaired functioning at work, school, or home
- Social or interpersonal conflicts
- Reduced recreational activities
- > 1 episode of use involving danger (eg, unsafe sex, driving while impaired)
- Continued use despite awareness of harm

In the case of appropriate medical treatment with prescribed medications (eg, opioid analgesics, sedatives, stimulants), symptoms of tolerance and withdrawal do not indicate a substance use disorder.

**Gambling disorder**

Persistent, recurrent, problematic gambling that cannot be better explained as a manic episode. Diagnosis made if patient meets ≥ 4 of the following criteria:
- Is preoccupied with gambling
- Requires more gambling to reach desired level of excitement
- Has failed efforts to limit, cut back, or stop gambling
- Becomes restless or irritable when limiting or attempting to stop gambling
- Gambles to escape or relieve feelings of helplessness, guilt, anxiety, or depression
- After losing money gambling, continues gambling in an attempt to recover losses
- Lies to conceal the extent of gambling
- Puts at risk or has lost significant relationship, career, or academic pursuits because of gambling
- Relies on money from others to fix financial collapse due to gambling

Treatment: psychotherapy.

## Transtheoretical model of change

| STAGE | FEATURES | MOTIVATIONAL STRATEGIES |
|---|---|---|
| Precontemplation | Denies problem and its consequences. | Encourage introspection. Use patient's personal priorities in explaining risks. Affirm your availability to the patient. |
| Contemplation | Acknowledges problem but is ambivalent or unwilling to change. | Discuss pros of changing and cons of maintaining current behavior. Suggest means to support behavior changes. |
| Preparation/ determination | Committed to and planning for behavior change. | Employ motivational interviewing. Encourage initial changes, promote expectations for positive results, provide resources to assist in planning. |
| Action/willpower | Executes a plan and demonstrates a change in behavior. | Assist with strategies for self-efficacy, contingency management, and coping with situations that trigger old behaviors. |
| Maintenance | New behaviors become sustained, integrate into personal identity and lifestyle. | Reinforce developing habits. Evaluate and mitigate relapse risk. Praise progress. |
| Relapse | Regression to prior behavior (does not always occur). | Varies based on degree of regression. Encourage return to changes. Provide reassurance that change remains possible. |

## Psychiatric emergencies

| | CAUSE | MANIFESTATION | TREATMENT |
|---|---|---|---|
| **Serotonin syndrome** | Any drug that ↑ 5-HT. Psychiatric drugs: MAO inhibitors, SSRIs, SNRIs, TCAs, vilazodone, vortioxetine, buspirone Nonpsychiatric drugs: tramadol, ondansetron, triptans, linezolid, MDMA, dextromethorphan, meperidine, St. John's wort | **3 A's:** ↑ **a**ctivity (neuromuscular; eg, clonus, hyperreflexia, hypertonia, tremor, seizure), **a**utonomic instability (eg, hyperthermia, diaphoresis, diarrhea), **a**ltered mental status | Benzodiazepines and supportive care; cyproheptadine (5-HT$_2$ receptor antagonist) if no improvement Prevention: avoid simultaneous serotonergic drugs, and allow a washout period between them |
| **Hypertensive crisis** | Eating tyramine-rich foods (eg, aged cheeses, cured meats, wine, chocolate) while taking MAO inhibitors, insufficient washout period when switching antidepressants to or from MAO inhibitors | Hypertensive crisis (tyramine displaces other neurotransmitters [eg, NE] in the synaptic cleft → ↑ sympathetic stimulation) | Phentolamine |
| **Neuroleptic malignant syndrome** | Antipsychotics (typical > atypical) + genetic predisposition | Malignant **FEVER**: **M**yoglobinuria, **F**ever, **E**ncephalopathy, **V**itals unstable, ↑ **E**nzymes (eg, CK), muscle **R**igidity ("lead pipe") | Dantrolene, dopaminergics (eg, bromocriptine, amantadine), benzodiazepines; discontinue causative agent |
| **Delirium tremens** | Alcohol withdrawal; occurs 2–4 days after last drink Classically seen in hospital setting when inpatient cannot drink | Altered mental status, hallucinations, autonomic hyperactivity, anxiety, seizures, tremors, psychomotor agitation, insomnia, nausea | Longer-acting benzodiazepines |
| **Acute dystonia** | Typical antipsychotics, anticonvulsants (eg, carbamazepine), metoclopramide | Sudden onset of muscle spasms, stiffness, and/or oculogyric crisis occurring hours to days after medication use; can lead to laryngospasm requiring intubation | Benztropine or diphenhydramine |
| **Lithium toxicity** | ↑ lithium dosage, ↓ renal elimination (eg, acute kidney injury), medications affecting clearance (eg, ACE inhibitors, thiazide diuretics, NSAIDs) Narrow therapeutic window | Nausea, vomiting, slurred speech, hyperreflexia, seizures, ataxia, nephrogenic diabetes insipidus | Discontinue lithium, hydrate aggressively with isotonic sodium chloride, consider hemodialysis |
| **Tricyclic antidepressant toxicity** | TCA overdose | Sedation, anticholinergic effects, prolonged QT and QRS **Tricyclic's:** **c**onvulsions, **c**oma, **c**ardiotoxicity (arrhythmia due to Na$^+$ channel inhibition) | Supportive treatment, monitor ECG, NaHCO$_3$ (prevents arrhythmia), activated charcoal |

## Psychoactive drug intoxication and withdrawal

| DRUG | MECHANISM | INTOXICATION | WITHDRAWAL |
|---|---|---|---|
| **Depressants** | | | |
| | | Nonspecific: mood elevation, ↓ anxiety, sedation, behavioral disinhibition, respiratory depression. | Nonspecific: anxiety, tremor, seizures, insomnia. |
| **Alcohol** | GABA-A receptor positive allosteric modulator. Inhibits glutamate-induced excitation of NMDA. | Emotional lability, slurred speech, ataxia, coma, blackouts. **AST** value is 2× **ALT** value ("ToAST 2 ALcohol"). Treatment: supportive (eg, fluids, antiemetics). | Adaptation causes ↑ glutamate receptors; symptoms result from unregulated excess excitation. Treatment: longer-acting benzodiazepines. |
| **Barbiturates** | GABA-A receptor positive allosteric modulator. | Low safety margin, marked respiratory depression. Treatment: symptom management (eg, assist respiration, ↑ BP). | Delirium, life-threatening cardiovascular collapse. |
| **Benzodiazepines** | GABA-A receptor positive allosteric modulator. | Greater safety margin. Ataxia, minor respiratory depression. Treatment: flumazenil (benzodiazepine receptor antagonist). | Seizures, sleep disturbance, depression. |
| **Opioids** | Opioid receptor modulator. | Activation of μ receptors causes the prototypic effect of miosis (pinpoint pupils), ↓ GI motility, respiratory and CNS depression, euphoria, ↓ gag reflex, seizures. Most common cause of drug overdose death. Overdose treatment: naloxone. | Mydriasis, diarrhea, flulike symptoms, rhinorrhea, yawning, nausea, sweating, piloerection ("cold turkey"), lacrimation. Treatment: symptom management, methadone, buprenorphine. |
| **Inhalants** | Enhanced GABA signaling. | Disinhibition, euphoria, slurred speech, ataxia, disorientation, drowsiness, periorifical rash. Rapid onset and resolution. | Irritability, dysphoria, sleep disturbance, headache. |
| **Stimulants** | | | |
| | Nonspecific. | Mood elevation, ↓ appetite, psychomotor agitation, insomnia, cardiac arrhythmias, ↑ HR, anxiety. | Post-use "crash," including depression, lethargy, ↑ appetite, sleep disturbance, vivid nightmares. |
| **Amphetamines** | Induces reversal of monoamine transporters (VMAT, DAT, SERT, NET), ↑ neurotransmitter release. | Euphoria, grandiosity, mydriasis, prolonged wakefulness, hyperalertness, hypertension, paranoia, fever. Skin excoriations with methamphetamine use. Severe: cardiac arrest, seizures. Treatment: benzodiazepines for agitation and seizures. | Meth mites (tactile hallucinations) |

**Psychoactive drug intoxication and withdrawal** *(continued)*

| DRUG | MECHANISM | INTOXICATION | WITHDRAWAL |
|---|---|---|---|
| Caffeine | Adenosine receptor antagonist. | Palpitation, agitation, tremor, insomnia. | Headache, difficulty concentrating, flulike symptoms. |
| Cocaine | Blocks reuptake by dopamine (DAT), serotonin (SERT), and norepinephrine (NET) transporters. | Impaired judgment, mydriasis, diaphoresis, hallucinations (including formication), paranoia, angina, sudden cardiac death. Chronic use may lead to perforated nasal septum due to vasoconstriction and resulting ischemic necrosis. Treatment: benzodiazepines. | Restlessness, hunger, severe depression, sleep disturbance. |
| Nicotine | Stimulates central nicotinic acetylcholine receptors. | Restlessness. | Irritability, anxiety, restlessness, ↓ concentration, ↑ appetite/weight. Treatment: nicotine replacement therapy (eg, patch, gum, lozenge); bupropion/varenicline. |
| **Hallucinogens** | | | |
| **Lysergic acid diethylamide** | 5-HT$_{2A}$ receptor agonist. | Perceptual distortion (visual, auditory), depersonalization, anxiety, paranoia, psychosis, flashbacks, mydriasis. | |
| **Cannabis/ cannabinoids** | CB1 receptor agonist. | Euphoria, anxiety, paranoid delusions, perception of slowed time, impaired judgment, social withdrawal, ↑ appetite, dry mouth, conjunctival injection, hallucinations. | Irritability, anxiety, depression, insomnia, restlessness, ↓ appetite. |
| **MDMA (ecstasy)** | Induces reversal of transporters for monoamines (SERT > DAT, NET), → ↑ neurotransmitter release. | Euphoria, hallucinations, disinhibition, hyperactivity, ↑ thirst, bruxism, distorted perceptions, mydriasis. Life-threatening effects include hypertension, tachycardia, hyperthermia, hyponatremia, serotonin syndrome. | Depression, fatigue, change in appetite, difficulty concentrating, anxiety. |
| **Phencyclidine** | NMDA receptor antagonist. | Violence, nystagmus, impulsivity, psychomotor agitation, tachycardia, hypertension, analgesia, psychosis, delirium, seizures. | |

| | |
|---|---|
| **Alcohol use disorder** | Diagnosed using criteria for substance use disorder.<br>Complications: vitamin $B_1$ (thiamine) deficiency, alcoholic cirrhosis, hepatitis, pancreatitis, peripheral neuropathy, testicular atrophy.<br>Treatment: naltrexone (reduces cravings; avoid in liver failure), acamprosate (contraindicated in renal failure), disulfiram (to condition the patient to abstain from alcohol use). Support groups such as Alcoholics Anonymous are helpful in sustaining abstinence and supporting patient and family. |
| **Wernicke-Korsakoff syndrome** | Results from vitamin $B_1$ deficiency. Symptoms can be precipitated by administering dextrose before vitamin $B_1$. Triad of confusion, ophthalmoplegia, ataxia (Wernicke encephalopathy). May progress to irreversible memory loss, confabulation, personality change (Korsakoff syndrome).<br>Treatment: IV vitamin $B_1$ (before dextrose). |

## ▶ PSYCHIATRY—PHARMACOLOGY

### Psychotherapy

| | |
|---|---|
| **Behavioral therapy** | Teaches patients how to identify and change maladaptive behaviors or reactions to stimuli (eg, systematic desensitization for specific phobia). |
| **Cognitive behavioral therapy** | Teaches patients to recognize distortions in their thought processes, develop constructive coping skills, and ↓ maladaptive coping behaviors → greater emotional control and tolerance of distress (eg, recognizing triggers for alcohol consumption). |
| **Dialectical behavioral therapy** | Designed for use in borderline personality disorder, but can be used in other psychiatric conditions as well (eg, depression). |
| **Interpersonal therapy** | Focused on improving interpersonal relationships and communication skills. |
| **Motivational interviewing** | Enhances intrinsic motivation to change by exploring and resolving ambivalence. Used in substance use disorder and weight loss. |
| **Supportive therapy** | Utilizes empathy to help individuals during a time of hardship to maintain optimism or hope. |

| | |
|---|---|
| **Central nervous system stimulants** | Methylphenidate, dextroamphetamine, methamphetamine, lisdexamfetamine. |
| MECHANISM | ↑ catecholamines in the synaptic cleft, especially norepinephrine and dopamine. |
| CLINICAL USE | ADHD, narcolepsy, binge-eating disorder. |
| ADVERSE EFFECTS | Nervousness, agitation, anxiety, insomnia, anorexia, tachycardia, hypertension, weight loss, tics, bruxism. |

| | |
|---|---|
| **Antipsychotics** | Typical (1st-generation) antipsychotics—haloperidol, pimozide, trifluoperazine, fluphenazine, thioridazine, chlorpromazine.<br>Atypical (2nd-generation) antipsychotics—aripiprazole, asenapine, clozapine, olanzapine, quetiapine, iloperidone, paliperidone, risperidone, lurasidone, ziprasidone. |
| MECHANISM | Block dopamine $D_2$ receptor ($\uparrow$ cAMP). Atypical antipsychotics also block serotonin 5-HT$_2$ receptor. Aripiprazole is a $D_2$ partial agonist. |
| CLINICAL USE | Schizophrenia (typical antipsychotics primarily treat positive symptoms; atypical antipsychotics treat both positive and negative symptoms), disorders with concomitant psychosis (eg, bipolar disorder), Tourette syndrome, OCD, Huntington disease. Clozapine is used for treatment-resistant psychotic disorders or those with persistent suicidality (cloze to the edge). |
| ADVERSE EFFECTS | Antihistaminic (sedation), anti-$\alpha_1$-adrenergic (orthostatic hypotension), antimuscarinic (dry mouth, constipation) (anti-**HAM**). Use with caution in dementia.<br>Metabolic: weight gain, hyperglycemia, dyslipidemia. $\uparrow$ risk with clozapine and olanzapine (obesity).<br>Endocrine: hyperprolactinemia → galactorrhea, oligomenorrhea, gynecomastia.<br>Cardiac: QT prolongation.<br>Neurologic: neuroleptic malignant syndrome.<br>Ophthalmologic: chlorpromazine—corneal deposits; thioridazine—retinal deposits.<br>Clozapine—agranulocytosis (monitor WBCs clozely), seizures (dose related), myocarditis.<br>Extrapyramidal symptoms—**ADAPT**:<ul><li>Hours to days: **A**cute **D**ystonia (muscle spasm, stiffness, oculogyric crisis). Treatment: benztropine, diphenhydramine.</li><li>Days to months:<ul><li>**A**kathisia (restlessness). Treatment: β-blockers, benztropine, benzodiazepines.</li><li>**P**arkinsonism (bradykinesia). Treatment: benztropine, amantadine.</li></ul></li><li>Months to years: **T**ardive dyskinesia (chorea, especially orofacial). Treatment: benzodiazepines, botulinum toxin injections, valbenazine, deutetrabenazine.</li></ul> |
| NOTES | Lipid soluble → stored in body fat → slow to be removed from body.<br>Typical antipsychotics have greater affinity for $D_2$ receptor than atypical antipsychotics → $\uparrow$ risk for hyperprolactinemia, extrapyramidal symptoms, neuroleptic malignant syndrome.<br>High-potency typical antipsychotics: haloperidol, trifluoperazine, pimozide, fluphenazine (**Hal** tries pie to fly high)—more neurologic adverse effects (eg, extrapyramidal symptoms).<br>Low-potency typical antipsychotics: chlorpromazine, thioridazine (cheating thieves are low)—more antihistaminic, anti-$\alpha_1$-adrenergic, antimuscarinic effects. |

## Lithium

| MECHANISM | Affects neurotransmission (↓ excitatory, ↑ inhibitory) and second messenger systems (eg, G proteins). |
|---|---|
| CLINICAL USE | Mood stabilizer for bipolar disorder; treats acute manic episodes and prevents relapse. |
| ADVERSE EFFECTS | Tremor, hypothyroidism, hyperthyroidism, mild hypercalcemia, polyuria (causes nephrogenic diabetes insipidus), teratogenesis (causes Ebstein anomaly). Narrow therapeutic window requires close monitoring of serum levels. Almost exclusively excreted by kidneys; most is reabsorbed at PCT via Na⁺ channels. Thiazides, ACE inhibitors, NSAIDs, and other drugs affecting clearance are implicated in lithium toxicity. |

LiTHIUM:
Low Thyroid (hypothyroidism)
Heart (Ebstein anomaly)
Insipidus (nephrogenic diabetes insipidus)
Unwanted Movements (tremor)

## Buspirone

| MECHANISM | Partial 5-HT$_{1A}$ receptor agonist. |
|---|---|
| CLINICAL USE | Generalized anxiety disorder. Does not cause sedation, addiction, or tolerance. Begins to take effect after 1–2 weeks. Does not interact with alcohol (vs barbiturates, benzodiazepines). |

I get anxious if the bus doesn't arrive at one, so I take buspirone.

## Antidepressants

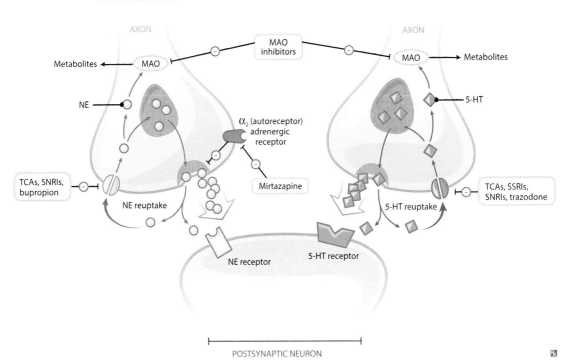

| **Selective serotonin reuptake inhibitors** | Fluoxetine, fluvoxamine, paroxetine, sertraline, escitalopram, citalopram. | |
| --- | --- | --- |
| MECHANISM | Inhibit 5-HT reuptake. | It normally takes 4–8 weeks for antidepressants to show appreciable effect. |
| CLINICAL USE | Depression, generalized anxiety disorder, panic disorder, OCD, bulimia, binge-eating disorder, social anxiety disorder, PTSD, premature ejaculation, premenstrual dysphoric disorder. | |
| ADVERSE EFFECTS | Fewer than TCAs. Serotonin syndrome, GI distress, SIADH, sexual dysfunction (anorgasmia, erectile dysfunction, ↓ libido), mania precipitation if underlying bipolar disorder. | |

| **Serotonin-norepinephrine reuptake inhibitors** | Venlafaxine, desvenlafaxine, duloxetine, levomilnacipran, milnacipran. |
| --- | --- |
| MECHANISM | Inhibit 5-HT and NE reuptake. |
| CLINICAL USE | Depression, generalized anxiety disorder, diabetic neuropathy. Venlafaxine is also indicated for social anxiety disorder, panic disorder, PTSD, OCD. Duloxetine and milnacipran are also indicated for fibromyalgia. |
| ADVERSE EFFECTS | ↑ BP, stimulant effects, sedation, sexual dysfunction, nausea. |

| **Tricyclic antidepressants** | Amitriptyline, nortriptyline, imipramine, desipramine, clomipramine, doxepin, amoxapine. |
| --- | --- |
| MECHANISM | TCAs inhibit 5-HT and NE reuptake. |
| CLINICAL USE | MDD, peripheral neuropathy, chronic neuropathic pain, migraine prophylaxis, OCD (clomipramine), nocturnal enuresis (imipramine). |
| ADVERSE EFFECTS | Sedation, $\alpha_1$-blocking effects including postural hypotension, and atropine-like (anticholinergic) adverse effects (tachycardia, urinary retention, dry mouth). 3° TCAs (amitriptyline) have more anticholinergic effects than 2° TCAs (nortriptyline). Can prolong QT interval.<br>Tri-CyCliC's: Convulsions, Coma, Cardiotoxicity (arrhythmia due to $Na^+$ channel inhibition); also respiratory depression, hyperpyrexia. Confusion and hallucinations are more common in older adults due to anticholinergic adverse effects (2° amines [eg, nortriptyline] better tolerated). Treatment: $NaHCO_3$ to prevent arrhythmia. |

| **Monoamine oxidase inhibitors** | Tranylcypromine, phenelzine, isocarboxazid, selegiline (selective MAO-B inhibitor). (**MAO** takes pride in Shanghai). |
| --- | --- |
| MECHANISM | Nonselective MAO inhibition → ↑ levels of amine neurotransmitters (norepinephrine, 5-HT, dopamine). |
| CLINICAL USE | Atypical depression, anxiety. Parkinson disease (selegiline). |
| ADVERSE EFFECTS | CNS stimulation; hypertensive crisis, most notably with ingestion of tyramine. Contraindicated with SSRIs, TCAs, St. John's wort, meperidine, dextromethorphan, pseudoephedrine, linezolid (to avoid precipitating serotonin syndrome).<br>Wait 2 weeks after stopping MAO inhibitors before starting serotonergic drugs (risk for serotonin syndrome) or stopping dietary restrictions (risk for tyramine induced hypertensive crisis). |

## Atypical antidepressants

| | |
|---|---|
| Bupropion | Inhibits NE and DA reuptake. Also used for smoking cessation. Adverse effects: stimulant effects (tachycardia, insomnia), headache, seizures in patients with bulimia and anorexia nervosa. ↓ risk of sexual adverse effects and weight gain compared to other antidepressants. |
| Mirtazapine | $\alpha_2$-antagonist (↑ release of NE and 5-HT), potent 5-HT$_2$ and 5-HT$_3$ receptor antagonist, and H$_1$ antagonist. Adverse effects: sedation (which may be desirable in depressed patients with insomnia), ↑ appetite, weight gain (which may be desirable in underweight patients), dry mouth. |
| Trazodone | Primarily blocks 5-HT$_2$, $\alpha_1$-adrenergic, and H$_1$ receptors; also weakly inhibits 5-HT reuptake. Used primarily for insomnia, as high doses are needed for antidepressant effects. Adverse effects: sedation, nausea, priapism, postural hypotension. Think tra**ZZZ**obone due to sedative and male-specific adverse effects. |
| Vilazodone | Inhibits 5-HT reuptake; 5-HT$_{1A}$ receptor partial agonist. Used for MDD. Adverse effects: headache, diarrhea, nausea, anticholinergic effects. May cause serotonin syndrome if taken with other serotonergic agents. |
| Vortioxetine | Inhibits 5-HT reuptake; 5-HT$_{1A}$ receptor agonist and 5-HT$_3$ receptor antagonist. Used for MDD. Adverse effects: nausea, sexual dysfunction, sleep disturbances, anticholinergic effects. May cause serotonin syndrome if taken with other serotonergic agents. |

## Pharmacotherapies for smoking cessation

| | |
|---|---|
| Nicotine replacement therapy | Binds to nicotinic ACh receptors. Aim to relieve withdrawal symptoms upon stopping smoking. Long-acting patch and short-acting products (ie, gum, lozenge) can be used in combination. Adverse effects: headache, oral irritation. |
| Varenicline | Nicotinic ACh receptor partial agonist. Diminishes effect on reward system, but also reduces withdrawal. Adverse effects: GI discomfort, sleep disturbance. Varenicline helps nicotine cravings decline. |

| | |
|---|---|
| **Medically supervised opioid withdrawal and relapse prevention** | Injection drug use ↑ risk for HBV, HCV, HIV, skin and soft tissue infections, bacteremia, right-sided infective endocarditis. |
| Methadone | Long-acting oral opioid used for medically supervised opioid (eg, heroin) withdrawal or long-term maintenance therapy. |
| Buprenorphine | Partial opioid agonist. Sublingual form (film) used to suppress withdrawal and for maintenance therapy. Partial agonists can precipitate withdrawal symptoms in opioid-dependent individuals or when administered shortly after use of a full agonist. |
| Naloxone | Short-acting opioid antagonist given IM, IV, or as a nasal spray to treat acute opioid overdose, particularly to reverse respiratory and CNS depression. |
| Naltrexone | Long-acting oral opioid antagonist used after detoxification to prevent relapse. May help alcohol and nicotine cessation, weight loss. Use nal**trex**one for the long **trex** back to sobriety. |

# Renal

"But I know all about love already. I know precious little still about kidneys."

—Aldous Huxley, *Antic Hay*

"This too shall pass. Just like a kidney stone."

—Hunter Madsen

"Playing dead is difficult with a full bladder."

—Diane Lane

Being able to understand and apply renal physiology will be critical for the exam. Important topics include electrolyte disorders, acid-base derangements, glomerular disorders (including histopathology), acute and chronic kidney disease, urine casts, diuretics, ACE inhibitors, and AT II receptor blockers. Renal anomalies associated with various congenital defects are also high-yield associations to think about when evaluating pediatric vignettes.

▸ RENAL—EMBRYOLOGY

**Kidney embryology**

Pronephros—week 4 of development; then degenerates.

Mesonephros—week 4 of development; functions as interim kidney for 1st trimester; persists in the male genital system as Wolffian duct, forming ductus deferens and epididymis.

Metanephros—permanent; first appears in week 5 of development; nephrogenesis is normally completed by week 36 of gestation.

- Ureteric bud (metanephric diverticulum)— fully canalized by week 10 of development; derived from mesonephric duct to form ureters, pelvises, calyces, and collecting ducts
- Metanephric mesenchyme (ie, metanephric blastema)—ureteric bud interacts with this tissue to induce differentiation and formation of glomerulus through distal convoluted tubule (DCT)
- Aberrant interaction between these 2 tissues may result in several congenital malformations of the kidney (eg, renal agenesis, multicystic dysplastic kidney)

Ureteropelvic junction → last part of ureter to canalize; if doesn't fully canalize → congenital obstruction. Can be unilateral or bilateral. Most common pathologic cause of prenatal hydronephrosis. Detected by prenatal ultrasound.

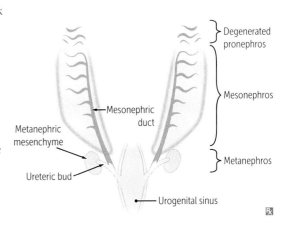

**Potter sequence**

Oligohydramnios → compression of developing fetus → limb deformities, facial anomalies (eg, low-set ears and retrognathia, flattened nose), compression of chest and lack of amniotic fluid aspiration into fetal lungs → pulmonary hypoplasia (cause of death).

Caused by chronic placental insufficiency or reduced fetal urine output, including ARPKD, obstructive uropathy (eg, posterior urethral valves), bilateral renal agenesis.

Babies who can't "Pee" in utero develop Potter sequence.

POTTER sequence associated with:
Pulmonary hypoplasia
Oligohydramnios (trigger)
Twisted face
Twisted skin
Extremity defects
Renal failure (in utero)

## Horseshoe kidney

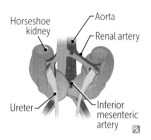

Inferior poles of both kidneys fuse abnormally . As they ascend from pelvis during fetal development, horseshoe kidneys get trapped under inferior mesenteric artery and remain low in the abdomen. Kidneys can function normally, but associated with hydronephrosis (eg, ureteropelvic junction obstruction), renal stones, infection, ↑ risk of renal cancer.

Higher incidence in chromosomal aneuploidy (eg, Turner syndrome, trisomies 13, 18, 21).

## Congenital solitary functioning kidney

Condition of being born with only one functioning kidney. Majority asymptomatic with compensatory hypertrophy of contralateral kidney, but anomalies in contralateral kidney are common. Often diagnosed prenatally via ultrasound bilateral agenesis or dysplasia leads to Potter sequence.

### Unilateral renal agenesis

Ureteric bud fails to develop and induce differentiation of metanephric mesenchyme → complete absence of kidney and ureter.

### Multicystic dysplastic kidney

Ureteric bud develops, but fails to induce differentiation of metanephric mesenchyme → nonfunctional kidney consisting of cysts and connective tissue. Predominantly nonhereditary and usually unilateral.

## Duplex collecting system

Bifurcation of ureteric bud before it enters the metanephric blastema creates a Y-shaped bifid ureter. Duplex collecting system can alternatively occur through two ureteric buds reaching and interacting with metanephric blastema. Strongly associated with vesicoureteral reflux and/or ureteral obstruction, ↑ risk for UTIs. Frequently presents with hydronephrosis.

## Posterior urethral valves

Membrane remnant in posterior (prostatic) urethra in males; its persistence can lead to urethral obstruction. Diagnosed prenatally by bilateral hydronephrosis and dilated or thick-walled bladder on ultrasound. Severe obstruction in fetus associated with oligohydramnios. Most common cause of bladder outlet obstruction in male infants.

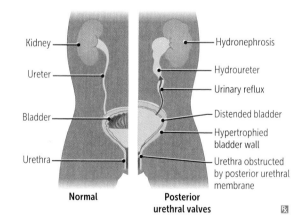

| **Vesicoureteral reflux** | Retrograde flow of urine from bladder toward upper urinary tract. Can be 1° due to abnormal/ insufficient insertion of the ureter within the vesicular wall (ureterovesical junction [UVJ]) or 2° due to abnormally high bladder pressure resulting in retrograde flow via the UVJ. ↑ risk of recurrent UTIs. |
|---|---|

## ▶ RENAL—ANATOMY

### Renal blood flow

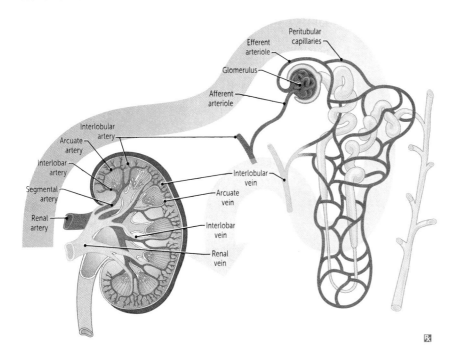

Left renal vein receives two additional veins: left suprarenal and left gonadal veins.

Renal medulla receives significantly less blood flow than the renal cortex. This makes medulla very sensitive to hypoxia and vulnerable to ischemic damage (eg, ATN).

Left kidney is taken during living donor transplantation because it has a longer renal vein.

### Glomerular anatomy

## Course of ureters

Course of ureter **A**: arises from renal pelvis, travels under gonadal arteries → **over** common iliac artery → **under** uterine artery/vas deferens (retroperitoneal).

Gynecologic procedures (eg, ligation of uterine or ovarian vessels) may damage ureter → ureteral obstruction or leak.

Bladder contraction compresses the intramural ureter, preventing urine reflux.

3 common points of ureteral obstruction: ureteropelvic junction, pelvic inlet, ureterovesical junction.

Water (ureters) flows **over** the iliacs and **under** the bridge (uterine artery or vas deferens).

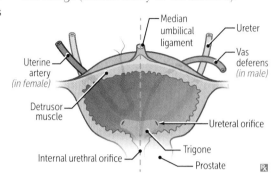

## ▶ RENAL—PHYSIOLOGY

### Fluid compartments

Salty banana: Na⁺ (**salt**) on the outside, K⁺ (**banana**) on the inside.

60–40–20 rule (% of body weight for average person):
- 60% total body water
- 40% ICF, mainly composed of $K^+$, $Mg^{2+}$, organic phosphates (eg, ATP)
- 20% ECF, mainly composed of $Na^+$, $Cl^-$, $HCO_3^-$, albumin

Plasma volume can be measured by radiolabeling albumin.

Extracellular volume can be measured by inulin or mannitol.

Serum osmolality = 275–295 mOsm/kg $H_2O$.

Plasma volume = TBV × (1 − Hct).

### Glomerular filtration barrier

Responsible for filtration of plasma according to size and charge selectivity.

Composed of
- Fenestrated capillary endothelium
- Basement membrane with type IV collagen chains and heparan sulfate
- Visceral epithelial layer consisting of podocyte foot processes (FPs) **A**

Charge barrier—glomerular filtration barrier contains ⊖ charged glycoproteins that prevent entry of ⊖ charged molecules (eg, albumin).

Size barrier—fenestrated capillary endothelium (prevents entry of > 100 nm molecules/blood cells); podocyte foot processes interpose with glomerular basement membrane (GBM); slit diaphragm (prevents entry of molecules > 40–50 nm).

| | |
|---|---|
| **Renal clearance** | $C_x = (U_x V)/P_x$ = volume of plasma from which the substance is completely cleared in the urine per unit time.<br>If $C_x$ < GFR: net tubular reabsorption and/or not freely filtered.<br>If $C_x$ > GFR: net tubular secretion of X.<br>If $C_x$ = GFR: no net secretion or reabsorption. | $C_x$ = clearance of X (mL/min).<br>$U_x$ = urine concentration of X (eg, mg/mL).<br>$P_x$ = plasma concentration of X (eg, mg/mL).<br>V = urine flow rate (mL/min). |

**Glomerular filtration rate**

Inulin clearance can be used to calculate GFR because it is freely filtered and is neither reabsorbed nor secreted.

$$C_{inulin} = GFR = U_{inulin} \times V/P_{inulin}$$
$$= K_f [(P_{GC} - P_{BS}) - (\pi_{GC} - \pi_{BS})]$$

$P_{GC}$ = glomerular capillary hydrostatic pressure; $P_{BS}$ = Bowman space hydrostatic pressure; $\pi_{GC}$ = glomerular capillary oncotic pressure; $\pi_{BS}$ = Bowman space oncotic pressure; $\pi_{BS}$ normally equals zero; $K_f$ = filtration coefficient.
Normal GFR ≈ 100 mL/min.
Creatinine clearance is an approximate measure of GFR. Slightly overestimates GFR because creatinine is moderately secreted by proximal renal tubules.

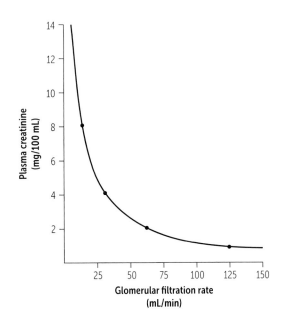

**Renal blood flow autoregulation**

Autoregulatory mechanisms help maintain a constant RBF and GFR to protect the kidney from rapid fluctuations in renal perfusion pressure that could cause renal injury leading to reduced glomerular filtration. Mechanisms:

**Myogenic**: ↑ arterial pressure → stretch of afferent arteriole → mechanical activation of vascular smooth muscle → vasoconstriction of afferent arteriole → ↓ RBF.

**Tubuloglomerular**: ↑ NaCl of the filtrate sensed by macula densa cells → paracrine-driven vasoconstriction of afferent arteriole → ↓ RBF.

**Effective renal plasma flow**

Effective renal plasma flow (eRPF) can be estimated using *para*-aminohippuric acid (PAH) clearance. Between filtration and secretion, there is nearly complete excretion of all PAH that enters the kidney.
$eRPF = U_{PAH} \times V/P_{PAH} = C_{PAH}$.
Renal blood flow (RBF) = RPF/(1 − Hct).
Usually 20–25% of cardiac output.
eRPF underestimates true renal plasma flow (RPF) slightly.

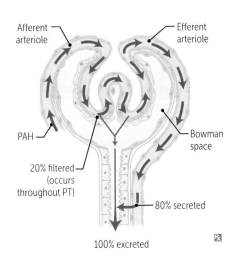

## Filtration

Filtration fraction (FF) = GFR/RPF.
Normal FF = 20%.
Filtered load (mg/min) = GFR (mL/min) × plasma concentration (mg/mL).

GFR can be estimated with creatinine clearance.
RPF is best estimated with PAH clearance.
Prostaglandins Dilate Afferent arteriole (PDA).
Angiotensin II Constricts Efferent arteriole (ACE).

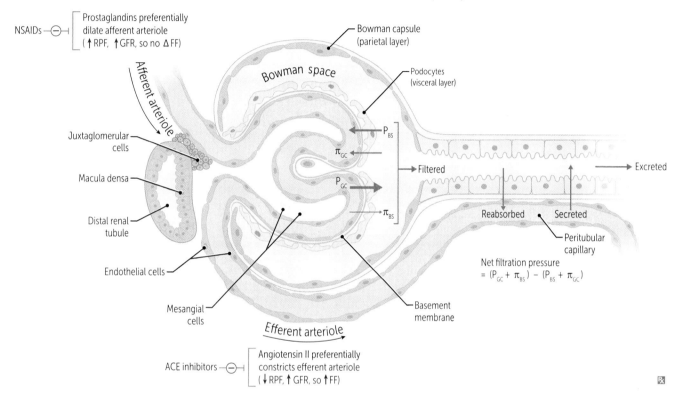

NSAIDs — ⊖ ⊢ [ Prostaglandins preferentially dilate afferent arteriole (↑RPF, ↑GFR, so no ΔFF)

Afferent arteriole

Bowman capsule (parietal layer)

Bowman space

Podocytes (visceral layer)

Juxtaglomerular cells

$P_{BS}$
$\pi_{GC}$
$P_{GC}$
$\pi_{BS}$

Filtered

Excreted

Macula densa

Distal renal tubule

Reabsorbed   Secreted

Peritubular capillary

Endothelial cells

Net filtration pressure
$= (P_{GC} + \pi_{BS}) - (P_{BS} + \pi_{GC})$

Mesangial cells

Basement membrane

Efferent arteriole

ACE inhibitors — ⊖ ⊢ [ Angiotensin II preferentially constricts efferent arteriole (↓RPF, ↑GFR, so ↑FF)

## Changes in glomerular dynamics

| | GFR | RPF | FF (GFR/RPF) |
|---|---|---|---|
| Afferent arteriole constriction | ↓ | ↓ | — |
| Efferent arteriole constriction | ↑ | ↓ | ↑ |
| ↑ plasma protein concentration | ↓ | — | ↓ |
| ↓ plasma protein concentration | ↑ | — | ↑ |
| Constriction of ureter | ↓ | — | ↓ |
| Dehydration | ↓ | ↓↓ | ↑ |

Notably for patients undergoing nephrectomy, there is a proportionate decline in renal function (↓ nephron number) → ↓ remaining kidney renal function to ~50% of prenephrectomy value until long-term compensations like hypertrophy develop.

| **Calculation of reabsorption and secretion rate** | Filtered load = $GFR \times P_x$. |
|---|---|

Excretion rate = $V \times U_x$.
Reabsorption rate = filtered – excreted.
Secretion rate = excreted – filtered.
$Fe_{Na}$ = fractional excretion of sodium.

$$Fe_{Na} = \frac{Na^+ \text{ excreted}}{Na^+ \text{ filtered}} = \frac{V \times U_{Na}}{GFR \times P_{Na}} = \frac{P_{Cr} \times U_{Na}}{U_{Cr} \times P_{Na}} \quad \text{where GFR} = \frac{U_{Cr} \times V}{P_{Cr}}$$

---

**Glucose clearance**

Glucose at a normal plasma level (range 60–120 mg/dL) is completely reabsorbed in proximal convoluted tubule (PCT) by $Na^+$/glucose cotransport.

In adults, at plasma glucose of ~ 200 mg/dL, glucosuria begins (threshold). At rate of ~ 375 mg/min, all transporters are fully saturated ($T_m$).

Normal pregnancy is associated with ↑ GFR. With ↑ filtration of all substances, including glucose, the glucose threshold occurs at lower plasma glucose concentrations → glucosuria at normal plasma glucose levels.

Sodium-glucose cotransporter 2 (SGLT2) inhibitors (eg, -flozin drugs) lead to glucosuria at plasma concentrations < 200 mg/dL.

Glucosuria is an important clinical clue to diabetes mellitus.

Splay phenomenon—$T_m$ for glucose is reached gradually rather than sharply due to the heterogeneity of nephrons (ie, different $T_m$ points); represented by the portion of the titration curve between threshold and $T_m$.

## Nephron transport physiology

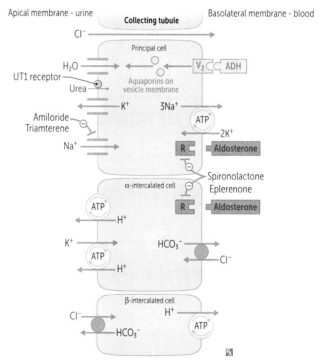

**Early PCT**—contains brush border. Reabsorbs all glucose and amino acids and most $HCO_3^-$, $Na^+$, $Cl^-$, $PO_4^{3-}$, $K^+$, $H_2O$, and uric acid. Isotonic absorption. Generates and secretes $NH_3$, which enables the kidney to excrete (via secretion) more $H^+$.

PTH—inhibits $Na^+/PO_4^{3-}$ cotransport → ↑ $PO_4^{3-}$ excretion.
AT II—stimulates $Na^+/H^+$ exchange → ↑ $Na^+$, $H_2O$, and $HCO_3^-$ reabsorption (permitting contraction alkalosis). 65–80% $Na^+$ and $H_2O$ reabsorbed.

**Thin descending loop of Henle**—passively reabsorbs $H_2O$ via medullary hypertonicity (impermeable to $Na^+$). Concentrating segment. Makes urine hypertonic.

**Thick ascending loop of Henle**—reabsorbs $Na^+$, $K^+$, and $Cl^-$. Indirectly induces paracellular reabsorption of $Mg^{2+}$ and $Ca^{2+}$ through ⊕ lumen potential generated by $K^+$ backleak. Impermeable to $H_2O$. Makes urine less concentrated as it ascends.
10–20% $Na^+$ reabsorbed.

**Early DCT**—reabsorbs $Na^+$, $Cl^-$. Impermeable to $H_2O$. Makes urine fully dilute (hypotonic).
PTH—↑ $Ca^{2+}/Na^+$ exchange → ↑ $Ca^{2+}$ reabsorption.
5–10% $Na^+$ reabsorbed.

**Collecting tubule**—reabsorbs $Na^+$ in exchange for secreting $K^+$ and $H^+$ (regulated by aldosterone).
Aldosterone—acts on mineralocorticoid receptor → mRNA → protein synthesis. In principal cells: ↑ apical $K^+$ conductance, ↑ $Na^+/K^+$ pump, ↑ epithelial $Na^+$ channel (ENaC) activity → lumen negativity → $K^+$ secretion. In α-intercalated cells: lumen negativity → ↑ $H^+$ ATPase activity → ↑ $H^+$ secretion → ↑ $HCO_3^-/Cl^-$ exchanger activity.
ADH—acts at $V_2$ receptor → insertion of aquaporin $H_2O$ channels on apical side.
3–5% $Na^+$ reabsorbed.

**Renal tubular defects**    Order: Fanconi's BaGeLS

| | DEFECTS | EFFECTS | CAUSES | NOTES |
|---|---|---|---|---|
| **Fanconi syndrome** | Generalized reabsorption defect in PCT → ↑ excretion of amino acids, glucose, $HCO_3^-$, and $PO_4^{3-}$, and all substances reabsorbed by the PCT | Metabolic acidosis (proximal RTA), hypophosphatemia, hypokalemia | Hereditary defects (eg, Wilson disease, tyrosinemia, glycogen storage disease), ischemia, multiple myeloma, drugs (eg, ifosfamide, cisplatin, tenofovir, lead poisoning | Growth retardation and rickets/osteopenia common due to hypophosphatemia Volume depletion also common |
| **Bartter syndrome** | Reabsorption defect in thick ascending loop of Henle (affects $Na^+/K^+/2Cl^-$ cotransporter) | Metabolic alkalosis, hypokalemia, hypercalciuria | Autosomal recessive | Presents similarly to chronic loop diuretic use |
| **Gitelman syndrome** | Reabsorption defect of NaCl in DCT | Metabolic alkalosis, hypomagnesemia, hypokalemia, hypocalciuria | Autosomal recessive | Presents similarly to chronic thiazide diuretic use Less severe than Bartter syndrome |
| **Liddle syndrome** | Gain of function mutation → ↓ $Na^+$ channel degradation → ↑ $Na^+$ reabsorption in collecting tubules | Metabolic alkalosis, hypokalemia, hypertension, ↓ serum aldosterone | Autosomal dominant | Presents similarly to hyperaldosteronism, but aldosterone is nearly undetectable Treatment: amiloride |
| **Syndrome of Apparent Mineralocorticoid Excess** | Cortisol activates mineralocorticoid receptors; 11β-HSD converts cortisol to cortisone (inactive on these receptors) Hereditary 11β-HSD deficiency → ↑ cortisol → ↑ mineralocorticoid receptor activity | Metabolic alkalosis, hypokalemia, hypertension ↓ serum aldosterone level; cortisol tries to be the **SAME** as aldosterone | Autosomal recessive Can acquire disorder from glycyrrhetinic acid (present in licorice), which blocks activity of 11β-hydroxysteroid dehydrogenase | Treatment: $K^+$-sparing diuretics (↓ mineralocorticoid effects) or corticosteroids (exogenous corticosteroid ↓ endogenous cortisol production → ↓ mineralocorticoid receptor activation) |

## Features of renal disorders

| CONDITION | BLOOD PRESSURE | PLASMA RENIN | ALDOSTERONE | SERUM Mg²⁺ | URINE Ca²⁺ |
|---|---|---|---|---|---|
| SIADH | —/↑ | —/↓ | —/↓ | — | — |
| Bartter syndrome | — | ↑ | ↑ | — | ↑ |
| Gitelman syndrome | — | ↑ | ↑ | ↓ | ↓ |
| Renin-secreting tumor | ↑ | ↑ | ↑ | — | — |
| Primary hyperaldosteronism | ↑ | ↓ | ↑ | — | — |
| Liddle syndrome, syndrome of apparent mineralocorticoid excess | ↑ | ↓ | ↓ | — | — |

↑↓ = important differentiating feature.

**Relative concentrations along proximal tubule**

[TF/P] > 1 when solute is reabsorbed less quickly than water or when solute is secreted

[TF/P] = 1 when solute and water are reabsorbed at the same rate

[TF/P] < 1 when solute is reabsorbed more quickly than water

$\frac{[\text{Tubular fluid}]}{[\text{Plasma}]}$

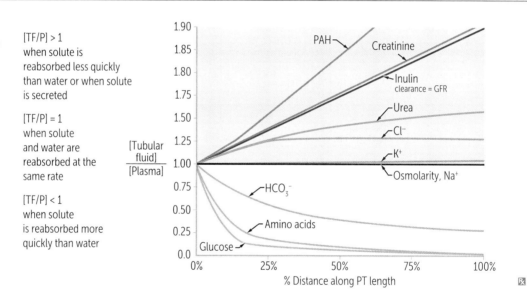

Tubular inulin ↑ in concentration (but not amount) along the PT as a result of water reabsorption. Cl⁻ reabsorption occurs at a slower rate than Na⁺ in early PCT and then matches the rate of Na⁺ reabsorption more distally. Thus, its relative concentration ↑ before it plateaus.

## Renin-angiotensin-aldosterone system

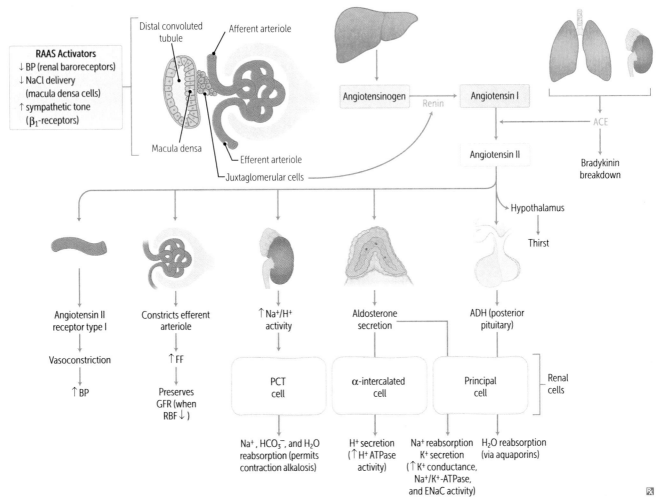

| Renin | Secreted by JG cells in response to ↓ renal perfusion pressure (detected in afferent arteriole), ↑ renal sympathetic discharge (β₁ effect), and ↓ NaCl delivery to macula densa cells. |
|---|---|
| ACE | Catalyzes conversion of angiotensin I to angiotensin II. Located in many tissues but conversion occurs most extensively in the lung. Produced by vascular endothelial cells in the lung. |
| AT II | Helps maintain blood volume and blood pressure. Affects baroreceptor function; limits reflex bradycardia, which would normally accompany its pressor effects. |
| ANP, BNP | Released from atria (ANP) and ventricles (BNP) in response to ↑ volume; relaxes vascular smooth muscle via cGMP → ↑ GFR; ↓ renin → angiotensin-aldosterone inhibition. Dilates afferent arteriole, promotes natriuresis. |
| ADH (vasopressin) | Primarily regulates serum osmolality; also responds to low blood volume states. Stimulates reabsorption of water in collecting ducts. Also stimulates reabsorption of urea in medullary collecting ducts to maximize corticopapillary osmotic gradient. |
| Aldosterone | Primarily regulates ECF volume and Na⁺ content; ↑ release in hypovolemic states. Responds to hyperkalemia by ↑ K⁺ excretion. |

| **Juxtaglomerular apparatus** | Consists of mesangial cells, JG cells (modified smooth muscle of afferent arteriole), and the macula densa (NaCl sensor located at the DCT). JG cells secrete renin in response to ↓ renal blood pressure and ↑ sympathetic tone ($\beta_1$). Macula densa cells sense ↓ NaCl delivery to DCT → ↑ renin release → efferent arteriole vasoconstriction → ↑ GFR. | JGA prevents short-term changes in GFR through autoregulation and maintains GFR long-term through regulation of the renin-angiotensin-aldosterone system. $\beta$-blockers ↓ BP by ↓ CO and inhibiting $\beta_1$-receptors of the JGA → ↓ renin release. |

### Kidney endocrine/paracrine functions

| | | |
|---|---|---|
| Erythropoietin | Released by interstitial cells in peritubular capillary bed in response to hypoxia. | Stimulates RBC proliferation in bone marrow. Administered for anemia secondary to chronic kidney disease. Adverse effect: ↑ risk of HTN in some individuals. |
| Calciferol (vitamin D) | PCT cells convert 25-OH vitamin $D_3$ to 1,25-$(OH)_2$ vitamin $D_3$ (calcitriol, active form). Increases calcium absorption in small bowel. | 25-OH $D_3$ (calcidiol) $\xrightarrow{1\alpha\text{-hydroxylase}}$ 1,25-$(OH)_2$ $D_3$ (calcitriol)  <br> ⊕ PTH |
| Prostaglandins | Paracrine secretion vasodilates afferent arterioles to ↑ RBF. | NSAIDs block renal-protective prostaglandin synthesis → constriction of afferent arteriole and ↓ GFR; this may result in acute kidney injury in low renal blood flow states. |
| Dopamine | Secreted by PT cells, promotes natriuresis. At low doses; dilates interlobular arteries, afferent arterioles, efferent arterioles → ↑ RBF, little or no change in GFR. At higher doses; acts as vasoconstrictor. | |

## Hormones acting on kidney

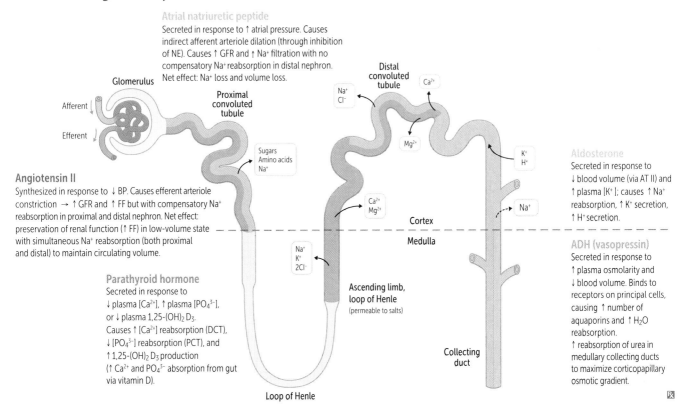

**Atrial natriuretic peptide**
Secreted in response to ↑ atrial pressure. Causes indirect afferent arteriole dilation (through inhibition of NE). Causes ↑ GFR and ↑ Na⁺ filtration with no compensatory Na⁺ reabsorption in distal nephron. Net effect: Na⁺ loss and volume loss.

Glomerulus
Afferent
Efferent

Proximal convoluted tubule

Sugars
Amino acids
Na⁺

Distal convoluted tubule

Na⁺
Cl⁻

Ca²⁺

Mg²⁺

K⁺
H⁺

Na⁺

Ca²⁺
Mg²⁺

Cortex
Medulla

Na⁺
K⁺
2Cl⁻

Ascending limb, loop of Henle
(permeable to salts)

Collecting duct

Loop of Henle

**Angiotensin II**
Synthesized in response to ↓ BP. Causes efferent arteriole constriction → ↑ GFR and ↑ FF but with compensatory Na⁺ reabsorption in proximal and distal nephron. Net effect: preservation of renal function (↑ FF) in low-volume state with simultaneous Na⁺ reabsorption (both proximal and distal) to maintain circulating volume.

**Parathyroid hormone**
Secreted in response to ↓ plasma $[Ca^{2+}]$, ↑ plasma $[PO_4^{3-}]$, or ↓ plasma $1,25-(OH)_2 D_3$. Causes ↑ $[Ca^{2+}]$ reabsorption (DCT), ↓ $[PO_4^{3-}]$ reabsorption (PCT), and ↑ $1,25-(OH)_2 D_3$ production (↑ $Ca^{2+}$ and $PO_4^{3-}$ absorption from gut via vitamin D).

**Aldosterone**
Secreted in response to ↓ blood volume (via AT II) and ↑ plasma $[K^+]$; causes ↑ Na⁺ reabsorption, ↑ K⁺ secretion, ↑ H⁺ secretion.

**ADH (vasopressin)**
Secreted in response to ↑ plasma osmolarity and ↓ blood volume. Binds to receptors on principal cells, causing ↑ number of aquaporins and ↑ $H_2O$ reabsorption. ↑ reabsorption of urea in medullary collecting ducts to maximize corticopapillary osmotic gradient.

---

## Potassium shifts

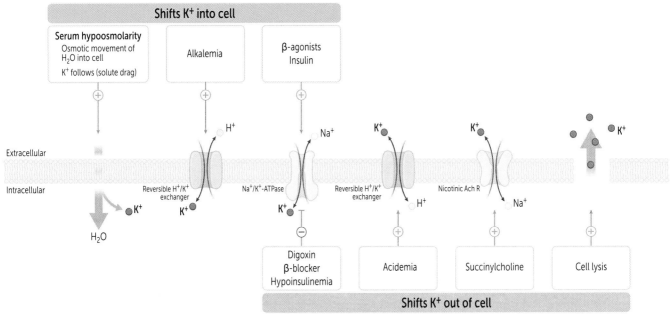

**Shifts K⁺ into cell**

**Serum hypoosmolarity**
Osmotic movement of $H_2O$ into cell
K⁺ follows (solute drag)

**Alkalemia**

**β-agonists**
**Insulin**

Extracellular

Intracellular

H⁺
Reversible H⁺/K⁺ exchanger
K⁺

$H_2O$    K⁺

Na⁺
Na⁺/K⁺-ATPase
K⁺

K⁺
Reversible H⁺/K⁺ exchanger
H⁺

K⁺
Nicotinic Ach R
Na⁺

K⁺

K⁺

**Digoxin**
**β-blocker**
**Hypoinsulinemia**

**Acidemia**

**Succinylcholine**

**Cell lysis**

**Shifts K⁺ out of cell**

## Electrolyte disturbances

| ELECTROLYTE | LOW SERUM CONCENTRATION | HIGH SERUM CONCENTRATION |
|---|---|---|
| Sodium | Nausea, malaise, stupor, coma, seizures | Irritability, stupor, coma |
| Potassium | U waves and flattened T waves on ECG, arrhythmias, muscle cramps, spasm, weakness | Wide QRS and peaked T waves on ECG, arrhythmias, muscle weakness |
| Calcium | Tetany, seizures, QT prolongation, twitching (eg, Chvostek sign), spasm (eg, Trousseau sign) | Stones (renal), bones (pain), groans (abdominal pain), thrones (↑ urinary output frequency), psychiatric overtones (anxiety, altered mental status) |
| Magnesium | Tetany, torsades de pointes, hypokalemia, hypocalcemia (when $[Mg^{2+}] < 1.0$ mEq/L) | ↓ DTRs, lethargy, bradycardia, hypotension, cardiac arrest, hypocalcemia |
| Phosphate | Bone loss, osteomalacia (adults), rickets (children) | Renal stones, metastatic calcifications, hypocalcemia |

## Acid-base physiology

Metabolic acid-base disorders cause $HCO_3^-$ alterations. Respiratory acid-base disorders cause $P_{CO_2}$ alterations.

| | pH | $P_{CO_2}$ | $[HCO_3^-]$ | COMPENSATORY RESPONSE |
|---|---|---|---|---|
| **Metabolic acidosis** | ↓ | ↓ | ↓ | Hyperventilation (immediate) |
| **Metabolic alkalosis** | ↑ | ↑ | ↑ | Hypoventilation (immediate) |
| **Respiratory acidosis** | ↓ | ↑ | ↑ | ↑ renal $[HCO_3^-]$ reabsorption (delayed) |
| **Respiratory alkalosis** | ↑ | ↓ | ↓ | ↓ renal $[HCO_3^-]$ reabsorption (delayed) |

Key: ↓ ↑ = compensatory response.

Henderson-Hasselbalch equation: $pH = 6.1 + \log \dfrac{[HCO_3^-]}{0.03\ P_{CO_2}}$

Predicted respiratory compensation for a simple metabolic acidosis can be calculated using the Winters formula. If measured $P_{CO_2}$ > predicted $P_{CO_2}$ → concomitant respiratory acidosis; if measured $P_{CO_2}$ < predicted $P_{CO_2}$ → concomitant respiratory alkalosis:

$$P_{CO_2} = 1.5\ [HCO_3^-] + 8 \pm 2$$

## Acidosis and alkalosis

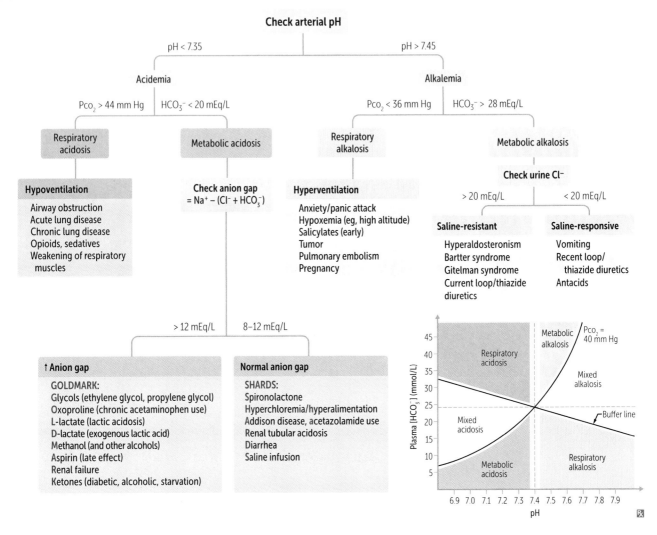

**Check arterial pH**

pH < 7.35 → **Acidemia**

Pco$_2$ > 44 mm Hg → **Respiratory acidosis**

HCO$_3^-$ < 20 mEq/L → **Metabolic acidosis**

pH > 7.45 → **Alkalemia**

Pco$_2$ < 36 mm Hg → **Respiratory alkalosis**

HCO$_3^-$ > 28 mEq/L → **Metabolic alkalosis**

**Respiratory acidosis**

**Hypoventilation**
Airway obstruction
Acute lung disease
Chronic lung disease
Opioids, sedatives
Weakening of respiratory
  muscles

**Metabolic acidosis**

**Check anion gap**
$= Na^+ - (Cl^- + HCO_3^-)$

**Respiratory alkalosis**

**Hyperventilation**
Anxiety/panic attack
Hypoxemia (eg, high altitude)
Salicylates (early)
Tumor
Pulmonary embolism
Pregnancy

**Metabolic alkalosis**

**Check urine Cl$^-$**

> 20 mEq/L → **Saline-resistant**
Hyperaldosteronism
Bartter syndrome
Gitelman syndrome
Current loop/thiazide
  diuretics

< 20 mEq/L → **Saline-responsive**
Vomiting
Recent loop/
  thiazide diuretics
Antacids

> 12 mEq/L → **↑ Anion gap**

**GOLDMARK:**
Glycols (ethylene glycol, propylene glycol)
Oxoproline (chronic acetaminophen use)
L-lactate (lactic acidosis)
D-lactate (exogenous lactic acid)
Methanol (and other alcohols)
Aspirin (late effect)
Renal failure
Ketones (diabetic, alcoholic, starvation)

8–12 mEq/L → **Normal anion gap**

**SHARDS:**
Spironolactone
Hyperchloremia/hyperalimentation
Addison disease, acetazolamide use
Renal tubular acidosis
Diarrhea
Saline infusion

## Renal tubular acidosis

| | Distal renal tubular acidosis (RTA type 1) | Proximal renal tubular acidosis (RTA type 2) | Hyperkalemic tubular acidosis (RTA type 4) |
|---|---|---|---|
| DEFECT | Inability of α-intercalated cells to secrete $H^+$ → no new $HCO_3^-$ is generated → metabolic acidosis | Defect in PCT $HCO_3^-$ reabsorption → ↑ excretion of $HCO_3^-$ in urine → metabolic acidosis<br>Urine can be acidified by α-intercalated cells in collecting duct, but not enough to overcome ↑ $HCO_3^-$ excretion | Hypoaldosteronism or aldosterone resistance; hyperkalemia → ↓ $NH_3$ synthesis in PCT → ↓ $NH_4^+$ excretion |
| URINE pH | > 5.5 | < 5.5 when plasma $HCO_3^-$ below reduced resorption threshold<br>> 5.5 when filtered $HCO_3^-$ exceeds resorptive threshold | Variable |
| SERUM K⁺ | ↓ | ↓ | ↑ |
| CAUSES | Amphotericin B toxicity, analgesic nephropathy, congenital anomalies (obstruction) of urinary tract, autoimmune diseases (eg, SLE) | Fanconi syndrome, multiple myeloma, carbonic anhydrase inhibitors | ↓ aldosterone production (eg, diabetic hyporeninism, ACE inhibitors, ARB, NSAIDs, heparin, cyclosporine, adrenal insufficiency) or aldosterone resistance (eg, K⁺-sparing diuretics, nephropathy due to obstruction, TMP-SMX) |
| ASSOCIATIONS | ↑ risk for calcium phosphate kidney stones (due to ↑ urine pH and ↑ bone turnover related to buffering) | ↑ risk for hypophosphatemic rickets (in Fanconi syndrome) | |

## ▶ RENAL—PATHOLOGY

| | |
|---|---|
| **Casts in urine** | Presence of casts indicates that hematuria/pyuria is of glomerular or renal tubular origin. Bladder cancer, kidney stones → hematuria, no casts. Acute cystitis → pyuria, no casts. All casts contain a matrix composed primarily of Tamm-Horsfall mucoprotein (uromodulin), secreted by renal tubular cells to prevent UTIs. |
| **RBC casts A** | Glomerulonephritis, hypertensive emergency. |
| **WBC casts B** | Tubulointerstitial inflammation, acute pyelonephritis, transplant rejection. |
| **Granular casts C** | Acute tubular necrosis (ATN). Can be "muddy brown" in appearance. |
| **Fatty casts ("oval fat bodies")** | Nephrotic syndrome. Associated with "Maltese cross" sign D. |
| **Waxy casts** | End-stage renal disease/chronic kidney disease. |
| **Hyaline casts E** | Nonspecific, can be a normal finding with dehydration, exercise, or diuretic therapy. |

### Nomenclature of glomerular disorders

| TYPE | CHARACTERISTICS | EXAMPLE |
|---|---|---|
| **Focal** | < 50% of glomeruli are involved | Focal segmental glomerulosclerosis |
| **Diffuse** | > 50% of glomeruli are involved | Diffuse proliferative glomerulonephritis |
| **Proliferative** | Hypercellular glomeruli | Membranoproliferative glomerulonephritis |
| **Membranous** | Thickening of glomerular basement membrane (GBM) | Membranous nephropathy |
| **Primary glomerular disease** | 1° disease of the kidney specifically impacting the glomeruli | Minimal change disease |
| **Secondary glomerular disease** | Systemic disease or disease of another organ system that also impacts the glomeruli | SLE, diabetic nephropathy |

## Glomerular diseases

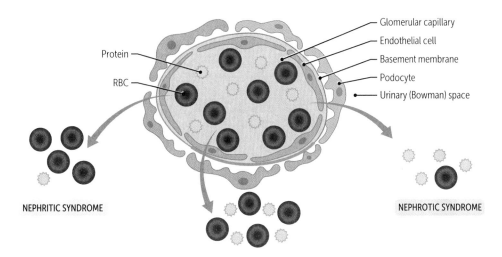

| TYPE | ETIOLOGY | CLINICAL PRESENTATION | EXAMPLES |
|---|---|---|---|
| **Nephritic syndrome** | Glomerular inflammation → GBM damage → loss of RBCs into urine → dysmorphic RBCs, hematuria | Hematuria, RBC casts in urine ↓ GFR → oliguria, azotemia ↑ renin release, HTN Proteinuria often in the subnephrotic range (< 3.5 g/day) but in severe cases may be in nephrotic range | ▪ Infection-associated glomerulonephritis ▪ Goodpasture syndrome ▪ IgA nephropathy (Berger disease) ▪ Alport syndrome ▪ Membranoproliferative glomerulonephritis |
| **Nephrotic syndrome** | Podocyte damage → impaired charge barrier → proteinuria | Massive proteinuria (> 3.5 g/day) with edema, hypoalbuminemia → ↑ hepatic lipogenesis → hypercholesterolemia Frothy urine with fatty casts Associated with hypercoagulable state due to antithrombin loss in urine and ↑ risk of infection (loss of IgGs in urine and soft tissue compromise by edema) | May be 1° (eg, direct podocyte damage) or 2° (podocyte damage from systemic process): ▪ Focal segmental glomerulosclerosis (1° or 2°) ▪ Minimal change disease (1° or 2°) ▪ Membranous nephropathy (1° or 2°) ▪ Amyloidosis (2°) ▪ Diabetic glomerulonephropathy (2°) |
| **Nephritic-nephrotic syndrome** | Severe GBM damage → loss of RBCs into urine + impaired charge barrier → hematuria + proteinuria | Nephrotic-range proteinuria (> 3.5 g/day) and concomitant features of nephritic syndrome | Can occur with any form of nephritic syndrome, but is most common with: ▪ Diffuse proliferative glomerulonephritis ▪ Membranoproliferative glomerulonephritis |

**Nephritic syndrome**

| | MECHANISM | LIGHT MICROSCOPY | IMMUNOFLUORESCENCE | ELECTRON MICROSCOPY |
|---|---|---|---|---|
| **Infection-related glomerulonephritis** | Type III hypersensitivity reaction with consumptive hypocomplementemia Children: seen ~2–4 weeks after group A streptococcal pharyngitis or skin infection Adults: *Staphylococcus* is additional causative agent | Enlarged and hypercellular glomeruli A | Granular ("starry sky") appearance ("lumpy-bumpy") B due to IgG, IgM, and C3 deposition along GBM and mesangium | Subepithelial IC humps |
| **IgA nephropathy (Berger disease)** | Occurs concurrently with respiratory or GI tract infections (IgA is secreted by mucosal linings) Renal pathology of IgA vasculitis | Mesangial proliferation | IgA-based IC deposits in mesangium | Mesangial IC deposition |
| **Rapidly progressive (crescentic) glomerulonephritis** | Poor prognosis Multiple causes: Type II HSR in Goodpasture syndrome | Crescent moon shape C; crescents consist of fibrin and plasma proteins (eg, C3b) with glomerular parietal cells, monocytes, macrophages | Linear IF due to antibodies to GBM and alveolar basement membrane: Goodpasture syndrome— hematuria/ hemoptysis Negative IF/Pauci-immune (no IgC3 deposition): granulomatosis with polyangiitis—PR3-ANCA/c-ANCA, eosinophilic granulomatosis with polyangiitis, or Microscopic polyangiitis—MPO-ANCA/p-ANCA Granular IF—PSGN or DPGN | Goodpasture syndrome: breaks in GBM, necrosis and crescent formation with no deposits Pauci-immune: usually no deposits EM features depend on underlying cause |
| **Diffuse proliferative glomerulonephritis** | Often due to SLE (think "wire lupus"); DPGN and MPGN often present as nephritic and nephrotic syndromes concurrently | "Wire looping" of capillaries D | Granular | Subendothelial, sometimes subepithelial or intramembranous IgG-based ICs often with C3 deposition |

## Nephritic syndrome (continued)

| | | | | |
|---|---|---|---|---|
| **Alport syndrome** | Type IV collagen mutation → glomerular basement membrane alterations; mostly X-linked dominant. Eye problems (eg, retinopathy, anterior lenticonus), glomerulonephritis, SNHL (can't see, can't pee, can't hear a bee) | Irregular thinning and thickening and splitting of glomerular basement membrane | Initially negative; non-specific staining (usually stays negative) | "Basket-weave" appearance due to irregular thickening and longitudinal splitting of GBM |
| **Membrano- proliferative glomerulonephritis** | Type I may be 2° to HBV or HCV infection; type II associated with C3 nephritic factor (IgG autoantibody that stabilizes C3 convertase → persistent complement activation → ↓ C3) | Mesangial ingrowth → GBM splitting → "tram-track" on H&E and PAS  stains | Granular | Type I—subendothelial IC deposits Type II— intramembranous deposits, also called dense deposit disease |

## Nephrotic syndrome

| | MECHANISM | LIGHT MICROSCOPY | IMMUNOFLUORESCENCE | ELECTRON MICROSCOPY |
|---|---|---|---|---|
| **Minimal change disease** | Also called lipoid nephrosis. Often 1° (idiopathic), triggered by recent infection, immunization, immune stimulus (4 Is); rarely 2° to lymphoma (eg, cytokine-mediated damage). Loss of antithrombin → renal vein thrombosis. | Normal glomeruli (lipid may be seen in PT cells) | ⊖ | Effacement of podocyte foot processes  |
| **Focal segmental glomerulosclerosis** | Can be 1° (idiopathic) or 2° (eg, HIV infection, sickle cell disease, obesity, or congenital malformations); may progress to CKD. More common in Black people. | Segmental sclerosis and hyalinosis B | Often ⊖ but may be ⊕ for nonspecific focal deposits of IgM, C3, C1 | Effacement of podocyte foot processes |
| **Membranous nephropathy** | Also called membranous glomerulonephritis. Can be 1° (eg, antibodies to phospholipase $A_2$ receptor) or 2° to drugs (eg, NSAIDs, penicillamine, gold), infections (eg, HBV, HCV, syphilis), SLE, or solid tumors. ↑ risk of thromboembolism (eg, DVT, renal vein thrombosis). | Diffuse capillary and GBM thickening C | Granular due to immune complex (IC) deposition | "Spike and dome" appearance of subepithelial deposits |
| **Amyloidosis** | Kidney most commonly involved organ. Associated with chronic conditions that predispose to amyloid deposition (eg, AL amyloid, AA amyloid, prolonged dialysis). | Congo red stain shows apple-green birefringence under polarized light due to amyloid deposition in the mesangium | AL amyloidosis: may be positive for lambda and kappa light chains<br><br>AA amyloidosis: positive for AA protein | Mesangial expansion by amyloid fibrils |
| **Diabetic glomerulo-nephropathy** | Most common cause of ESRD in United States. Hyperglycemia → nonenzymatic glycation of tissue proteins → mesangial expansion → GBM thickening and ↑ permeability. Hyperfiltration (glomerular HTN and ↑ GFR) → glomerular hypertrophy and glomerular scarring (glomerulosclerosis) → further progression of nephropathy. Look for albuminuria with ↑ urine albumin-to-creatinine ratio. ACE inhibitors and ARBs are renoprotective. | Mesangial expansion, GBM thickening, eosinophilic nodular glomerulo-sclerosis (Kimmelstiel-Wilson lesions D) | Non-specific staining. Usually negative. | Prominent thickening of GBM with expanded mesangium, predominantly due to increased mesangial matrix, segmental podocyte effacement |

**Kidney stones**

Can lead to severe complications such as hydronephrosis, pyelonephritis, and acute kidney injury. Obstructed stone presents with unilateral flank tenderness, colicky pain radiating to groin, hematuria. Treat and prevent by encouraging fluid intake. Radiolucent stones: I can't c (see) u (you) (cystine and uric acid).

| CONTENT | PRECIPITATES WITH | X-RAY FINDINGS | CT FINDINGS | URINE CRYSTAL | NOTES |
|---|---|---|---|---|---|
| Calcium | Calcium oxalate: hypocitraturia | Radiopaque | Hyperdense | Shaped like envelope  or dumbbell | Calcium stones most common (80%); calcium oxalate more common than calcium phosphate stones. Can result from ethylene glycol (antifreeze) ingestion, vitamin C overuse, hypocitraturia (usually associated with ↓ urine pH), malabsorption (eg, Crohn disease). Treatment: thiazides, citrate, low-sodium diet. |
| | Calcium phosphate: ↑ pH | Radiopaque | Hyperdense | Wedge-shaped prism | Treatment: low-sodium diet, thiazides. |
| Ammonium magnesium phosphate (struvite) | ↑ pH | Radiopaque | Hyperdense | Coffin lid ("sarcophagus") | Account for 15% of stones. Caused by infection with urease ⊕ bugs (eg, *Proteus mirabilis*, *Staphylococcus saprophyticus*, *Klebsiella*) that hydrolyze urea to ammonia → urine alkalinization. Commonly form staghorn calculi **B**. Treatment: eradication of underlying infection, surgical removal of stone. |
| Uric acid | ↓ pH | Radiolucent | Visible | Rhomboid **C** or rosettes | About 5% of all stones. Risk factors: arid climates, acidic pH. Strong association with hyperuricemia (eg, gout). Often seen in diseases with ↑ cell turnover (eg, leukemia). Treatment: alkalinization of urine, allopurinol. |
| Cystine | ↓ pH | Faintly radiopaque | Moderately radiodense | Hexagonal **D** | Hereditary (autosomal recessive) condition in which Cystine-reabsorbing PCT transporter loses function, causing cystinuria. Transporter defect also results in poor reabsorption of Ornithine, Lysine, Arginine (COLA). Cystine is poorly soluble, thus stones form in urine. Usually begins in childhood. Can form staghorn calculi. Sodium cyanide nitroprusside test ⊕. "Sixtine" stones have six sides. Treatment: low sodium diet, alkalinization of urine, chelating agents (eg, tiopronin, penicillamine) if refractory. |

**Hydronephrosis**

Distention/dilation of renal pelvis and/or calyces ◼. Mostly caused by urinary tract obstruction (eg, renal stones, severe BPH, congenital obstructions, locally advanced cervical cancer, injury to ureter); other causes include retroperitoneal fibrosis, vesicoureteral reflux. Dilation occurs proximal to site of pathology. Serum creatinine becomes elevated if obstruction is bilateral or if patient has an obstructed solitary kidney. Leads to compression and possible atrophy of renal cortex and medulla.

**Urinary incontinence**

Mixed incontinence has features of both stress and urgency incontinence.

| | Stress incontinence | Urgency incontinence | Overflow incontinence |
|---|---|---|---|
| MECHANISM | Outlet incompetence (urethral hypermobility or intrinsic sphincter deficiency) → leak with ↑ intra-abdominal pressure (eg, sneezing, lifting) ⊕ bladder stress test (directly observed leakage from urethra upon coughing or Valsalva maneuver) | Detrusor overactivity → leak with urge to void immediately | Incomplete emptying (detrusor underactivity or outlet obstruction) → leak with overfilling, ↑ postvoid residual on catheterization or ultrasound |
| ASSOCIATIONS | Obesity, pregnancy, vaginal delivery, prostate surgery | UTI | Polyuria (eg, diabetes), bladder outlet obstruction (eg, BPH), spinal cord injury |
| TREATMENT | Pelvic floor muscle strengthening (Kegel) exercises, weight loss, pessaries | Kegel exercises, bladder training (timed voiding, distraction or relaxation techniques), antimuscarinics (eg, oxybutynin for overactive bladder), mirabegron | Catheterization, relieve obstruction (eg, α-blockers for BPH) |

**Acute cystitis**

Inflammation of urinary bladder. Presents as suprapubic pain, dysuria, urinary frequency, urgency. Systemic signs (eg, high fever, chills) are usually absent.

Risk factors include female sex (short urethra), sexual intercourse, indwelling catheter, diabetes mellitus, impaired bladder emptying.

Causes:
- *E coli* (most common)
- *Staphylococcus saprophyticus*—seen in sexually active young women (*E coli* is still more common in this group)
- *Klebsiella*
- *Proteus mirabilis*—urine has ammonia scent

Labs: ⊕ leukocyte esterase. ⊕ nitrites (indicates presence of Enterobacteriaceae). Sterile pyuria (pyuria with ⊖ urine cultures) could suggest urethritis by *Neisseria gonorrhoeae* or *Chlamydia trachomatis*.

Treatment: antibiotics (eg, TMP-SMX, nitrofurantoin).

**Pyelonephritis**

**Acute pyelonephritis**

Neutrophils infiltrate renal interstitium . Affects cortex with relative sparing of glomeruli/vessels. Presents with fevers, flank pain (costovertebral angle tenderness), nausea/vomiting, chills.

Causes include ascending UTI (*E coli* is most common), hematogenous spread to kidney. Presents with WBCs in urine +/– WBC casts. CT would show striated parenchymal enhancement.

Risk factors include indwelling urinary catheter, urinary tract obstruction, vesicoureteral reflux, diabetes mellitus, pregnancy (progesterone-mediated ↓ in ureter tone and compression by gravid uterus).

Complications include chronic pyelonephritis, renal papillary necrosis, perinephric abscess (with possible posterior spread to adjacent psoas muscle), urosepsis.

Treatment: antibiotics.

**Chronic pyelonephritis**

The result of recurrent or inadequately treated episodes of acute pyelonephritis. Typically requires predisposition to infection such as vesicoureteral reflux or chronically obstructing kidney stones.

Coarse, asymmetric corticomedullary scarring, blunted calyces. Tubules can contain eosinophilic casts resembling thyroid tissue  (thyroidization of kidney).

## Acute kidney injury

|  | Prerenal azotemia | Intrinsic renal failure | Postrenal azotemia |
|---|---|---|---|
| ETIOLOGY | Hypovolemia<br>↓ cardiac output<br>↓ effective circulating volume<br>(eg, HF, liver failure) | Tubules and interstitium:<br>▪ Acute tubular necrosis<br>  (ischemia, nephrotoxins)<br>▪ Acute interstitial nephritis<br>Glomerulus:<br>▪ Acute glomerulonephritis<br>Vascular:<br>▪ Vasculitis<br>▪ Hypertensive emergency<br>▪ TTP-HUS | Stones<br>BPH<br>Neoplasm<br>Congenital anomalies |
| PATHOPHYSIOLOGY | ↓ RBF → ↓ GFR<br>  → ↑ reabsorption of $Na^+/H_2O$<br>  and urea | In ATN, patchy necrosis<br>  → debris obstructing tubules<br>  and fluid backflow → ↓ GFR | Outflow obstruction (bilateral) |
| URINE OSMOLALITY (mOsm/kg) | >500 | <350 | Varies |
| URINE $Na^+$ (mEq/L) | <20 | >40 | Varies |
| $FE_{Na}$ | <1% | >2% | Varies |
| SERUM BUN/Cr | >20 | <15 | Varies |

## Acute interstitial nephritis

Also called tubulointerstitial nephritis. Acute interstitial renal inflammation. Pyuria (classically eosinophils) and azotemia occurring after administration of drugs that act as haptens, inducing hypersensitivity (eg, diuretics, NSAIDs, penicillin derivatives, proton pump inhibitors, rifampin, quinolones, sulfonamides). Less commonly may be 2° to other processes such as systemic infections (eg, *Mycoplasma*) or autoimmune diseases (eg, Sjögren syndrome, SLE, sarcoidosis).

Associated with fever, rash, pyuria, hematuria, and costovertebral angle tenderness, but can be asymptomatic.
Remember the causes of inflammation to your **DRAINS**:
▪ **D**iuretics
▪ **R**ifampin
▪ **A**ntibiotics (penicillins and cephalosporins)
▪ **P**roton pump **I**nhibitors
▪ **N**SAIDs
▪ **S**ulfa drugs

**Acute tubular necrosis**

Most common cause of intrinsic acute kidney injury in hospitalized patients. Spontaneously resolves in many cases. Can be fatal, especially during initial oliguric phase. ↑ $FE_{Na}$.

Key finding: granular casts (often muddy brown in appearance) A.

3 stages:
1. Inciting event
2. Maintenance phase—oliguric; lasts 1–3 weeks; risk of hyperkalemia, metabolic acidosis, uremia
3. Recovery phase—polyuric; BUN and serum creatinine fall; risk of hypokalemia and renal wasting of other electrolytes and minerals

Can be caused by ischemic or nephrotoxic injury:
- Ischemic—2° to ↓ renal blood flow (eg, prerenal azotemia). Results in death of tubular cells that may slough into tubular lumen B (PT and thick ascending limb are highly susceptible to injury).
- Nephrotoxic—2° to injury resulting from toxic substances (eg, aminoglycosides, radiocontrast agents, lead, cisplatin, ethylene glycol, uric acid in tumor lysis syndrome), myoglobinuria (rhabdomyolysis), hemoglobinuria. PTs are particularly susceptible to injury.

**Diffuse cortical necrosis**

Acute generalized cortical infarction of both kidneys. Likely due to a combination of vasospasm and DIC.

Associated with obstetric catastrophes (eg, placental abruption), septic shock.

**Renal papillary necrosis**

Sloughing of necrotic renal papillae A → gross hematuria. May be triggered by recent infection or immune stimulus.

Associated with:
- Sickle cell disease or trait
- Acute pyelonephritis
- Analgesics (eg, NSAIDs)
- Diabetes mellitus

**SAAD papa** with papillary necrosis.

**Consequences of renal failure**

Decline in renal filtration can lead to excess retained nitrogenous waste products and electrolyte disturbances.

Consequences (**MAD HUNGER**):
- Metabolic Acidosis
- Dyslipidemia (especially ↑ triglycerides)
- High potassium
- Uremia
- $Na^+/H_2O$ retention (HF, pulmonary edema, hypertension)
- Growth retardation and developmental delay
- Erythropoietin deficiency (anemia)
- Renal osteodystrophy

2 forms of renal failure: acute (eg, ATN) and chronic (eg, hypertension, diabetes mellitus, congenital anomalies).

Incremental reductions in GFR define the stages of chronic kidney disease.

Normal phosphate levels are maintained during early stages of CKD due to ↑ levels of fibroblast growth factor 23 (FGF23), which promotes renal excretion of phosphate. "FGF23 fights f(ph)osphate."

**Ure**mia—syndrome resulting from high serum urea. Can present with Pericarditis, Encephalopathy (seen with asterixis), Anorexia, Nausea (pronounce "Ure-PEAN" [European]).

| | |
|---|---|
| **Renal osteodystrophy** | Hypocalcemia, hyperphosphatemia, and failure of vitamin D hydroxylation associated with chronic kidney disease → 2° hyperparathyroidism → 3° hyperparathyroidism (if 2° poorly managed). High serum phosphate can bind with $Ca^{2+}$ → tissue deposits → ↓ serum $Ca^{2+}$.<br>↓ 1,25-$(OH)_2D_3$ → ↓ intestinal $Ca^{2+}$ absorption. Causes subperiosteal thinning of bones. |

### Renal cyst disorders

| | |
|---|---|
| **Autosomal dominant polycystic kidney disease**<br> | Numerous cysts in cortex and medulla  causing bilateral enlarged kidneys ultimately destroy kidney parenchyma. Presents with combinations of flank pain, hematuria, hypertension, urinary infection; progressive renal failure in ~ 50% of individuals.<br>Mutation in genes encoding polycystin protein: PKD1 (85% of cases, chromosome 16) or PKD2 (15% of cases, chromosome 4). Complications include chronic kidney disease and hypertension (caused by ↑ renin production). Associated with berry aneurysms, mitral valve prolapse, benign hepatic cysts, diverticulosis.<br>Treatment: If hypertension or proteinuria develops, treat with ACE inhibitors or ARBs. |
| **Autosomal recessive polycystic kidney disease**<br> | Mutation in *PKHD1* encoding fibrocystin. Cystic dilation of collecting ducts B. Often presents in infancy, and may be seen on prenatal ultrasound. Associated with congenital hepatic fibrosis. Significant oliguric renal failure in utero can lead to Potter sequence. Concerns beyond neonatal period include systemic hypertension, progressive renal insufficiency, and portal hypertension from congenital hepatic fibrosis. |
| **Autosomal dominant tubulointerstitial kidney disease** | Also called medullary cystic kidney disease. Causes tubulointerstitial fibrosis and progressive renal insufficiency with inability to concentrate urine. Medullary cysts usually not visualized; smaller kidneys on ultrasound. Poor prognosis. |
| **Simple vs complex renal cysts** | Simple cysts are filled with ultrafiltrate (anechoic on ultrasound). Very common and account for majority of all renal masses. Found incidentally and typically asymptomatic.<br>Complex cysts, including those that are septated, enhanced, or have solid components on imaging require follow-up or removal due to possibility of renal cell carcinoma. |

## Renovascular disease

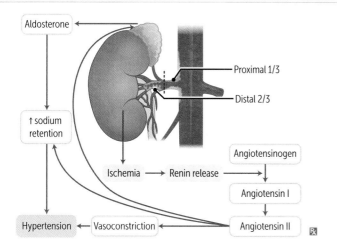

Unilateral or bilateral renal artery stenosis (RAS) → ↓ renal perfusion → ↑ renin → ↑ angiotensin → HTN. Most common cause of 2° HTN in adults.

Main causes of RAS:
- Atherosclerotic plaques: proximal 1/3 of renal artery, usually in older males, smokers.
- Fibromuscular dysplasia: distal 2/3 of renal artery or segmental branches, usually young or middle-aged females

For unilateral RAS, affected kidney can atrophy → asymmetric kidney size. Renal venous sampling will show ↑ renin in affected kidney, ↓ renin in unaffected kidney.

For bilateral RAS, patients can have a sudden rise in creatinine after starting an ACE inhibitor, ARB, or renin inhibitor, due to their interference on RAAS-mediated renal perfusion.

Can present with severe/refractory HTN, flash pulmonary edema, epigastric/flank bruit. Patients with RAS may also have stenosis in other large vessels.

## Renal cell carcinoma

Polygonal clear cells A filled with accumulated lipids and carbohydrate. Often golden-yellow B on gross pathology, due to ↑ lipid content.

Originates from PCT → invades renal vein (may develop varicocele if left sided) → IVC → hematogenous spread → metastasis to lung, bone, and liver.

Manifests with flank pain, palpable mass, hematuria (classic triad) as well as anemia, 2° polycythemia (less common), fever, weight loss.

Treatment: surgery/ablation for localized disease. Immunotherapy (eg, ipilimumab) or targeted therapy for metastatic disease, rarely curative. Resistant to radiation and chemotherapy.

Most common 1° renal malignancy C.

Most common in males 50–70 years old, ↑ incidence with tobacco smoking and obesity.

Associated with paraneoplastic syndromes, eg, PTHrP, Ectopic EPO, ACTH, Renin ("PEAR"-aneoplastic).

Clear cell (most common subtype) associated with gene deletion on chromosome 3 (sporadic, or inherited as von Hippel-Lindau syndrome).

RCC = 3 letters = chromosome 3 = associated with VHL (also 3 letters).

**Renal oncocytoma**

Benign epithelial cell tumor arising from collecting ducts (arrows in  point to well-circumscribed mass with central scar). Large eosinophilic cells with abundant mitochondria without perinuclear clearing  (vs chromophobe renal cell carcinoma). Presents with painless hematuria, flank pain, abdominal mass.

Often resected to exclude malignancy (eg, renal cell carcinoma).

**Nephroblastoma**

Also called Wilms tumor. Most common renal malignancy of early childhood (ages 2–4). Contains embryonic glomerular structures. Most often present with large, palpable, unilateral flank mass 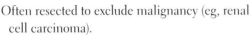 and/or hematuria and possible HTN.

Can be associated with loss-of-function mutations of tumor suppressor genes *WT1* or *WT2* on chromosome 11 (W11ms tumor).

May be a part of several syndromes:

- **WAGR** complex—Wilms tumor, Aniridia (absence of iris), Genitourinary malformations, Range of developmental delays (*WT1* deletion)
- **Denys-D**rash syndrome—Wilms tumor, Diffuse mesangial sclerosis (early-onset nephrotic syndrome), Dysgenesis of gonads (male pseudohermaphroditism), *WT1* mutation
- Beckwith-**W**iedemann syndrome—Wilms tumor, macroglossia, organomegaly, hemihyperplasia (imprinting defect causing genetic overexpression, associated with *WT2* mutation), omphalocele

**Urothelial carcinoma of the bladder**

Also called transitional cell carcinoma. Most common tumor of urinary tract system (can occur in renal calyces, renal pelvis, ureters, and bladder) . Can be suggested by Painless hematuria (no casts).

Associated with problems in your Pee SAC: Tobacco **S**moking, **A**romatic amines (found in dyes), **C**yclophosphamide.

**Squamous cell carcinoma of the bladder**

Chronic irritation of urinary bladder → squamous metaplasia → dysplasia and squamous cell carcinoma.

Risk factors include 4 S's: *Schistosoma haematobium* infection (Middle East), chronic cystitis ("systitis"), smoking, chronic nephrolithiasis (stones). Presents with painless hematuria (no casts).

## ▶ RENAL—PHARMACOLOGY

### Diuretics: site of action

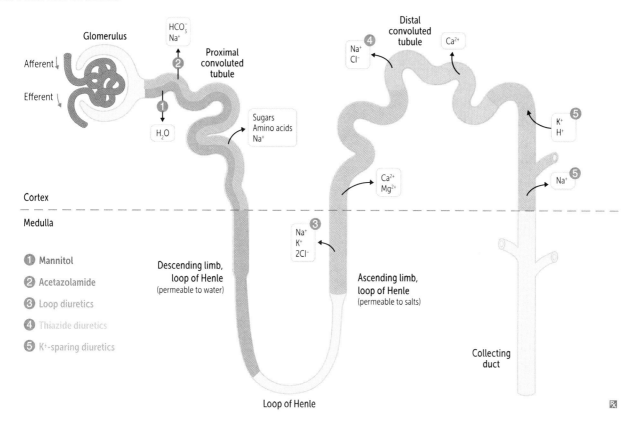

Cortex

Medulla

**1** Mannitol

**2** Acetazolamide

**3** Loop diuretics

**4** Thiazide diuretics

**5** K⁺-sparing diuretics

Glomerulus

Afferent

Efferent

$HCO_3^-$ / $Na^+$ **2**

$H_2O$ **1**

Proximal convoluted tubule

Sugars / Amino acids / $Na^+$

Distal convoluted tubule

$Na^+$ / $Cl^-$ **4**

$Ca^{2+}$

$Ca^{2+}$ / $Mg^{2+}$

$K^+$ / $H^+$ **5**

$Na^+$ **5**

Descending limb, loop of Henle (permeable to water)

$Na^+$ / $K^+$ / $2Cl^-$ **3**

Ascending limb, loop of Henle (permeable to salts)

Collecting duct

Loop of Henle

### Diuretics: effects on electrolyte excretion

| | $Na^+$ | $HCO_3^-$ | $K^+$ | $Cl^-$ | $Ca^{2+}$ | $Mg^{2+}$ | $H^+$ |
|---|---|---|---|---|---|---|---|
| Carbonic anhydrase inhibitors | ↑ | ↑↑ | ↑↑ | –/↑ | – | – | ↓ |
| Loop diuretics | ↑↑ | ↑ | ↑↑ | ↑↑ | ↑↑ | ↑↑ | ↑ |
| Thiazide diuretics | ↑ | ↑ | ↑↑ | ↑ | ↓↓ | –/↑ | ↑ |
| K⁺-sparing diuretics | ↑ | – | ↓ | ↑ | ↓/– | ↓/– | ↓ |

Blood pH ↓ (**acidemia**): carbonic anhydrase inhibitors: ↓ $HCO_3^-$ reabsorption. K⁺ sparing: aldosterone blockade prevents K⁺ secretion and H⁺ secretion. Additionally, hyperkalemia leads to K⁺ entering all cells (via H⁺/K⁺ exchanger) in exchange for H⁺ exiting cells.

↑ (**alkalemia**): loop diuretics and thiazides cause alkalemia through several mechanisms:
  ▪ Volume contraction → ↑ AT II → ↑ $Na^+$/$H^+$ exchange in PCT → ↑ $HCO_3^-$ reabsorption ("contraction alkalosis")
  ▪ K⁺ loss leads to K⁺ exiting all cells (via H⁺/K⁺ exchanger) in exchange for H⁺ entering cells
  ▪ In low K⁺ state, H⁺ (rather than K⁺) is exchanged for $Na^+$ in cortical collecting tubule → alkalosis and "paradoxical aciduria"

## Mannitol

| | |
|---|---|
| MECHANISM | Osmotic diuretic. ↑ serum osmolality → fluid shift from interstitium to intravascular space → ↑ urine flow, ↓ intracranial/intraocular pressure. |
| CLINICAL USE | Drug overdose, elevated intracranial/intraocular pressure. |
| ADVERSE EFFECTS | Dehydration, hypo- or hypernatremia, pulmonary edema. Contraindicated in anuria, HF. |

## Acetazolamide

| | | |
|---|---|---|
| MECHANISM | Carbonic anhydrase inhibitor. Causes self-limited $NaHCO_3$ diuresis and ↓ total body $HCO_3^-$ stores. Alkalinizes urine. | |
| CLINICAL USE | Glaucoma, metabolic alkalosis, altitude sickness (by offsetting respiratory alkalosis), idiopathic intracranial hypertension (pseudotumor cerebri). | |
| ADVERSE EFFECTS | Proximal renal tubular acidosis (type 2 RTA), paresthesias, $NH_3$ toxicity, sulfa allergy, hypokalemia. Promotes calcium phosphate stones (insoluble at high urine pH). | "Acid"azolamide causes acidosis. |

## Loop diuretics

### Furosemide, bumetanide, torsemide

| | | |
|---|---|---|
| MECHANISM | Sulfonamide loop diuretics. Inhibit cotransport system ($Na^+/K^+/2Cl^-$) of thick ascending limb of loop of Henle. Abolish hypertonicity of medulla, preventing concentration of urine. Associated with ↑ PGE (vasodilatory effect on afferent arteriole); inhibited by NSAIDs. ↑ $Ca^{2+}$ excretion. Loops lose $Ca^{2+}$. | |
| CLINICAL USE | Edematous states (HF, cirrhosis, nephrotic syndrome, pulmonary edema), hypertension, hypercalcemia. | |
| ADVERSE EFFECTS | Ototoxicity, Hypokalemia, Hypomagnesemia, Dehydration, Allergy (sulfa), metabolic Alkalosis, Nephritis (interstitial), Gout. | OHH DAANG! |

### Ethacrynic acid

| | | |
|---|---|---|
| MECHANISM | Nonsulfonamide inhibitor of cotransport system ($Na^+/K^+/2Cl^-$) of thick ascending limb of loop of Henle. | |
| CLINICAL USE | Diuresis in patients allergic to sulfa drugs. | |
| ADVERSE EFFECTS | Similar to furosemide, but more ototoxic. | Loop earrings hurt your ears. |

| **Thiazide diuretics** | Hydrochlorothiazide, chlorthalidone, metolazone. | |
|---|---|---|
| MECHANISM | Inhibit NaCl reabsorption in early DCT → ↓ diluting capacity of nephron. ↓ Ca$^{2+}$ excretion. | |
| CLINICAL USE | Hypertension, HF, idiopathic hypercalciuria, nephrogenic diabetes insipidus, osteoporosis. | |
| ADVERSE EFFECTS | Hypokalemic metabolic alkalosis, hyponatremia, hyperglycemia, hyperlipidemia, hyperuricemia, hypercalcemia. Sulfa allergy. | Hypergluc. |

| **Potassium-sparing diuretics** | Spironolactone, Eplerenone, Amiloride, Triamterene. | Keep your SEAT. |
|---|---|---|
| MECHANISM | Spironolactone and eplerenone are competitive aldosterone receptor antagonists in cortical collecting tubule. Triamterene and amiloride block Na$^+$ channels at the same part of the tubule. | |
| CLINICAL USE | Hyperaldosteronism, HF, hepatic ascites (spironolactone), nephrogenic DI (amiloride), antiandrogen (spironolactone). | |
| ADVERSE EFFECTS | Hyperkalemia (can lead to arrhythmias), endocrine effects with spironolactone (eg, gynecomastia, antiandrogen effects), metabolic acidosis. | |

| **Angiotensin-converting enzyme inhibitors** | Captopril, enalapril, lisinopril, ramipril. | |
| --- | --- | --- |
| MECHANISM | Inhibit ACE → ↓ AT II → ↓ GFR by preventing constriction of efferent arterioles. ↑ renin due to loss of negative feedback. Inhibition of ACE also prevents inactivation of bradykinin, a potent vasodilator. | |
| CLINICAL USE | Hypertension, HF (↓ mortality), proteinuria, diabetic nephropathy. Prevent unfavorable heart remodeling as a result of chronic hypertension. | In chronic kidney disease (eg, diabetic nephropathy), ↓ intraglomerular pressure, slowing GBM thickening. |
| ADVERSE EFFECTS | Cough, Angioedema (both due to ↑ bradykinin; contraindicated in C1 esterase inhibitor deficiency), Teratogen (fetal renal malformations), ↑ Creatinine (↓ GFR), Hyperkalemia, and Hypotension. Used with caution in bilateral renal artery stenosis because ACE inhibitors will further ↓ GFR → renal failure. | Captopril's CATCHH. |

| **Angiotensin II receptor blockers** | Losartan, candesartan, valsartan. |
| --- | --- |
| MECHANISM | Selectively block binding of angiotensin II to $AT_1$ receptor. Effects similar to ACE inhibitors, but ARBs do not increase bradykinin. |
| CLINICAL USE | Hypertension, HF, proteinuria, or chronic kidney disease (eg, diabetic nephropathy) with intolerance to ACE inhibitors (eg, cough, angioedema). |
| ADVERSE EFFECTS | Hyperkalemia, ↓ GFR, hypotension; teratogen. |

| **Aliskiren** | |
| --- | --- |
| MECHANISM | Direct renin inhibitor, blocks conversion of angiotensinogen to angiotensin I. Aliskiren kills renin. |
| CLINICAL USE | Hypertension. |
| ADVERSE EFFECTS | Hyperkalemia, ↓ GFR, hypotension, angioedema. Relatively contraindicated in patients already taking ACE inhibitors or ARBs and contraindicated in pregnancy. |

# Reproductive

*"Life is always a rich and steady time when you are waiting for something to happen or to hatch."*

—E.B. White, *Charlotte's Web*

*"Love is only a dirty trick played on us to achieve continuation of the species."*

—W. Somerset Maugham

*"I liked that in obstetrics you end up with twice the number of patients you started with."*

—Adam Kay

*"Life is a sexually transmitted disease and the mortality rate is one hundred percent."*

—R.D. Laing

Organizing the reproductive system by key concepts such as embryology, endocrinology, pregnancy, and oncology can help with understanding this complex topic. Study the endocrine and reproductive chapters together, because mastery of the hypothalamic-pituitary-gonadal axis is key to answering questions on ovulation, menstruation, disorders of sexual development, contraception, and many pathologies.

Embryology is a nuanced subject that spans multiple organ systems. Approach it from a clinical perspective. For instance, make the connection between the presentation of DiGeorge syndrome and the 3rd/4th pharyngeal pouch, and between the Müllerian/Wolffian systems and disorders of sexual development.

As for oncology, don't worry about remembering screening or treatment guidelines. It is more important to recognize the clinical presentation (eg, signs and symptoms) of reproductive cancers and their associated labs, histopathology, and risk factors. In addition, some of the testicular and ovarian cancers have distinct patterns of hCG, AFP, LH, or FSH derangements that serve as helpful clues in exam questions.

### Early embryonic development

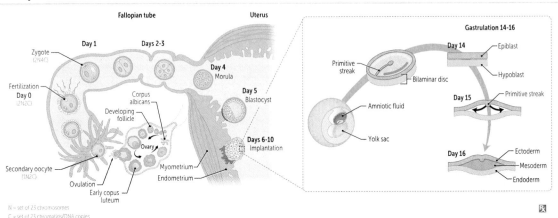

| Week 1 | hCG secretion begins around the time of blastocyst implantation. Blastocyst "sticks" on day six. |
|---|---|
| Week 2 | Formation of **bi**laminar embryonic disc; **two** layers = epiblast, hypoblast. |
| Week 3 | Formation of **tri**laminar embryonic disc via gastrulation (epiblast cell invagination through primitive streak); **three** layers = endoderm, mesoderm, ectoderm.<br>Notochord arises from midline mesoderm and induces overlying ectoderm (via SHH) to become neural plate, which gives rise to neural tube via neurulation. |
| Week 4 | Heart begins to beat (**four** chambers). Cardiac activity visible by transvaginal ultrasound.<br>Upper and lower limb buds begin to form (**four** limbs). |
| Week 8 | Genitalia have male/female characteristics (pronounce "gen**eight**alia"). |

## Embryologic derivatives

| Ectoderm | | External/outer layer |
|---|---|---|
| Surface ectoderm | Epidermis; adenohypophysis (from Rathke pouch); lens of eye; epithelial linings of oral cavity, sensory organs of ear, and olfactory epithelium; anal canal below the pectinate line; parotid, sweat, mammary glands. | Craniopharyngioma—benign Rathke pouch tumor with cholesterol crystals, calcifications. |
| Neural tube | Brain (neurohypophysis, CNS neurons, oligo-dendrocytes, astrocytes, ependymal cells, pineal gland), retina, spinal cord. | Neuroectoderm—think CNS. |
| Neural crest | Enterochromaffin cells, Melanocytes, Odontoblasts, PNS ganglia (cranial, dorsal root, autonomic), Adrenal medulla, Schwann cells, Spiral membrane (aorticopulmonary septum), Endocardial cushions (also derived partially from mesoderm), Skull bones. | **EMO PASSES** Neural crest—think PNS and non-neural structures nearby. |
| **Mesoderm** | Muscle, bone, connective tissue, serous linings of body cavities (eg, peritoneum, pericardium, pleura), spleen (develops within foregut mesentery), cardiovascular structures, lymphatics, blood, wall of gut tube, proximal vagina, kidneys, adrenal cortex, dermis, testes, ovaries, microglia, tracheal cartilage. Notochord induces ectoderm to form neuroectoderm (neural plate); its only postnatal derivative is the nucleus pulposus of the intervertebral disc. | Middle/"meat" layer. Mesodermal defects = VACTERL association: Vertebral defects Anal atresia Cardiac defects Tracheo-Esophageal fistula Renal defects Limb defects (bone and muscle) |
| **Endoderm** | Gut tube epithelium (including anal canal above the pectinate line), most of urethra and distal vagina (derived from urogenital sinus), luminal epithelial derivatives (eg, lungs, liver, gallbladder, pancreas, eustachian tube, thymus, parathyroid, thyroid follicular and parafollicular [C] cells). | "Enternal" layer. |

| **Teratogens** | Most susceptible during organogenesis in embryonic period (before week 8 of development). Before implantation, "all-or-none" effect. After week 8 (fetal period), growth and function affected. |
|---|---|

| TERATOGEN | EFFECT ON FETUS |
|---|---|
| **Medications** | |
| **ACE inhibitors** | Renal failure, oligohydramnios, hypocalvaria. |
| **Alkylating agents** | Multiple anomalies (eg, ear/facial abnormalities, absence of digits). |
| **Aminoglycosides** | Ototoxicity. "**A** mean **g**uy hit the baby in the ear." |
| **Antiepileptic drugs** | Neural tube defects, cardiac defects, cleft palate, skeletal abnormalities (eg, phalanx/nail hypoplasia, facial dysmorphism). Most commonly due to valproate, carbamazepine, phenytoin, phenobarbital; high-dose folate supplementation recommended. |
| **Diethylstilbestrol** | Vaginal clear cell adenocarcinoma, congenital Müllerian anomalies. |
| **Fluoroquinolones** | Cartilage damage. |
| **Folate antagonists** | Neural tube defects. Most commonly due to trimethoprim, methotrexate. |
| **Isotretinoin** | Craniofacial (eg, microtia, dysmorphism), CNS, cardiac, and thymic defects. Contraception mandatory. Pronounce "isoteratinoin" for its **ter**atogenicity. |
| **Lithium** | Ebstein anomaly. |
| **Methimazole** | Aplasia cutis congenita (congenital absence of skin, typically on scalp). |
| **Tetracyclines** | Discolored **teeth**, inhibited bone growth. Pronounce "**teeth**racyclines." |
| **Thalidomide** | **Limb** defects (eg, phocomelia—flipperlike limbs). Pronounce "tha**limb**domide." |
| **Warfarin** | Bone and cartilage deformities (stippled epiphyses, nasal and limb hypoplasia), optic nerve atrophy, cerebral hemorrhage. Use heparin during pregnancy (does not cross placenta). |
| **Substance use** | |
| **Alcohol** | Fetal alcohol syndrome. |
| **Cocaine** | Preterm birth, low birth weight, fetal growth restriction (FGR). Cocaine → vasoconstriction. |
| **Tobacco smoking** | Preterm birth, low birth weight (leading cause in resource-rich countries), FGR, sudden infant death syndrome (SIDS), ADHD. Nicotine → vasoconstriction, CO → impaired $O_2$ delivery. |
| **Other** | |
| **Iodine lack or excess** | Congenital hypothyroidism. |
| **Maternal diabetes** | Caudal regression syndrome, cardiac defects (eg, transposition of great arteries, VSD), neural tube defects, macrosomia, neonatal hypoglycemia (due to islet cell hyperplasia), polycythemia, respiratory distress syndrome. |
| **Maternal PKU** | Fetal growth restriction, microcephaly, intellectual disability, congenital heart defects. |
| **Methylmercury** | Neurotoxicity. ↑ concentration in top-predator fish (eg, shark, swordfish, king mackerel, tilefish). |
| **X-rays** | Microcephaly, intellectual disability. Effects minimized by use of lead shielding. |

## Types of errors in morphogenesis

| | |
|---|---|
| Agenesis | Absent organ due to absent primordial tissue. |
| Aplasia | Absent organ despite presence of primordial tissue. |
| Hypoplasia | Incomplete organ development; primordial tissue present. |
| Disruption | 2° breakdown of tissue with normal developmental potential (eg, amniotic band syndrome). |
| Deformation | Extrinsic mechanical distortion (eg, congenital torticollis); occurs during fetal period. |
| Malformation | Intrinsic developmental defect (eg, cleft lip/palate); occurs during embryonic period. |
| Sequence | Abnormalities result from a single 1° embryologic event (eg, oligohydramnios → Potter sequence). |
| Field defect | Disturbance of tissues that develop in a contiguous physical space (eg, holoprosencephaly). |

| | | |
|---|---|---|
| **Fetal alcohol syndrome** | One of the leading preventable causes of intellectual disability in the US. 2° to maternal alcohol use during pregnancy. Newborns may present with developmental delay, microcephaly, facial abnormalities (eg, smooth philtrum, thin vermillion border, small palpebral fissures, flat nasal bridge), limb dislocation, heart defects. Holoprosencephaly may occur in more severe presentations. One mechanism is due to impaired migration of neuronal and glial cells. | 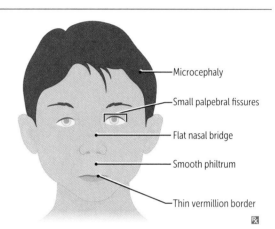 |

Microcephaly
Small palpebral fissures
Flat nasal bridge
Smooth philtrum
Thin vermillion border

| | |
|---|---|
| **Neonatal abstinence syndrome** | Complex disorder involving CNS, ANS, and GI systems. 2° to maternal substance use (most commonly opioids) during pregnancy. Newborns may present with uncoordinated sucking reflexes, irritability, high-pitched crying, tremors, tachypnea, sneezing, diarrhea, and possibly seizures.<br>Treatment (for opioid use): methadone, morphine, buprenorphine.<br>Universal screening for substance use is recommended in all pregnant patients. |

| **Placenta** | 1° site of nutrient and gas exchange between mother and fetus. |
| --- | --- |
| Fetal component | |
| **Cytotrophoblast** | Inner layer of chorionic villi; creates cells. |
| **Syncytiotrophoblast** | Outer layer of chorionic villi; synthesizes and secretes hormones, eg, hCG (structurally similar to LH; stimulates corpus luteum to secrete progesterone during first trimester). Lacks MHC I expression → ↓ chance of attack by maternal immune system. |
| Maternal component | |
| **Decidua basalis** | Derived from endometrium. Maternal blood in lacunae. |

## Amniotic fluid

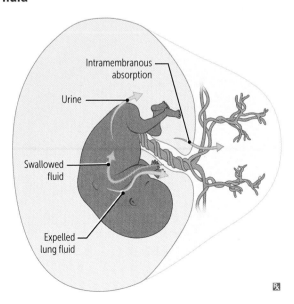

Derived from fetal urine (mainly) and fetal lung liquid.

Cleared by fetal swallowing (mainly) and intramembranous absorption.

**Polyhydramnios**—too much amniotic fluid. May be idiopathic or associated with fetal malformations (eg, esophageal/duodenal atresia, anencephaly; both result in inability to swallow amniotic fluid), maternal diabetes, fetal anemia, multifetal gestation.

**Oligohydramnios**—too little amniotic fluid. Associated with placental insufficiency, bilateral renal agenesis, posterior urethral valves (in males); these result in inability to excrete urine. Profound oligohydramnios can cause Potter sequence.

| **Twinning** | Dizygotic ("fraternal") twins arise from 2 eggs that are separately fertilized by 2 different sperm (always 2 zygotes) and will have 2 separate amniotic sacs and 2 separate placentas (chorions). Monozygotic ("identical") twins arise from 1 fertilized egg (1 egg + 1 sperm) that splits in early pregnancy. The timing of splitting determines chorionicity (number of chorions) and amnionicity (number of amnions) (take **separate** cars or **share** a **CAB**):<br>▪ Splitting 0–4 days: **separate** chorion and amnion (di-di)<br>▪ Splitting 4–8 days: **shared** Chorion (mo-di)<br>▪ Splitting 8–12 days: **shared** chorion and Amnion (mo-mo)<br>▪ Splitting 13+ days: **shared** chorion, amnion, and Body (mo-mo; conjoined) |
|---|---|

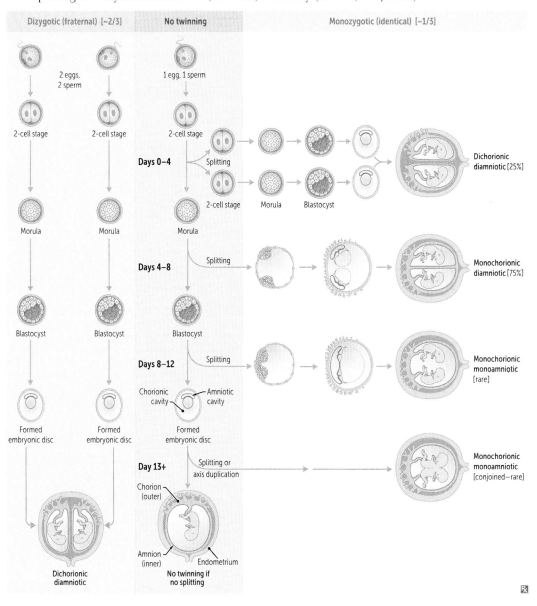

| **Twin-twin transfusion syndrome** | Occurs in monochorionic twin gestations. Unbalanced arteriovenous anastomoses between twins in shared placenta → net blood flow from one twin to the other.<br>Donor twin → hypovolemia and oligohydramnios ("stuck twin" appearance).<br>Recipient twin → hypervolemia and polyhydramnios. |
|---|---|

| | | |
|---|---|---|
| **Umbilical cord** | Two umbilical arteries return deoxygenated blood from fetal internal iliac arteries to placenta. One umbilical vein supplies oxygenated blood from placenta to fetus; drains into IVC via liver or via ductus venosus. | Single umbilical artery (2-vessel cord) is associated with congenital and chromosomal anomalies. Umbilical arteries and vein are derived from allantois. |

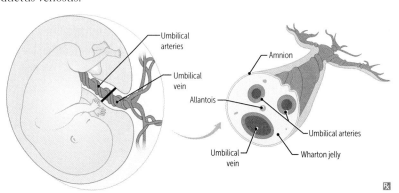

| | |
|---|---|
| **Urachus** | Allantois forms from yolk sac and extends into cloaca. Intra-abdominal remnant of allantois is called the urachus, a duct between fetal bladder and umbilicus. Failure of urachus to involute can lead to anomalies that may increase risk of infection and/or malignancy (eg, adenocarcinoma) if not treated. Obliterated urachus is represented by the median umbilical ligament after birth, which is covered by median umbilical fold of the peritoneum. |
| Patent urachus | Total failure of urachus to obliterate → urine discharge from umbilicus. |
| Urachal cyst | Partial failure of urachus to obliterate; fluid-filled cavity lined with uroepithelium, between umbilicus and bladder. Cyst can become infected and present as painful mass below umbilicus. |
| Vesicourachal diverticulum | Slight failure of urachus to obliterate → outpouching of bladder. |

Normal    Patent urachus    Urachal cyst    Vesicourachal diverticulum

| | |
|---|---|
| **Vitelline duct** | Also called omphalomesenteric duct. Connects yolk sac to midgut lumen. Obliterates during week 7 of development. |
| Patent vitelline duct | Total failure of vitelline duct to obliterate → meconium discharge from umbilicus. |
| Vitelline duct cyst | Partial failure of vitelline duct to obliterate. ↑ risk for volvulus. |
| Meckel diverticulum | Slight failure of vitelline duct to obliterate → outpouching of ileum (true diverticulum, arrow in ). Usually asymptomatic. May have heterotopic gastric and/or pancreatic tissue → melena, hematochezia, abdominal pain. |

Normal    Patent vitelline duct    Vitelline duct cyst    Meckel diverticulum

| | | |
|---|---|---|
| **Pharyngeal apparatus** | Composed of pharyngeal (branchial) clefts, arches, pouches.<br>Pharyngeal clefts—derived from ectoderm. Also called pharyngeal grooves.<br>Pharyngeal arches—derived from mesoderm (muscles, arteries) and neural crest (bones, cartilage).<br>Pharyngeal pouches—derived from endoderm. | CAP covers outside to inside:<br>  Clefts = ectoderm<br>  Arches = mesoderm + neural crest<br>  Pouches = endoderm<br> |

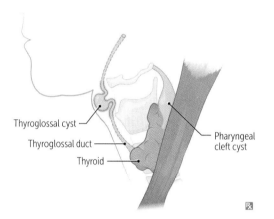

| | | |
|---|---|---|
| **Pharyngeal cleft derivatives** | 1st cleft develops into external auditory meatus. 2nd through 4th clefts form temporary cervical sinuses, which are obliterated by proliferation of 2nd arch mesenchyme.<br><br>**Pharyngeal cleft cyst**—persistent cervical sinus; presents as lateral neck mass anterior to sternocleidomastoid muscle that does not move with swallowing (vs thyroglossal duct cyst). | |

**Pharyngeal pouch derivatives**

Ear, tonsils, bottom-to-top: 1 (ear), 2 (**tonsils**), 3 dorsal (**bottom = inferior** parathyroids), 3 ventral (**to = thymus**), 4 (**top = superior** parathyroids).

| POUCH | DERIVATIVES | NOTES |
|---|---|---|
| **1st pharyngeal pouch** | Middle ear cavity, eustachian tube, mastoid air cells | 1st pouch contributes to endoderm-lined structures of ear |
| **2nd pharyngeal pouch** | Epithelial lining of palatine tonsil | |
| **3rd pharyngeal pouch** | Dorsal wings → **inferior** parathyroids<br>Ventral wings → thymus | Third pouch contributes to **thymus** and both inferior parathyroids.<br>Structures from 3rd pouch end up **below** those from 4th pouch |
| **4th pharyngeal pouch** | Dorsal wings → **superior** parathyroids<br>Ventral wings → ultimopharyngeal body<br>  → parafollicular (C) cells of thyroid | 4th pharyngeal pouch forms para"4"llicular cells |

**Pharyngeal arch derivatives**    When at the restaurant of the golden **arches**, children tend to first **chew** (1), then **smile** (2), then **swallow stylishly** (3) or **simply swallow** (4), and then **speak** (6).

| ARCH | NERVES[a] | MUSCLES | CARTILAGE | NOTES |
|---|---|---|---|---|
| **1st pharyngeal arch** | CN V$_3$ **chew** | Muscles of mastication (temporalis, masseter, lateral and medial pterygoids), mylohyoid, anterior belly of digastric, tensor tympani, anterior 2/3 of tongue, tensor veli palatini | Maxillary process → maxilla, zygomatic bone<br>Mandibular process → meckel cartilage → mandible, malleus and incus, sphenomandibular ligament | Pierre Robin sequence—micrognathia, glossoptosis, cleft palate, airway obstruction<br>Treacher Collins syndrome—autosomal dominant neural crest dysfunction → craniofacial abnormalities (eg, zygomatic bone and mandibular hypoplasia), hearing loss, airway compromise |
| **2nd pharyngeal arch** | CN VII (seven) **smile** (facial expression) | Muscles of facial expression, stapedius, stylohyoid, platysma, posterior belly of digastric | Reichert cartilage: stapes, styloid process, lesser horn of hyoid, stylohyoid ligament | |
| **3rd pharyngeal arch** | CN IX **swallow stylishly** | Stylopharyngeus | Greater horn of hyoid | |
| **4th and 6th pharyngeal arches** | 4th arch: CN X (superior laryngeal branch) **simply swallow**<br>6th arch: CN X (recurrent/ inferior laryngeal branch) **speak** | 4th arch: most pharyngeal constrictors; cricothyroid, levator veli palatini<br>6th arch: all intrinsic muscles of larynx except cricothyroid | Arytenoids, Cricoid, Corniculate, Cuneiform, Thyroid (used to sing and **ACCCT**) | Arches 3 and 4 form posterior 1/3 of tongue<br>Arch 5 makes no major developmental contributions |

[a]Sensory and motor nerves are not pharyngeal arch derivatives. They grow into the arches and are derived from neural crest (sensory) and neuroectoderm (motor).

| **Orofacial clefts** | Cleft lip and cleft palate have distinct, multifactorial etiologies, but often occur together. | |
| --- | --- | --- |
| Cleft lip | Due to failure of fusion of the intermaxillary segment (merged medial nasal processes) with the maxillary process (formation of 1° palate). | |
| Cleft palate | Due to failure of fusion of the two lateral palatine shelves or failure of fusion of lateral palatine shelf with the nasal septum and/or 1° palate (formation of 2° palate). | |

**Genital embryology**

| Female | Default development. Mesonephric duct degenerates and paramesonephric duct develops. | |
| --- | --- | --- |
| Male | *SRY* gene on Y chromosome—produces testis-determining factor → testes development. Sertoli cells secrete Müllerian-inhibiting substance (MIS, also called anti-Müllerian hormone) that suppresses development of paramesonephric ducts. Leydig cells secrete androgens that stimulate development of mesonephric ducts. | |
| Paramesonephric (Müllerian) duct | Develops into female internal structures—fallopian tubes, uterus, proximal vagina (distal vagina from urogenital sinus). Male remnant is appendix testis. Müllerian agenesis (Mayer-Rokitansky-Küster-Hauser syndrome)—1° amenorrhea with absent uterus, blind vaginal pouch, normal female external genitalia and 2° sexual characteristics (functional ovaries). Associated with urinary tract anomalies (eg, renal agenesis). | |
| Mesonephric (Wolffian) duct | Develops into male internal structures (except prostate)—Seminal vesicles, Epididymis, Ejaculatory duct, Ductus deferens (SEED). Female remnant is Gartner duct. | |

## Sexual differentiation

Absence of Sertoli cells or lack of Müllerian-inhibiting substance → develop both male and female internal genitalia and male external genitalia (streak gonads)

5α-reductase deficiency—inability to convert testosterone into DHT → male internal genitalia, atypical external genitalia until puberty (when ↑ testosterone levels cause masculinization)

In the testes:

Leydig leads to male (internal and external) sexual differentiation.

Sertoli shuts down female (internal) sexual differentiation.

| | |
|---|---|
| **Uterine (Müllerian duct) anomalies** | ↓ fertility and ↑ risk of complicated pregnancy (eg, spontaneous abortion, prematurity, FGR, malpresentation). Hysterosalpigogram of normal uterus demonstrates normal uterine cavity and intraperitoneal spill of contrast (indicative of patent fallopian tubes). |
| **Septate uterus** | Incomplete resorption of septum **A**. Common anomaly. Treat with septoplasty. |
| **Bicornuate uterus** | Incomplete fusion of Müllerian ducts **B**. |
| **Uterus didelphys** | Complete failure of fusion → double uterus, cervix, vagina. |

Normal

Septate

Bicornuate

Didelphys

## Male/female genital homologs

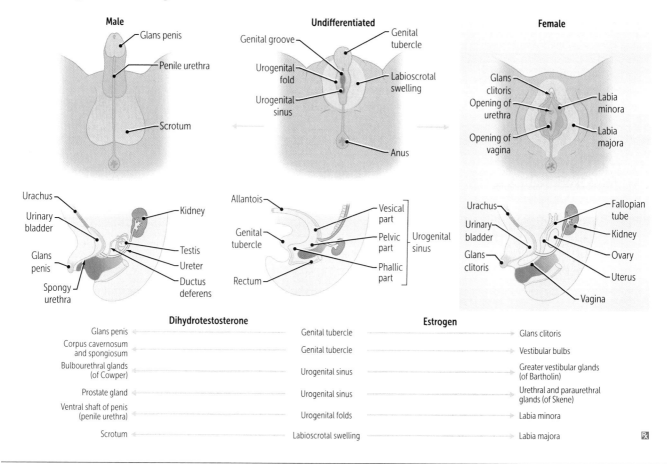

| Dihydrotestosterone | | Estrogen | |
| --- | --- | --- | --- |
| Glans penis | Genital tubercle | | Glans clitoris |
| Corpus cavernosum and spongiosum | Genital tubercle | | Vestibular bulbs |
| Bulbourethral glands (of Cowper) | Urogenital sinus | | Greater vestibular glands (of Bartholin) |
| Prostate gland | Urogenital sinus | | Urethral and paraurethral glands (of Skene) |
| Ventral shaft of penis (penile urethra) | Urogenital folds | | Labia minora |
| Scrotum | Labioscrotal swelling | | Labia majora |

## Congenital penile abnormalities

| Hypospadias | | |
| --- | --- | --- |
|  | Abnormal opening of penile urethra on ventral (under) surface due to failure of urethral folds to fuse. | Hypospadias is more common than epispadias. Associated with inguinal hernia, cryptorchidism, chordee (downward or upward bending of penis). Can be seen in 5α-reductase deficiency. |
| **Epispadias** | | |
|  | Abnormal opening of penile urethra on dorsal (top) surface due to faulty positioning of genital tubercle. | Exstrophy of the bladder is associated with epispadias. |

## Descent of testes and ovaries

|  | DESCRIPTION | MALE REMNANT | FEMALE REMNANT |
| --- | --- | --- | --- |
| Gubernaculum | Band of fibrous tissue | Anchors testes within scrotum | Ovarian ligament + round ligament of uterus |
| Processus vaginalis | Evagination of peritoneum | Forms tunica vaginalis<br>Persistent patent processus vaginalis → hydrocele | Obliterated |

## ▶ REPRODUCTIVE—ANATOMY

### Drainage of reproductive organs

| Venous drainage | Right ovary/testis → right gonadal vein → IVC.<br>Left ovary/testis → left gonadal vein → left renal vein → IVC (takes the longer way).<br>Left testicular vein enters left renal vein at 90° angle → flow is less laminar on the left than on the right → left venous pressure > right venous pressure → varicocele is more common on the left. |
| --- | --- |

### Lymphatic drainage

**PARA-AORTIC**
- ♀ Ovaries, fallopian tubes, uterine fundus
- ♂ Testes

**EXTERNAL ILIAC**
- Superior part of bladder
- ♀ Body of uterus, cervix

**INTERNAL ILIAC**
- Inferior part of bladder
- ♀ Cervix, proximal vagina
- ♂ Prostate, corpus cavernosum

**SUPERFICIAL INGUINAL**
- Distal anal canal
- ♀ Distal vagina, vulva
- ♂ Scrotum

**DEEP INGUINAL**
- ♀ Glans clitoris
- ♂ Glans penis

Fallopian tube
Uterus
Ovary
Bladder
Vagina
Glans clitoris
Vulva
Anus

Inferior vena cava
Left renal vein
Gonadal vein
Bladder
Prostate
Pampiniform plexus
Scrotum
Testis
Corpus cavernosum
Glans penis
Anus

## Female reproductive anatomy

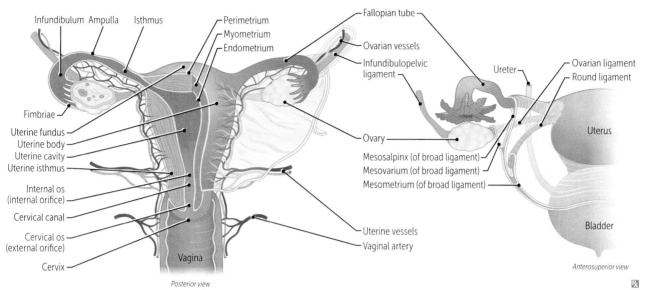

Infundibulum  Ampulla  Isthmus

Perimetrium
Myometrium
Endometrium

Fimbriae

Uterine fundus
Uterine body
Uterine cavity
Uterine isthmus

Internal os
(internal orifice)

Cervical canal

Cervical os
(external orifice)

Cervix

Vagina

*Posterior view*

Fallopian tube

Ovarian vessels

Infundibulopelvic
ligament

Ovary

Mesosalpinx (of broad ligament)
Mesovarium (of broad ligament)
Mesometrium (of broad ligament)

Uterine vessels
Vaginal artery

Ureter

Ovarian ligament
Round ligament

Uterus

Bladder

*Anterosuperior view*

| LIGAMENT | CONNECTS | STRUCTURES CONTAINED | NOTES |
|---|---|---|---|
| **Infundibulopelvic ligament** | Ovary to lateral pelvic wall | Ovarian vessels | Also called suspensory ligament of ovary<br>Ovarian vessel ligation during oophorectomy risks damaging the ureter |
| **Ovarian ligament** | Ovary to uterine horn | | Derivative of gubernaculum |
| **Round ligament** | Uterine horn to labia majora | | Travels through inguinal canal<br>Derivative of gubernaculum |
| **Broad ligament** | Uterus to lateral pelvic wall | Ovary, fallopian tube, round ligament | Fold of peritoneum comprising the mesometrium, mesovarium, and mesosalpinx |
| **Cardinal ligament** | Cervix to lateral pelvic wall | Uterine vessels | Condensation at the base of broad ligament<br>Uterine vessel ligation during hysterectomy risks damaging the ureter |
| **Uterosacral ligament** | Cervix to sacrum | | |

## Adnexal torsion

Torsion

Twisting of ovary and fallopian tube around infundibulopelvic ligament and ovarian ligament → compression of ovarian vessels in infundibulopelvic ligament → blockage of lymphatic and venous outflow. Continued arterial perfusion → ovarian edema → complete blockage of arterial inflow → necrosis, local hemorrhage. Associated with ovarian masses/cysts. Presents with acute pelvic pain, adnexal mass, nausea/vomiting. Surgical emergency.

## Pelvic organ prolapse

Herniation of pelvic organs to or beyond the vaginal walls (anterior, posterior) or apex. Associated with multiparity, ↑ age, obesity. Presents with pelvic pressure, bulging sensation or tissue protrusion from vagina, urinary frequency, constipation, sexual dysfunction.
- Anterior compartment prolapse—bladder (cystocele). Most common type.
- Posterior compartment prolapse—rectum (rectocele) or small bowel (enterocele).
- Apical compartment prolapse—uterus, cervix, or vaginal vault.

Uterine procidentia—herniation involving all 3 compartments.

**Female reproductive epithelial histology**

| TISSUE | HISTOLOGY/NOTES |
|---|---|
| Vulva | Stratified squamous epithelium |
| Vagina | Stratified squamous epithelium, nonkeratinized |
| Ectocervix | Stratified squamous epithelium, nonkeratinized |
| Transformation zone | Squamocolumnar junction (most common area for cervical cancer; sampled in Pap test) |
| Endocervix | Simple columnar epithelium |
| Uterus | Simple columnar epithelium with long tubular glands in proliferative phase; coiled glands in secretory phase |
| Fallopian tube | Simple columnar epithelium, ciliated |
| Ovary, outer surface | Simple cuboidal epithelium (germinal epithelium covering surface of ovary) |

## Male reproductive anatomy

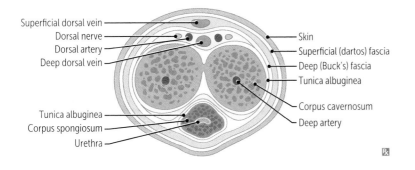

Pathway of sperm during ejaculation—
SEVEN UP:
Seminiferous tubules
Epididymis
Vas deferens
Ejaculatory ducts
(Nothing)
Urethra
Penis

| | |
|---|---|
| **Genitourinary trauma** | Most commonly due to blunt trauma (eg, motor vehicle collision). |
| **Renal injury** | Presents with bruises, flank pain, hematuria. Caused by direct blows or lower rib fractures. |
| **Bladder injury** | Presents with hematuria, suprapubic pain, difficulty voiding.<br>▪ Superior bladder wall (dome) injury—direct trauma to full bladder (eg, seatbelt) → abrupt ↑ intravesical pressure → dome rupture (weakest part) → intraperitoneal urine accumulation. Peritoneal absorption of urine → ↑ BUN, ↑ creatinine.<br>▪ Anterior bladder wall or neck injury—pelvic fracture → perforation by bony spicules → extraperitoneal urine accumulation (retropubic space). |
| **Urethral injury** | Occurs almost exclusively in males. Presents with blood at urethral meatus, hematuria, difficulty voiding. Urethral catheterization is relatively contraindicated.<br>▪ Anterior urethral injury—perineal straddle injury → disruption of bulbar (spongy) urethra → scrotal hematoma. If Buck fascia is torn, urine escapes into perineal space.<br>▪ Posterior urethral injury—pelvic fracture → disruption at bulbomembranous junction (weakest part) → urine leakage into retropubic space and high-riding prostate. |

Anterior urethral injury

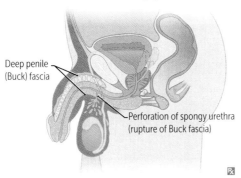

Deep penile (Buck) fascia

Perforation of spongy urethra (rupture of Buck fascia)

Posterior urethral injury

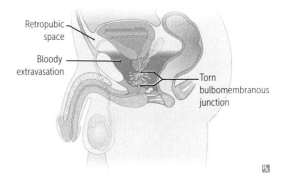

Retropubic space

Bloody extravasation

Torn bulbomembranous junction

| | | |
|---|---|---|
| **Autonomic innervation of male sexual response** | Erection—parasympathetic nervous system (pelvic splanchnic nerves, S2-S4):<br>▪ NO → ↑ cGMP → smooth muscle relaxation → vasodilation → proerectile.<br>▪ Norepinephrine → ↑ $[Ca^{2+}]_{in}$ → smooth muscle contraction → vasoconstriction → antierectile.<br>Emission—sympathetic nervous system (hypogastric nerve, T11-L2).<br>Expulsion—visceral and somatic nerves (pudendal nerve). | Point, squeeze, and shoot.<br>S2, 3, 4 keep the penis off the floor.<br>PDE-5 inhibitors (eg, sildenafil) → ↓ cGMP breakdown. |

## Seminiferous tubules

| CELL | FUNCTION | LOCATION/NOTES |
|---|---|---|
| Spermatogonia | Maintain germ cell pool and produce 1° spermatocytes | Line seminiferous tubules 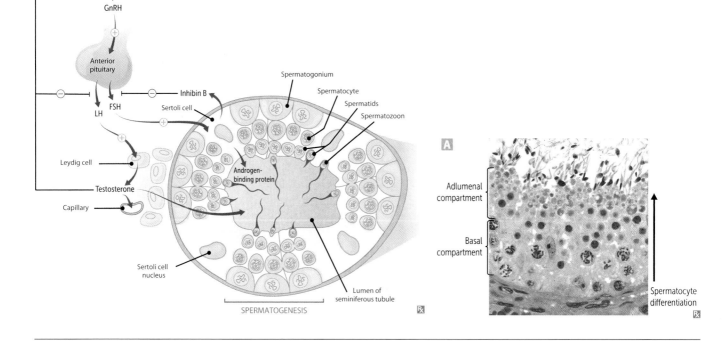 Germ cells |
| Sertoli cells | Secrete inhibin B → inhibit FSH<br>Secrete androgen-binding protein → maintain local levels of testosterone<br>Produce MIF<br>Tight junctions between adjacent Sertoli cells form blood-testis barrier → isolate gametes from autoimmune attack<br>Support and nourish developing spermatozoa<br>Regulate spermatogenesis<br>Temperature sensitive; ↓ sperm production and ↓ inhibin B with ↑ temperature | Line seminiferous tubules<br>Non–germ cells<br>Convert testosterone and androstenedione to estrogens via aromatase<br>Sertoli cells are temperature sensitive, line seminiferous tubules, support sperm synthesis, and inhibit FSH<br>Homolog of female granulosa cells<br>↑ temperature seen in varicocele, cryptorchidism |
| Leydig cells | Secrete testosterone in the presence of LH; testosterone production unaffected by temperature | Interstitium<br>Endocrine cells<br>Homolog of female theca interna cells |

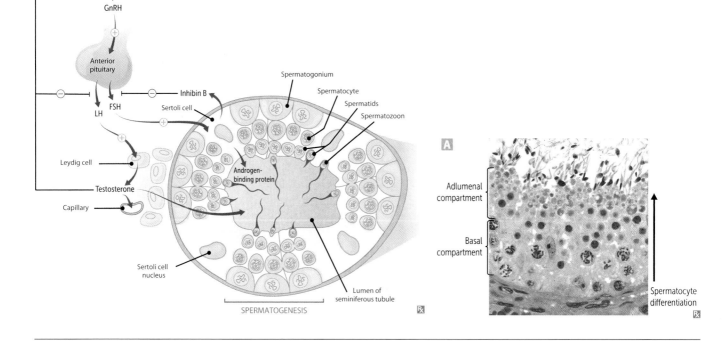

## ▶ REPRODUCTIVE—PHYSIOLOGY

**Spermatogenesis**

Begins at puberty with spermatogonia. Full development takes 2 months. Occurs in seminiferous tubules. Produces spermatids that undergo spermiogenesis (loss of cytoplasmic contents, gain of acrosomal cap) to form mature spermatozoa.

"Gonium" is going to be a sperm; "zoon" is "zooming" to egg.

Tail mobility impaired in ciliary dyskinesia/ Kartagener syndrome → infertility.

Tail mobility normal in cystic fibrosis (in CF, absent vas deferens → infertility).

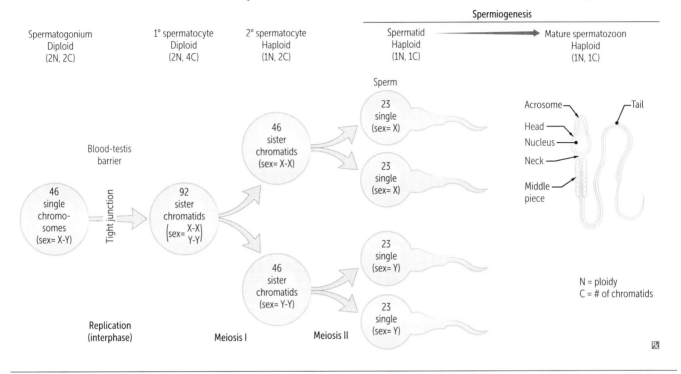

## Estrogen

| | | |
|---|---|---|
| SOURCE | Ovary (estradiol), placenta (estriol), adipose tissue (estrone via aromatization). | Potency: estradiol > estrone > estriol. Estradiol is produced from 2 ovaries. |
| FUNCTION | Development of internal/external genitalia, breasts, female fat distribution. Growth of follicle, endometrial proliferation, ↑ myometrial excitability. Upregulation of estrogen, LH, and progesterone receptors; feedback inhibition of FSH and LH, then LH surge; stimulation of prolactin secretion, ↓ prolactin action on breasts. ↑ transport proteins, SHBG; ↑ HDL; ↓ LDL. | Pregnancy: <br> ▪ 50-fold ↑ in estradiol and estrone <br> ▪ 1000-fold ↑ in estriol (indicator of fetal well-being) <br> Estrogen receptors expressed in cytoplasm; translocate to nucleus when bound by estrogen. |

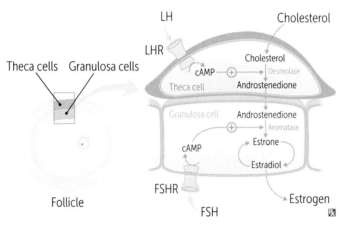

## Progesterone

| | | |
|---|---|---|
| SOURCE | Corpus luteum, placenta, adrenal cortex, testes. | Fall in estrogen and progesterone after delivery disinhibits prolactin → lactation. ↑ progesterone is indicative of ovulation. Progesterone is **pro-gestation**. Prolactin is **pro-lactation**. |
| FUNCTION | During luteal phase, prepares uterus for implantation of fertilized egg: <br> ▪ Stimulation of endometrial glandular secretions and spiral artery development <br> ▪ Production of thick cervical mucus → inhibits sperm entry into uterus <br> ▪ Prevention of endometrial hyperplasia <br> ▪ ↑ body temperature <br> ▪ ↓ estrogen receptor expression <br> ▪ ↓ gonadotropin (LH, FSH) secretion <br> During pregnancy: <br> ▪ Maintenance of endometrial lining and pregnancy <br> ▪ ↓ myometrial excitability → ↓ contraction frequency and intensity <br> ▪ ↓ prolactin action on breasts | |

**Oogenesis**

1° oocytes begin meiosis I during fetal life and complete meiosis I just prior to ovulation. Meiosis I is arrested in prophase I (one) for years until ovulation (1° oocytes). Meiosis II is arrested in metaphase II (two) until fertilization (2° oocytes). If fertilization does not occur within 1 day, the 2° oocyte degenerates.

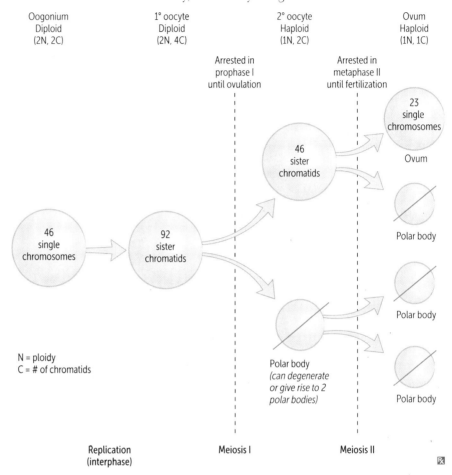

**Ovulation**

Follicular rupture and 2° oocyte release. Caused by sudden LH release (LH surge) at midcycle. Estrogen normally inhibits LH release, but high estrogen at midcycle transiently stimulates LH release → LH surge → ovulation.

**Mittel**schmerz ("middle hurts")—pain with ovulation. Associated with peritoneal irritation from normal bleeding upon follicular rupture. Typically unilateral and mild, but can mimic acute appendicitis.

| Menstrual cycle | Regular cyclic changes periodically preparing the female reproductive system for fertilization and pregnancy. Occurs in phases based on events taking place in ovaries and uterus. | |
| --- | --- | --- |
| | 1ST DAY OF MENSES TO OVULATION | OVULATION TO 1ST DAY OF NEXT MENSES |
| Ovarian cycle | Follicular phase—follicular development; late stages are stimulated by FSH; can fluctuate in length. | Luteal phase—corpus luteum formation from follicular remnants; stimulated by LH; lasts a fixed 14 days. |
| Uterine cycle | Proliferative phase—endometrial development; stimulated by estrogen. Straight, narrow endometrial glands. | Secretory phase—endometrial preparation for implantation; stimulated by progesterone. Tortuous, dilated endometrial glands. |

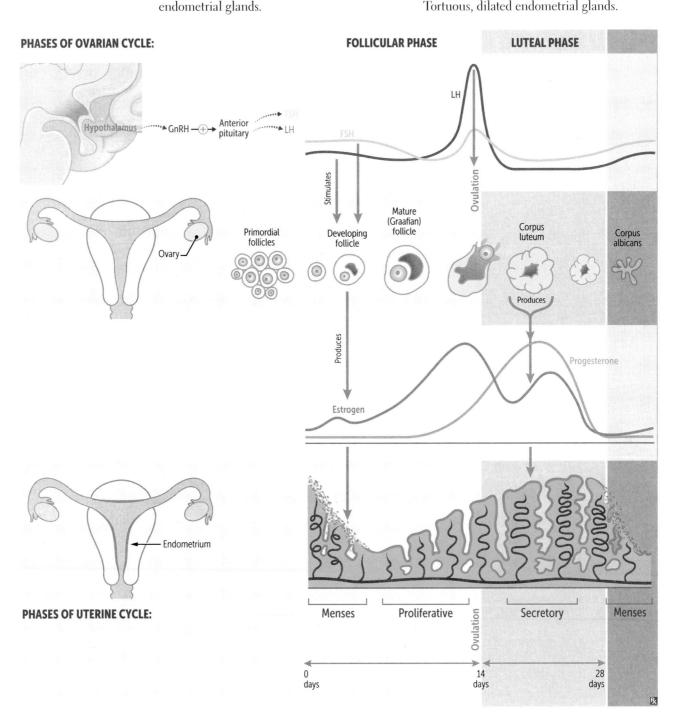

PHASES OF OVARIAN CYCLE:

FOLLICULAR PHASE  LUTEAL PHASE

Hypothalamus ······▸ GnRH ─⊕─▸ Anterior pituitary ······▸ FSH
······▸ LH

LH

FSH

Stimulates

Ovulation

Ovary

Primordial follicles

Developing follicle

Mature (Graafian) follicle

Corpus luteum

Corpus albicans

Produces

Produces

Estrogen

Progesterone

Endometrium

PHASES OF UTERINE CYCLE:

Menses  Proliferative  Ovulation  Secretory  Menses

0 days  14 days  28 days

| Abnormal uterine bleeding | Deviation from normal menstruation volume, duration, frequency, regularity, or intermenstrual bleeding.<br>Causes (**PALM-COEIN**):<br>  ▪ Structural: **P**olyp, **A**denomyosis, **L**eiomyoma, **M**alignancy/hyperplasia<br>  ▪ Nonstructural: **C**oagulopathy, **O**vulatory, **E**ndometrial, **I**atrogenic, **N**ot yet classified | Terms such as dysfunctional uterine bleeding, menorrhagia, metrorrhagia, polymenorrhea, and oligomenorrhea are no longer recommended. |
|---|---|---|
| Pregnancy | Fertilization (conception) most commonly occurs in upper end of fallopian tube (the ampulla). Occurs within 1 day of ovulation.<br>Implantation in the uterine wall occurs 6 days after fertilization. Syncytiotrophoblasts secrete hCG, which is detectable in blood 1 week after fertilization and on home urine tests 2 weeks after fertilization.<br>Embryonic/developmental age—time since fertilization. Used in embryology.<br>Gestational age—time since first day of last menstrual period. Used clinically.<br>Gravidity ("gravida")—number of pregnancies.<br>Parity ("para")—number of pregnancies that resulted in live births. | Placental hormone secretion generally increases over the course of pregnancy, but hCG peaks at 8–10 weeks of gestation.<br> |

## Physiologic changes in pregnancy

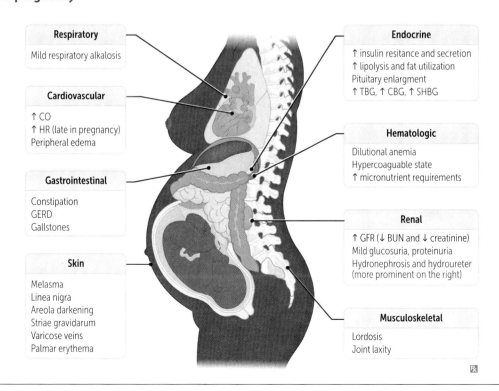

**Respiratory**
Mild respiratory alkalosis

**Cardiovascular**
↑ CO
↑ HR (late in pregnancy)
Peripheral edema

**Gastrointestinal**
Constipation
GERD
Gallstones

**Skin**
Melasma
Linea nigra
Areola darkening
Striae gravidarum
Varicose veins
Palmar erythema

**Endocrine**
↑ insulin resitance and secretion
↑ lipolysis and fat utilization
Pituitary enlargment
↑ TBG, ↑ CBG, ↑ SHBG

**Hematologic**
Dilutional anemia
Hypercoaguable state
↑ micronutrient requirements

**Renal**
↑ GFR (↓ BUN and ↓ creatinine)
Mild glucosuria, proteinuria
Hydronephrosis and hydroureter (more prominent on the right)

**Musculoskeletal**
Lordosis
Joint laxity

## Human chorionic gonadotropin

| | |
|---|---|
| SOURCE | Syncytiotrophoblast of placenta. |
| FUNCTION | Maintains corpus luteum (and thus progesterone) for first 8–10 weeks of gestation by acting like LH (otherwise no luteal cell stimulation → abortion). Luteal-placental shift is complete after 8–10 weeks; placenta synthesizes its own estriol and progesterone and corpus luteum degenerates. Used to detect pregnancy because it appears early in urine (see above). |
| | Has identical α subunit as LH, FSH, TSH. β subunit is unique (detected by pregnancy tests) but structurally similar to that of TSH (states of ↑ hCG can cause hyperthyroidism). hCG is ↑ in multifetal gestation, hydatidiform moles, choriocarcinomas, and Down syndrome; hCG is ↓ in ectopic/failing pregnancy, Edwards syndrome, and Patau syndrome. |

## Human placental lactogen

Also called human chorionic somatomammotropin.

| | |
|---|---|
| SOURCE | Syncytiotrophoblast of placenta. |
| FUNCTION | Promotes insulin resistance to supply growing fetus with glucose and amino acids. Concurrently stimulates insulin secretion; inability to overcome insulin resistance → gestational diabetes. |

## Apgar score

| | Score 2 | Score 1 | Score 0 |
|---|---|---|---|
| **A**ppearance | Pink | Extremities blue | Pale or blue |
| **P**ulse | ≥ 100 bpm | < 100 bpm | No pulse |
| **G**rimace | Cries and pulls away | Grimaces or weak cry | No response to stimulation |
| **A**ctivity | Active movement | Arms, legs flexed | No movement |
| **R**espiration | Strong cry | Slow, irregular | No breathing |

Assessment of newborn vital signs following delivery via a 10-point scale evaluated at 1 minute and 5 minutes. **Apgar** score is based on **appearance**, **pulse**, **grimace**, **activity**, and **respiration**. Apgar scores < 7 may require further evaluation. If Apgar score remains low at later time points, there is ↑ risk the child will develop long-term neurologic damage.

## Neonatal birth weight

| | Low birth weight | High birth weight (macrosomia) |
|---|---|---|
| DEFINITION | Birth weight < 2500 g | Birth weight > 4000 g |
| RISK FACTORS | Prematurity, FGR | Fetal: constitutional/genetic<br>Maternal: obesity, diabetes mellitus |
| COMPLICATIONS | ↑ mortality (SIDS), ↑ morbidity | ↑ risk of maternal or fetal trauma (eg, shoulder dystocia) |

| | |
|---|---|
| **Lactation** | After parturition and delivery of placenta, rapid ↓ in estrogen and progesterone disinhibits prolactin → initiation of lactation. Suckling is required to maintain milk production and ejection, since ↑ nerve stimulation → ↑ oxytocin and prolactin.<br><br>Prolactin—induces and maintains lactation and ↓ reproductive function.<br>Oxytocin—assists in milk letdown; also promotes uterine contractions.<br>Breast milk is the ideal nutrition for infants < 6 months old. Contains immunoglobulins (conferring passive immunity; mostly IgA), macrophages, lymphocytes. Breast milk reduces infant infections and is associated with ↓ risk for child to develop asthma, allergies, diabetes mellitus, and obesity. Exclusively breastfed infants should get vitamin D +/– iron supplementation.<br>Breastfeeding ↓ maternal risk of breast and ovarian cancer and facilitates mother-child bonding. |

| | | |
|---|---|---|
| **Menopause** | Diagnosed by amenorrhea for 12 months. ↓ estrogen production due to age-linked decline in number of ovarian follicles. Average age at onset is 51 years (earlier in people who smoke tobacco).<br>Usually preceded by 4–5 years of abnormal menstrual cycles. Source of estrogen (estrone) after menopause becomes peripheral conversion of androgens, ↑ androgens → hirsutism.<br>↑↑ FSH is specific for menopause (loss of negative feedback on FSH due to ↓ estrogen). | Hormonal changes: ↓ estrogen, ↑↑ FSH, ↑ LH (no surge), ↑ GnRH.<br>Causes **HAVOCS**: Hot flashes (most common), Atrophy of the Vagina, Osteoporosis (↑ osteoclast activity), Coronary artery disease, Sleep disturbances.<br>Hormone replacement therapy is used to ameliorate menopausal symptoms. Estrogen-only treatment is associated with ↑ risk of endometrial cancer (progesterone is added).<br>Menopause before age 40 suggests 1° ovarian insufficiency (premature ovarian failure); may occur in females who have received chemotherapy and/or radiation therapy. |

| | | |
|---|---|---|
| **Androgens** | Testosterone, dihydrotestosterone (DHT), androstenedione. | |
| SOURCE | DHT and testosterone (testis), androstenedione (adrenal) | Potency: DHT > testosterone > androstenedione. |
| FUNCTION | Testosterone:<br>  ▪ Differentiation of epididymis, vas deferens, seminal vesicles (internal genitalia, except prostate)<br>  ▪ Growth spurt: penis, seminal vesicles, sperm, muscle, RBCs<br>  ▪ Deepening of voice<br>  ▪ Closing of epiphyseal plates (via estrogen converted from testosterone)<br>  ▪ Libido<br>DHT:<br>  ▪ Early—differentiation of penis, scrotum, prostate<br>  ▪ Late—prostate growth, balding, sebaceous gland activity | Testosterone is converted to DHT by 5α-reductase, which is inhibited by finasteride.<br>In the male, androgens are converted to estrogens by aromatase (primarily in adipose tissue and testes).<br><br>Anabolic-androgenic steroid use—↑ fat-free mass, muscle strength, performance. Suspect in males who present with changes in behavior (eg, aggression), acne, gynecomastia, erythrocytosis (↑ risk of thromboembolism), small testes (exogenous testosterone → hypothalamic-pituitary-gonadal axis inhibition → ↓ intratesticular testosterone → ↓ testicular size, ↓ sperm count, azoospermia). Females may present with virilization (eg, hirsutism, acne, breast atrophy, male pattern baldness). |

**Tanner stages of sexual development**

Tanner stage is assigned independently to genitalia, pubic hair, and breast (eg, a person can have Tanner stage 2 genitalia, Tanner stage 3 pubic hair). Earliest detectable secondary sexual characteristic is breast bud development in females, testicular enlargement in males.

| Stage I | Stage II | Stage III | Stage IV | Stage V |
|---|---|---|---|---|
| No sexual hair ♂ ♀ Flat-appearing chest with raised nipple ♀ | Pubic hair appears ♂ ♀ (pubarche) Testicular enlargement ♂ Breast bud forms (thelarche), mound forms ♀ | Coarsening of pubic hair ♂ ♀ Penis size/length ↑ ♂ Breast enlarges ♀ | Coarse hair across pubis, sparing thigh ♂ ♀ Penis width/glans ↑ ♂ Breast enlarges, raised areola, mound on mound ♀ | Coarse hair across pubis and medial thigh ♂ ♀ Penis and testis enlarge to adult size ♂ Adult breast contour, areola flattens ♀ |
| Pre-pubertal | ~ 8–11.5 years | ~ 11.5–13 years | ~ 13–15 years | Usually > 15 years |

**Precocious puberty**

Appearance of 2° sexual characteristics (eg, pubarche, thelarche) before age 8 years in females and 9 years in males. ↑ sex hormone exposure or production → ↑ linear growth, somatic and skeletal maturation (eg, premature closure of epiphyseal plates → short stature). Types include:
- Central precocious puberty (↑ GnRH secretion): idiopathic (most common; early activation of hypothalamic-pituitary gonadal axis), CNS tumors.
- Peripheral precocious puberty (GnRH-independent; ↑ sex hormone production or exposure to exogenous sex steroids): congenital adrenal hyperplasia, estrogen-secreting ovarian tumor (eg, granulosa cell tumor), Leydig cell tumor, McCune-Albright syndrome.

**Delayed puberty**

Absence of 2° sexual characteristics by age 13 years in females and 14 years in males. Causes:
- Hypergonadotropic (1°) hypogonadism: Klinefelter syndrome, Turner syndrome, gonadal injury (eg, chemotherapy, radiotherapy, infection).
- Hypogonadotropic (2°) hypogonadism: constitutional delay of growth and puberty ("late blooming"), Kallmann syndrome, CNS lesions.

## ▶ REPRODUCTIVE—PATHOLOGY

| | | |
|---|---|---|
| **Sex chromosome disorders** | Aneuploidy most commonly due to meiotic nondisjunction. | |
| **Klinefelter syndrome**<br> | Male, 47,XXY.<br>Small, firm testes; infertility (azoospermia); tall stature with eunuchoid proportions (delayed epiphyseal closure → ↑ long bone length); gynecomastia **A**; female hair distribution. May present with developmental delay. Presence of inactivated X chromosome (Barr body). Common cause of hypogonadism seen in infertility workup. ↑ risk of breast cancer. | Dysgenesis of seminiferous tubules → ↓ inhibin B → ↑ FSH.<br>Abnormal Leydig cell function → ↓ testosterone → ↑ LH. |
| **Turner syndrome**<br> | Female, 45,XO.<br>Short stature (preventable with GH therapy), ovarian dysgenesis (streak ovary), broad chest with widely spaced nipples, bicuspid aortic valve, coarctation of the aorta (femoral < brachial pulse), lymphatic defects (result in webbed neck **B** or cystic hygroma; lymphedema in feet, hands), horseshoe kidney, high-arched palate, shortened 4th metacarpals. Most common cause of 1° amenorrhea. No Barr body. | Menopause before menarche.<br>↓ estrogen leads to ↑ LH, FSH.<br>Sex chromosome (X, or rarely Y) loss often due to nondisjunction during meiosis or mitosis.<br>Meiosis errors usually occur in paternal gametes → sperm missing the sex chromosome.<br>Mitosis errors occur after zygote formation → loss of sex chromosome in some but not all cells → mosaic karyotype (eg. 45,X/46,XX).<br>(45,X/46,XY) mosaicism associated with increased risk for gonadoblastoma.<br>Pregnancy is possible in some cases (IVF, exogenous estradiol-17β and progesterone). |
| **Double Y males** | 47,XYY.<br>Phenotypically normal (usually undiagnosed), very tall. Normal fertility. May be associated with severe acne, learning disability, autism spectrum disorders. | |

| | |
|---|---|
| **Other disorders of sex development** | Formerly called intersex states. Discrepancy between phenotypic sex (external genitalia, influenced by hormonal levels) and gonadal sex (testes vs ovaries, corresponds with Y chromosome). |
| **46,XX DSD** | Ovaries present, but external genitalia are virilized or atypical. Most commonly due to congenital adrenal hyperplasia (excessive exposure to androgens early in development). |
| **46,XY DSD** | Testes present, but external genitalia are feminized or atypical. Most commonly due to androgen insensitivity syndrome (defect in androgen receptor). |
| **Ovotesticular DSD** | 46,XX > 46,XY. Both ovarian and testicular tissue present (ovotestis); atypical genitalia. |

| **Diagnosing disorders by sex hormones** | Testosterone | LH | Diagnosis |
|---|---|---|---|
| | ↑ | ↑ | Androgen insensitivity syndrome |
| | ↑ | ↓ | Testosterone-secreting tumor, exogenous androgenic steroids |
| | ↓ | ↑ | Hypergonadotropic (1°) hypogonadism |
| | ↓ | ↓ | Hypogonadotropic (2°) hypogonadism |

| **Diagnosing disorders by physical characteristics** | Uterus | Breasts | Diagnosis |
|---|---|---|---|
| | ⊕ | ⊖ | Hypergonadotropic (1°) hypogonadism in genotypic female <br> Hypogonadotropic (2°) hypogonadism in genotypic female |
| | ⊖ | ⊕ | Müllerian agenesis in genotypic female <br> Androgen insensitivity syndrome in genotypic male |

| **Aromatase deficiency** | Inability to synthesize endogenous estrogens. Autosomal recessive. During fetal life, DHEA produced by fetal adrenal glands cannot be converted to estrogen by the placenta and is converted to testosterone peripherally → virilization of both female infant (atypical genitalia) and mother (acne, hirsutism; fetal androgens can cross placenta). |
|---|---|

| **Androgen insensitivity syndrome** | Defect in androgen receptor resulting in female-appearing genetic male (46,XY DSD); breast development and female external genitalia with scant axillary and pubic hair, rudimentary vagina; uterus and fallopian tubes absent due to persistence of anti-Müllerian hormone from testes. Patients develop normal functioning testes (often found in labia majora; surgically removed to prevent malignancy). ↑ testosterone, estrogen, LH (vs sex chromosome disorders). |
|---|---|

| **5α-reductase deficiency** | Autosomal recessive; sex limited to genetic males (46,XY DSD). Inability to convert testosterone to DHT. Atypical genitalia until puberty, when ↑ testosterone causes masculinization/↑ growth of external genitalia. Testosterone/estrogen levels are normal; LH is normal or ↑. Internal genitalia are normal. |
|---|---|

| **Kallmann syndrome** | Failure to complete puberty; a form of hypogonadotropic hypogonadism. Defective migration of neurons and subsequent failure of olfactory bulbs to develop → ↓ synthesis of GnRH in the hypothalamus; hyposmia/anosmia; ↓ GnRH, FSH, LH, testosterone. Infertility (low sperm count in males; amenorrhea in females). |
|---|---|

## Placental disorders

### Placenta accreta spectrum

Abnormal invasion of trophoblastic tissue into uterine wall 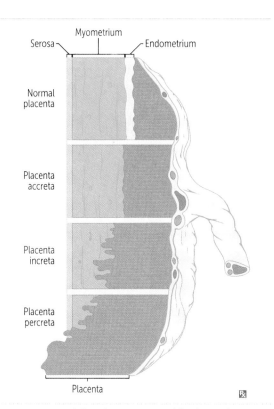. Risk factors: prior C-section or other uterine surgery (areas of uterine scarring impair normal decidualization), placenta previa, ↑ maternal age, multiparity. Three types depending on depth of trophoblast invasion:

- Placenta accreta—attaches to myometrium (instead of overlying decidua basalis) without invading it. Most common type.
- Placenta increta—partially invades into myometrium.
- Placenta percreta—completely invades ("**perforates**") through myometrium and serosa, sometimes extending into adjacent organs (eg, bladder → hematuria).

Presents with difficulty separating placenta from uterus after fetal delivery and severe postpartum hemorrhage upon attempted manual removal of placenta (often extracted in pieces). Treatment: hysterectomy.

### Placenta previa

Attachment of placenta over internal cervical os (a "**preview**" of the placenta is visible through cervix). Risk factors: prior C-section, multiparity.

Presents with painless vaginal bleeding in third trimester.

Low-lying placenta—located < 2 cm from, but not covering, the internal cervical os.

### Vasa previa

Fetal vessels run over, or < 2 cm from, the internal cervical os. Risk factors: velamentous insertion of umbilical cord (inserts in chorioamniotic membrane rather than placenta → fetal vessels travel to placenta unprotected by Wharton jelly), bilobed or succenturiate placenta.

Presents with painless vaginal bleeding (fetal blood from injured vessels) upon rupture of membranes accompanied by fetal heart rate abnormalities (eg, bradycardia). May lead to fetal death from exsanguination.

### Placental abruption

Also called abruptio placentae. Premature separation of placenta from uterus prior to fetal delivery. Risk factors: maternal hypertension, preeclampsia, smoking, cocaine use, abdominal trauma.

Presents with abrupt, painful vaginal bleeding in third trimester; can lead to maternal hypovolemic shock (due to hemorrhage) and DIC (due to release of tissue factor from injured placenta), fetal distress (eg, hypoxia). May be life threatening for both mother and fetus.

Normal placenta

Placenta previa

Vasa previa

Placental abruption

**Uterine rupture**

Full-thickness disruption of uterine wall. Risk factors: prior C-section (usually occurs during labor in a subsequent pregnancy), abdominal trauma.

Presents with painful vaginal bleeding, fetal heart rate abnormalities (eg, bradycardia), easily palpable fetal parts, loss of fetal station. May be life threatening for both mother and fetus.

---

**Postpartum hemorrhage**

Greater-than-expected blood loss after delivery. Leading cause of maternal mortality worldwide.

Etiology (4 T's): Tone (uterine atony → soft, boggy uterus; most common), Trauma (eg, lacerations, incisions, uterine rupture), Tissue (retained products of conception), Thrombin (coagulopathy).

Treatment: uterine massage, oxytocin. If refractory, surgical ligation of uterine or internal iliac arteries (fertility is preserved since ovarian arteries provide collateral circulation).

---

**Ectopic pregnancy**

Implantation of fertilized ovum in a site other than the uterus, most often in ampulla of fallopian tube . Risk factors: tubal pathologies (eg, scarring from salpingitis [PID] or surgery), previous ectopic pregnancy, IUD, IVF.

Presents with first-trimester bleeding and/ or lower abdominal pain. Often clinically mistaken for appendicitis. Suspect in patients with history of amenorrhea, lower-than-expected rise in hCG based on dates. Confirm with ultrasound, which may show extraovarian adnexal mass.

Treatment: methotrexate, surgery.

## Hydatidiform mole

Cystic swelling of chorionic villi and proliferation of chorionic epithelium (only trophoblast). Presents with vaginal bleeding, emesis, uterine enlargement more than expected, pelvic pressure/ pain. Associated with hCG-mediated sequelae: hyperthyroidism, theca lutein cysts, hyperemesis gravidarum, early preeclampsia (before 20 weeks of gestation).
Treatment: dilation and curettage +/– methotrexate. Monitor hCG.

|  | Complete mole | Partial mole |
|---|---|---|
| KARYOTYPE | 46,XX (most common); 46,XY | 69,XXX; 69,XXY; 69,XYY |
| COMPONENTS | Most commonly enucleated egg + single sperm (subsequently duplicates paternal DNA) | 2 sperm + 1 egg |
| HISTOLOGY | Hydropic villi, circumferential and diffuse trophoblastic proliferation | Only some villi are hydropic, focal/minimal trophoblastic proliferation |
| FETAL PARTS | No | Yes (partial = fetal parts) |
| STAINING FOR P57 PROTEIN | ⊖ (paternally imprinted) | ⊕ (maternally expressed) Partial mole is P57 positive |
| UTERINE SIZE | ↑ | — |
| hCG | ↑↑↑↑ | ↑ |
| IMAGING | "Honeycombed" uterus or "clusters of grapes" A, "snowstorm" B on ultrasound | Fetal parts |
| RISK OF INVASIVE MOLE | 15–20% | < 5% |
| RISK OF CHORIOCARCINOMA | 2% | Rare |

**Choriocarcinoma**

Rare malignancy of trophoblastic tissue  (cytotrophoblasts, syncytiotrophoblasts), without chorionic villi present. Most commonly occurs after an abnormal pregnancy (eg, hydatidiform mole, abortion); can occur nongestationally in gonads.

Presents with abnormal uterine bleeding, hCG-mediated sequelae, dyspnea, hemoptysis. Hematogenous spread to lungs → "cannonball" metastases .

Treatment: methotrexate.

## Hypertension in pregnancy

| | |
|---|---|
| **Gestational hypertension** | BP > 140/90 mm Hg after 20 weeks of gestation. No preexisting hypertension. No proteinuria or end-organ damage. Hypertension prior to 20 weeks of gestation suggests chronic hypertension. Treatment: antihypertensives (Hydralazine, α-methyldopa, labetalol, nifedipine), deliver at 37–39 weeks. Hypertensive moms love nifedipine. |
| **Preeclampsia** | New-onset hypertension with either proteinuria or end-organ dysfunction after 20 weeks of gestation (onset of preeclampsia < 20 weeks of gestation may suggest molar pregnancy). Caused by abnormal placental spiral arteries → endothelial dysfunction, vasoconstriction, ischemia. Risk factors: history of preeclampsia, multifetal gestation, nulliparity, chronic hypertension, diabetes, chronic kidney disease, autoimmune disorders (eg, antiphospholipid syndrome), obesity. Complications: placental abruption, coagulopathy, renal failure, pulmonary edema, uteroplacental insufficiency; may lead to eclampsia and/or HELLP syndrome. Treatment: antihypertensives, IV magnesium sulfate (to prevent seizure); definitive is delivery. Prophylaxis: aspirin. |
| **Eclampsia** | Preeclampsia with seizures. Death due to stroke, intracranial hemorrhage, ARDS. Treatment: IV magnesium sulfate, antihypertensives, immediate delivery. |
| **HELLP syndrome** | Preeclampsia with thrombotic microangiopathy of the liver. Hemolysis, Elevated Liver enzymes, Low Platelets. May occur in the absence of hypertension and proteinuria. Blood smear shows schistocytes. Can lead to hepatic subcapsular hematomas (rupture → severe hypotension) and DIC (due to release of tissue factor from injured placenta). Treatment: immediate delivery. |

| **Supine hypotensive syndrome** | Also called aortocaval compression syndrome. Seen at > 20 weeks of gestation. Supine position → compression of abdominal aorta and IVC by gravid uterus → ↓ placental perfusion (can lead to pregnancy loss) and ↓ venous return (hypotension). Relieved by left lateral decubitus position. | |
|---|---|---|
| **Gynecologic tumor epidemiology** | Incidence (US)—endometrial > ovarian > cervical; cervical cancer is more common worldwide due to lack of screening or HPV vaccination.<br>Prognosis: Cervical (best prognosis, diagnosed < 45 years old) > Endometrial (middle-aged, about 55 years old) > Ovarian (worst prognosis, > 65 years). | CEOs often go from best to worst as they get older. |

### Vulvar pathology

**Non-neoplastic**

| **Bartholin cyst and abscess** | Due to blockage of Bartholin gland duct causing accumulation of gland fluid. May lead to abscess 2° to obstruction and inflammation . Usually in reproductive-age females. |
|---|---|
| **Lichen sclerosus** | Chronic, progressive inflammatory disease characterized by porcelain-white plaques  that can be hemorrhagic, eroded, or ulcerated. May extend to anus producing figure-eight appearance. ↑ incidence in prepubertal and peri-/postmenopausal females. Presents with intense pruritus, dyspareunia, dysuria, dyschezia. Benign, but slightly ↑ risk for SCC. |
| **Lichen simplex chronicus** | Hyperplasia of vulvar squamous epithelium. Presents with leathery, thick vulvar skin with enhanced skin markings due to chronic rubbing or scratching. Benign, no risk of SCC. |

**Neoplastic**

| **Vulvar carcinoma** | Carcinoma from squamous epithelial lining of vulva . Usually seen in postmenopausal females. Presents with leukoplakia, biopsy often required to distinguish carcinoma from other causes.<br>HPV-related vulvar carcinoma—associated with high-risk HPV types 16, 18.<br>Non-HPV vulvar carcinoma—usually from long-standing lichen sclerosus. |
|---|---|
| **Extramammary Paget disease** | Intraepithelial adenocarcinoma. Carcinoma in situ, low risk of underlying carcinoma (vs Paget disease of the breast, which is always associated with underlying carcinoma). Presents with pruritus, erythema, crusting, ulcers . |

| | |
|---|---|
| **Imperforate hymen** | Incomplete degeneration of the central portion of the hymen. Accumulation of vaginal mucus at birth → self-resolving bulge in introitus. If untreated, leads to 1° amenorrhea, cyclic abdominal pain, hematocolpos (accumulation of menstrual blood in vagina → bulging and bluish hymenal membrane). |

**Vaginal tumors**

| | |
|---|---|
| Squamous cell carcinoma | Usually 2° to cervical SCC; 1° vaginal carcinoma rare. |
| Clear cell adenocarcinoma | Arises from vaginal adenosis (persistence of glandular columnar epithelium in proximal vagina), found in females who had exposure to diethylstilbestrol in utero. |
| Sarcoma botryoides | Embryonal rhabdomyosarcoma variant. Affects females < 4 years old; spindle-shaped cells; desmin ⊕. Presents with clear, grapelike, polypoid mass emerging from vagina. |

| | | |
|---|---|---|
| **Anovulatory infertility** | Infertility 2° to lack of ovulation. Causes:<br>▪ PCOS (most common)<br>▪ Primary ovarian insufficiency<br>▪ Hypogonadotropic hypogonadism<br>▪ Hyperprolactinemia | Anovulation is normal during pregnancy, breastfeeding, and near menarche or menopause. |

| | |
|---|---|
| **Polycystic ovary syndrome**<br> | Unknown cause; associated with dysregulation of ovarian steroidogenesis. ↑ LH:FSH, ↑ androgens (eg, testosterone) from theca interna cells, ↓ rate of follicular maturation → unruptured follicles (cysts) + anovulation. Common cause of ↓ fertility in females.<br>Diagnosed based on ≥ 2 of the following: cystic/enlarged ovaries on ultrasound (arrows in Ⓐ), oligo-/anovulation, hyperandrogenism (eg, hirsutism, acne). Associated with obesity, insulin resistance, acanthosis nigricans. ↑ risk of endometrial cancer 2° to unopposed estrogen from repeated anovulatory cycles.<br>Treatment: cycle regulation via weight reduction (↓ peripheral estrone formation), OCPs (prevent endometrial hyperplasia due to unopposed estrogen); ovulation induction for infertility; spironolactone, finasteride, flutamide to treat hirsutism. |

| | |
|---|---|
| **Primary ovarian insufficiency** | Also called premature ovarian failure.<br>Premature atresia of ovarian follicles in females of reproductive age. Most often idiopathic; associated with chromosomal abnormalities (eg, Turner syndrome, fragile X syndrome premutation), autoimmunity. Need karyotype screening. Patients present with signs of menopause after puberty but before age 40. ↓ estrogen, ↑ LH, ↑ FSH. |

| | |
|---|---|
| **Functional hypothalamic amenorrhea** | Also called exercise-induced amenorrhea. Severe caloric restriction, ↑ energy expenditure, and/or stress → functional disruption of pulsatile GnRH secretion → ↓ LH, FSH, estrogen. Pathogenesis includes ↓ leptin (due to ↓ fat) and ↑ cortisol (stress, excessive exercise).<br><br>Associated with eating disorders and "female athlete triad" (↓ calorie availability/excessive exercise, ↓ bone mineral density, menstrual dysfunction). |

### Cervical pathology

| | |
|---|---|
| **Dysplasia and carcinoma in situ**  | Disordered squamous epithelial growth; begins at basal layer of squamocolumnar junction (transformation zone) and extends outward. Classified as CIN 1, CIN 2, or CIN 3 (severe, irreversible dysplasia or carcinoma in situ), depending on extent of dysplasia. Associated with HPV-16 and HPV-18, which produce both the E6 gene product (inhibits *TP53*) and E7 gene product (inhibits *pRb*) (6 before 7; P before R). Koilocytes (cells with wrinkled "raisinoid" nucleus and perinuclear halo Ⓐ) are pathognomonic of HPV infection. May progress slowly to invasive carcinoma if left untreated. Typically asymptomatic (detected with Pap smear) or presents as abnormal vaginal bleeding (often postcoital).<br><br>Risk factors: multiple sexual partners, HPV, smoking, early coitarche, DES exposure, immunocompromise (eg, HIV, transplant). |
| **Invasive carcinoma** | Often squamous cell carcinoma. Pap smear can detect cervical dysplasia before it progresses to invasive carcinoma. Diagnose via colposcopy and biopsy. Lateral invasion can block ureters → hydronephrosis → renal failure. |

| | |
|---|---|
| **Primary dysmenorrhea** | Painful menses, caused by uterine contractions to ↓ blood loss → ischemic pain. Mediated by prostaglandins. Treatment: NSAIDs, acetaminophen, hormonal contraceptives. |

| | |
|---|---|
| **Ovarian cysts** | Usually asymptomatic, but may rupture, become hemorrhagic, or lead to adnexal torsion. |
| **Follicular cyst** | Functional (physiologic) cyst. Most common ovarian mass in young females. Caused by failure of mature follicle to rupture and ovulate. May produce excess estrogen. Usually resolves spontaneously. |
| **Corpus luteal cyst** | Functional cyst. Caused by failure of corpus luteum to involute after ovulation. May produce excess progesterone. Usually resolves spontaneously. |
| **Theca lutein cyst** | Also called hyperreactio luteinalis. Caused by hCG overstimulation. Often bilateral/multiple. Associated with gestational trophoblastic disease (eg, hydatidiform mole, choriocarcinoma). |

**Ovarian tumors**

Most common adnexal mass in females > 55 years old. Present with abdominal distention, bowel obstruction, pleural effusion.

Risk ↑ with advanced age, ↑ number of lifetime ovulations (early menarche, late menopause, nulliparity), endometriosis, genetic predisposition (eg, *BRCA1/BRCA2* mutations, Lynch syndrome).

Risk ↓ with previous pregnancy, history of breastfeeding, OCPs, tubal ligation.

Epithelial tumors are typically serous (lined by serous epithelium natively found in fallopian tubes, and often bilateral) or mucinous (lined by mucinous epithelium natively found in cervix). Monitor response to therapy/relapse by measuring CA 125 levels (not good for screening).

Germ cell tumors can differentiate into somatic structures (eg, teratomas), or extra-embryonic structures (eg, yolk sac tumors), or can remain undifferentiated (eg, dysgerminoma).

Sex cord stromal tumors develop from embryonic sex cord (develops into theca and granulosa cells of follicle, Sertoli and Leydig cells of seminiferous tubules) and stromal (ovarian cortex) derivatives.

| TYPE | CHARACTERISTICS |
| --- | --- |
| **Epithelial tumors** | |
| **Serous cystadenoma** | Benign. Most common ovarian neoplasm. Lined by fallopian tube–like epithelium. |
| **Mucinous cystadenoma** | Benign. Multiloculated, large. Lined by mucus-secreting epithelium A. |
| **Brenner tumor** | Usually benign. Nests of urothelial-like (bladderlike) epithelium with "coffee bean" nuclei. |
| **Serous carcinoma** | Most common malignant ovarian neoplasm. Psammoma bodies. |
| **Mucinous carcinoma** | Malignant. Rare. May be metastatic from appendiceal or other GI tumors. Can result in pseudomyxoma peritonei (intraperitoneal accumulation of mucinous material). |
| **Germ cell tumors** | |
| **Mature cystic teratoma** | Also called dermoid cyst. Benign. Most common ovarian tumor in young females. Cystic mass with elements from all 3 germ layers (eg, teeth, hair, sebum) B. May be painful 2° to ovarian enlargement or torsion. Monodermal form with thyroid tissue (struma ovarii C) may present with hyperthyroidism. Malignant transformation rare (usually to squamous cell carcinoma). |
| **Immature teratoma** | Malignant, aggressive. Contains fetal tissue, neuroectoderm. Commonly diagnosed before age 20. Typically represented by immature/embryoniclike neural tissue. |
| **Dysgerminoma** | Malignant. Most common in adolescents. Equivalent to male seminoma but rarer. Sheets of uniform "fried egg" cells D. Tumor markers: ↑ hCG, ↑ LDH. |
| **Yolk sac tumor** | Also called endodermal sinus tumor. Malignant, aggressive. Yellow, friable (hemorrhagic) mass. 50% have Schiller-Duval bodies (resemble glomeruli E). Tumor marker: ↑ AFP. Occurs in children and young adult females. |

## Ovarian tumors *(continued)*

| TYPE | CHARACTERISTICS |
|------|-----------------|
| **Sex cord stromal tumors** | |
| Fibroma | Benign. Bundle of spindle-shaped fibroblasts.<br>Meigs syndrome—triad of ovarian fibroma, ascites, pleural effusion. "Pulling" sensation in groin. |
| Thecoma | Benign. May produce estrogen. Usually presents as abnormal uterine bleeding in a postmenopausal female. |
| Sertoli-Leydig cell tumor | Benign. Gray to yellow-brown mass. Resembles testicular histology with tubules/cords lined by pink Sertoli cells. May produce androgens → virilization (eg, hirsutism, male pattern baldness, clitoral enlargement). |
| Granulosa cell tumor | Most common malignant sex cord stromal tumor. Predominantly occurs in females in their 50s. Often produces estrogen and/or progesterone. Presents with postmenopausal bleeding, endometrial hyperplasia, sexual precocity (in preadolescents), breast tenderness. Histology shows Call-Exner bodies (granulosa cells arranged haphazardly around collections of eosinophilic fluid, resembling primordial follicles; arrow in **F**). Tumor marker: ↑ inhibin. "Give Granny a Call." |

## Uterine conditions

| TYPE | CHARACTERISTICS |
| --- | --- |
| **Non-neoplastic** | |
| **Adenomyosis** | Presence of endometrial tissue (glands and stroma) in myometrium. May be due to invagination of basal layer of endometrium or metaplasia of remnant progenitor cells. Presents with abnormal uterine bleeding, dysmenorrhea. Diffusely enlarged ("globular"), soft ("boggy") uterus on exam. |
| **Endometriosis** | Presence of endometrial tissue (glands and stroma) outside uterus. May be due to ectopic implantation of endometrial tissue (via retrograde menses, blood vessels, lymphatics) or metaplasia of remnant progenitor cells. Typically involves pelvic sites, such as superficial peritoneum (yellow-brown "powder burn" lesions ) and ovaries (forms blood-filled "chocolate" cyst called endometrioma). Presents with chronic pelvic pain (eg, dysmenorrhea, dyspareunia), abnormal uterine bleeding, infertility. Normal-sized uterus on exam. |
| **Endometrial hyperplasia** | Abnormal endometrial gland proliferation. Usually caused by excess estrogen unopposed by progesterone. Associated with obesity, anovulation (eg, PCOS), hormone replacement therapy, tamoxifen. Presents with abnormal uterine bleeding. ↑ risk for endometrial carcinoma (especially with nuclear atypia). |
| **Endometritis** | Inflammation of endometrium . Usually occurs after delivery due to inoculation of uterine cavity by vaginal microbiota. C-section is the most important risk factor (sutures and necrotic tissue act as nidus for polymicrobial infection). Presents with fever, uterine tenderness, purulent lochia. |
| **Intrauterine adhesions** | Fibrous bands/tissue within endometrial cavity. Caused by damage to basal layer of endometrium, usually after dilation and curettage. Presents with abnormal uterine bleeding (↓ menses), infertility, recurrent pregnancy loss, dysmenorrhea. Also called Asherman syndrome when symptomatic. |
| **Neoplastic** | |
| **Leiomyoma** | Benign tumor of myometrium (also called fibroid). Most common gynecological tumor. Arises in reproductive-age females. ↑ incidence in Black population. Typically multiple; subtypes based on location: submucosal, intramural, or subserosal. Usually asymptomatic, but may present with abnormal uterine bleeding, pelvic pressure/pain, reproductive dysfunction. Estrogen sensitive; tumor size ↑ with pregnancy and ↓ with menopause. Enlarged uterus with nodular contour on exam . Histology: whorled pattern of smooth muscle bundles  and well-demarcated borders. |
| **Endometrial carcinoma** | Malignant tumor of endometrium. Most common gynecological cancer in resource-rich countries. Usually arises in postmenopausal females. Presents with abnormal uterine bleeding. Endometrioid carcinoma—most common subtype of endometrial carcinoma. Associated with long-term exposure to unopposed estrogen. Histology: confluent endometrial glands without intervening stroma . |

## Breast pathology

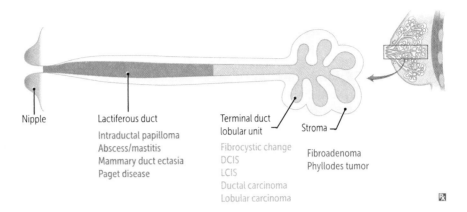

Nipple

Lactiferous duct
Intraductal papilloma
Abscess/mastitis
Mammary duct ectasia
Paget disease

Terminal duct
lobular unit
Fibrocystic change
DCIS
LCIS
Ductal carcinoma
Lobular carcinoma

Stroma

Fibroadenoma
Phyllodes tumor

## Benign breast diseases

| | |
|---|---|
| **Fibrocystic changes** | Most common in premenopausal females 20–50 years old. Present with premenstrual breast pain or lumps; often bilateral and multifocal. Nonproliferative lesions include simple cysts (fluid-filled duct dilation, blue dome), papillary apocrine change/metaplasia, stromal fibrosis. Risk of cancer is usually not increased. Proliferative lesions include<br>▪ Sclerosing adenosis—acini and stromal fibrosis, associated with calcifications. Slight ↑ risk for cancer.<br>▪ Epithelial hyperplasia—cells in terminal ductal or lobular epithelium. ↑ risk of carcinoma with atypical cells. |
| **Inflammatory processes** | Fat necrosis—benign, usually painless, lump due to injury to breast tissue. Calcified oil cyst on mammography; necrotic fat and giant cells on biopsy. Up to 50% of patients may not report trauma.<br>Lactational mastitis—occurs during breastfeeding, ↑ risk of bacterial infection through cracks in nipple. S aureus is most common pathogen. Treat with antibiotics and continue breastfeeding.<br>Mammary duct ectasia—dilation of subareolar ducts with inflammation and fibrosis. Associated with smoking. Presents with areolar pain, multicolored discharge, inverted nipple, periareolar mass. |
| **Benign tumors**<br> | Fibroadenoma—most common in females < 35 years old. Small, well-defined, mobile mass. Tumor composed of fibrous tissue and glands. ↑ size and tenderness with ↑ estrogen (eg, pregnancy, prior to menstruation). Risk of cancer is usually not increased.<br>Intraductal papilloma—small fibroepithelial tumor within lactiferous ducts, typically beneath areola. Most common cause of nipple discharge (serous or bloody). Slight ↑ risk for cancer.<br>Phyllodes tumor—large mass of connective tissue and cysts with "leaflike" lobulations A. Most common in 5th decade. Some may become malignant. |
| **Gynecomastia** | Breast enlargement in males due to ↑ estrogen compared with androgen activity. Physiologic in newborn, pubertal, and older males, but may persist after puberty. Other causes include cirrhosis, hypogonadism (eg, Klinefelter syndrome), testicular tumors, drugs (eg, spironolactone). |

| **Breast cancer** | Commonly postmenopausal. Often presents as a palpable hard mass most often in upper outer quadrant. Invasive cancer can become fixed to pectoral muscles, deep fascia, Cooper ligaments, and overlying skin → nipple retraction/skin dimpling.<br>Usually arises from terminal duct lobular unit. Amplification/overexpression of estrogen/progesterone receptors or HER2 (an EGF receptor) is common; triple negative (ER ⊖, PR ⊖, and HER2 ⊖) form more aggressive. | Risk factors in females: ↑ age; history of atypical hyperplasia; family history of breast cancer; race (White patients at highest risk, Black patients at ↑ risk for triple ⊖ breast cancer); *BRCA1/BRCA2* mutations; ↑ estrogen exposure (eg, nulliparity); postmenopausal obesity (adipose tissue converts androstenedione to estrone); ↑ total number of menstrual cycles; absence of breastfeeding; later age of first pregnancy; alcohol intake. In males: *BRCA2* mutation, Klinefelter syndrome.<br>Axillary lymph node metastasis most important prognostic factor in early-stage disease. |
| --- | --- | --- |

| TYPE | CHARACTERISTICS | NOTES |
| --- | --- | --- |
| Noninvasive carcinomas | | |
| **Ductal carcinoma in situ** | Fills ductal lumen (black arrow in indicates neoplastic cells in duct; blue arrow shows engorged blood vessel). Arises from ductal atypia. Often seen early as microcalcifications on mammography. | Early malignancy without basement membrane penetration. Usually does not produce a mass. |
| **Paget disease** | Extension of underlying DCIS/invasive breast cancer up the lactiferous ducts and into the contiguous skin of nipple → eczematous patches over nipple and areolar skin . | Paget cells = intraepithelial adenocarcinoma cells. |
| **Lobular carcinoma in situ** | ↓ E-cadherin expression. No mass or calcifications → incidental biopsy finding. | ↑ risk of cancer in either breast (vs DCIS, same breast and quadrant). |
| Invasive carcinomas | | |
| **Invasive ductal** | Firm, fibrous, "rock-hard" mass with sharp margins and small, glandular, ductlike cells in desmoplastic stroma. | Most common type of invasive breast cancer. |
| **Invasive lobular** | ↓ E-cadherin expression → orderly row of cells ("single file" ) and no duct formation. Often lacks desmoplastic response. | Often bilateral with multiple lesions in the same location.<br>Lobular carcinoma lacks cadherin and forms lines of cells. |
| **Inflammatory** | Dermal lymphatic space invasion → breast pain with warm, swollen, erythematous skin around exaggerated hair follicles (peau d'orange) . | Poor prognosis (50% survival at 5 years).<br>Often mistaken for mastitis or Paget disease.<br>Usually lacks a palpable mass. |

## Penile pathology

### Peyronie disease

Abnormal curvature of penis A due to fibrous plaque within tunica albuginea. Associated with repeated minor trauma during intercourse. Can cause pain, anxiety, erectile dysfunction. Consider surgical repair or treatment with collagenase injections once curvature stabilizes. Distinct from penile fracture (rupture of tunica albuginea due to forced bending).

### Ischemic priapism

Painful sustained erection lasting > 4 hours. Associated with sickle cell disease (sickled RBCs block venous drainage of corpus cavernosum vascular channels), medications (eg, sildenafil, trazodone). Treat immediately with corporal aspiration, intracavernosal phenylephrine, or surgical decompression to prevent ischemia.

### Squamous cell carcinoma

Seen in the US, but more common in Asia, Africa, South America. Most common type of penile cancer B. Precursor in situ lesions: Bowen disease (in penile shaft, presents as leukoplakia "white plaque"), erythroplasia of Queyrat (carcinoma in situ of the glans, presents as erythroplakia "red plaque"), Bowenoid papulosis (carcinoma in situ of unclear malignant potential, presenting as reddish papules). Associated with uncircumcised males and HPV-16.

### Cryptorchidism

Descent failure of one A or both testes. Impaired spermatogenesis (since sperm develop best at temperatures < 37°C) → subfertility. Can have normal testosterone levels (Leydig cells are mostly unaffected by temperature). Associated with ↑ risk of germ cell tumors. Prematurity ↑ risk of cryptorchidism. ↓ inhibin B, ↑ FSH, ↑ LH; testosterone ↓ in bilateral cryptorchidism, normal in unilateral. Most cases resolve spontaneously; otherwise, orchiopexy performed before 2 years of age.

### Testicular torsion

Rotation of testicle around spermatic cord and vascular pedicle. Commonly presents in males 12–18 years old. Associated with congenital inadequate fixation of testis to tunica vaginalis → horizontal positioning of testes ("bell clapper" deformity). May occur after an inciting event (eg, trauma) or spontaneously. Characterized by acute, severe pain, high-riding testis, and absent cremasteric reflex. ⊖ Prehn sign.

Treatment: surgical correction (orchiopexy) within 6 hours, manual detorsion if surgical option unavailable in timeframe. If testis is not viable, orchiectomy. Orchiopexy, when performed, should be bilateral because the contralateral testis is at risk for subsequent torsion.

### Varicocele

Dilated veins in pampiniform plexus due to ↑ venous pressure; most common cause of scrotal enlargement in adult males. Most often on left side because of ↑ resistance to flow from left gonadal vein drainage into left renal vein. Right-sided varicocele may indicate IVC obstruction (eg, from RCC invading right renal vein). Can cause infertility because of ↑ temperature. Diagnosed by standing clinical exam/Valsalva maneuver (distension on inspection and "bag of worms" on palpation; augmented by Valsalva) or ultrasound A. Does not transilluminate. Treatment: consider surgical ligation or embolization if associated with pain or infertility.

| **Extragonadal germ cell tumors** | Arise in midline locations. In adults, most commonly in retroperitoneum, mediastinum, pineal, and suprasellar regions. In infants and young children, sacrococcygeal teratomas are most common. |
| --- | --- |

| **Benign scrotal lesions** | Testicular masses that can be transilluminated  (vs solid testicular tumors). |
| --- | --- |

| **Hydrocele** | Accumulation of serous fluid within tunica vaginalis. Types: |
| --- | --- |

- Congenital (communicating)—due to incomplete obliteration of processus vaginalis. Common cause of scrotal swelling in infants. Most resolve spontaneously within 1 year.
- Acquired (noncommunicating)—due to infection, trauma, tumor. Termed hematocele if bloody.

| **Spermatocele** | Cyst due to dilated epididymal duct or rete testis. Paratesticular fluctuant nodule on palpation. |
| --- | --- |

Pampiniform plexus

Testicular artery

Vas deferens

Epididymis

Testes

Tunica vaginalis

Normal    Hydrocele    Spermatocele    Varicocele    Testicular torsion ℞

| **Testicular tumors** | Germ cell tumors account for ~ 95% of all testicular tumors. Arise from germ cells that produce sperm. Most often occur in young males. Risk factors: cryptorchidism, Klinefelter syndrome. Can present as mixed germ cell tumors. Do not transilluminate. Usually not biopsied (risk of seeding scrotum), removed via radical orchiectomy.<br>Sex cord stromal tumors develop from embryonic sex cord (develops into Sertoli and Leydig cells of seminiferous tubules, theca and granulosa cells of follicle) derivatives. 5% of all testicular tumors. Mostly benign. |
| --- | --- |

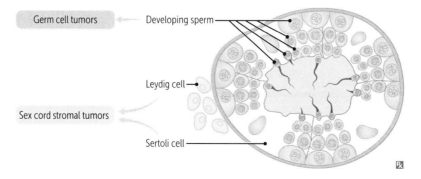

Germ cell tumors ⟵ Developing sperm

Leydig cell

Sex cord stromal tumors ⟵

Sertoli cell

℞

## Testicular tumors (continued)

| TYPE | CHARACTERISTICS |
|---|---|
| **Germ cell tumors** | |
| Seminoma | Malignant. Painless, homogenous testicular enlargement. Most common testicular tumor. Analogous to ovarian dysgerminoma. Does not occur in infancy. Large cells in lobules with watery cytoplasm and "fried egg" appearance on histology, ↑ placental alkaline phosphatase (PLAP). Highly radiosensitive. Late metastasis, excellent prognosis. |
| Embryonal carcinoma | Malignant. Painful, hemorrhagic mass with necrosis. Often glandular/papillary morphology. "Pure" embryonal carcinoma is rare; most commonly mixed with other tumor types. May present with metastases. May be associated with ↑ hCG and normal AFP levels when pure (↑ AFP when mixed). Worse prognosis than seminoma. |
| Teratoma | Mature teratoma may be malignant in adult males. Benign in children and females. |
| Yolk sac tumor | Also called endodermal sinus tumor. Malignant, aggressive. Yellow, mucinous. Analogous to ovarian yolk sac tumor. Schiller-Duval bodies resemble primitive glomeruli. ↑ AFP is highly characteristic. Most common testicular tumor in children < 3 years old. |
| Choriocarcinoma | Malignant. Disordered syncytiotrophoblastic and cytotrophoblastic elements. Hematogenous metastases to lungs and brain. ↑ hCG. May produce gynecomastia, symptoms of hyperthyroidism (hCG and TSH share an identical $\alpha$ subunit and a similar $\beta$ subunit, which determines their hormonal function). |
| **Non–germ cell tumors** | |
| Leydig cell tumor | Mostly benign. Golden brown color; contains Reinke crystals (eosinophilic cytoplasmic inclusions). Produces androgens or estrogens → precocious puberty, gynecomastia. |
| Sertoli cell tumor | Also called androblastoma (arises from sex cord stroma). Mostly benign. |
| Primary testicular lymphoma | Malignant, aggressive. Typically diffuse large B-cell lymphoma. Often bilateral. Most common testicular cancer in males > 60 years old. |

## Hormone levels in germ cell tumors

| | SEMINOMA | YOLK SAC TUMOR | CHORIOCARCINOMA | TERATOMA | EMBRYONAL CARCINOMA |
|---|---|---|---|---|---|
| PLAP | ↑ | – | – | – | – |
| AFP | – | ↑↑ | – | –/↑ | –/↑ (when mixed) |
| $\beta$-hCG | –/↑ | –/↑ | ↑↑ | – | ↑ |

| | |
|---|---|
| **Epididymitis and orchitis** | Most common causes: <br> ▪ *C trachomatis* and *N gonorrhoeae* (young males) <br> ▪ *E coli* and *Pseudomonas* (older males, associated with UTI and BPH) <br> ▪ Autoimmune (eg, granulomas involving seminiferous tubules) |
| Epididymitis | Inflammation of epididymis. Presents with localized pain and tenderness over posterior testis. ⊕ Prehn sign (pain relief with scrotal elevation). May progress to involve testis. |
| Orchitis | Inflammation of testis. Presents with testicular pain and swelling. Mumps orchitis ↑ infertility risk. Rare in males < 10 years old. |

**Benign prostatic hyperplasia**

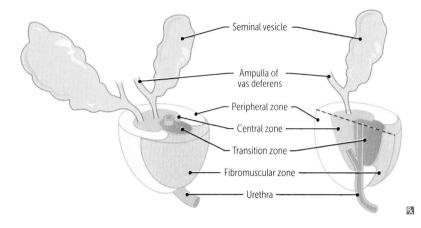

Seminal vesicle

Ampulla of vas deferens

Peripheral zone

Central zone

Transition zone

Fibromuscular zone

Urethra

Common in males > 50 years old. Characterized by smooth, elastic, firm nodular enlargement (hyperplasia not hypertrophy) of transition zone, which compress the urethra into a vertical slit. Not premalignant.

Often presents with ↑ frequency of urination, nocturia, difficulty starting and stopping urine stream, dysuria. May lead to distention and hypertrophy of bladder, hydronephrosis, UTIs. ↑ total PSA, with ↑ fraction of free PSA. PSA is made by prostatic epithelium stimulated by androgens.

Treatment: $\alpha_1$-antagonists (terazosin, tamsulosin), which cause relaxation of smooth muscle; $5\alpha$-reductase inhibitors (eg, finasteride); PDE-5 inhibitors (eg, tadalafil); surgical resection (eg, TURP, ablation).

**Prostatitis**

Characterized by dysuria, frequency, urgency, low back pain. Warm, tender, enlarged prostate.
Acute bacterial prostatitis—in older males most common bacterium is *E coli*; in young males consider *C trachomatis*, *N gonorrhoeae*.
Chronic prostatitis—either bacterial or nonbacterial (eg, 2° to previous infection, nerve problems, chemical irritation).

**Prostatic adenocarcinoma**

Common in males > 50 years old. Arises most often from posterior lobe (peripheral zone) of prostate gland and is most frequently diagnosed by ↑ PSA and subsequent needle core biopsies (transrectal, ultrasound-guided). Histologically graded using Gleason grade, which is based on glandular architecture and correlates closely with metastatic potential. Prostatic acid phosphatase (PAP) and PSA are useful tumor markers (↑ total PSA, with ↓ fraction of free PSA). Osteoblastic metastases in bone may develop in late stages, as indicated by lower back pain and ↑ serum ALP and PSA. Metastasis to the spine often occurs via Batson (vertebral) venous plexus.

### Control of reproductive hormones

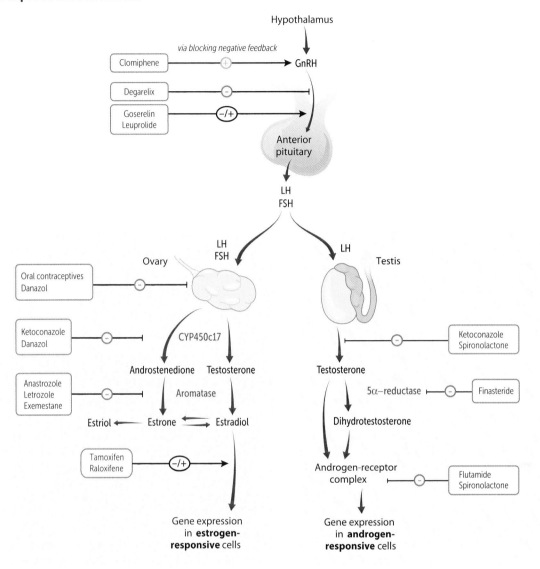

| Gonadotropin-releasing hormone analogs | Leuprolide, goserelin, nafarelin, histrelin. |
|---|---|
| MECHANISM | Act as GnRH agonists when used in pulsatile fashion. When used in continuous fashion, first transiently act as GnRH agonists (tumor flare), but subsequently act as GnRH antagonists (downregulate GnRH receptor in pituitary → ↓ FSH and ↓ LH → ↓ estrogen in females and ↓ testosterone in males). Can be used in lieu of GnRH. |
| CLINICAL USE | Uterine fibroids, endometriosis, precocious puberty, prostate cancer, infertility. Pulsatile for pregnancy, continuous for cancer. |
| ADVERSE EFFECTS | Hypogonadism, ↓ libido, erectile dysfunction, nausea, vomiting. |

| **Degarelix** | |
|---|---|
| MECHANISM | GnRH antagonist. No start-up flare. |
| CLINICAL USE | Prostate cancer. |
| ADVERSE EFFECTS | Hot flashes, liver toxicity. |

| **Ethinyl estradiol** | |
|---|---|
| MECHANISM | Binds estrogen receptors. |
| CLINICAL USE | Hypogonadism or ovarian failure, contraception (combined with progestins), hormone replacement therapy in postmenopausal females. |
| ADVERSE EFFECTS | ↑ risk of endometrial cancer (when given without progesterone), bleeding in postmenopausal patients, hepatic adenoma, breast tenderness, ↑ risk of thrombi. Contraindications—people > 35 years old who smoke tobacco (↑ risk of cardiovascular events), patients with ↑ risk of cardiovascular disease (including history of venous thromboembolism, coronary artery disease, stroke), migraine (especially with aura), breast cancer, liver disease. |

| **Selective estrogen receptor modulators** | |
|---|---|
| Clomiphene | Antagonist at estrogen receptors in hypothalamus. Prevents normal feedback inhibition and ↑ release of LH and FSH from pituitary, which stimulates ovulation. Used to treat infertility due to anovulation (eg, PCOS). May cause hot flashes, ovarian enlargement, multiple simultaneous pregnancies, visual disturbances. |
| Tamoxifen | Antagonist at breast, partial agonist at uterus, bone. Hot flashes, ↑ risk of thromboembolic events (especially with tobacco smoking), and endometrial cancer. Used to treat and prevent recurrence of ER/PR ⊕ breast cancer and to prevent gynecomastia in patients undergoing prostate cancer therapy. |
| Raloxifene | Antagonist at breast, uterus; agonist at bone; hot flashes, ↑ risk of thromboembolic events (especially with tobacco smoking), but no increased risk of endometrial cancer (vs tamoxifen, so you can "**relax**"); used primarily to treat osteoporosis. |

| **Aromatase inhibitors** | Anastrozole, letrozole, exemestane. |
|---|---|
| MECHANISM | Inhibit peripheral conversion of androgens to estrogen. |
| CLINICAL USE | ER ⊕ breast cancer in postmenopausal females. |

| **Progestins** | Levonorgestrel, medroxyprogesterone, etonogestrel, norethindrone, megestrol. |
|---|---|
| MECHANISM | Bind progesterone receptors, ↓ growth and ↑ vascularization of endometrium, thicken cervical mucus. |
| CLINICAL USE | Contraception (forms include pill, intrauterine device, implant, depot injection), endometrial cancer, abnormal uterine bleeding. Progestin challenge: presence of bleeding upon withdrawal of progestins excludes anatomic defects (eg, Asherman syndrome) and chronic anovulation without estrogen. |

| **Antiprogestins** | Mifepristone, ulipristal. |
|---|---|
| MECHANISM | Competitive inhibitors of progestins at progesterone receptors. |
| CLINICAL USE | Termination of pregnancy (mifepristone with misoprostol); emergency contraception (ulipristal). |

**Contraception**  Birth control.

| | METHOD | MECHANISM | NOTES |
|---|---|---|---|
| **Hormonal** | Estrogen combined with progestins<br>Progestin-only | Prevent ovulation by ↓ GnRH → ↓ LH/FSH → no estrogen surge → no LH surge<br>Progestins also thicken cervical mucus (↓ sperm entry) and thin endometrium (less suitable for implantation) | Forms include pill (OCPs), transdermal patch, vaginal ring |
| **Intrauterine device** | Copper IUD (hormone free) | Copper IUD causes local inflammation that is toxic to sperm and ova preventing fertilization and implantation | IUDs ↑ risk for abnormal uterine bleeding; insertion contraindicated in patients with active STI |
| | Progesterone IUD | Same as progestins | |
| **Surgical** | Males—vasectomy<br>Females—tubal ligation | No sperm in ejaculate<br>Sperm cannot reach ova | Irreversible |

| **Tocolytics** | Medications that relax the uterus; include terbutaline ($\beta_2$-agonist action), nifedipine ($Ca^{2+}$ channel blocker), indomethacin (NSAID). Used to ↓ contraction frequency in preterm labor and allow time for administration of glucocorticoids (to promote fetal lung maturity) or transfer to appropriate medical center with obstetrical care. |
|---|---|

## Danazol

| | |
|---|---|
| MECHANISM | Synthetic androgen that acts as partial agonist at androgen receptors. |
| CLINICAL USE | Endometriosis, hereditary angioedema. |
| ADVERSE EFFECTS | Weight gain, edema, acne, hirsutism, masculinization, ↓ HDL levels, hepatotoxicity, idiopathic intracranial hypertension. |

## Testosterone, methyltestosterone

| | |
|---|---|
| MECHANISM | Agonists at androgen receptors. |
| CLINICAL USE | Treat hypogonadism and promote development of 2° sex characteristics. |
| ADVERSE EFFECTS | Virilization in females; testicular atrophy in males. Premature closure of epiphyseal plates. ↑ LDL, ↓ HDL. |

## Antiandrogens

| DRUG | MECHANISM | CLINICAL USE | ADVERSE EFFECTS |
|---|---|---|---|
| **Abiraterone** | 17$\alpha$-hydroxylase/17,20-lyase inhibitor (↓ steroid synthesis) | Prostate cancer | Hypertension, hypokalemia (↑ mineralocorticoids) |
| **Finasteride** | 5$\alpha$-reductase inhibitor (↓ conversion of testosterone to DHT) | BPH, male-pattern baldness | Gynecomastia, sexual dysfunction |
| **Flutamide, bicalutamide** | Nonsteroidal competitive inhibitors at androgen receptor (↓ steroid binding) | Prostate cancer | Gynecomastia, sexual dysfunction |
| **Ketoconazole** | 17$\alpha$-hydroxylase/17,20-lyase inhibitor | Prostate cancer | Gynecomastia |
| **Spironolactone** | Androgen receptor and 17$\alpha$-hydroxylase/17,20-lyase inhibitor | PCOS | Amenorrhea |

## Tamsulosin

| | |
|---|---|
| MECHANISM | $\alpha_1$-antagonist selective for $\alpha_{1A/D}$ receptors in prostate (vs vascular $\alpha_{1B}$ receptors) → ↓ smooth muscle tone → ↑ urine flow. |
| CLINICAL USE | BPH. |

## Minoxidil

| | |
|---|---|
| MECHANISM | Direct arteriolar vasodilator. |
| CLINICAL USE | Androgenetic alopecia (pattern baldness), severe refractory hypertension. |

# Respiratory

*"Whenever I feel blue, I start breathing again."*

—L. Frank Baum

*"Until I feared I would lose it, I never loved to read. One does not love breathing."*

—Scout, *To Kill a Mockingbird*

*"Love is anterior to life, posterior to death, initial of creation, and the exponent of breath."*

—Emily Dickinson

*"Love and a cough cannot be concealed."*

—Anne Sexton

Group key respiratory, cardiovascular, and renal concepts together for study whenever possible. Respiratory physiology is challenging but high yield, especially as it relates to the pathophysiology of respiratory diseases. Develop a thorough understanding of normal respiratory function. Get familiar with obstructive vs restrictive lung disorders, ventilation/perfusion mismatch, lung volumes, mechanics of respiration, and hemoglobin physiology. Lung cancers and other causes of lung masses are also high yield. Be comfortable reading basic chest x-rays, CT scans, and PFTs.

▶ RESPIRATORY—EMBRYOLOGY

**Lung development**

Occurs in five stages. Begins with the formation of lung bud from distal end of respiratory diverticulum during week 4 of development. Every pulmonologist can see alveoli.

| STAGE | STRUCTURAL DEVELOPMENT | NOTES |
|---|---|---|
| Embryonic (weeks 4–7) | Lung bud → trachea → bronchial buds → mainstem bronchi → secondary (lobar) bronchi → tertiary (segmental) bronchi. | Errors at this stage can lead to tracheoesophageal fistula. |
| Pseudoglandular (weeks 5–17) | Endodermal tubules → terminal bronchioles. Surrounded by modest capillary network. | Respiration impossible, incompatible with life. |
| Canalicular (weeks 16–25) | Terminal bronchioles → respiratory bronchioles → alveolar ducts. Surrounded by prominent capillary network. | Airways increase in diameter. Pneumocytes develop starting at week 20. Respiration capable at week 25. |
| Saccular (week 24–birth) | Alveolar ducts → terminal sacs. Terminal sacs separated by 1° septae. | |
| Alveolar (week 36–8 years) | Terminal sacs → adult alveoli (due to 2° septation). | In utero, "breathing" occurs via aspiration and expulsion of amniotic fluid → ↑ pulmonary vascular resistance through gestation. At birth, air replaces fluid → ↓ pulmonary vascular resistance. |

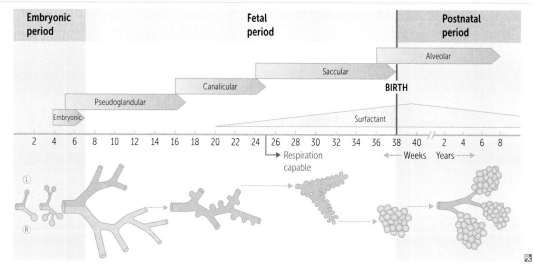

**Choanal atresia**

Blockage of posterior nasal opening. Often associated with bony abnormalities of the midface. Most often unilateral. When bilateral, represents an emergency and presents with upper airway obstruction, noisy breathing, and/or cyanosis that worsens during feeding and improves with crying. Diagnosed by failure to pass nasopharyngeal tube and confirmed with CT scan.

Often part of multiple malformation syndromes, such as **CHARGE** syndrome:
- **C**oloboma of eye
- **H**eart defects
- **A**tresia of choanae
- **R**estricted growth and development
- **G**enitourinary defects
- **E**ar defects

## Lung malformations

| | |
|---|---|
| Pulmonary hypoplasia | Poorly developed bronchial tree with abnormal histology. Associated with congenital diaphragmatic hernia (usually left-sided), bilateral renal agenesis (Potter sequence). |
| Bronchogenic cysts | Caused by abnormal budding of the foregut and dilation of terminal or large bronchi. Discrete, round, sharply defined, fluid-filled densities on CXR (air-filled if infected). Generally asymptomatic but can drain poorly → airway compression, recurrent respiratory infections. |

| | |
|---|---|
| **Club cells** | Nonciliated; low columnar/cuboidal with secretory granules. Located in bronchioles. Degrade toxins via cytochrome P-450; secrete component of surfactant; progenitor cells for club and ciliated cells. |

## Alveolar cell types

| | | |
|---|---|---|
| Type I pneumocytes | Squamous. 97% of alveolar surfaces. Thinly line the alveoli **A** for optimal gas exchange. | Pores of Kohn—anatomical communications between alveoli that allow for passing of air, fluid, phagocytes, and bacteria (in pneumonia). |
| Type II pneumocytes | Cuboidal and clustered **B**. 2 functions:<br>1. Serve as stem cell precursors for 2 cell types (type I and type II pneumocytes); proliferate during lung damage.<br>2. Secrete surfactant from lamellar bodies (arrowheads in **B**).<br>Application of Law of Laplace in alveoli–alveoli have ↑ tendency to collapse on expiration as radius ↓. | Surfactant—↓ alveolar surface tension, ↓ alveolar collapse, ↓ lung recoil, and ↑ compliance. Composed of multiple lecithins, mainly dipalmitoylphosphatidylcholine (DPPC). Synthesis begins ~20 weeks of gestation and achieves mature levels ~35 weeks of gestation. Glucocorticoids are important for fetal surfactant synthesis and lung development.<br>Collapsing pressure = 2 (surface tension)/radius |
| Alveolar macrophages | Phagocytose foreign materials; release cytokines and alveolar proteases. | Hemosiderin-laden macrophages may be found (eg, pulmonary edema, alveolar hemorrhage). |

## Neonatal respiratory distress syndrome

Surfactant deficiency → ↑ surface tension → alveolar collapse ("ground-glass" appearance of lung fields) **A**.

Risk factors: prematurity, diabetes during pregnancy (due to ↑ fetal insulin), C-section delivery (↓ release of fetal glucocorticoids; less stressful than vaginal delivery).

Treatment: maternal glucocorticoids before birth; exogenous surfactant for infant.

Therapeutic supplemental $O_2$ can result in Retinopathy of prematurity, Intraventricular hemorrhage, Bronchopulmonary dysplasia (RIB).

Screening tests for fetal lung maturity: lecithin-sphingomyelin (L/S) ratio in amniotic fluid (≥ 2 is healthy; < 1.5 predictive of NRDS), foam stability index, surfactant-albumin ratio.

Persistently low $O_2$ tension → risk of PDA.

## ▶ RESPIRATORY—ANATOMY

### Respiratory tree

| | |
|---|---|
| Conducting zone | Large airways consist of nose, pharynx, larynx, trachea, and bronchi. Airway resistance highest in the large- to medium-sized bronchi. Small airways consist of bronchioles that further divide into terminal bronchioles (large numbers in parallel → least airway resistance).<br><br>Warms, humidifies, and filters air but does not participate in gas exchange → "anatomic dead space."<br><br>Cartilage and goblet cells extend to the end of bronchi.<br><br>Pseudostratified ciliated columnar cells primarily make up epithelium of bronchus and extend to beginning of terminal bronchioles, then transition to cuboidal cells. Clear mucus and debris from lungs (mucociliary escalator).<br><br>Airway smooth muscle cells extend to end of terminal bronchioles (sparse beyond this point). |
| Respiratory zone | Lung parenchyma; consists of respiratory bronchioles, alveolar ducts, and alveoli. Participates in gas exchange.<br><br>Mostly cuboidal cells in respiratory bronchioles, then simple squamous cells up to alveoli. Cilia terminate in respiratory bronchioles. Alveolar macrophages clear debris and participate in immune response. |

**Conducting zone**

Trachea

Bronchi

Goblet cell — Basal cell — Ciliated cell
Pseudostratified ciliated columnar epithelium
Smooth muscle
Cartilage

Bronchioles

Club cell — Ciliated cell
Simple ciliated columnar epithelium
Smooth muscle

Terminal bronchioles

Cuboidal ciliated cells — Club cell
Simple ciliated cuboidal epithelium
Smooth muscle

**Respiratory zone**

Respiratory bronchioles

Cuboidal cells — Club cell — Squamous cell
Simple cuboidal and squamous epithelium
Smooth muscle (sparse)

Alveolar sacs

Type I pneumocyte
Type II pneumocyte
Alveolar macrophage
Capillary

## Lung anatomy

Trachea

Carina

Right bronchus   Left bronchus

Right lung has 3 lobes; Left has less lobes (2) and lingula (homolog of right middle lobe). Instead of a middle lobe, left lung has a space occupied by the heart **A**.

Relation of the pulmonary artery to the bronchus at each lung hilum is described by **RALS**—Right **A**nterior; **L**eft **S**uperior. Carina is posterior to ascending aorta and anteromedial to descending aorta **B**.

Right lung is a more common site for inhaled foreign bodies because right main stem bronchus is wider, more vertical, and shorter than the left. If you aspirate a peanut:

- While supine—usually enters superior segment of right lower lobe or sometimes enters posterior segment of right upper lobe.
- While lying on right side or prone—usually enters right upper lobe.
- While upright—usually enters right lower lobe.

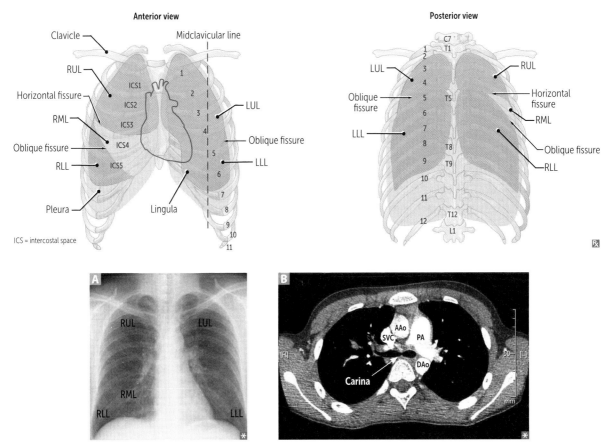

**Anterior view**

Clavicle — Midclavicular line

RUL

Horizontal fissure

RML

Oblique fissure

RLL

Pleura

ICS1, ICS2, ICS3, ICS4, ICS5

Lingula

LUL

Oblique fissure

LLL

ICS = intercostal space

**Posterior view**

C7, T1, T5, T8, T9, T12, L1

LUL

Oblique fissure

LLL

RUL

Horizontal fissure

RML

Oblique fissure

RLL

**A** — RUL, LUL, RML, RLL, LLL

**B** — AAo, SVC, PA, DAo, Carina

## Diaphragm structures

Inferior vena cava (T8)

Central tendon

Esophagus (T10)

Rib

Aorta (T12)

Vertebra

Inferior view

Structures perforating diaphragm:

- At T8: IVC, right phrenic nerve
- At T10: esophagus, vagus (CN 10; 2 trunks)
- At T12: aorta (red), thoracic duct (white), azygos vein (blue) ("At T-1-2 it's the red, white, and blue")

Diaphragm innervated by C3-5 (phrenic). Pain from diaphragm irritation can be referred to shoulder (C5) and trapezius ridge (C3, 4). Phrenic nerve injury causes elevation of the ipsilateral hemidiaphragm on x-ray.

Number of letters = T level:

T8: vena cava (IVC)
T10: (O)esophagus
T12: aortic hiatus

I ate (8) ten eggs at twelve.

C3, 4, 5 keeps the diaphragm alive.

Other bifurcations:

- The Common Carotid bifurcates at C4.
- The Trachea bifurcates at T4.
- The abdominal aorta bifurcates at L4.

## ▶ RESPIRATORY—PHYSIOLOGY

| **Lung volumes and capacities** | Note: a capacity is a sum of ≥ 2 physiologic volumes. There are 4 volumes and 4 capacities. |
|---|---|
| Tidal volume | Air that moves into lung with each quiet inspiration, 6–8 mL/kg, typically ~500 mL. |
| Inspiratory reserve volume | Air that can still be breathed in after normal inspiration |
| Expiratory reserve volume | Air that can still be breathed out after normal expiration |
| Residual volume | Air in lung after maximal expiration; RV and any lung capacity that includes RV cannot be measured by spirometry |
| Inspiratory capacity | $IRV + V_T$<br>Air that can be breathed in after normal exhalation |
| Functional residual capacity | $RV + ERV$<br>Volume of gas in lungs after normal expiration; outward pulling force of chest wall is balanced with inward collapsing force of lungs |
| Vital capacity | $IRV + V_T + ERV$<br>Maximum volume of gas that can be expired after a maximal inspiration |
| Total lung capacity | $IRV + V_T + ERV + RV = VC + RV$<br>Volume of gas present in lungs after a maximal inspiration |

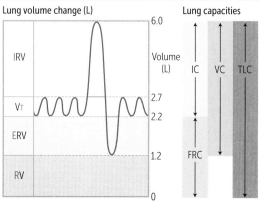

Lung volume change (L)    Lung capacities

IRV = inspiratory reserve volume    IC = inspiratory capacity
$V_T$ = tidal volume    FRC = functional residual capacity
ERV = expiratory reserve volume    VC = vital capacity
RV = residual volume    TLC = total lung capacity

| **Work of breathing** | Refers to the energy expended or $O_2$ consumed by respiratory muscles to produce the ventilation needed to meet the body's metabolic demand. Comprises the work needed to overcome both elastic recoil and airway resistance (ie, work = force × distance = pressure × volume). Minimized by optimizing respiratory rate (RR) and $V_T$. ↑ in restrictive diseases (↑ work to overcome elastic recoil achieved with ↑ RR and ↓ $V_T$) and obstructive diseases (↑ work to overcome airway resistance achieved with ↓ RR and ↑ $V_T$). |
|---|---|

| **Determination of physiologic dead space** | $V_D = V_T \times \dfrac{P_{aCO_2} - P_{ECO_2}}{P_{aCO_2}}$<br>$V_D$ = physiologic dead space = anatomic dead space of conducting airways plus alveolar dead space; apex of healthy lung is largest contributor of alveolar dead space. $V_D$ = volume of inspired air that does not take part in gas exchange.<br>$P_{aCO_2}$ = arterial $P_{CO_2}$.<br>$P_{ECO_2}$ = expired air $P_{CO_2}$. | Physiologic dead space—approximately equivalent to anatomic dead space in normal lungs. May be greater than anatomic dead space in lung diseases with ventilation/perfusion mismatch. |
|---|---|---|

## Ventilation

| | | |
|---|---|---|
| **Minute ventilation** | Abbreviated as $V_E$. Total volume of gas entering lungs per minute.<br>$V_E = V_T \times RR$ | Normal values:<br>▪ RR = 12–20 breaths/min<br>▪ $V_T$ = 500 mL/breath<br>▪ $V_D$ = 150 mL/breath |
| **Alveolar ventilation** | Abbreviated as $V_A$. Volume of gas that reaches alveoli each minute.<br>$V_A = (V_T - V_D) \times RR$ | |

| | | |
|---|---|---|
| **Lung and chest wall properties** | Because of historical reasons and small pressures, pulmonary pressures are always presented in cm $H_2O$. | |
| **Elastic recoil** | Tendency for lungs to collapse inward and chest wall to spring outward.<br>At FRC, airway and alveolar pressures equal atmospheric pressure ($P_B$; called zero), and intrapleural pressure is negative (preventing atelectasis). The inward pull of the lung is balanced by the outward pull of the chest wall. System pressure is atmospheric. Pulmonary vascular resistance (PVR) is at a minimum. | |
| **Compliance** | Change in lung volume for a change in pressure ($\Delta V/\Delta P$). Inversely proportional to wall stiffness and increased by surfactant.<br>▪ ↑ compliance = lung easier to fill (eg, emphysema, older adults)<br>▪ ↓ compliance = lung more difficult to fill (eg, pulmonary fibrosis, pneumonia, ARDS, pulmonary edema) | |
| **Hysteresis** | Lung inflation follows a different pressure-volume curve than lung deflation due to need to overcome surface tension forces in inflation. | |

**Pulmonary circulation**

Normally a low-resistance, high-compliance system. A ↓ in $P_{AO_2}$ causes hypoxic vasoconstriction that shifts blood away from poorly ventilated regions of lung to well-ventilated regions of lung.

Perfusion limited—$O_2$ (normal health), $CO_2$, $N_2O$. Gas equilibrates early along the length of the capillary. Exchange can be ↑ only if blood flow ↑.

Diffusion limited—$O_2$ (emphysema, fibrosis), CO. Gas does not equilibrate by the time blood reaches the end of the capillary.

$O_2$ diffuses slowly, while $CO_2$ diffuses very rapidly across the alveolar membrane. Disease states that lead to diffusion limitation (eg, pulmonary fibrosis) are more likely to cause early hypoxia than hypercapnia.

Chronic hypoxic vasoconstriction may lead to pulmonary hypertension +/− cor pulmonale.

$$\text{Diffusion } (J) = A \times D_k \times \frac{P_1 - P_2}{\Delta_x} \text{ where}$$

A = area, $\Delta_x$ = alveolar wall thickness,
  $D_k$ = diffusion coefficient of gas,
  $P_1 - P_2$ = difference in partial pressures.
  ▪ A ↓ in emphysema.
  ▪ $\Delta_x$ ↑ in pulmonary fibrosis.

DLCO is the extent to which CO passes from air sacs of lungs into blood.

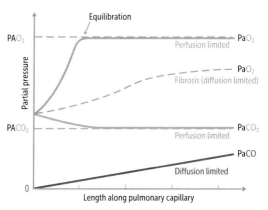

Pa = partial pressure of gas in pulmonary capillary blood
PA = partial pressure of gas in alveolar air

---

**Pulmonary vascular resistance**

$$PVR = \frac{P_{\text{pulm artery}} - P_{\text{L atrium}}}{\dot{Q}}$$

Remember: $\Delta P = \dot{Q} \times R$, so $R = \Delta P / \dot{Q}$

$$R = \frac{8\eta l}{\pi r^4}$$

$P_{\text{pulm artery}}$ = pressure in pulmonary artery
$P_{\text{L atrium}} \approx$ pulmonary artery occlusion pressure (also called pulmonary capillary wedge pressure)
$\dot{Q}$ = cardiac output (mL/min)
R = resistance
$\eta$ = viscosity of blood ("stickiness")
l = vessel length
r = vessel radius

**Ventilation/perfusion mismatch**

Ideally, ventilation (V) is matched to perfusion (Q) per minute (ie, $\dot{V}/\dot{Q}$ ratio = 1) for adequate gas exchange.

Lung zones:
- $\dot{V}/\dot{Q}$ at apex of lung = 3 (wasted ventilation)
- $\dot{V}/\dot{Q}$ at base of lung = 0.6 (wasted perfusion)

Both ventilation and perfusion are greater at the base of the lung than at the apex of the lung.

With exercise (↑ cardiac output), there is vasodilation of apical capillaries → $\dot{V}/\dot{Q}$ ratio approaches 1.

Certain organisms that thrive in high $O_2$ (eg, TB) flourish in the apex.

$\dot{V}/\dot{Q}$ = 0 = "oirway" obstruction (shunt). In shunt, 100% $O_2$ does not improve $Pa_{O_2}$ (eg, foreign body aspiration).

$\dot{V}/\dot{Q}$ = ∞ = blood flow obstruction (physiologic dead space). Assuming < 100% dead space, 100% $O_2$ improves $Pa_{O_2}$ (eg, pulmonary embolus).

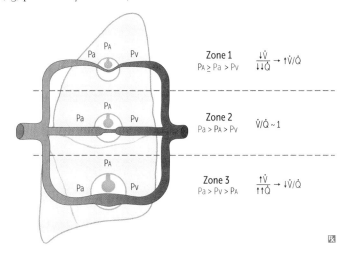

**Alveolar gas equation**

$$P_{A_{O_2}} = P_{I_{O_2}} - \frac{Pa_{CO_2}}{RQ}$$

$$\approx 150 \text{ mm Hg}^a - \frac{Pa_{CO_2}}{0.8}$$

[a]At sea level breathing room air

$P_{A_{O_2}}$ = alveolar $P_{O_2}$ (mm Hg)

$P_{I_{O_2}}$ = $P_{O_2}$ in inspired air (mm Hg)

$Pa_{CO_2}$ = arterial $P_{CO_2}$ (mm Hg)

RQ = respiratory quotient = $CO_2$ produced/ $O_2$ consumed

A-a gradient = $P_{A_{O_2}} - Pa_{O_2}$. Normal A-a gradient estimated as (age/4) + 4 (eg, for a person < 40 years old, gradient should be < 14).

## Carbon dioxide transport

$CO_2$ is transported from tissues to lungs in 3 forms:

❶ $HCO_3^-$ (70%–90%). $HCO_3^-/Cl^-$ transporter on RBC membrane allows $HCO_3^-$ to diffuse out to plasma and $Cl^-$ to diffuse into RBC (chloride shift) via facilitated diffusion countertransport

❷ Carbaminohemoglobin or $HbCO_2$ (10%–20%). $CO_2$ bound to Hb at N-terminus of globin (not heme). $CO_2$ favors deoxygenated form ($O_2$ unloaded).

❸ Dissolved $CO_2$ (~ 10%).

In lungs, oxygenation of Hb promotes dissociation of $H^+$ from Hb. This shifts equilibrium toward $CO_2$ formation; therefore, $CO_2$ is released from RBCs (Haldane effect).

Majority of blood $CO_2$ is carried as $HCO_3^-$ in the plasma.

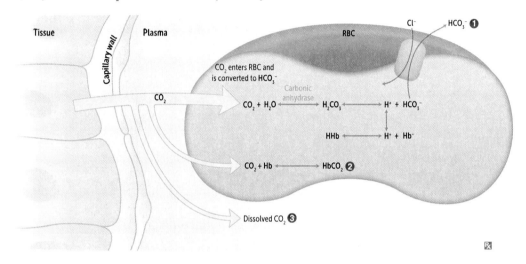

## Hypoxia and hypoxemia

### Hypoxia

↓ $O_2$ delivery to tissues. Commonly due to ↓ cardiac output, hypoxemia (insufficient oxygenation of blood with ↓ $PaO_2$), ischemia, anemia, CO/ cyanide poisoning.

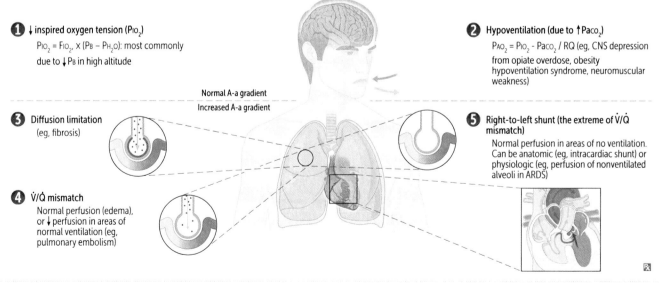

❶ ↓ inspired oxygen tension ($PIO_2$)

$PIO_2 = FIO_2 \times (PB - PH_2O)$: most commonly due to ↓ $PB$ in high altitude

❷ Hypoventilation (due to ↑$Paco_2$)

$PAO_2 = PIO_2 - Paco_2 / RQ$ (eg, CNS depression from opiate overdose, obesity hypoventilation syndrome, neuromuscular weakness)

Normal A-a gradient
Increased A-a gradient

❸ Diffusion limitation (eg, fibrosis)

❺ Right-to-left shunt (the extreme of V̇/Q̇ mismatch)

Normal perfusion in areas of no ventilation. Can be anatomic (eg, intracardiac shunt) or physiologic (eg, perfusion of nonventilated alveoli in ARDS)

❹ V̇/Q̇ mismatch

Normal perfusion (edema), or ↓ perfusion in areas of normal ventilation (eg, pulmonary embolism)

### Hypoxemia

Insufficient oxygenation of blood (↓ $Pao_2$).

**Hemoglobin**

Normal adult hemoglobin (Hb) is composed of 4 polypeptide subunits (2 α and 2 β) that each bind one $O_2$ molecule. Hb is an allosteric protein that exhibits positive cooperativity when binding to $O_2$, such that:
- Oxygenated Hb has high affinity for $O_2$ (300×).
- Deoxygenated Hb has low affinity for $O_2$ → promotes release/unloading of $O_2$.

The protein component of hemoglobin acts as buffer for $H^+$ ions.
Myoglobin is composed of a single polypeptide chain associated with one heme moiety. Higher affinity for oxygen than Hb.

**Oxygen content of blood**

$O_2$ content = ($O_2$ bound to hemoglobin) + ($O_2$ solubilized in plasma) = ($1.34 \times Hb \times Sao_2$) + ($0.003 \times Pao_2$).
$Sao_2$ = percent saturation of arterial blood with $O_2$.
$0.003$ = solubility constant of $O_2$; $Pao_2$ = partial pressure of $O_2$ in arterial blood.

Normally 1 g Hb can bind 1.34 mL $O_2$; normal Hb amount in blood is 15 g/dL.
$O_2$ binding (carrying) capacity ≈ 20 mL $O_2$/dL of blood.
With ↓ Hb there is ↓ $O_2$ content of arterial blood, but no change in $O_2$ saturation and $Pao_2$.
$O_2$ delivery to tissues = cardiac output × $O_2$ content of blood.

| | Hb CONCENTRATION | $Sao_2$ | $Pao_2$ | TOTAL $O_2$ CONTENT |
|---|---|---|---|---|
| CO poisoning | Normal | ↓ (CO competes with $O_2$) | Normal | ↓ |
| Anemia | ↓ | Normal | Normal | ↓ |
| Polycythemia | ↑ | Normal | Normal | ↑ |
| Methemoglobinemia | Normal | ↓ ($Fe^{3+}$ poor at binding $O_2$) | Normal | ↓ |
| Cyanide toxicity | Normal | Normal | Normal | Normal |

**Oxyhemoglobin dissociation curve**

Shifts in oxyhemoglobin dissociation curve (ODC) reflect local tissue oxygen needs. Can be helpful (meets metabolic needs) or harmful (in toxicities, pathophysiologic situations).
Right shift in ODC reflects ↓ Hb affinity for $O_2$ → ↑ $O_2$ unloading at tissue. Physiologically occurs with ↑ $O_2$ needs: exercise, ↓ pH, ↑ temperature/fever, hypoxia (↑ 2,3-BPG); at the cellular level, caused by ↑ $H^+$ and ↑ $CO_2$ created by tissue metabolism (Bohr effect).
Left shift in ODC reflects ↑ Hb affinity for $O_2$ → ↓ $O_2$ unloading at tissue. Physiologically occurs with ↓ $O_2$ needs (↓ temperature) and pregnancy (fetal Hb has higher $O_2$ affinity than adult Hb, and ↑ $O_2$ binding due to ↓ affinity for 2,3-BPG → left shift, driving $O_2$ across placenta to fetus). Pathologically occurs with ↑ CO, ↑ MetHb, genetic mutation (↓ 2,3-BPG). **Left is lower.**

ODC has sigmoidal shape due to positive cooperativity (ie, tetrameric Hb molecule can bind 4 $O_2$ molecules and has higher affinity for each subsequent $O_2$ molecule bound). Myoglobin is monomeric and thus does not show positive cooperativity; curve lacks sigmoidal appearance.

| | |
|---|---|
| **Response to high altitude** | Constant $F_{IO_2}$ but ↓ $P_B$ → ↓ atmospheric oxygen ($P_{IO_2}$) → ↓ $Pa_{O_2}$ → ↑ ventilation → ↓ $Pa_{CO_2}$ → respiratory alkalosis → altitude sickness (headaches, nausea, fatigue, lightheadedness, sleep disturbance). |

Chronic ↑ in ventilation.

↑ erythropoietin → ↑ Hct and Hb (due to chronic hypoxia).

↑ 2,3-BPG (binds to Hb → rightward shift of oxyhemoglobin dissociation curve → ↑ $O_2$ release).

Cellular changes (↑ mitochondria).

↑ renal excretion of $HCO_3^-$ to compensate for respiratory alkalosis (can augment with acetazolamide).

Chronic hypoxic pulmonary vasoconstriction → ↑ pulmonary vascular resistance → pulmonary hypertension, right ventricular hypertrophy (RVH).

---

**Response to exercise**

↑ HR and ↑ SV → ↑ $\dot{Q}$ → ↑ pulmonary blood flow → ↑ $\dot{V}/\dot{Q}$ ratio from base to apex (becoming more uniform).

↑ cellular respiration → ↑ $CO_2$ production and ↓ pH at tissues → right shift of ODC → tissue offloading of more $O_2$ → ↑ $O_2$ consumption. ↑ RR to meet ↑ $O_2$ demand and remove excess $CO_2$ → ↑ pulmonary blood flow.

$Pa_{O_2}$ and $Pa_{CO_2}$ are maintained by homeostatic mechanisms.

↓ $P\bar{v}_{O_2}$ due to ↑ $O_2$ consumption.

↑ $P\bar{v}_{CO_2}$ due to ↑ $CO_2$ production.

---

**Methemoglobin**

Iron in Hb is normally in a reduced state (ferrous $Fe^{2+}$; "just the 2 of us"). Oxidized form of Hb (ferric, $Fe^{3+}$) does not bind $O_2$ as readily as $Fe^{2+}$, but has ↑ affinity for cyanide → tissue hypoxia from ↓ $O_2$ saturation and ↓ $O_2$ content.

This $Fe^{3+}$ form is called methemoglobinemia. While typical concentrations are 1–2%, methemoglobinemia will occur at higher levels and may present with cyanosis (does not improve with supplemental $O_2$) and with chocolate-colored blood.

Dapsone, local anesthetics (eg, benzocaine), and nitrites (eg, from dietary intake or polluted water sources) cause poisoning by oxidizing $Fe^{2+}$ to $Fe^{3+}$.

Methemoglobinemia can be treated with methylene blue and vitamin C.

| | Cyanide | Carbon monoxide |
|---|---|---|
| **Cyanide vs carbon monoxide poisoning** | Both inhibit aerobic metabolism via inhibition of complex IV of ETC (cytochrome c oxidase) → hypoxia that does not fully correct with supplemental $O_2$ and ↑ anaerobic metabolism. | |
| EXPOSURE | Synthetic product combustion, amygdalin ingestion (found in apricot seeds), cyanide ingestion (eg, in suicide attempts), fire victims. | Motor exhaust, gas heaters, fire victims. |
| PRESENTATION | Headache, dyspnea, drowsiness, seizure, coma. Skin may appear flushed ("cherry red"). Venules in retina appear bright red. Breath may have bitter almond odor. | Headache, vomiting, confusion, visual disturbances, coma. May have cherry-red skin with bullous skin lesions. Multiple victims may be involved (eg, family due to faulty furnace). |
| LABS | Normal $Pao_2$. Elevated lactate → anion gap metabolic acidosis. | Normal $Pao_2$. Elevated carboxyhemoglobin on co-oximetry. Classically associated with bilateral globus pallidus lesions on MRI A, although can rarely be seen with cyanide toxicity. |
| EFFECT ON OXYGEN-HEMOGLOBIN CURVE | Curve normal. Oxygen saturation may appear normal initially. Despite ample $O_2$ supply, it cannot be used due to ineffective oxidative phosphorylation. | Left shift in ODC → ↑ affinity for $O_2$ → ↓ $O_2$ unloading in tissues. Binds competitively to Hb with > 200× greater affinity than $O_2$ to form carboxyhemoglobin → ↓ %$O_2$ saturation of Hb. |
| TREATMENT | Decontamination (eg, remove clothing). Hydroxocobalamin (binds cyanide → cyanocobalamin → renal excretion). Nitrites (oxidize Hb → methemoglobin → binds cyanide → cyanomethemoglobin → ↓ toxicity). Sodium thiosulfate (↑ cyanide conversion to thiocyanate → renal excretion). | 100% $O_2$. Hyperbaric oxygen if severe. |

## ▶ RESPIRATORY—PATHOLOGY

**Rhinosinusitis**

Obstruction of sinus drainage into nasal cavity → inflammation and pain over affected area.
  Typically affects maxillary sinuses, which drain against gravity due to ostia located superomedially
  (red arrow points to fluid-filled right maxillary sinus in ).
Superior meatus—drains posterior ethmoid; middle meatus—drains frontal, maxillary, and anterior
  ethmoid; inferior meatus—drains nasolacrimal duct.
Acute rhinosinusitis is most commonly caused by viruses (eg, rhinovirus); may lead to superimposed
  bacterial infection, most commonly nontypeable *H influenzae*, *S pneumoniae*, *M catarrhalis*.
Paranasal sinus infections may extend to the orbits, cavernous sinus, and brain, causing
  complications (eg, orbital cellulitis, cavernous sinus syndrome, meningitis).

**Epistaxis**

Nose bleed. Most commonly occurs in anterior
segment of nostril (Kiesselbach plexus at
caudal septum). Life-threatening hemorrhages
occur in posterior segment (sphenopalatine
artery, a branch of maxillary artery). Common
causes include foreign body, trauma, allergic
rhinitis, and nasal angiofibromas (common in
adolescent males).

Kiesselbach drives his Lexus with his LEGS:
superior Labial artery, anterior and posterior
Ethmoidal arteries, Greater palatine artery,
Sphenopalatine artery.

**Head and neck cancer**

Mostly squamous cell carcinoma. Risk factors include tobacco, alcohol, HPV-16 (oropharyngeal),
  EBV (nasopharyngeal). Field cancerization: carcinogen damages wide mucosal area → multiple
  tumors that develop independently after exposure.
Nasopharyngeal carcinoma may present with unilateral nasal obstruction, discharge, epistaxis.
  Eustachian tube obstruction may lead to otitis media +/– effusion, hearing loss.
Laryngeal papillomatosis—also called recurrent respiratory papillomatosis. Benign laryngeal
  tumor, commonly affecting areas of stratified squamous epithelium such as the true vocal
  cords, especially in children (possibly from HPV transmitted from mother to baby during labor).
  Associated with HPV-6 and HPV-11. Symptoms can guide location of pathology (supraglottic →
  dysphagia, infraglottic/glottic → hoarseness).

**Deep venous thrombosis**

Blood clot within a deep vein → swelling,
redness , warmth, pain. Predisposed by
Virchow triad (SHE):
  ▪ Stasis (eg, post-op, long drive/flight)
  ▪ Hypercoagulability (eg, defect in coagulation
    cascade proteins, such as factor V Leiden;
    oral contraceptive use; pregnancy)
  ▪ Endothelial damage (exposed collagen
    triggers clotting cascade)
DVT of proximal deep veins of lower extremity
(iliac, femoral, popliteal) → embolic source.

D-dimer test may be used clinically to rule out
  DVT if disease probability is low or moderate
  (high sensitivity, low specificity). Imaging
  test of choice is compression ultrasound with
  Doppler.
Use unfractionated heparin or low-molecular
  weight heparins (eg, enoxaparin) for
  prophylaxis and acute management. Use direct
  anticoagulants (eg, rivaroxaban, apixaban) for
  treatment and long-term prevention.

| | |
|---|---|
| **Pulmonary emboli** | Obstruction of the pulmonary artery or its branches by foreign material (usually thrombus) that originated elsewhere. Affected alveoli are ventilated but not perfused ($\dot{V}/\dot{Q}$ mismatch). May present with sudden-onset dyspnea, pleuritic chest pain, tachypnea, tachycardia, hypoxemia, respiratory alkalosis. Large emboli or saddle embolus (red arrows show filling defects in ) may cause sudden death due to clot preventing blood from filling LV and increased RV size further compromising LV filling (obstructive shock). CT pulmonary angiography is imaging test of choice for PE (look for filling defects) . ECG may show sinus tachycardia or, less commonly, S1Q3T3 abnormality. |

Lines of Zahn  are interdigitating areas of pink (platelets, fibrin) and red (RBCs) found only in thrombi formed before death; help distinguish pre- and postmortem thrombi.

Treatment: anticoagulation (eg, heparin, direct thrombin/factor Xa inhibitors), IVC filter (if anticoagulation is contraindicated).

Types: Fat, Air, Thrombus, Bacteria, Amniotic fluid, Tumor. An embolus moves like a **FAT BAT**.

Fat emboli—associated with long bone fractures and liposuction; classic triad of hypoxemia, neurologic abnormalities, petechial rash.

Air emboli—nitrogen bubbles precipitate in ascending divers (caisson disease/decompression sickness); treat with hyperbaric $O_2$; or, can be iatrogenic 2° to invasive procedures (eg, central line placement).

Amniotic fluid emboli—typically occurs during labor or postpartum, but can be due to uterine trauma. Can lead to DIC. Rare, but high mortality.

| | |
|---|---|
| **Mediastinal pathology** | Normal mediastinum contains heart, thymus, lymph nodes, esophagus, and aorta. |
| **Mediastinal masses** | Some pathologies (eg, lymphoma, lung cancer, abscess) can occur in any compartment, but there are common associations: <br> ▪ Anterior—4 T's: thyroid (substernal goiter), thymic neoplasm, teratoma, "terrible" lymphoma. <br> ▪ Middle—metastases, hiatal hernia, bronchogenic cysts. <br> ▪ Posterior—esophageal cancer (may present as mass in, or spread to, middle mediastinum), neurogenic tumor (eg, neurofibroma), multiple myeloma. |
| **Mediastinitis** | Inflammation of mediastinal tissues. Commonly due to postoperative complications of cardiothoracic procedures (≤ 14 days), esophageal perforation, or contiguous spread of odontogenic/retropharyngeal infection. <br> Chronic mediastinitis—also called fibrosing mediastinitis; due to ↑ proliferation of connective tissue in mediastinum. *Histoplasma capsulatum* is common cause. <br> Clinical features: fever, tachycardia, leukocytosis, chest pain, and sternal wound drainage. |
| **Pneumomediastinum** | Presence of gas (usually air) in the mediastinum. Can either be spontaneous (due to rupture of pulmonary bleb) or 2° (eg, trauma, iatrogenic, Boerhaave syndrome). <br> Ruptured alveoli allow tracking of air into the mediastinum via peribronchial and perivascular sheaths. <br> Clinical features: chest pain, dyspnea, voice change, subcutaneous emphysema, ⊕ Hamman sign (crepitus on cardiac auscultation). |

## Flow-volume loops

| FLOW-VOLUME PARAMETER | Normal | Obstructive lung disease | Restrictive lung disease |
| --- | --- | --- | --- |
| RV | | ↑ | ↓ |
| FRC | | ↑ | ↓ |
| TLC | | ↑ | ↓ |
| $FEV_1$ | >80% predicted | ↓↓ | ↓ |
| FVC | >80% predicted | ↓ | ↓ |
| $FEV_1/FVC$ | >70% | ↓ <br> $FEV_1$ decreased more than FVC | Normal or ↑ <br> $FEV_1$ decreased proportionately to FVC |

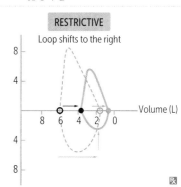

| | | |
| --- | --- | --- |
| **NORMAL** | **OBSTRUCTIVE** <br> Loop shifts to the left | **RESTRICTIVE** <br> Loop shifts to the right |

| Obstructive lung diseases | Obstruction of air flow (↓↓ $FEV_1$, ↓ FVC ↓ $FEV_1/FVC$ ratio) → air trapping in lungs (↑ RV, →↑ FRC and ↑ TLC) due to premature airway closure at high lung volumes. Includes COPD (chronic bronchitis and emphysema), asthma, and bronchiectasis. |
| --- | --- |
| **Chronic obstructive pulmonary disease** | Often due to tobacco use (most important risk factor), pollutants, or allergens. Includes chronic bronchitis and emphysema, which often co-exist. Exacerbation: acute worsening of symptoms, often associated with viral or bacterial upper respiratory tract infection. |
| **Chronic bronchitis** | |
| DIAGNOSIS | Clinical diagnosis. Criteria: productive cough for ≥ 3 months in ≥ 2 consecutive years. <br> May also have dyspnea, wheezes, crackles (due to mucus), cyanosis (hypoxemia due to shunting), 2° polycythemia. Leads to metaplasia of pseudostratified ciliated columnar epithelium into stratified squamous epithelium. |
| MECHANISMS | Hypertrophy and hyperplasia of mucus-secreting glands in bronchi. |
| NOTES | ↑ Reid index (thickness of mucosal gland layer to thickness of wall between epithelium and cartilage) > 50%. |
| **Emphysema** | |
| DIAGNOSIS | Radiologic or biopsy diagnosis. CXR: barrel chest, ↑ AP diameter (best seen in lateral A), flattened diaphragm, ↑ lung field lucency. |
| MECHANISMS | Alveolar wall destruction B → ↑ compliance of lung, ↓ recoil, and damage to alveolar capillary membrane → ↓ DLCO; results in ↑ air space. <br> Centriacinar—spares distal alveoli, frequently in upper lobes. Associated with tobacco smoking C D. <br> Panacinar—affects respiratory bronchioles and alveoli, frequently in lower lobes. Associated with $\alpha_1$-antitrypsin deficiency. |

## Obstructive lung diseases *(continued)*

| | |
|---|---|
| NOTES | Mediated by oxidative stress, chronic inflammation (CD8+ T cells, neutrophils, and macrophages), and imbalance of proteases and antiproteases (↑ elastase activity → ↑ loss of elastic fibers → alveolar destruction). Defect/deficiency/absence of $\alpha_1$-antitrypsin (antiprotease that inhibits neutrophil elastase) leads to unopposed elastase activity |

### Asthma

| | |
|---|---|
| | Intermittent obstructive lung disease often triggered by allergens, viral URIs, stress. Associated with atopy.<br>NSAID- or aspirin-exacerbated respiratory disease—asthma, nasal polyps, and COX-inhibitor sensitivity (leukotriene overproduction → airway constriction) (Samter's triad). |
| DIAGNOSIS | Clinical diagnosis. Intermittent episodes of dyspnea, coughing, wheezing, tachypnea.<br>Diagnosis supported by spirometry (obstructive pattern with bronchodilator response, but may be normal when not in exacerbation) +/– methacholine challenge. |
| MECHANISMS | Type I hypersensitivity reaction → smooth muscle hypertrophy and hyperplasia. Hyperresponsive bronchi → reversible bronchoconstriction. Mucus plugging E. |
| OTHER | Curschmann spirals F—shed epithelium forms whorled mucus plugs. Charcot-Leyden crystals G—eosinophilic, hexagonal, double-pointed crystals formed from breakdown of eosinophils in sputum. |

### Bronchiectasis

| | |
|---|---|
| | Obstructive lung disease. Most commonly associated with cystic fibrosis. |
| DIAGNOSIS | Characterized by chronic cough and daily purulent sputum production. Often have recurrent pulmonary infections. Confirmed by imaging demonstrating airway dilation and bronchial thickening. Supported by obstructive PFT pattern. |
| PATHOPHYSIOLOGY | Initial insult of pulmonary infection combined with obstruction or impaired clearance → dysregulated host response → bronchial inflammation → permanently dilated airways. |
| NOTES | Many etiologies, including airway obstruction (eg, foreign body aspiration, mass), poor ciliary motility (eg, tobacco smoking, Kartagener syndrome), cystic fibrosis (H shows a coughed up inspissated mucus plug), allergic bronchopulmonary aspergillosis, pulmonary infections (eg, *Mycobacterium avium*). |

| | |
|---|---|
| **Restrictive lung diseases** | May lead to ↓ lung volumes (↓ FVC and TLC). PFTs: normal or ↑ $FEV_1$/FVC ratio. Patient presents with short, shallow breaths.<br><br>Types:<br><ul><li>Altered respiratory mechanics (extrapulmonary, normal $D_{LCO}$, normal A-a gradient):<ul><li>Respiratory muscle weakness—polio, myasthenia gravis, Guillain-Barré syndrome, ALS</li><li>Chest wall abnormalities—scoliosis, severe obesity</li></ul></li><li>Diffuse parenchymal lung diseases, also called interstitial lung diseases (pulmonary, ↓ $D_{LCO}$, ↑ A-a gradient):<ul><li>Pneumoconioses (eg, coal workers' pneumoconiosis, silicosis, asbestosis)</li><li>Sarcoidosis: bilateral hilar lymphadenopathy, noncaseating granulomas; ↑ ACE and $Ca^{2+}$</li><li>Idiopathic pulmonary fibrosis</li><li>Granulomatosis with polyangiitis</li><li>Pulmonary Langerhans cell histiocytosis (eosinophilic granuloma)</li><li>Hypersensitivity pneumonitis</li><li>Drug toxicity (eg, bleomycin, busulfan, amiodarone, methotrexate)</li><li>Acute respiratory distress syndrome</li><li>**Radiation-induced lung injury**—associated with proinflammatory cytokine release (eg, TNF-α, IL-1, IL-6). May be asymptomatic but most common symptoms are dry cough and dyspnea +/– low-grade fever. Acute radiation pneumonitis develops within 3–12 weeks (exudative phase); radiation fibrosis may develop after 6–12 months.</li></ul></li></ul> |
| **Idiopathic pulmonary fibrosis** | Progressive fibrotic lung disease of unknown etiology. May involve multiple cycles of lung injury, inflammation, and fibrosis. Associated with tobacco smoking, environmental pollutants, genetic defects.<br>Findings: progressive dyspnea, fatigue, nonproductive cough, crackles, clubbing. Imaging shows peripheral reticular opacities with traction bronchiectasis +/– "honeycomb" appearance of lung (advanced disease). Histologic pattern: usual interstitial pneumonia. ↓ type 1 pneumocytes, ↑ type 2 pneumocytes, ↑ fibroblasts.<br>Complications: pulmonary hypertension, right heart failure, arrhythmias, coronary artery disease, respiratory failure, lung cancer. |
| **Hypersensitivity pneumonitis** | Mixed type III/IV hypersensitivity reaction to environmental antigens such as thermophilic *Actinomyces* and *Aspergillus*. Often seen in farmers and bird-fanciers. Acutely, causes dyspnea, cough, chest tightness, fever, headache. Often self-limiting if stimulus is removed. Chronically, leads to irreversible fibrosis with noncaseating granuloma, alveolar septal thickening, traction bronchiectasis. |

**Sarcoidosis**

Characterized by immune-mediated, widespread noncaseating granulomas , elevated serum ACE levels, and elevated CD4/CD8 ratio in bronchoalveolar lavage fluid. More common in Black females. Often asymptomatic except for enlarged lymph nodes. CXR shows bilateral adenopathy and coarse reticular opacities B; CT of the chest better demonstrates the extensive hilar and mediastinal adenopathy C.

Associated with Bell palsy, parotid enlargement, granulomas (noncaseating epithelioid, containing microscopic Schaumann and Asteroid bodies), Rheumatoid arthritis–like arthropathy, ↑ Calcium, Ocular uveitis, Interstitial fibrosis, vitamin D activation (due to ↑ 1α-hydroxylase in macrophages), Skin changes (eg, lupus pernio, erythema nodosum) (SARCOIDS).

Treatment: glucocorticoids (if symptomatic).

**Mesothelioma**

Malignancy of the pleura associated with asbestosis. May result in hemorrhagic pleural effusion (exudative), pleural thickening.

Histology may show psammoma bodies. EM may show polygonal tumor cells with microvilli, desmosomes, tonofilaments.

Calretinin and cytokeratin 5/6 ⊕ in almost all mesotheliomas, ⊖ in most carcinomas.

Tobacco smoking is not a risk factor.

| | | |
|---|---|---|
| **Pneumoconioses** | Asbestos is from the roof (was common in insulation), but affects the base (lower lobes). Silica, coal, and berries are from the base (earth), but affect the roof (upper lobes). | |
| **Asbestos-related disease** | Asbestos causes asbestosis (pulmonary fibrosis), pleural disease, malignancies. Associated with shipbuilding, roofing, plumbing. "Ivory white," calcified, supradiaphragmatic and pleural  plaques are pathognomonic.<br>Risk of bronchogenic carcinoma > risk of mesothelioma. ↑ risk of Caplan syndrome (rheumatoid arthritis and pneumoconioses with intrapulmonary nodules). | Affects lower lobes.<br>Asbestos (ferruginous) bodies are golden-brown fusiform rods resembling dumbbells, found in alveolar sputum sample, visualized using Prussian blue stain , often obtained by bronchoalveolar lavage.<br>↑ risk of pleural effusions. |
| **Berylliosis** | Associated with exposure to beryllium in aerospace and manufacturing industries. Granulomatous (noncaseating)  on histology and therefore occasionally responsive to glucocorticoids. ↑ risk of cancer and cor pulmonale. | Affects upper lobes. |
| **Coal workers' pneumoconiosis** | Prolonged coal dust exposure → macrophages laden with carbon → inflammation and fibrosis.<br>Also called black lung disease. ↑ risk of Caplan syndrome. | Affects upper lobes.<br>Small, rounded nodular opacities seen on imaging.<br>Anthracosis—asymptomatic condition found in many urban dwellers exposed to sooty air. |
| **Silicosis** | Associated with sandblasting, foundries, mines. Macrophages respond to silica and release fibrogenic factors, leading to fibrosis. It is thought that silica may disrupt phagolysosomes and impair macrophages, increasing susceptibility to TB. ↑ risk of lung cancer, cor pulmonale, and Caplan syndrome. | Affects upper lobes.<br>"Eggshell" calcification of hilar lymph nodes on CXR.<br>The silly egg sandwich I found is mine! |

## Acute respiratory distress syndrome

| | |
|---|---|
| PATHOPHYSIOLOGY | Alveolar insult → release of pro-inflammatory cytokines → neutrophil recruitment, activation, and release of toxic mediators (eg, reactive oxygen species, proteases, etc) → capillary endothelial damage and ↑ vessel permeability → leakage of protein-rich fluid into alveoli → formation of intra-alveolar hyaline membranes (arrows in ) and noncardiogenic pulmonary edema (normal PCWP) → ↓ compliance and V̇/Q̇ mismatch → hypoxic vasoconstriction → ↑ pulmonary vascular resistance.<br>Loss of surfactant also contributes to alveolar collapse (eg, preterm infants, drowning). |
| CAUSES | Sepsis (most common), aspiration pneumonia, burns, trauma, pancreatitis, drowning injuries. |
| DIAGNOSIS | Diagnosis of exclusion with the following criteria (**ARDS**):<br>▪ Abnormal chest X-ray (bilateral lung opacities) <br>▪ Respiratory failure within 1 week of alveolar insult<br>▪ Decreased $Pao_2/Fio_2$ (ratio < 300, hypoxemia due to ↑ intrapulmonary shunting and diffusion abnormalities)<br>▪ Symptoms of respiratory failure are not due to HF/fluid overload |
| CONSEQUENCES | Impaired gas exchange, ↓ lung compliance; pulmonary hypertension. |
| MANAGEMENT | Treat the underlying cause.<br>Mechanical ventilation: ↓ tidal volume, ↑ PEEP (keeps alveoli open during expiration). |

Endotracheal tube
Right internal jugular line
Diffuse opacities    Diffuse opacities

## Sleep apnea

Repeated cessation of breathing > 10 seconds during sleep → disrupted sleep → daytime somnolence. Diagnosis confirmed by sleep study.

Nocturnal hypoxia → systemic and pulmonary hypertension, arrhythmias (atrial fibrillation/flutter), sudden death.

Hypoxia → ↑ EPO release → ↑ erythropoiesis.

### Obstructive sleep apnea

Respiratory effort against airway obstruction. $Pao_2$ is usually normal during the day. Associated with obesity, loud snoring, daytime sleepiness. Usually caused by excess parapharyngeal/oropharyngeal tissue in adults, adenotonsillar hypertrophy in children. Treatment: weight loss, CPAP, dental devices, hypoglossal nerve stimulation, upper airway surgery.

### Central sleep apnea

Impaired respiratory effort due to CNS injury/toxicity, Congestive HF, opioids. May be associated with Cheyne-Stokes respirations (oscillations between apnea and hyperpnea). Treatment: positive airway pressure.

### Obesity hypoventilation syndrome

Also called Pickwickian syndrome. Obesity (BMI ≥ 30 $kg/m^2$) → hypoventilation → ↑ $Paco_2$ during waking hours (retention); ↓ $Pao_2$ and ↑ $Paco_2$ during sleep. Treatment: weight loss, positive airway pressure.

| Pulmonary hypertension | Elevated mean pulmonary artery pressure (> 20 mm Hg) at rest. Results in arteriosclerosis, medial hypertrophy, intimal fibrosis of pulmonary arteries, plexiform lesions. ↑ pulmonary vascular resistance → ↑ RV pressure → RVH (parasternal heave on examination), RV failure. |
|---|---|

**ETIOLOGIES**

| Pulmonary arterial hypertension (group 1) | Often idiopathic. Females > males. Heritable PAH can be due to an inactivating mutation in *BMPR2* gene (normally inhibits vascular smooth muscle proliferation); poor prognosis. Pulmonary vasculature endothelial dysfunction results in ↑ vasoconstrictors (eg, endothelin) and ↓ vasodilators (eg, NO and prostacyclins). Other causes include drugs (eg, amphetamines, cocaine), connective tissue disease, HIV infection, portal hypertension, congenital heart disease, schistosomiasis. |
|---|---|
| Left heart disease (group 2) | Causes include systolic/diastolic dysfunction and valvular disease. |
| Lung diseases or hypoxia (group 3) | Destruction of lung parenchyma (eg, COPD), lung inflammation/fibrosis (eg, interstitial lung diseases), hypoxemic vasoconstriction (eg, obstructive sleep apnea, living in high altitude). |
| Chronic thromboembolic (group 4) | Recurrent microthrombi → ↓ cross-sectional area of pulmonary vascular bed. |
| Multifactorial (group 5) | Causes include hematologic, systemic, and metabolic disorders, along with compression of the pulmonary vasculature by a tumor. |

### Physical findings in select lung diseases

| ABNORMALITY | BREATH SOUNDS | PERCUSSION | FREMITUS | TRACHEAL DEVIATION |
|---|---|---|---|---|
| Pleural effusion | ↓ | Dull | ↓ | None if small<br>Away from side of lesion if large |
| Atelectasis | ↓ | Dull | ↓ | Toward side of lesion |
| Simple pneumothorax | ↓ | Hyperresonant | ↓ | None |
| Tension pneumothorax | ↓ | Hyperresonant | ↓ | Away from side of lesion |
| Consolidation (lobar pneumonia, pulmonary edema) | Bronchial breath sounds; late inspiratory crackles, egophony, whispered pectoriloquy | Dull | ↑ | None |

| Digital clubbing | Increased angle between nail bed and nail plate (> 180°) . Pathophysiology not well understood; in patients with intrapulmonary shunt, platelets and megakaryocytes become lodged in digital vasculature → local release of PDGF and VEGF. Can be hereditary or acquired. Causes include respiratory diseases (eg, idiopathic pulmonary fibrosis, cystic fibrosis, bronchiectasis, lung cancer), cardiovascular diseases (eg, cyanotic congenital heart disease), infections (eg, lung abscess, TB), and others (eg, IBD). Not typically associated with COPD or asthma. |
|---|---|

## Atelectasis

Alveolar collapse (right upper lobe collapse against mediastinum in 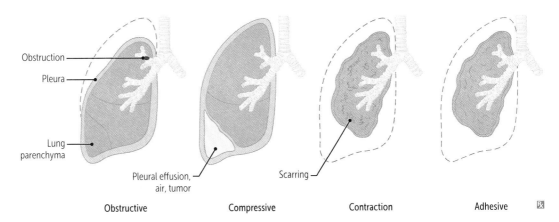). Multiple causes:

- Obstructive—airway obstruction prevents new air from reaching distal airways, old air is resorbed (eg, foreign body, mucous plug, tumor)
- Compressive—external compression on lung decreases lung volumes (eg, space-occupying lesion, pleural effusion)
- Contraction (cicatrization)—scarring of lung parenchyma that distorts alveoli (eg, sarcoidosis)
- Adhesive—due to lack of surfactant (eg, NRDS in premature infants)

Decreased via incentive spirometry or ↑ PEEP during mechanical ventilation.

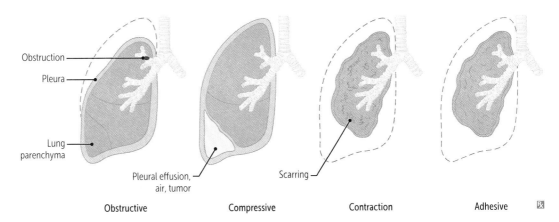

Obstruction
Pleura
Lung parenchyma
Pleural effusion, air, tumor
Scarring

Obstructive  Compressive  Contraction  Adhesive

## Pleural effusions

Excess accumulation of fluid 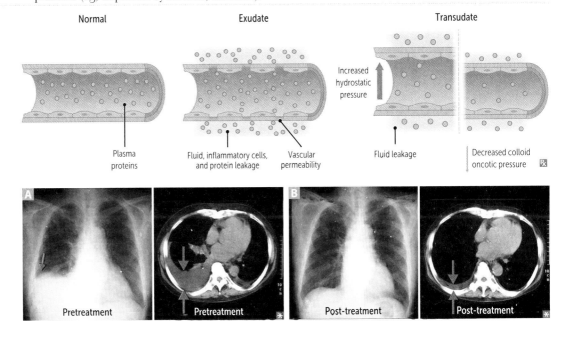 between pleural layers → restricted lung expansion during inspiration. Can be treated with thoracentesis to remove/reduce fluid B. Based on the Light's criteria, fluid is consistent with an exudate if pleural fluid protein/serum protein > 0.5, pleural fluid LDH/serum LDH > 0.6, or pleural fluid LDH > 2/3 upper limit of normal serum LDH.

### Exudate

Cloudy fluid (cellular). Due to infection (eg, pneumonia, tuberculosis), malignancy, connective tissue disease, lymphatic (chylothorax), trauma. Often requires drainage due to ↑ risk of infection.

### Transudate

Clear fluid (hypocellular). Due to ↑ hydrostatic pressure (eg, HF, Na⁺ retention) and/or ↓ oncotic pressure (eg, nephrotic syndrome, cirrhosis).

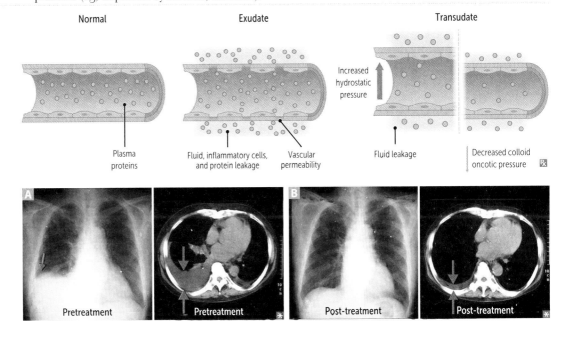

Normal  Exudate  Transudate

Increased hydrostatic pressure

Plasma proteins

Fluid, inflammatory cells, and protein leakage

Vascular permeability

Fluid leakage

Decreased colloid oncotic pressure

Pretreatment  Pretreatment  Post-treatment  Post-treatment

| | |
|---|---|
| **Pneumothorax** | Accumulation of air in pleural space . Dyspnea, uneven chest expansion. Chest pain, ↓ tactile fremitus, hyperresonance, and diminished breath sounds, all on the affected side. |
| Primary spontaneous pneumothorax | Due to rupture of apical subpleural bleb or cysts. Occurs most frequently in tall, thin, young males. Associated with tobacco smoking. |
| Secondary spontaneous pneumothorax | Due to diseased lung (eg, bullae in emphysema, Marfan syndrome, infections), mechanical ventilation with use of high pressures → barotrauma. |
| Traumatic pneumothorax | Caused by blunt (eg, rib fracture), penetrating (eg, gunshot), or iatrogenic (eg, central line placement, lung biopsy, barotrauma due to mechanical ventilation) trauma. |
| Tension pneumothorax | Can be from any of the above. Air enters pleural space but cannot exit. Increasing trapped air → tension pneumothorax. Trachea deviates away from affected lung . May lead to increased intrathoracic pressure → mediastinal displacement → kinking of IVC → ↓ venous return → ↓ cardiac output, obstructive shock (hypotension, tachycardia), jugular venous distention. Needs immediate needle decompression and chest tube placement. |

## Pneumonia

| TYPE | TYPICAL ORGANISMS | CHARACTERISTICS |
| --- | --- | --- |
| **Lobar pneumonia** | *S pneumoniae* (most common), *Legionella*, *Klebsiella* | Intra-alveolar exudate → consolidation A; may involve entire lobe or the whole lung. |
| **Bronchopneumonia** | *S pneumoniae*, *S aureus*, *H influenzae*, *Klebsiella* | Acute inflammatory infiltrates from bronchioles into adjacent alveoli; patchy distribution involving ≥ 1 lobe. |
| **Interstitial (atypical) pneumonia** | *Mycoplasma*, *Chlamydophila pneumoniae*, *Chlamydophila psittaci*, *Legionella*, *Coxiella burnetii*, viruses (RSV, CMV, influenza, adenovirus) | Diffuse patchy inflammation localized to interstitial areas at alveolar walls; CXR shows bilateral multifocal opacities B. Generally follows a more indolent course ("walking" pneumonia). |
| **Cryptogenic organizing pneumonia** | Etiology unknown. ⊖ sputum and blood cultures, often responds to glucocorticoids but not to antibiotics. | Formerly called bronchiolitis obliterans organizing pneumonia (BOOP). Noninfectious pneumonia characterized by inflammation of bronchioles and surrounding structure. |
| **Aspiration pneumonia** | Aspiration of oropharyngeal or gastric contents → pulmonary infection. Risk factors: altered mental status (↓ cough reflex or glottic closure), dysphagia, neurologic disorders (eg, stroke), invasive tubes (eg, nasogastric tube). | Presents days after aspiration event in dependent lung segment. More common in RLL if sitting up and RUL if lying down (recumbent) due to bronchial anatomy. Can progress to abscess. Aspiration (chemical) pneumonitis—presents hours after aspiration event. Due to gastric acid–mediated inflammation. Presents with infiltrates in lower lobe(s) and resolves with supportive treatment. |

## Natural history of lobar pneumonia

|  | Congestion | Red hepatization | Gray hepatization | Resolution |
|---|---|---|---|---|
| DAYS | 1–2 | 3–4 | 5–7 | 8+ |
| FINDINGS | Red-purple, partial consolidation of parenchyma<br>Exudate with mostly bacteria | Red-brown consolidation<br>Exudate with fibrin, bacteria, RBCs, WBCs<br>Reversible | Uniformly gray<br>Exudate full of WBCs, lysed RBCs, and fibrin | Enzymatic digestion of exudate by macrophages |

Healthy alveolus
Macrophage
Capillary
WBC

Bacteria
Exudate

RBC — Fibrin

Lysed RBC — Exudate

Normal | Congestion | Red hepatization | Gray hepatization | Resolution

## Lung abscess

Localized collection of pus within parenchyma. Caused by aspiration of oropharyngeal contents (especially in patients predisposed to loss of consciousness [eg, alcohol overuse, epilepsy]) or bronchial obstruction (eg, cancer).

Air-fluid levels often seen on CXR; presence suggests cavitation. Due to anaerobes (eg, *Bacteroides, Fusobacterium, Peptostreptococcus*) or *S aureus*.

Treatment: antibiotics, drainage, or surgery.

Lung abscess **A** 2° to aspiration is most often found in right lung. Location depends on patient's position during aspiration: RLL if upright, RUL or RML if recumbent.

| Lung cancer | | |
|---|---|---|
| Leading cause of cancer death. Presentation: cough, hemoptysis, bronchial obstruction, wheezing, pneumonic "coin" lesion on CXR or noncalcified nodule on CT. Sites of metastases from lung cancer: liver (jaundice, hepatomegaly), adrenals, **bone** (pathologic fracture), **brain**; "Lung 'mets' Love affective boneheads and brainiacs." In the lung, metastases (usually multiple lesions) are more common than 1° neoplasms. Most often from breast, colon, prostate, and bladder cancer. | **SPHERE** of complications: **S**uperior vena cava/ thoracic outlet syndromes, **P**ancoast tumor, **H**orner syndrome, **E**ndocrine (paraneoplastic), **R**ecurrent laryngeal nerve compression (hoarseness), **E**ffusions (pleural or pericardial). Risk factors include tobacco smoking, secondhand smoke, radiation, environmental exposures (eg, radon, asbestos), pulmonary fibrosis, family history. **S**quamous and **s**mall cell carcinomas are **s**entral (central) and often caused by tobacco smoking. Hamartomas are found incidentally on imaging, appearing as well-circumscribed mass. | |

| TYPE | LOCATION | CHARACTERISTICS | HISTOLOGY |
|---|---|---|---|
| **Small cell** | | | |
| **Small cell (oat cell) carcinoma** | Central | Undifferentiated → very aggressive. May cause **neurologic** paraneoplastic syndromes (eg, Lambert-Eaton myasthenic syndrome, paraneoplastic myelitis, encephalitis, subacute cerebellar degeneration) and **endocrine** paraneoplastic syndromes (Cushing syndrome, SIADH). Amplification of *myc* oncogenes common. Managed with chemotherapy +/– radiation. | Neoplasm of **neuroendocrine** Kulchitsky cells → small dark blue cells . Chromogranin A ⊕, neuron-specific enolase ⊕, synaptophysin ⊕. |
| **Non–small cell** | | | |
| **Adenocarcinoma** | Peripheral | Most common 1° lung cancer. Most common subtype in people who do not smoke. More common in females than males. Activating mutations include *KRAS*, *EGFR*, and *ALK*. Associated with hypertrophic osteoarthropathy (clubbing). Bronchioloalveolar subtype (adenocarcinoma in situ): CXR often shows hazy infiltrates similar to pneumonia; better prognosis. | Glandular pattern, often stains mucin ⊕ . Bronchioloalveolar subtype: grows along alveolar septa → apparent "thickening" of alveolar walls. Tall, columnar cells containing mucus. |
| **Squamous cell carcinoma** | Central | Hilar mass  arising from bronchus; cavitation; cigarettes; hypercalcemia (produces PTHrP). | Keratin pearls  and intercellular bridges (desmosomes). |
| **Large cell carcinoma** | Peripheral | Highly anaplastic undifferentiated tumor. Strong association with tobacco smoking. May produce hCG → gynecomastia (en**larg**ed breasts). Less responsive to chemotherapy; removed surgically. Poor prognosis. | Pleomorphic **giant** cells . |
| **Bronchial carcinoid tumor** | Central or peripheral | Excellent prognosis; metastasis rare. Symptoms due to mass effect (wheezing) or carcinoid syndrome (flushing, diarrhea). | Nests of neuroendocrine cells; chromogranin A ⊕. |

**Pancoast tumor**

Also called superior sulcus tumor. Carcinoma that occurs in the apex of lung  may cause Pancoast syndrome by invading/compressing local structures.

Compression of locoregional structures may cause array of findings:
- Recurrent laryngeal nerve → hoarseness
- Stellate ganglion → Horner syndrome (ipsilateral ptosis, miosis, anhidrosis)
- Superior vena cava → SVC syndrome
- Brachiocephalic vein → brachiocephalic syndrome (unilateral symptoms)
- Brachial plexus → shoulder pain, sensorimotor deficits (eg, atrophy of intrinsic muscles of the hand)
- Phrenic nerve → hemidiaphragm paralysis (hemidiaphragm elevation on CXR)

**Superior vena cava syndrome**

Obstruction of the SVC (eg, thrombus, tumor) impairs blood drainage from the head ("facial plethora"; note blanching after fingertip pressure in ), neck (jugular venous distension, laryngeal/pharyngeal edema), and upper extremities (edema). Commonly caused by malignancy (eg, mediastinal mass, Pancoast tumor) and thrombosis from indwelling catheters. Medical emergency. Can raise intracranial pressure (if obstruction is severe) → headaches, dizziness, ↑ risk of aneurysm/rupture of intracranial arteries.

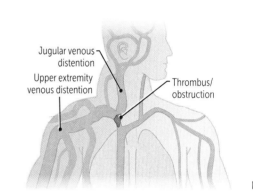

Jugular venous distention
Upper extremity venous distention
Thrombus/obstruction

---

▶ **RESPIRATORY—PHARMACOLOGY**

| **H₁-blockers** | Also called antihistamines. Reversible inhibitors of H₁ histamine receptors. May function as neutral antagonists or inverse agonists. | |
|---|---|---|
| **First generation** | Diphenhydramine, dimenhydrinate, chlorpheniramine, doxylamine. | Names usually contain "-en/-ine" or "-en/-ate." |
| CLINICAL USE | Allergy, motion sickness, vomiting in pregnancy, sleep aid. | |
| ADVERSE EFFECTS | Sedation, antimuscarinic, anti-α-adrenergic. | |
| **Second generation** | Loratadine, fexofenadine, desloratadine, cetirizine. | Names usually end in "-adine." Setirizine (cetirizine) is second-generation agent. |
| CLINICAL USE | Allergy. | |
| ADVERSE EFFECTS | Far less sedating than 1st generation because of ↓ entry into CNS. | |

---

**Dextromethorphan**

Antitussive (antagonizes NMDA glutamate receptors can act as a hallucinogenic dissociative agent similar to ketamine at high doses (and may be combined with bupropion as a fast acting antidepressant). Synthetic codeine analog. Has mild opioid effect when used in excess. Naloxone can be given for overdose. Mild abuse potential. May cause serotonin syndrome if combined with other serotonergic agents.

## Pseudoephedrine, phenylephrine

| | |
|---|---|
| MECHANISM | Activation of α-adrenergic receptors in nasal mucosa → local vasoconstriction. |
| CLINICAL USE | Reduce hyperemia, edema (used as nasal decongestants); open obstructed eustachian tubes. |
| ADVERSE EFFECTS | Hypertension. Rebound congestion (rhinitis medicamentosa) if used more than 4–6 days. Associated with tachyphylaxis. Can also cause CNS stimulation/anxiety (pseudoephedrine). |

## Pulmonary hypertension drugs

| DRUG | MECHANISM | CLINICAL NOTES |
|---|---|---|
| Endothelin receptor antagonists | Competitively antagonizes endothelin-1 receptors → ↓ pulmonary vascular resistance. | Hepatotoxic (monitor LFTs). Example: bosentan. |
| PDE-5 inhibitors | Inhibits PDE-5 → ↑ cGMP → prolonged vasodilatory effect of NO. | Also used to treat erectile dysfunction. Contraindicated when taking nitroglycerin or other nitrates (due to risk of severe hypotension). Example: sildenafil. |
| Prostacyclin analogs | $PGI_2$ (prostacyclin) with direct vasodilatory effects on pulmonary and systemic arterial vascular beds. Inhibits platelet aggregation. | Adverse effects: flushing, jaw pain. Examples: epoprostenol, iloprost. |

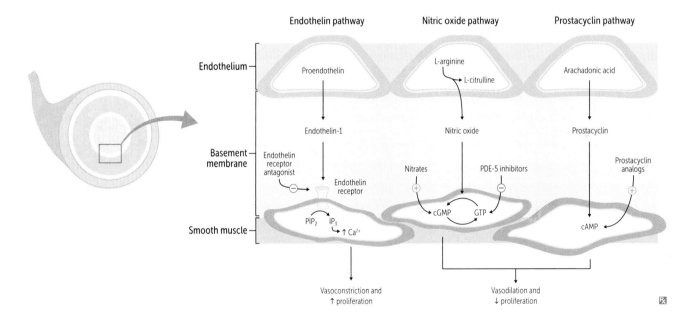

| | |
|---|---|
| **Asthma drugs** | Bronchoconstriction is mediated by (1) inflammatory processes and (2) parasympathetic tone; therapy is directed at these 2 pathways. |
| **Inhaled β₂-agonists** | **Albuterol, salmeterol, formoterol**—relax bronchial smooth muscle. Can cause tremor, arrhythmia. Albuterol is short-acting, used for acute symptoms. Salmeterol and formoterol are long-acting. |
| **Inhaled or oral glucocorticoids** | **Fluticasone, budesonide**—inhibit the synthesis of virtually all cytokines. Inactivate NF-κB, the transcription factor that induces production of TNF-α and other inflammatory agents. 1st-line therapy for chronic asthma. Use a spacer or rinse mouth after use to prevent oral thrush. |
| **Muscarinic antagonists** | **Tiotropium, ipratropium**—competitively block muscarinic receptors, preventing bronchoconstriction. Also used for COPD. Tiotropium is long acting. |
| **Antileukotrienes** | **Montelukast, zafirlukast**—block leukotriene receptors (CysLT1). Especially good for aspirin-induced and exercise-induced asthma.<br>**Zileuton**—5-lipoxygenase inhibitor. ↓ conversion of arachidonic acid to leukotrienes. Hepatotoxic. |
| **Anti-IgE monoclonal therapy** | **Omalizumab**—binds mostly unbound serum IgE and blocks binding to FcεRI. Used in allergic asthma with ↑ IgE levels resistant to inhaled glucocorticoids and long-acting β₂-agonists. |
| **Methylxanthines** | **Theophylline**—likely causes bronchodilation by inhibiting phosphodiesterase → ↑ cAMP levels due to ↓ cAMP hydrolysis. Limited use due to narrow therapeutic index (cardiotoxicity, neurotoxicity); metabolized by cytochrome P-450. Blocks actions of adenosine. |
| **PDE-4 Inhibitors** | **Roflumilast**—inhibits phosphodiesterase → ↑ cAMP → bronchodilation, ↓ airway inflammation. Used in COPD to reduce exacerbations. |
| **Chromones** | **Cromolyn**—prevents mast cell degranulation. Prevents acute asthma symptoms. Rarely used. |
| **Anti-IL-5 monoclonal therapy** | Prevents eosinophil differentiation, maturation, activation, and survival mediated by IL-5 stimulation. For maintenance therapy in severe eosinophilic asthma.<br>**Mepolizumab, reslizumab**—against IL-5. **Benralizumab**—against IL-5 receptor α. |

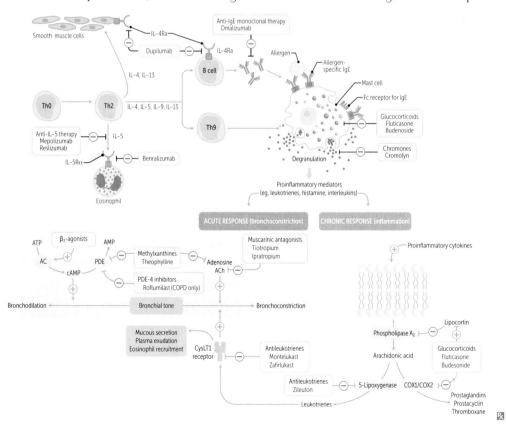

# Rapid Review

*"Study without thought is vain: thought without study is dangerous."*
—Confucius

*"It is better, of course, to know useless things than to know nothing."*
—Lucius Annaeus Seneca

*"For every complex problem there is an answer that is clear, simple, and wrong."*
—H. L. Mencken

The following tables represent a collection of high-yield associations between diseases and their clinical findings, treatments, and key associations. They can be quickly reviewed in the days before the exam.

We have added a high-yield Pathophysiology of Important Diseases section for review of disease mechanisms and removed the Classic/Relevant Treatments section to accommodate the change in focus of the USMLE from pharmacology to pathophysiology.

## ▶ PATHOPHYSIOLOGY OF IMPORTANT DISEASES

| CONDITION | MECHANISM | PAGE |
|---|---|---|
| Lesch-Nyhan syndrome | Absent HGPRT → ↑ de novo purine synthesis → ↑ uric acid production | 35 |
| β-thalassemia | Mutation at splice site or promoter sequences → retained intron in mRNA | 38, 424 |
| Lynch syndrome | Failure of mismatch repair during the S phase → microsatellite instability | 37, 395 |
| I-cell disease | N-acetylglucosaminyl-1-phosphotransferase defect → Golgi mediated mannose residues phosphorylation failure (↓ mannose-6-phosphate) → ↑ cellular debris in lysosomes | 45 |
| Osteogenesis imperfecta | Type 1 collagen defect due to inability to form triple helices; mutation in COL1A1 and COL1A2 genes | 49 |
| Menkes disease | Defective ATP7A protein → impaired copper absorption and transport → ↓ lysyl oxidase activity → ↓ collagen cross-linking | 49 |
| Marfan syndrome | FBN1 mutation on chromosome 15 → defective fibrillin (normally forms sheath around elastin) | 50 |
| Prader-Willi syndrome | Uniparental disomy or imprinting leading to silencing of maternal gene. Disease expressed when paternal allele deleted or mutated | 56 |
| Angelman syndrome | Silenced paternal gene leading to mutation, lack of expression, or deletion of UBE3A on maternal chromosome 15 | 56 |
| Cystic fibrosis | Autosomal recessive ΔF508 deletion in CFTR gene on chromosome 7 → impaired ATP-gated Cl⁻ channel (secretes Cl⁻ in lungs and GI tract and reabsorbs Cl⁻ in sweat glands) | 58 |
| Duchenne muscular dystrophy | Dystrophin gene frameshift mutations → loss of anchoring protein to ECM (dystrophin) → myonecrosis | 59 |
| Myotonic dystrophy | CTG trinucleotide repeat expansion in DMPK gene → abnormal expression of myotonin protein kinase → myotonia | 59 |
| Fragile X syndrome | CGG trinucleotide repeat in FMR1 gene → hypermethylation → ↓ expression | 60 |
| Bitot spots in vitamin A deficiency | ↓ differentiation of epithelial cells into specialized tissue → squamous metaplasia | 64 |
| Wernicke encephalopathy in alcoholic patient given glucose | Thiamine deficiency → impaired glucose breakdown → ATP depletion worsened by glucose infusion | 64 |
| Pellagra in malignant carcinoid syndrome | Tryptophan is diverted towards serotonin synthesis by tumor → $B_3$ deficiency ($B_3$ is derived from tryptophan) | 65 |
| Kwashiorkor | Protein malnutrition → ↓ oncotic pressure (→ edema), ↓ apolipoprotein synthesis (→ liver fatty change) | 69 |
| Lactic acidosis, fasting hypoglycemia, hepatic steatosis in alcoholism | ↑ NADH/NAD⁺ ratio due to ethanol metabolism | 70 |
| Aspirin-induced hyperthermia | ↑ permeability of mitochondrial membrane → ↓ proton [H⁺] gradient and ↑ $O_2$ consumption → uncoupling | 76 |
| Hereditary fructose intolerance | Aldolase B deficiency → Fructose-1-phosphate accumulates → ↓ available phosphate → inhibition of glycogenolysis and gluconeogenesis | 78 |
| Classic galactosemia | Galactose-1-phosphate uridyltransferase deficiency → accumulation of toxic substances (eg, galactitol in eyes) | 78 |

| CONDITION | MECHANISM | PAGE |
|---|---|---|
| Cataracts, retinopathy, peripheral neuropathy in DM | Lens, retina, Schwann cells lack sorbitol dehydrogenase → intracellular sorbitol accumulation → osmotic damage | 79 |
| Recurrent *Neisseria* bacteremia | Terminal complement deficiencies (C5–C9) → failure of MAC formation | 105 |
| Hereditary angioedema | C1 esterase inhibitor deficiency → unregulated activation of kallikrein → ↑ bradykinin | 105 |
| Paroxysmal nocturnal hemoglobinuria | *PIGA* gene mutation → ↓ GPI anchors for complement inhibitors (DAF/CD55, MIRL/CD59) → complement-mediated intravascular hemolysis | 105 |
| Type I hypersensitivity | Immediate (minutes): antigen cross links IgE on mast cells → degranulation → release of histamine and tryptase <br> Late (hours): mast cells secrete chemokines (attract eosinophils) and leukotrienes → inflammation, tissue damage | 110 |
| Type II hypersensitivity | Antibodies bind to cell-surface antigens → cellular destruction, inflammation, cellular dysfunction | 110 |
| Type III hypersensitivity | Antigen-antibody complexes → activate complement → attracts neutrophils | 111 |
| Type IV hypersensitivity | T cell-mediated (no antibodies involved). CD8$^+$ directly kills target cells, CD4$^+$ releases cytokines | 111 |
| Acute hemolytic transfusion reaction | Type II hypersensitivity reaction against donor RBCs (usually ABO antigens) | 112 |
| X-linked (Bruton) agammaglobulinemia | Defect in *BTK* gene (tyrosine kinase) → no B-cell maturation → absent B cells in peripheral blood, ↓ Ig of all classes | 114 |
| DiGeorge syndrome | 22q11 microdeletion → failure to develop 3rd and 4th branchial (pharyngeal) pouches | 114 |
| Hyper-IgM syndrome | Defective CD40L on Th cells → class switching defect | 115 |
| Leukocyte adhesion deficiency (type 1) | LFA-1 integrin (CD18) defect → impaired phagocyte migration and chemotaxis | 115 |
| Chédiak-Higashi syndrome | *LYST* mutation → microtubule dysfunction → phagosome-lysosome fusion defect | 115 |
| Chronic granulomatous disease | NADPH oxidase defect → ↓ ROS, ↓ respiratory burst in neutrophils | 115 |
| *Candida* infection in immunodeficiency | ↓ granulocytes (systemic), ↓ T cells (local) | 114, 116 |
| Graft-versus-host disease | Type IV hypersensitivity reaction; HLA mismatch → donor T cells attack host cells | 117 |
| Recurrent *S aureus, Serratia, B cepacia* infections in CGD | Catalase ⊕ organisms degrade $H_2O_2$ before it can be converted to microbicidal products by the myeloperoxidase system | 126 |
| Hemolytic uremic syndrome | Shiga/Shiga-like toxins inactivate 60S ribosome → ↑ cytokine release | 130, 432 |
| Tetanus | Tetanospasmin prevents release of inhibitory neurotransmitters (GABA and glycine) from Renshaw cells | 130 |
| Botulism | Toxin (protease) cleaves SNARE → ↓ neurotransmitter (ACh) release at NMJ | 130 |
| Gas gangrene | Alpha toxin (phospholipase/lecithinase) degrades phospholipids → myonecrosis | 131 |
| Toxic shock syndrome, scarlet fever | TSST-1 and erythrogenic exotoxin A (scarlet) cross-link β region of TCR to MHC class II on APCs outside of antigen binding site → ↑↑ IL-1, IL-2, IFN-γ, TNF-α | 131 |

| CONDITION | MECHANISM | PAGE |
|---|---|---|
| Shock and DIC by gram ⊖ bacteria | Lipid A of LPS → macrophage activation (TLR4/CD14), complement activation, tissue factor activation | 131 |
| Prosthetic device infection by *S epidermidis* | Biofilm production | 126, 133 |
| Endocarditis 2° to *S sanguinis* | Dextrans (biofilm) production that bind to fibrin-platelet aggregates on damaged heart valves | 126, 134 |
| Pseudomembranous colitis 2° to *C difficile* | Toxins A and B damage enterocytes → watery diarrhea | 136 |
| Diphtheria | Exotoxin inhibits protein synthesis via ADP-ribosylation of EF-2 | 137 |
| Virulence of *M tuberculosis* | Cord factor activates macrophages (promoting granuloma formation), induces release of TNF-α; sulfatides (surface glycolipids) inhibit phagolysosomal fusion | 138 |
| Tuberculoid leprosy | Th1 immune response → mild symptoms | 139 |
| No effective vaccine for N *gonorrhoeae* | Antigenic variation of pilus proteins | 140 |
| Cystitis and pyelonephritis by *E coli* | Fimbriae (P pili) | 143 |
| Pneumonia, neonatal meningitis by *E coli* | K capsule | 143 |
| Chlamydiae resistance to β-lactam antibiotics | Lack of classic peptidoglycan due to reduced muramic acid | 146 |
| Influenza pandemics | RNA segment reassortment → antigenic shift | 166 |
| Influenza epidemics | Mutations in hemagglutinin, neuraminidase → antigenic drift | 166 |
| CNS invasion by rabies | Binds to ACh receptors → retrograde transport (dynein) | 169 |
| HIV infection | Virus binds CD4 along with CCR5 on macrophages (early), or CXCR4 on T cells (late) | 173 |
| Granuloma | Macrophages present antigens to CD4$^+$ and secrete IL-12 → CD4$^+$ differentiation into Th1 which secrete IFN-γ → macrophage activation | 213 |
| Limitless replicative potential of cancer cells | Reactivation of telomerase → maintains and lengthens telomeres → prevention of chromosome shortening and aging | 217 |
| Tissue invasion by cancer | ↓ E-cadherin function → ↓ intercellular junctions → basement membrane and ECM degradation by metalloproteinases → cell attachment to ECM proteins (laminin, fibronectin) → locomotion → vascular dissemination | 217 |
| Persistent truncus arteriosus | Failure of aorticopulmonary septum formation | 302 |
| D-transposition of great arteries | Failure of the aorticopulmonary septum to spiral | 302 |
| Tet spells in tetralogy of Fallot | Crying, fever, exercise → ↑ RV outflow obstruction → ↑ right-to-left flow across VSD; squatting → ↑ SVR → ↓ right-to-left shunt → ↓ cyanosis | 302 |
| Eisenmenger syndrome | Uncorrected left-to-right shunt → ↑ pulmonary blood flow → remodeling of vasculature → pulmonary hypertension → RVH → right to left shunting | 303 |
| Atherosclerosis | Endothelial cell dysfunction → macrophage and LDL accumulation → foam cell formation → fatty streaks → smooth muscle cell migration, extracellular matrix deposition → fibrous plaque → complex atheromas | 305 |
| Thoracic aortic aneurysm | Cystic medial degeneration | 306 |
| Myocardial infarction | Rupture of coronary artery atherosclerotic plaque → acute thrombosis | 308 |

| CONDITION | MECHANISM | PAGE |
|---|---|---|
| Non–ST-segment elevation MI | Subendocardial infarcts (subendocardium vulnerable to ischemia) | 308 |
| ST-segment elevation MI | Transmural infarcts | 308 |
| Death within 0-24 hours post MI | Ventricular arrhythmia | 309, 314 |
| Death or shock within 3-14 days post MI | Macrophage-mediated ruptures: papillary muscle (2-7 days), interventricular septum (3-5 days), free wall (5-14 days) | 309, 314 |
| Wolff-Parkinson-White | Abnormal accessory pathway from atria to ventricle bypasses the AV node → ventricles begin to partially depolarize earlier → delta wave. Reentrant circuit → supraventricular tachycardia | 311 |
| Hypertrophic obstructive cardiomyopathy | Sarcomeric proteins gene mutations (myosin binding protein C and β-myosin heavy chain) → concentric hypertrophy (sarcomeres added in parallel). Death due to arrhythmia | 315 |
| Syncope, dyspnea in HOCM | Asymmetric septal hypertrophy, systolic anterior motion of mitral valve → outflow obstruction | 315 |
| Hypovolemic shock | ↓ preload → ↓ CO | 317 |
| Cardiogenic shock | ↓ CO due to left heart dysfunction | 317 |
| Distributive shock | ↓ SVR (afterload) | 317 |
| Rheumatic fever | Antibodies against M protein cross react with self antigens; type II hypersensitivity reaction | 319 |
| Most common form of congenital adrenal hyperplasia | 21-hydroxylase deficiency→ ↓ mineralocorticoids, ↓ cortisol, ↑ sex hormones, ↑ 17-hydroxyprogesterone | 339 |
| Heat intolerance, weight loss in hyperthyroidism | ↑ $Na^+$-$K^+$ ATPase → ↑ basal metabolic rate → ↑ calorigenesis | 344 |
| Myxedema in hypothyroidism | ↑ GAGs in interstitial space → ↑ osmotic pressure → ↑ water retention | 344 |
| Graves ophthalmopathy | Lymphocytic infiltration, fibroblast secretion of GAGs → ↑ osmotic muscle swelling, inflammation | 346 |
| 1° hyperparathyroidism | Parathyroid adenoma or hyperplasia → ↑ PTH | 349 |
| 2° hyperparathyroidism | ↓ $Ca^{2+}$ and/or ↑ $PO_4^{3-}$ → parathyroid hyperplasia → ↑ PTH, ↑ ALP | 349 |
| Euvolemic hyponatremia in SIADH | ↑ ADH → water retention → ↓ aldosterone, ↑ ANB, ↑ BNP → ↑ urinary $Na^+$ secretion | 342 |
| Small/large vessel disease in DM | Nonenzymatic glycation of proteins; small vessels → hyaline arteriosclerosis; large vessels → atherosclerosis | 350 |
| Diabetic ketoacidosis | ↓ Insulin or ↑ insulin requirement → ↑ fat breakdown → ↑ free fatty acids → ↑ ketogenesis | 351 |
| Hyperosmolar hyperglycemic state | Hyperglycemia → ↑ serum osmolality, excessive osmotic diuresis | 351 |
| Zollinger-Ellison syndrome | Gastrin-secreting tumor (gastrinoma) of pancreas or duodenum → recurrent ulcers in duodenum/jejunum and malabsorption | 357 |
| Duodenal atresia | Failure to recanalize | 366 |
| Jejunal/ileal atresia | Disruption of SMA → ischemic necrosis of fetal intestine | 366 |
| Superior mesenteric artery syndrome | Diminished mesenteric fat → compression of transverse (third) portion of duodenum by SMA and aorta | 370 |
| Achalasia | Loss of postganglionic inhibitory neurons (contain NO and VIP) in myenteric plexus → failure of LES relaxation | 383 |

| CONDITION | MECHANISM | PAGE |
|---|---|---|
| Barrett esophagus | Chronic GERD → replacement (metaplasia) of nonkeratinized stratified squamous epithelium with intestinal epithelium (nonciliated columnar with goblet cells) | 385 |
| Acute gastritis 2° to NSAIDs | ↓ $PGE_2$ → ↓ gastric protection | 386 |
| Celiac disease | Autoimmune-mediated intolerance of gliadin (found in wheat) → malabsorption (distal duodenum, proximal jejunum), steatorrhea | 388 |
| Fistula formation in Crohn | Transmural inflammation | 389 |
| Meckel diverticulum | Persistence of the vitelline (omphalomesenteric) duct | 391 |
| Hirschsprung disease | Loss of function mutation in *RET* → failure of neural crest migration → lack of ganglion cells/enteric nervous plexuses in distal colon | 391 |
| Adenoma-carcinoma sequence in colorectal cancer | Loss of *APC* (↓ intercellular adhesion, ↑ proliferation) → *KRAS* mutation (unregulated intracellular signaling) → loss of tumor suppressor genes (*TP53, DCC*) | 395 |
| Fibrosis in cirrhosis | Stellate cells | 396 |
| Reye syndrome | Aspirin ↓ β-oxidation by reversible inhibition of mitochondrial enzymes | 398 |
| Hepatic encephalopathy | Cirrhosis → portosystemic shunts → ↓ $NH_3$ metabolism | 399 |
| $\alpha_1$-antitrypsin deficiency | Misfolded proteins aggregate in hepatocellular ER → cirrhosis. In lungs, ↓ $\alpha_1$-antitrypsin → uninhibited elastase in alveoli → panacinar emphysema | 400 |
| Wilson disease | Mutated hepatocyte copper-transporting ATPase (*ATP7B* on chromosome 13) → ↓ copper incorporation into apoceruloplasmin, excretion into bile → ↓ serum ceruloplasmin, ↑ copper in tissues and urine | 402 |
| Hemochromatosis | *HFE* mutation on chromosome 6 → ↓ hepcidin production, ↑ intestinal absorption → iron overload (↑ ferritin,↑ iron, ↓ TIBC → ↑ transferrin saturation) | 402 |
| Gallstone ileus | Fistula between gallbladder and GI tract → stone enters GI lumen → obstructing ileocecal valve (narrowest point) | 403 |
| Acute cholangitis | Biliary tree obstruction → stasis/bacterial overgrowth | 403 |
| Acute pancreatitis | Autodigestion of pancreas by pancreatic enzymes | 404 |
| Rh hemolytic disease of the newborn | Rh ⊖ mother form antibodies (maternal anti-D IgG) against RBCs of Rh ⊕ fetus | 411 |
| Anemia in lead poisoning | Lead inhibits ferrochelatase and ALA dehydratase → ↓ heme synthesis, ↑ RBC protoporphyrin. | 425 |
| Anemia of chronic disease | Inflammation → ↑ hepcidin → ↓ release of iron from macrophages, ↓ iron absorption from gut | 427 |
| G6PD deficiency | Defect in G6PD → ↓ NADPH → ↓ reduced glutathione → ↑ RBC susceptibility to oxidant stress | 428 |
| Sickle cell anemia | Point mutation → substitution of glutamic acid with valine in β chain → low $O_2$, high altitude, acidosis precipitates sickling (deoxygenated HbS polymerizes) → anemia, vaso-occlusive disease | 428 |
| Bernard-Soulier syndrome | ↓ GpIb → ↓ platelet-to-vWF adhesion | 432 |
| Glanzmann thrombasthenia | ↓ GpIIb/IIIa → ↓ platelet-to-platelet aggregation, defective platelet plug formation | 432 |
| Thrombotic thrombocytopenic purpura | ↓ *ADAMTS13* (a vWF metalloprotease) → ↓ degradation of vWF multimers → ↑ platelet adhesion and aggregation (microthrombi formation) | 432 |

| CONDITION | MECHANISM | PAGE |
|---|---|---|
| von Willebrand disease | ↓ vWF → ↓ platelet-to-vWF adhesion, possibly ↑ PTT (vWF protects factor VIII) | 433 |
| Factor V Leiden | Mutant factor V (Arg506Gln) that is resistant to degradation by protein C | 433 |
| Axillary nerve injury | Fractured surgical neck or anterior dislocation of humerus → flattened deltoid | 450 |
| Radial nerve injury ("Saturday night palsy") | Compression of axilla (use of crutches), midshaft humerus fracture, repetitive pronation/supination of forearm (use of screwdriver) → wrist/finger drop, decreased grip strength | 450 |
| Median nerve injury (Ape's hand/Pope's blessing) | Proximal lesion: supracondylar fracture → loss of sensation over thenar eminence, dorsal and palmar aspect of lateral 3½ fingers<br>Distal lesion: carpal tunnel syndrome | 450 |
| Ulnar nerve injury | Proximal lesion: fractured medial epicondyle → radial deviation of wrist on flexion<br>Distal lesion: fractured hook of hamate (fall on outstretched hand) → ulnar claw on digital extension | 450 |
| Erb palsy (waiter's tip) | Traction/tear of C5-C6 roots during delivery on the neck of the infant, and due to trauma in adults | 452 |
| Klumpke palsy | Traction/tear of C8-T1 roots during delivery on the arm of the infant, and on trying to grab a branch in adults | 452 |
| Winged scapula | Injury to long thoracic nerve (C5-C7), like on axillary node dissection during mastectomy | 452 |
| Common peroneal nerve injury | Trauma on lateral aspect of leg or fracture of fibular neck → foot drop with steppage gait | 457 |
| Superior gluteal nerve injury | Iatrogenic injury during IM injection at gluteal region → Trendelenburg sign: lesion contralateral to side of hip that drops due to adductor weakness | 457 |
| Pudendal nerve injury | Injury during horseback riding or prolonged cycling; can be blocked during delivery at the ischial spine → ↓ sensation in perineal and genital area ± fecal/urinary incontinence | 457 |
| Radial head subluxation (nursemaid's elbow) | Due to sudden pull on arm (in children; head slips out of immature annular ligament) | 466 |
| Slipped capital femoral epiphysis | Obese young adolescent with hip/knee pain. Increased axial force on femoral head → epiphysis displaces relative to femoral neck like a scoop of ice cream slips off a cone | 466 |
| Achondroplasia | Constitutive activation of FGFR3 → ↓ chondrocyte proliferation → failure of endochondral ossification → short limbs | 467 |
| Osteoporosis | ↑ osteoclast activity → ↓ bone mass secondary to 2° to ↓ estrogen levels, old age, and long term use of drugs like steroids | 467 |
| Osteopetrosis | Carbonic anhydrase II mutations → ↓ ability of osteoclasts to generate acidic environment → ↓ bone resorption leading to dense bones prone to fracture, pancytopenia (↓ marrow space) | 468 |
| Osteitis deformans (Paget disease) | ↑ osteoclast activity followed by ↑ osteoblast activity → poor quality bone formed that is prone to fractures | 468 |
| Osteoarthritis | Mechanical degeneration of articular cartilage causing inflammation with inadequate repair and osteophyte formation | 472 |
| Rheumatoid arthritis | Autoimmune inflammation due to HLA-DR4 causing pannus formation → errodes articular cartilage and bone. Type III hypersensitivity reaction | 111, 472 |

| CONDITION | MECHANISM | PAGE |
|---|---|---|
| Sjogren syndrome | Autoimmune type IV hypersensitivity reaction leading to lymphocyte mediated damage of exocrine glands | 474 |
| Systemic lupus erythematosus | Predominantly a type III hypersensitivity reaction with decreased clearance of immune complexes. Hematologic manifestations are a type II hypersensitivity reaction | 476 |
| Blindness in giant cell (temporal) arteritis | Ophthalmic artery occlusion | 478 |
| Myasthenia gravis | Autoantibodies to postsynaptic nicotinic (ACh) receptors | 480 |
| Lambert-Eaton myasthenic syndrome | Autoantibodies to presynaptic calcium channels → ↓ ACh release | 480 |
| Albinism | Normal melanocyte number, ↓ melanin production | 484 |
| Vitiligo | Autoimmune destruction of melanocytes | 484 |
| Atopic dermatitis | Epidermal barrier dysfunction, genetic factors (ie, loss-of-function mutations in the filaggrin [FLG] gene), immune dysregulation, altered skin microbiome, environmental triggers of inflammation | 485 |
| Allergic contact dermatitis | Type IV hypersensitivity reaction. During the sensitization phase, Allergen activates Th1 cells → memory CD4+ cells and CD8+ form. Upon reexposure → CD4+ cells release cytokines and CD8+ cells kill targeted cells | 485 |
| Pemphigus vulgaris | Type II hypersensitivity reaction. IgG autoantibodies form against desmoglein 1 and 3 in desmosomes → separation of keratinocytes in stratum spinosum from stratum basale | 489 |
| Bullous pemphigoid | Type II hypersensitivity reaction. IgG autoantibodies against hemidesmosomes → separation of epidermis from dermis | 489 |
| Spina bifida occulta, meningocele, myelomeningocele, myeloschisis | Failure of caudal neuropore to fuse by 4th week of development | 501 |
| Anencephaly | Failure of rostral neuropore to close → no forebrain, open calvarium | 501 |
| Holoprosencephaly | Failure of the forebrain (prosencephalon) to divide into 2 cerebral hemispheres; developmental field defect typically occurring at weeks 3-4 of development; associated with SHH mutations | 501 |
| Lissencephaly | Failure of neuronal migration → smooth brain surface lacking sulci and gyri | 501 |
| Chiari I malformation | Downward displacement of cerebellar tonsils inferior to foramen magnum | 502 |
| Chiari II malformation | Herniation of cerebellum (vermis and tonsils) and medulla through foramen magnum → noncommunicating hydrocephalus | 502 |
| Dandy-Walker malformation | Agenesis of cerebellar vermis → cystic enlargement of 4th ventricle that fills the enlarged posterior fossa; associated with noncommunicating hydrocephalus and spina bifida | 502 |
| Syringomyelia | Fluid-filled, gliosis-lined cavity within spinal cord, associated with Chiari I malformation (low-lying cerebellar tonsils), less commonly with infections, tumors, trauma; damages crossing spinothalamic tract | 502 |
| Gerstmann syndrome | Lesion in the dominant parietal cortex → agraphia, acalculia, finger agnosia, left-right disorientation | 524 |
| Hemispatial neglect syndrome | Lesion in the nondominant parietal cortex → agnosia of contralateral side | 524 |
| Klüver-Bucy syndrome | Bilateral lesions in the amygdala; seen in HSV-1 encephalitis → disinhibition, including hyperphagia, hypersexuality, hyperorality | 524 |

| CONDITION | MECHANISM | PAGE |
|---|---|---|
| Parinaud syndrome (inability to move eyes up and down) | Lesion in the dorsal midbrain; often due to pineal gland tumors | 524 |
| Cerebral edema | Fluid accumulation in the brain parenchyma → ↑ ICP; may be cytotoxic (intracellular fluid accumulation due to osmotic shift; associated with early ischemia, hyperammonemia, SIADH) or vasogenic (extracellular fluid accumulation due to increased permeability of BBB; associated with late ischemia, trauma, hemorrhage, inflammation, tumors) | 525 |
| Aphasia | Stroke in dominant (usually left) hemisphere, in either the superior temporal gyrus of temporal lobe (Wernicke; receptive aphasia) or inferior frontal gyrus of frontal lobe (Broca; expressive aphasia) | 526, 529 |
| Locked-in syndrome (loss of horizontal, but not vertical, eye movements) | Stroke of the basilar artery | 526 |
| Lateral pontine syndrome | Stroke of the anterior inferior cerebellar artery | 526 |
| Lateral medullary (Wallenberg) syndrome | Stroke of the posterior inferior cerebellar artery | 527 |
| Medial medullary syndrome | Stroke of the anterior spinal artery | 527 |
| Neonatal intraventricular hemorrhage | Reduced glial fiber support and impaired autoregulation of BP in premature infants → bleeding into the ventricles, originating in the germinal matrix (a highly vascularized layer within the subventricular zone) | 527 |
| Epidural hematoma | Rupture of middle meningeal artery, often secondary to skull fracture involving the pterion | 528 |
| Subdural hematoma | Rupture of bridging veins; acute (traumatic, high-energy impact, sudden deceleration injury) or chronic (mild trauma, cerebral atrophy, ↑ age, chronic alcohol overuse, shaken baby syndrome) | 528 |
| Subarachnoid hemorrhage | Trauma, rupture of aneurysm (such as a saccular aneurysm), or arteriovenous malformation → bleeding | 528 |
| Intraparenchymal hemorrhage | Systemic hypertension (most often occur in the putamen of basal ganglia, thalamus, pons, and cerebellum), amyloid angiopathy, arteriovenous malformation, vasculitis, neoplasm, or secondary to reperfusion injury in ischemic stroke → bleeding | 528 |
| Phantom limb pain | Most commonly following amputation → reorganization of primary somatosensory cortex → sensation of pain in a limb that is no longer present | 529 |
| Diffuse axonal injury | Traumatic shearing of white matter tracts during rapid acceleration and/or deceleration of the brain (eg, motor vehicle accident) → multiple punctate hemorrhages involving white matter tracts → neurologic injury, often causing coma or persistent vegetative state | 529 |
| Conduction aphasia | Damage to the arcuate fasciculus | 529 |
| Global aphasia | Damage to both Broca (inferior frontal gyrus of frontal lobe) and Wernicke (superior temporal gyrus of temporal lobe) areas | 529 |
| Heat stroke | Inability of body to dissipate heat (eg, exertion) → CNS dysfunction (eg, confusion), rhabdomyolysis, acute kidney injury, ARDS, DIC | 530 |
| Migraine | Irritation of CN V, meninges, or blood vessels (release of vasoactive neuropeptides [eg, substance P, calcitonin gene-related peptide]) | 532 |
| Parkinson disease | Loss of dopaminergic neurons of substantia nigra pars compacta | 534 |

| CONDITION | MECHANISM | PAGE |
|---|---|---|
| Huntington disease | Trinucleotide (CAG) repeat expansion in huntingtin (*HTT*) gene on chromosome 4 → toxic gain of function → atrophy of caudate and putamen with ex vacuo ventriculomegaly → ↑ dopamine, ↓ GABA, ↓ ACh in brain → neuronal death via glutamate excitotoxicity via NMDA receptor binding | 534 |
| Alzheimer disease | Widespread cortical atrophy, narrowing of gyri and widening of sulci; senile plaques in gray matter composed of beta-amyloid core (formed by cleavage of amyloid precursor protein); neurofibrillary tangles composed of intracellular, hyperphosphorylated tau protein; Hirano bodies (intracellular eosinophilic proteinaceous rods in hippocampus) | 534 |
| Frontotemporal dementia | Frontotemporal lobe degeneration → ↓ executive function and behavioral inhibition | 534 |
| Vascular dementia | Multiple arterial infarcts and/or chronic ischemia | 535 |
| HIV-associated dementia | Secondary to diffuse gray matter and subcortical atrophy | 535 |
| Idiopathic intracranial hypertension | Increased ICP, associated with dural venous sinus stenosis; impaired optic nerve axoplasmic flow → papilledema | 536 |
| Communicating hydrocephalus | Reduced CSF absorption by arachnoid granulations (eg, arachnoid scarring post-meningitis) → ↑ ICP, papilledema, herniation | 536 |
| Normal pressure hydrocephalus | Idiopathic, CSF pressure elevated only episodically, no ↑ subarachnoid space volume; expansion of ventricles distorts the fibers of the corona radiata | 536 |
| Noncommunicating hydrocephalus | Structural blockage of CSF circulation within ventricular system (eg, stenosis of aqueduct of Sylvius, colloid cyst blocking foramen of Monro, tumor) | 536 |
| Ex vacuo ventriculomegaly | Decreased brain tissue and neuronal atrophy → appearance of increased CSF on imaging | 536 |
| Multiple sclerosis | Autoimmune inflammation and demyelination of CNS (brain and spinal cord) → axonal damage | 537 |
| Osmotic demyelination syndrome | Rapid osmotic changes, most commonly iatrogenic correction of hyponatremia but also rapid shifts of other osmolytes (eg, glucose) → massive axonal demyelination in pontine white matter | 538 |
| Acute inflammatory demyelinating polyneuropathy (subtype of Guillain-Barré syndrome) | Autoimmune destruction of Schwann cells via inflammation and demyelination of motor and sensory fibers and peripheral nerves; likely facilitated by molecular mimicry and triggered by inoculations or stress | 538 |
| Charcot-Marie-Tooth disease | Defective production of proteins involved in the structure and function of peripheral nerves or the myelin sheath | 538 |
| Progressive multifocal leukoencephalopathy | Destruction of oligodendrocytes secondary to reactivation of latent JC virus infection → demyelination of CNS | 538 |
| Sturge-Weber syndrome | Somatic mosaicism of an activating mutation in one copy of the *GNAQ* gene → congenital anomaly of neural crest derivatives → capillary vascular malformation, ipsilateral leptomeningeal angioma with calcifications, episcleral hemangioma | 539 |
| Pituitary adenoma | Hyperplasia of only one type of endocrine cells found in pituitary (most commonly from lactotrophs, producing prolactin) | 540 |
| Spinal muscular atrophy | Congenital degeneration of anterior horns *SMN1* mutation → defective snRNP assembly → LMN apoptosis | 544 |
| Amyotrophic lateral sclerosis | Combined UMN and LMN degeneration; familial form associated with *SOD1* mutation | 544 |

| CONDITION | MECHANISM | PAGE |
|---|---|---|
| Tabes dorsalis | Degeneration/demyelination of dorsal columns and roots (in 3° syphilis) → progressive sensory ataxia (impaired proprioception → poor coordination) | 544 |
| Poliomyelitis | Poliovirus infection spreads from lymphoid tissue of oropharynx to small intestine and then to CNS via bloodstream → destruction of cells in anterior horn of spinal cord (LMN death) | 544 |
| Friedreich ataxia | Trinucleotide repeat disorder (GAA) on chromosome 9 in gene that encodes frataxin (iron-binding protein) → impairment in mitochondrial functioning → degeneration of lateral corticospinal tract, spinocerebellar tract, dorsal columns, and dorsal root ganglia | 545 |
| Noise-induced hearing loss | Damage to stereociliated cells in organ of Corti → loss of high-frequency hearing first; sudden extremely loud noises can lead to tympanic membrane rupture → hearing loss | 548 |
| Presbycusis | Destruction of hair cells at the cochlear base (preserved low-frequency hearing at apex) → aging-related progressive bilateral/symmetric sensorineural hearing loss (often of higher frequencies) | 548 |
| Cholesteatoma | Abnormal growth of keratinized squamous epithelium in middle ear; 1° acquired from tympanic membrane retraction pocket; 2° from tympanic membrane perforation | 548 |
| Ménière disease | Increased endolymph in inner ear → vertigo, sensorineural hearing loss, tinnitus and ear fullness | 548 |
| Hyperopia | Eye too short for refractive power of cornea and lens → light focused behind retina | 549 |
| Myopia | Eye too long for refractive power of cornea and lens → light focused in front of retina | 549 |
| Astigmatism | Abnormal curvature of cornea → different refractive power at different axes | 549 |
| Presbyopia | Aging-related impaired accommodation, likely due to primarily due to ↓ lens elasticity | 550 |
| Glaucoma | Optic neuropathy causing progressive vision loss (peripheral → central), usually accompanied by increased intraocular pressure | 551 |
| Open-angle glaucoma | Associated with increased resistance to aqueous humor drainage through trabecular meshwork | 551 |
| Angle-closure glaucoma | Anterior chamber angle is narrowed or closed; associated with anatomic abnormalities (eg, anteriorly displaced lens resting against central iris) → ↓ aqueous flow through pupil → ↑ pressure in posterior chamber → peripheral iris pushed against cornea → obstruction of drainage pathways by the iris | 551 |
| Diabetic retinopathy | Chronic hyperglycemia → ↑ permeability and occlusion of retinal vessels → microaneurysms, hemorrhages (nonproliferative); retinal neovascularization due to chronic hypoxia (proliferative) | 552 |
| Hypertensive retinopathy | Chronic hypertension → spasm, sclerosis, and fibrinoid necrosis of retinal vessels | 552 |
| Retinal artery occlusion | Blockage of central or branch retinal artery usually due to embolism (carotid artery atherosclerosis > cardiogenic); less commonly due to giant cell arteritis | 552 |

| CONDITION | MECHANISM | PAGE |
|---|---|---|
| Retinal vein occlusion | Primary thrombosis → central retinal vein occlusion; secondary thrombosis at arteriovenous crossings (sclerotic arteriole compresses adjacent venule causing turbulent blood flow) → branch retinal vein occlusion | 552 |
| Retinal detachment | Separation of neurosensory retina from underlying retinal pigment epithelium → loss of choroidal blood supply → hypoxia and degeneration of photoreceptors; due to retinal tears (rhegmatogenous) or tractional or exudative (fluid accumulation) (nonrhegmatogenous) | 552 |
| Retinitis pigmentosa | Progressive degeneration of photoreceptors and retinal pigment epithelium | 552 |
| Papilledema | ↑ ICP (eg, secondary to mass effect) → impaired axoplasmic flow in optic nerve → optic disc swelling (usually bilateral) | 552 |
| Relative afferent pupillary defect | Unilateral or asymmetric lesions of afferent limb of pupillary reflex (eg, retina, optic nerve) | 554 |
| Horner syndrome | Lesions along the sympathetic chain: 1st neuron (pontine hemorrhage, lateral medullary syndrome, spinal cord lesion above T1 like Brown-Sequard syndrome or late-stage syringomyelia); 2nd neuron (stellate ganglion compression by Pancoast tumor); 3rd neuron (carotid dissection) | 555 |
| Cavernous sinus syndrome | Secondary to pituitary tumor mass effect, carotid-cavernous fistula, or cavernous sinus thrombosis related to infection (spreads due to lack of valves in dural venous sinuses) | 557 |
| Delirium | Usually secondary to illnesses (eg, CNS disease, infection, trauma, substance use, metabolic/electrolyte imbalance, hemorrhage, urinary/fecal retention), or medications (eg, anticholinergics) | 575 |
| Schizophrenia | Altered dopaminergic activity, ↑ serotonergic activity, ↓ dendritic branching | 577 |
| Distal RTA (type 1) | Inability of $\alpha$-intercalated cells to secrete $H^+$ → no new $HCO_3^-$ generated → metabolic acidosis | 611 |
| Proximal RTA (type 2) | Defective PCT $HCO_3^-$ reabsorption → ↑ excretion of $HCO_3^-$ in urine → metabolic acidosis | 611 |
| Hyperkalemic tubular acidosis (type 4) | Hypoaldosteronism/aldosterone resistance → ↑ $K^+$ → $NH_3$ synthesis in PCT → ↓ $NH_4^+$ excretion | 611 |
| Nephritic syndrome | Glomerular inflammation → GBM damage → loss of RBCs in urine → dysmorphic RBCs, hematuria; ↓ GFR → oliguria, azotemia, ↑ renin release, HTN | 613 |
| Nephrotic syndrome | Podocyte damage → impaired charge barrier → proteinuria; hypoalbuminemia → ↑ hepatic lipogenesis → hypercholesterolemia; antithrombin loss → hypercoagulability; IgG loss → infections | 613 |
| Nephritic-nephrotic syndrome | Severe GBM damage → loss of RBCs in urine + impaired charge barrier → hematuria + proteinuria | 613 |
| Infection-related glomerulonephritis | Type III hypersensitivity reaction with consumptive hypocomplementemia | 614 |
| Alport syndrome | Type IV collagen mutation (X-linked dominant) → irregular thinning and thickening and splitting of GBM → nephritic syndrome | 615 |
| Stress incontinence | Outlet incompetence (urethral hypermobility/intrinsic sphincter deficiency) → leak on ↑ intraabdominal pressure (eg, sneezing, lifting) | 618 |
| Urge incontinence | Detrusor overactivity → leak with urge to void | 618 |
| Overflow incontinence | Incomplete emptying (detrusor underactivity or outlet obstruction) → leak with overfilling | 618 |

| CONDITION | MECHANISM | PAGE |
|---|---|---|
| Prerenal azotemia | ↓ RBF → ↓ GFR → ↑ reabsorption of $Na^+/H_2O$ and urea | 620 |
| Intrinsic renal failure | Patchy necrosis → debris obstructing tubules and fluid backflow → ↓ GFR | 620 |
| Postrenal azotemia | Outflow obstruction (bilateral) | 620 |
| Adnexal torsion | Twisting of ovary/fallopian tube around infundibulopelvic ligament and ovarian ligament → venous/lymphatic blockage → arterial inflow continued → edema → blockade of arterial inflow → necrosis | 643 |
| Preeclampsia | Abnormal placental spiral arteries → endothelial dysfunction, vasoconstriction, ischemia → new-onset HTN with proteinuria | 660 |
| Supine hypotensive syndrome | Supine position → compressed abdominal aorta and IVC by gravid uterus → ↓ placental perfusion and ↓ venous return | 661 |
| Polycystic ovary syndrome | Hyperinsulinemia and/or insulin resistance → altered hypothalamic feedback response → ↑ LH:FSH, ↑ androgens, ↓ rate of follicular maturation → unruptured follicles (cysts) + anovulation | 662 |
| Functional hypothalamic amenorrhea | Severe caloric restriction, ↑ energy expenditure, and/or stress → altered pulsatile GnRH secretion → ↓ LH, FSH, estrogen | 663 |
| Varicocele | Dilated veins in pampiniform plexus due to ↑ venous pressure → enlarged scrotum | 669 |
| Methemoglobin | Oxidized Hb secondary to dapsone, local anesthetics, nitrites → Hb oxidization ($Fe^{2+}$) → ↓ $O_2$ binding but ↑ cyanide affinity → tissue hypoxia | 688 |
| Deep venous thrombosis | Stasis, hypercoagulability, endothelial damage (Virchow triad) → blood clot within deep vein | 690 |
| Sarcoidosis associated hypercalcemia | Noncaseating granulomas → ↑ macrophage activity → ↑ 1α-hydroxylase activity in macrophage → vitamin D activation → ↑ $Ca^{2+}$ | 695 |
| Acute respiratory distress syndrome | Alveolar injury → inflammation → capillary endothelial damage and ↑ vessel permeability → leakage of protein-rich fluid into alveoli → intra-alveolar hyaline membranes and noncardiogenic pulmonary edema → ↓ compliance and V/Q mismatch → hypoxic vasoconstriction → ↑ pulmonary vascular resistance | 697 |
| Sleep apnea | Respiratory effort against airway obstruction (obstructive); impaired respiratory effort due to CNS injury/toxicity, CHF, opioids (central); obesity → hypoventilation → ↑ $PaCO_2$ during waking hours | 697 |

## ▸ CLASSIC PRESENTATIONS

| CLINICAL PRESENTATION | DIAGNOSIS/DISEASE | PAGE |
|---|---|---|
| Gout, intellectual disability, self-mutilating behavior in a boy | Lesch-Nyhan syndrome (HGPRT deficiency, X-linked recessive) | 35 |
| Situs inversus, chronic ear infections, sinusitis, bronchiectasis, infertility | Primary ciliary dyskinesia (Kartagener syndrome) | 47 |
| Blue sclera, multiple fractures, dental problems, conductive/mixed hearing loss | Osteogenesis imperfecta (type I collagen defect) | 49 |
| Elastic skin, hypermobility of joints, ↑ bleeding tendency | Ehlers-Danlos syndrome (type V collagen defect, type III collagen defect seen in vascular subtype of ED) | 49 |

| CLINICAL PRESENTATION | DIAGNOSIS/DISEASE | PAGE |
|---|---|---|
| Arachnodactyly, lens dislocation (upward and temporal), aortic dissection, hyperflexible joints | Marfan syndrome (fibrillin-1) | 50 |
| Arachnodactyly, pectus deformity, lens dislocation (downward) | Homocystinuria (autosomal recessive cystathionine synthase deficiency) | 50 |
| Café-au-lait spots (unilateral), polyostotic fibrous dysplasia, precocious puberty, multiple endocrine abnormalities | McCune-Albright syndrome ($G_s$-protein activating mutation) | 55 |
| Meconium ileus in neonate, recurrent pulmonary infections, nasal polyps, pancreatic insufficiency, infertility/subfertility, malabsorption/vitamin deficiencies | Cystic fibrosis (*CFTR* gene defect, chromosome 7, ΔF508) | 58 |
| Calf pseudohypertrophy | Muscular dystrophy (most commonly Duchenne, due to X-linked recessive frameshift mutation of dystrophin gene) | 59 |
| Child uses arms to stand up from squat | Duchenne muscular dystrophy (Gowers sign) | 59 |
| Slow, progressive muscle weakness in boys | Becker muscular dystrophy (X-linked non-frameshift deletions in dystrophin; less severe than Duchenne) | 59 |
| Infant with cleft lip/palate, microcephaly or holoprosencephaly, polydactyly, cutis aplasia | Patau syndrome (trisomy 13) | 61 |
| Infant with microcephaly, rocker-bottom feet, clenched hands, and structural heart defect | Edwards syndrome (trisomy 18) | 61 |
| Single palmar crease, flat facies, prominent epicanthal folds, congenital heart disease, intellectual disability | Down syndrome (trisomy 21) | 61 |
| Microcephaly, high-pitched cry, intellectual disability | Cri-du-chat (cry of the cat) syndrome | 62 |
| Confusion, ophthalmoplegia/nystagmus, ataxia | Wernicke encephalopathy (add confabulation/memory loss and personality changes for Korsakoff syndrome) | 64 |
| Dilated cardiomyopathy/high-output heart failure, edema, alcoholism or malnutrition | Wet beriberi (thiamine [vitamin $B_1$] deficiency) | 64 |
| Dermatitis, dementia, diarrhea | Pellagra (niacin [vitamin $B_3$] deficiency) | 65 |
| Burning feet syndrome, dermatitis, enteritis, alopecia | Pentothenic acid (vitamin $B_5$) deficiency | 65 |
| Megaloblastic anemia, subacute combined degeneration, paresthesias, cognitive changes | Cobalamin (vitamin B12) deficiency; malabsorption, decreased intrinsic factor, absent terminal ileum | 67 |
| Swollen gums, mucosal bleeding, poor wound healing, petechiae, corkscrew hairs, perifollicular hemorrhages | Scurvy (vitamin C deficiency: can't hydroxylate proline/lysine for collagen synthesis); tea and toast diet | 67 |
| Bowlegs (children), bone pain, and muscle weakness | Rickets (children), osteomalacia (adults); vitamin D deficiency | 68 |
| Hemorrhagic disease of newborn with aPTT, normal bleeding time | Vitamin K deficiency | 69 |
| Intellectual disability, musty body odor, hypopigmented skin, eczema | Phenylketonuria (tetrahydrobiopterin [$BH_4$] deficiency) | 82 |
| Bluish-black connective tissue, ear cartilage, sclerae; severe arthralgias; urine turns black on prolonged exposure to air | Alkaptonuria (homogentisate oxidase deficiency; ochronosis) | 82 |

| CLINICAL PRESENTATION | DIAGNOSIS/DISEASE | PAGE |
|---|---|---|
| Infant with hypoglycemia, hepatomegaly, cardiomyopathy | Cori disease (debranching enzyme deficiency) or von Gierke disease (glucose-6-phosphatase deficiency, more severe) | 85 |
| Chronic exercise intolerance with myalgia, fatigue, painful cramps, myoglobinuria | McArdle disease (skeletal muscle glycogen phosphorylase deficiency) | 85 |
| "Cherry-red spots" on macula | Tay-Sachs (ganglioside accumulation; no hepatosplenomegaly); Niemann-Pick disease (sphingomyelin accumulation; hepatosplenomegaly); central retinal artery occlusion | 86, 552 |
| Hepatosplenomegaly, pancytopenia, osteoporosis, avascular necrosis of femoral head, bone crises | Gaucher disease (glucocerebrosidase [β-glucosidase] deficiency) | 86 |
| Achilles tendon xanthoma, corneal arcus | Familial hypercholesterolemia (↓ LDL receptor signaling) | 92 |
| Male child, recurrent infections, no mature B cells | Bruton disease (X-linked agammaglobulinemia [BTK gene defect]) | 114 |
| Anaphylaxis following blood transfusion, atopy, airway/GI infections, autoimmune disease | Selective IgA deficiency | 114 |
| Recurrent cold (noninflamed) abscesses, eczema, high serum IgE, ↑ eosinophils | Hyper-IgE syndrome (Job syndrome: neutrophil chemotaxis abnormality; STAT3 mutation) | 114 |
| Late separation (>30 days) of umbilical cord, no pus, recurrent skin and mucosal bacterial infections | Leukocyte adhesion deficiency (type 1; defective LFA-1 [CD18] integrin) | 115 |
| Recurrent infections and granulomas with catalase ⊕ organisms | Chronic granulomatous disease (defect of NADPH oxidase) | 115 |
| Fever, vomiting, diarrhea, desquamating rash following prolonged use of nasal pack or tampon | Staphylococcal toxic shock syndrome | 133 |
| "Strawberry tongue" | Scarlet fever (sandpaper rash); Kawasaki disease (lymphadenopathy, high fever for 5 days) | 134, 478 |
| Colon cancer associated with infective endocarditis | Streptococcus gallolyticus (formerly S bovis) | 135 |
| Flaccid paralysis in newborn after ingestion of honey | Clostridium botulinum infection (floppy baby syndrome) | 136 |
| Abdominal pain, diarrhea, leukocytosis, recent antibiotic use | Clostridioides difficile infection | 136 |
| Tonsillar pseudomembrane with "bull's neck" appearance | Corynebacterium diphtheria infection | 137 |
| Back pain, fever, night sweats | Pott disease (vertebral TB) | 138 |
| Acute adrenal insufficiency, fever, bilateral adrenal hemorrhage | Waterhouse-Friderichsen syndrome (meningococcemia) | 140, 353 |
| Red "currant jelly" sputum in patients with alcohol overuse or diabetes | Klebsiella pneumoniae pneumonia | 143 |
| Fever, chills, headache, myalgia following antibiotic treatment for syphilis | Jarisch-Herxheimer reaction (due to host response to sudden release of bacterial antigens) | 144 |
| Large rash with bull's-eye appearance, flu-like symptoms | Erythema migrans from Ixodes tick bite (Lyme disease: Borrelia) | 144 |
| Ulcerated genital lesion | Nonpainful, indurated: chancre (1° syphilis, Treponema pallidum) <br> Painful, with exudate: chancroid (Haemophilus ducreyi) | 145, 180 |

| CLINICAL PRESENTATION | DIAGNOSIS/DISEASE | PAGE |
|---|---|---|
| Smooth, moist, painless, wartlike white lesions on genitals | Condylomata lata (2° syphilis) | 145 |
| Pupil accommodates but doesn't react to light | Neurosyphilis Argyll Robertson pupil (3° [neuro] syphilis) | 145 |
| Dog or cat bite resulting in infection (cellulitis, osteomyelitis) | *Pasteurella multocida* (cellulitis at inoculation site) | 147 |
| Atypical "walking pneumonia" with x-ray looking worse than the patient | *Mycoplasma pneumoniae* infection | 148 |
| Rash on palms and soles | Coxsackie A infection, 2° syphilis, Rocky Mountain spotted fever | 148 |
| Black eschar on face of patient with diabetic ketoacidosis and/or neutropenia | *Mucor* or *Rhizopus* fungal infection | 150 |
| Chorioretinitis, hydrocephalus, intracranial calcifications, +/– blueberry muffin rash | Congenital toxoplasmosis | 153, 181 |
| Pruritus, serpiginous rash after walking barefoot, microcytic anemia | Hookworm (*Ancylostoma* spp, *Necator americanus*) | 156 |
| Child with fever later develops red rash on face that spreads to body | Erythema infectiosum/fifth disease ("slapped cheeks" appearance, caused by parvovirus B19) | 161 |
| Fever, cough, conjunctivitis, coryza, diffuse rash | Measles | 167 |
| Small, irregular red spots on buccal/lingual mucosa with blue-white centers | Koplik spots (measles [rubeola] virus) | 167 |
| Hyperdynamic pulses, wide pulse pressure, early diastolic murmur (decrescendo), head bobbing | Aortic regurgitation | 296 |
| Systolic ejection murmur (crescendo-decrescendo), narrow pulse pressure, pulsus parvus et tardus | Aortic stenosis | 296 |
| Continuous "machinelike" heart murmur | PDA (close with indomethacin; keep open with PGE analogs) | 296 |
| Chest pain on exertion | Angina (stable: with moderate exertion; unstable: with minimal exertion or at rest) | 308 |
| Chest pain with ST depressions on ECG | Angina (⊖ troponins) or NSTEMI (⊕ troponins) | 308 |
| Chest pain, pericardial effusion/friction rub, persistent fever following MI | Postcardiac injury syndrome (autoimmune-mediated post-MI fibrinous pericarditis, 2 weeks to several months after acute episode) | 314 |
| Distant heart sounds, distended neck veins, hypotension | Beck triad of cardiac tamponade | 317 |
| Painful, raised red/purple lesions on pads of fingers/toes | Osler nodes (infective endocarditis, immune complex deposition) | 318 |
| Painless erythematous lesions on palms and soles | Janeway lesions (infective endocarditis, septic emboli/microabscesses) | 318 |
| Splinter hemorrhages in fingernails | Infective endocarditis | 318 |
| Retinal hemorrhages with pale centers | Roth spots (infective endocarditis) | 318 |
| Telangiectasias, recurrent epistaxis, skin discoloration, arteriovenous malformations, GI bleeding, hematuria | Hereditary hemorrhagic telangiectasia (Osler-Weber-Rendu syndrome) | 320 |
| Polyuria, polydipsia | Primary polydipsia, diabetes mellitus (types 1 and 2), diabetes insipidus (central, nephrogenic) | 342, 350 |
| No lactation postpartum, absent menstruation, cold intolerance | Sheehan syndrome (severe postpartum hemorrhage leading to pituitary infarction) | 343 |

| CLINICAL PRESENTATION | DIAGNOSIS/DISEASE | PAGE |
|---|---|---|
| Heat intolerance, weight loss, palpitations, fine tremor, hyperreflexia | Hyperthyroidism | 344 |
| Cold intolerance, weight gain, brittle hair, depressed mood, hyporeflexia | Hypothyroidism | 344 |
| Cutaneous/dermal edema due to deposition of mucopolysaccharides in connective tissue | Myxedema (caused by hypothyroidism or hyperthyroidism [Graves disease]) | 344 |
| Facial muscle spasm upon tapping | Chvostek sign (hypocalcemia) | 348 |
| Carpal spasm upon inflation of BP cuff | Trousseau sign (hypocalcemia) | 348 |
| Rapid, deep, labored breathing/hyperventilation | Diabetic ketoacidosis (Kussmaul respirations) | 351 |
| Skin hyperpigmentation, orthostatic hypotension, fatigue, weakness, muscle aches, weight loss, GI disturbances | Chronic 1° adrenal insufficiency (Addison disease) → ↑ ACTH, ↑ MSH | 353 |
| Shock, altered mental status, vomiting, abdominal pain, weakness, fatigue in patient under glucocorticoid therapy | Acute adrenal insufficiency (adrenal crisis) | 353 |
| Pancreatic, pituitary, parathyroid tumors | MEN1 (autosomal dominant *MEN1* mutation) | 356 |
| Medullary thyroid carcinoma, parathyroid hyperplasia, pheochromocytoma | MEN2A (autosomal dominant *RET* mutation) | 356 |
| Medullary thyroid carcinoma, pheochromocytoma, mucosal neuromas, marfanoid habitus | MEN2B (autosomal dominant *RET* mutation) | 356 |
| Cutaneous flushing, diarrhea, bronchospasm, heart murmur | Carcinoid syndrome (↑ urinary 5-HIAA); indicates systemic dissemination (eg, post liver metastases) | 357 |
| Jaundice, palpable distended nontender gallbladder | Courvoisier sign (distal obstruction of biliary tree by pancreatic head malignancy) | 375, 405 |
| Vomiting blood following gastroesophageal lacerations, +/– abdominal/back pain | Mallory-Weiss syndrome (alcohol use disorder, bulimia nervosa) | 384 |
| Dysphagia (esophageal webs), glossitis, iron deficiency anemia | Plummer-Vinson syndrome (may progress to esophageal squamous cell carcinoma) | 384 |
| Enlarged, hard left supraclavicular node | Virchow node (metastasis from abdominal malignancy) | 386 |
| Hematemesis, melena | Upper GI bleeding (eg, peptic ulcer disease) | 387 |
| Hematochezia | Lower GI bleeding (eg, colonic diverticulosis) | 387 |
| Arthralgias, cardiac and neurological symptoms, diarrhea | Whipple disease (*Tropheryma whipplei*) | 388 |
| Severe RLQ pain with palpation of LLQ | Rovsing sign (acute appendicitis) | 390 |
| Severe RLQ pain with deep tenderness | McBurney sign (acute appendicitis) | 390 |
| Hamartomatous GI polyps, hyperpigmented macules on mouth, feet, hands, genitalia | Peutz-Jeghers syndrome (inherited, benign polyposis can cause bowel obstruction; ↑ breast/GI cancer risk) | 394 |
| Multiple colon polyps, osteomas/soft tissue tumors, impacted/supernumerary teeth | Gardner syndrome (subtype of FAP) | 394 |
| Severe jaundice in neonate | Crigler-Najjar syndrome (congenital unconjugated hyperbilirubinemia) | 401 |
| Golden brown rings around peripheral cornea | Wilson disease (Kayser-Fleischer rings due to copper accumulation) | 402 |
| Female, fat (obese), fertile (multiparity), forty, fair, feeds (TPN), fasting (rapid weight loss) | Cholelithiasis (gallstones) | 403 |

| CLINICAL PRESENTATION | DIAGNOSIS/DISEASE | PAGE |
|---|---|---|
| Bluish line on gingiva | Burton line (lead poisoning) | 425 |
| Short stature, café-au-lait spots, thumb/radial defects, ↑ incidence of tumors/leukemia, aplastic anemia | Fanconi anemia (genetic loss of DNA crosslink repair; often progresses to AML) | 427 |
| Red/pink urine in the morning, pancytopenia, venous thrombosis | Paroxysmal nocturnal hemoglobinuria | 428 |
| Painful blue fingers/toes, hemolytic anemia | Cold autoimmune hemolytic anemia (caused by *Mycoplasma pneumoniae*, infectious mononucleosis, CLL) | 429 |
| Petechiae, mucosal bleeding, prolonged bleeding time | Platelet disorders (eg, Glanzmann thrombasthenia, Bernard Soulier, HUS, TTP, ITP, uremic platelet dysfunction) | 432 |
| Low-grade fever, night sweats, weight loss | B symptoms of malignancy | 434 |
| Skin patches/plaques, Pautrier microabscesses, atypical T cells | Mycosis fungoides (cutaneous T-cell lymphoma) or Sézary syndrome (mycosis fungoides + malignant T cells in blood) | 435 |
| Neonate with arm paralysis following difficult birth, arm in "waiter's tip" position | Erb palsy (superior trunk [C5–C6] brachial plexus injury) | 452 |
| Anterior drawer sign ⊕ | Anterior cruciate ligament injury | 455 |
| Bone pain, bone enlargement, long bone chalk-stick fractures | Osteitis deformans (Paget disease of bone, ↑ osteoblastic and osteoclastic activity) | 468 |
| Swollen, hard, painful finger joints in an elderly individual, pain worse with activity | Osteoarthritis (osteophytes on PIP [Bouchard nodes], DIP [Heberden nodes]) | 472 |
| Sudden swollen/painful big toe joint, tophi | Gout/podagra (hyperuricemia) | 473 |
| Dry eyes, dry mouth, arthritis, parotid enlargement | Sjögren syndrome (autoimmune destruction of exocrine glands) | 474 |
| Urethritis, conjunctivitis, arthritis | Reactive arthritis associated with HLA-B27 | 475 |
| "Butterfly" facial rash, arthritis, cytopenia, and fever in a female of reproductive age | Systemic lupus erythematosus | 476 |
| Cervical lymphadenopathy, desquamating rash, coronary aneurysms, red conjunctivae and tongue, hand-foot changes | Kawasaki disease (mucocutaneous lymph node syndrome, treat with IVIG and aspirin) | 478 |
| Palpable purpura on buttocks/legs, joint pain, abdominal pain, hematuria in a child | Immunoglobulin A vasculitis (Henoch-Schönlein purpura, affects skin and kidneys) | 479 |
| Painful fingers/toes changing color from white to blue to red with cold or stress | Raynaud phenomenon (vasospasm in extremities) | 480 |
| Dark purple skin/mouth nodules in a patient with AIDS | Kaposi sarcoma, associated with HHV-8 | 486 |
| Pruritic, purple, polygonal planar papules and plaques (6 P's) | Lichen planus | 491 |
| Dorsiflexion of large toe with fanning of other toes upon plantar scrape | Babinski sign (UMN lesion) | 523, 543 |
| Ataxia, nystagmus, head tilting, fall towards injured side | Cerebellar lesion (hemispheric affects voluntary movement of extremities; vermis affects axial and proximal movement) | 524 |

| CLINICAL PRESENTATION | DIAGNOSIS/DISEASE | PAGE |
|---|---|---|
| Hyperphagia, hypersexuality, hyperorality | Klüver-Bucy syndrome (bilateral amygdala lesion; HSV-1 encephalitis) | 524 |
| Resting tremor, athetosis, chorea | Basal ganglia lesion (eg, Huntington disease, Parkinson disease) | 524 |
| Dysphagia, hoarseness, ↓ gag reflex, nystagmus, ipsilateral Horner syndrome | Lateral medullary (Wallenberg) syndrome (posterior inferior cerebellar artery lesion) | 527 |
| Lucid interval after traumatic brain injury | Epidural hematoma (middle meningeal artery rupture; branch of maxillary artery) | 528 |
| "Worst headache of my life" | Subarachnoid hemorrhage | 528 |
| Resting tremor, rigidity, akinesia, postural instability, shuffling gait, micrographia | Parkinson disease (loss of dopaminergic neurons in substantia nigra pars compacta) | 534 |
| Chorea, dementia, caudate degeneration, dementia | Huntington disease (autosomal dominant CAG repeat expansion) | 534 |
| Urinary incontinence, gait apraxia, cognitive dysfunction | Normal pressure hydrocephalus | 536 |
| Relapsing and remitting nystagmus, intention tremor, optic neuritis, scanning speech, bilateral internuclear ophthalmoplegia | Multiple sclerosis | 537 |
| Rapidly progressive, symmetric limb weakness and hyporeflexia that ascends following GI/upper respiratory infection | Guillain-Barré syndrome (acute inflammatory demyelinating polyneuropathy) | 538 |
| Café-au-lait spots, Lisch nodules (iris hamartoma), cutaneous neurofibromas, pheochromocytomas, optic gliomas | Neurofibromatosis type I | 539 |
| Bilateral vestibular schwannomas | Neurofibromatosis type II | 539 |
| Vascular birthmark (port-wine stain) of the face | Nevus flammeus (benign, but associated with Sturge-Weber syndrome) | 539 |
| Renal cell carcinoma (bilateral), hemangioblastomas, angiomatosis, pheochromocytoma | von Hippel-Lindau disease (deletion of *VHL* on chromosome 3p) | 539 |
| Hyperreflexia, hypertonia, Babinski sign present | UMN damage | 543 |
| Hyporeflexia, hypotonia, atrophy, fasciculations | LMN damage | 543 |
| Staggering gait, frequent falls, nystagmus, hammer toes, diabetes mellitus, hypertrophic cardiomyopathy | Friedreich ataxia | 545 |
| Unilateral facial drooping involving forehead | LMN facial nerve (CN VII) palsy; UMN lesions spare the forehead | 546 |
| Episodic vertigo, tinnitus, sensorineural hearing loss | Ménière disease | 548 |
| Ptosis, miosis, anhidrosis | Horner syndrome (sympathetic chain lesion) | 555 |
| Conjugate horizontal gaze palsy, horizontal diplopia | Internuclear ophthalmoplegia (damage to MLF; may be unilateral or bilateral) | 558 |
| "Waxing and waning" level of consciousness (acute onset), ↓ attention span, ↓ level of arousal | Delirium (usually 2° to other cause) | 575 |
| Polyuria, renal tubular acidosis type II, growth retardation, electrolyte imbalances, hypophosphatemic rickets | Fanconi syndrome (generalized reabsorption defect of the proximal convoluted tubule) | 604, 611 |

| CLINICAL PRESENTATION | DIAGNOSIS/DISEASE | PAGE |
|---|---|---|
| Periorbital and/or peripheral edema, proteinuria (> 3.5 g/day; frothy urine), hypoalbuminemia, hypercholesterolemia | Nephrotic syndrome | 613 |
| Hereditary nephritis, sensorineural hearing loss, retinopathy, anterior lenticonus | Alport syndrome (mutation in type IV collagen) | 615 |
| Wilms tumor, macroglossia, organomegaly, hemihyperplasia, omphalocele | Beckwith-Wiedemann syndrome (WT2 mutation) | 624 |
| Streak ovaries, congenital heart disease, horseshoe kidney, cystic hygroma, short stature, webbed neck, lymphedema | Turner syndrome (45,XO) | 655 |
| Ovarian fibroma, ascites, pleural effusion | Meigs syndrome | 665 |
| Red, itchy, swollen rash of nipple/areola | Paget disease of the breast (sign of underlying neoplasm) | 668 |
| Fibrous plaques in tunica albuginea of penis with abnormal curvature | Peyronie disease (connective tissue disorder) | 669 |
| Pink complexion, dyspnea, hyperventilation | Emphysema ("pink puffer," centriacinar [tobacco smoking] or panacinar [$\alpha_1$-antitrypsin deficiency]) | 692 |
| Hypoxemia, polycythemia, hypercapnia | Chronic bronchitis (hypertrophy and hyperplasia of mucus-secreting glands, "blue bloater") | 692 |
| Bilateral hilar adenopathy, uveitis, arthropathy, skin changes | Sarcoidosis (noncaseating granulomas) | 695 |

## ▶ CLASSIC LABS/FINDINGS

| LAB/DIAGNOSTIC FINDING | DIAGNOSIS/DISEASE | PAGE |
|---|---|---|
| Colonies of *Pseudomonas* in lungs ↑ Cl$^-$ on sweat test, ↑ immunoreactive trypsinogen | Cystic fibrosis (autosomal recessive mutation in *CFTR* gene → fat-soluble vitamin deficiency and mucous plugs) | 58 |
| ↓ AFP on second trimester screening | Down syndrome, Edwards syndrome | 61 |
| ↑ β-hCG, ↓ PAPP-A on first trimester screening | Down syndrome | 61 |
| ↑ serum homocysteine, ↑ methylmalonic acid, ↓ folate | Vitamin B$_{12}$ deficiency | 67 |
| Anti-histone antibodies | Drug-induced lupus | 113 |
| ↓ T cells, ↓ PTH, ↓ Ca$^{2+}$, absent thymic shadow on CXR | Thymic aplasia (22q11microdeletion: DiGeorge syndrome, velocardiofacial syndrome) | 114 |
| Recurrent infections, eczema, thrombocytopenia | Wiskott-Aldrich syndrome (WAS gene mutation) | 115 |
| Large granules in phagocytes, immunodeficiency | Chédiak-Higashi disease (LYST gene mutation: congenital failure of phagolysosome formation) | 115 |
| Optochin sensitivity | Sensitive: S pneumoniae; resistant: viridans streptococci (S mutans, S sanguis, S mitis) | 132 |
| Novobiocin response | Sensitive: S epidermidis; resistant: S saprophyticus | 132 |
| Bacitracin response | Sensitive: S pyogenes (group A); resistant: S agalactiae (group B) | 132 |
| Branching gram ⊕ rods with sulfur granules | *Actinomyces israelii* | 137 |

| LAB/DIAGNOSTIC FINDING | DIAGNOSIS/DISEASE | PAGE |
|---|---|---|
| Hilar lymphadenopathy, peripheral granulomatous lesion in middle or lower lung lobes (can calcify) | Ghon complex (1° TB: *Mycobacterium* bacilli) | 138 |
| "Thumb sign" on lateral neck x-ray | Epiglottitis (*Haemophilus influenzae*) | 140 |
| Bacteria-covered vaginal epithelial cells, ⊕ whiff test | "Clue cells" (*Gardnerella vaginalis*) | 147 |
| Ring-enhancing brain lesion on CT/MRI in AIDS | *Toxoplasma gondii* (multiple), CNS lymphoma (may be solitary) | 153, 174 |
| Dilated cardiomyopathy with apical atrophy, megacolon, megaesophagus | Chagas disease (*Trypanosoma cruzi*) | 155 |
| Atypical lymphocytes, heterophile antibodies | Infectious mononucleosis (EBV infection) | 162 |
| Narrowing of upper trachea and subglottis (Steeple sign) on x-ray | Croup (parainfluenza virus) | 167 |
| Eosinophilic inclusion bodies in cytoplasm of hippocampal and cerebellar neurons | Negri bodies of rabies | 169 |
| Concentrically laminated calcified spherules (psammoma bodies) | Meningiomas, papillary thyroid carcinoma, mesothelioma, papillary serous carcinoma of the endometrium and ovary | 207 |
| "Boot-shaped" heart on x-ray | Tetralogy of Fallot (due to RVH) | 302 |
| Rib notching (inferior surface, on x-ray) | Coarctation of the aorta | 304 |
| "Delta wave" on ECG, short PR interval, supraventricular tachycardia | Wolff-Parkinson-White syndrome (bundle of Kent bypasses AV node) | 311 |
| Electrical alternans (alternating amplitude on ECG) | Cardiac tamponade | 317 |
| Granuloma with giant cells after pharyngeal infection | Aschoff bodies (rheumatic fever) | 319 |
| Empty-appearing nuclei with central clearing of thyroid cells | "Orphan Annie" eyes nuclei (papillary carcinoma of the thyroid) | 347 |
| "Brown" tumor of bone | Hyperparathyroidism or osteitis fibrosa cystica (deposited hemosiderin from hemorrhage gives brown color) | 349, 469 |
| Hypertension, hypokalemia, metabolic alkalosis, ↑ aldosterone, ↓ renin | 1° hyperaldosteronism (eg, Conn syndrome) | 354 |
| Mucin-filled cell with peripheral nucleus | "Signet ring" cells (diffuse gastric carcinoma) | 386 |
| Anti-transglutaminase/anti-deamidated gliadin/anti-endomysial antibodies | Celiac disease (diarrhea, weight loss) | 388 |
| Narrowing of bowel lumen on barium x-ray | "String sign" (Crohn disease) | 389 |
| "Lead pipe" appearance of colon on abdominal imaging | Ulcerative colitis (loss of haustra) | 389 |
| Thousands of polyps on colonoscopy after puberty | Familial adenomatous polyposis (autosomal dominant, mutation of APC gene) | 394 |
| "Apple core" lesion on barium enema x-ray | Colorectal cancer (usually left-sided) | 395 |
| "Nutmeg" appearance of liver | Chronic passive congestion of liver due to right heart failure, Budd-Chiari syndrome | 397 |
| Eosinophilic cytoplasmic inclusion of damaged keratin within hepatocyte | Mallory body (alcoholic hepatitis) | 398 |
| Triglyceride accumulation in liver cell vacuoles | Fatty liver disease (alcoholic or metabolic syndrome) | 398 |
| Anti-smooth muscle antibodies (ASMAs), anti-liver/kidney microsomal-1 (anti-LKM1) antibodies | Autoimmune hepatitis | 399 |

| LAB/DIAGNOSTIC FINDING | DIAGNOSIS/DISEASE | PAGE |
|---|---|---|
| Antimitochondrial antibodies (AMAs) | 1° biliary cholangitis (female, cholestasis, portal hypertension) | 402 |
| Low serum ceruloplasmin | Wilson disease | 402 |
| Migratory thrombophlebitis (leading to migrating DVTs and vasculitis) | Trousseau syndrome (adenocarcinoma of pancreas) | 405 |
| Hypersegmented neutrophils | Megaloblastic anemia (vitamin $B_{12}$ deficiency: neurologic symptoms; folate deficiency: no neurologic symptoms) | 426 |
| Basophilic nuclear remnants in RBCs | Howell-Jolly bodies (due to splenectomy or nonfunctional spleen) | 422 |
| Basophilic stippling of RBCs | Sideroblastic anemias, thalassemias | 421 |
| Hypochromic, microcytic anemia | Iron deficiency anemia, lead poisoning, thalassemia (fetal hemoglobin sometimes present), sideroblastic anemia | 424, 425 |
| "Hair on end" ("crew cut") appearance on x-ray | β-thalassemia, sickle cell anemia (marrow expansion) | 425, 428 |
| Anti-GpIIb/IIIa antibodies | Immune thrombocytopenia | 432 |
| High level of fibrin degradation products (D-dimers) | DVT, DIC | 433, 690 |
| Giant B cells with bilobed nucleus with prominent inclusions ("owl's eye") | Reed-Sternberg cells (Hodgkin lymphoma) | 434 |
| Sheets of medium-sized lymphoid cells with scattered pale, tingible body–laden macrophages ("starry sky" histology) | Burkitt lymphoma (t[8:14] c-*myc* activation, associated with EBV; "starry sky" made up of malignant cells) | 435 |
| Lytic ("punched-out") bone lesions on x-ray | Multiple myeloma | 436 |
| Monoclonal spike on serum protein electrophoresis | Multiple myeloma (usually IgG or IgA) Waldenström macroglobulinemia (IgM) Monoclonal gammopathy of undetermined significance | 436 |
| Stacks of RBCs | Rouleaux formation (high ESR, multiple myeloma) | 436 |
| Myeloperoxidase ⊕ cytoplasmic inclusions in myeloblasts, with ↑↑↑ circulating myeloblasts | Auer rods (APL) | 437 |
| WBCs that look "smudged" | CLL | 437 |
| "Tennis racket"-shaped cytoplasmic organelles (EM) in Langerhans cells | Birbeck granules (Langerhans cell histiocytosis) | 439 |
| "Soap bubble" in femur or tibia on x-ray | Giant cell tumor of bone (generally benign) | 470 |
| Raised periosteum (creating a "Codman triangle") | Aggressive bone lesion (eg, osteosarcoma, Ewing sarcoma) | 471 |
| "Onion skin" periosteal reaction | Ewing sarcoma (malignant small blue cell tumor) | 471 |
| IgM antibody that targets IgG Fc region, anti-cyclic citrullinated peptide antibodies | Rheumatoid arthritis (systemic inflammation, joint pannus, boutonniere and swan neck deformities) | 472 |
| Needle-shaped, ⊖ birefringent crystals | Gout (monosodium urate crystals) | 473 |
| ↑ uric acid levels | Gout, Lesch-Nyhan syndrome, tumor lysis syndrome, loop and thiazide diuretics | 473 |
| Rhomboid crystals, ⊕ birefringent | Pseudogout (calcium pyrophosphate dihydrate crystals) | 473 |

| LAB/DIAGNOSTIC FINDING | DIAGNOSIS/DISEASE | PAGE |
|---|---|---|
| "Bamboo spine" on x-ray | Ankylosing spondylitis (chronic inflammatory arthritis: HLA-B27) | 475 |
| Antinuclear antibodies (ANAs: anti-Smith and anti-dsDNA) | SLE (type III hypersensitivity) | 476 |
| Antineutrophil cytoplasmic antibodies (ANCAs) | Microscopic polyangiitis, eosinophilic granulomatosis with polyangiitis, and primary sclerosing cholangitis (MPO-ANCA/p-ANCA); granulomatosis with polyangiitis (PR3-ANCA/c-ANCA) | 402, 479 |
| Anticentromere antibodies | Limited scleroderma (CREST syndrome) | 481 |
| Anti-Scl-70 (anti-DNA topoisomerase-I) and anti-RNA polymerase III antibodies | Diffuse scleroderma | 481 |
| Anti-desmoglein (anti-desmosome) antibodies | Pemphigus vulgaris | 489 |
| Antihemidesmosome antibodies | Bullous pemphigoid | 489 |
| Keratin pearls on a skin biopsy | Squamous cell carcinoma | 493 |
| ↑ AFP in maternal serum | Dating error, open neural tube defects. | 501 |
| Bloody or yellow CSF on lumbar puncture | Xanthochromia (due to subarachnoid hemorrhage) | 528 |
| Eosinophilic cytoplasmic inclusion in neuron | Lewy body (Parkinson disease and Lewy body dementia) | 534 |
| Extracellular amyloid deposition in gray matter of brain | Senile plaques (Alzheimer disease) | 534 |
| Loss of dopaminergic (pigmented) neurons in substantia nigra | Parkinson disease | 534 |
| Protein aggregates in neurons from hyperphosphorylation of tau protein | Neurofibrillary tangles (Alzheimer disease) and Pick bodies (frontotemporal dementia) | 534 |
| Pseudopalisading pleomorphic tumor cells on brain biopsy | Glioblastoma | 540 |
| Small blue cells surrounding central area of neuropil | Homer-Wright rosettes (neuroblastoma, medulloblastoma) | 354, 542 |
| RBC casts in urine | Glomerulonephritis, hypertensive emergency | 612 |
| WBC casts in urine | Acute pyelonephritis, transplant rejection, tubulointerstitial inflammation | 612 |
| Granular, "muddy-brown" casts in urine | Acute tubular necrosis (eg, ischemia or toxic injury) | 612 |
| "Waxy" casts with very low urine flow | End-stage renal disease/chronic kidney disease | 612 |
| "Lumpy bumpy" appearance of glomeruli on immunofluorescence | Infection-related glomerulonephritis (due to deposition of IgG, IgM, and C3) | 614 |
| Anti–glomerular basement membrane antibodies | Goodpasture syndrome (hematuria and hemoptysis) | 614 |
| Linear appearance of IgG deposition on glomerular and alveolar basement membranes | Goodpasture syndrome | 614 |
| Necrotizing vasculitis (lungs) and necrotizing glomerulonephritis | Granulomatosis with polyangiitis (PR3-ANCA/c-ANCA) and Goodpasture syndrome (anti–basement membrane antibodies) | 614, 479 |
| Cellular crescents in Bowman's space on light microscopy | Rapidly progressive (crescentic) glomerulonephritis | 614 |
| "Wire loop" glomerular capillary appearance on light microscopy | Diffuse proliferative glomerulonephritis (usually seen with lupus) | 614 |

| LAB/DIAGNOSTIC FINDING | DIAGNOSIS/DISEASE | PAGE |
|---|---|---|
| "Tram-track" appearance of capillary loops of glomerular basement membranes on light microscopy | Membranoproliferative glomerulonephritis | 615 |
| "Spikes" on basement membrane, "domelike" subepithelial deposits | Membranous nephropathy (nephrotic syndrome) | 616 |
| Effacement of podocyte foot processes on electron microscopy | Minimal change disease (child with nephrotic syndrome) | 616 |
| Eosinophilic nodular hyaline deposits in glomeruli | Kimmelstiel-Wilson nodules (diabetic glomerulonephropathy) | 616 |
| Thyroidlike appearance of kidney | Chronic pyelonephritis | 619 |
| hCG elevated | Multifetal gestation, hydatidiform moles, choriocarcinomas, Down syndrome | 652 |
| Dysplastic squamous cervical cells with "raisinoid" nuclei and perinuclear halo | Koilocytes (HPV infection: predisposes to cervical cancer) | 663 |
| Sheets of uniform "fried egg" cells, ↑ hCG, ↑ LDH | Dysgerminoma | 664 |
| Schiller-Duval bodies (resemble glomeruli), ↑AFP | Yolk sac tumor | 664 |
| Disarrayed granulosa cells arranged around collections of eosinophilic fluid | Call-Exner bodies (granulosa cell tumor of the ovary) | 665 |
| "Chocolate cyst" in ovary | Endometriosis | 666 |
| Mammary gland ("blue domed") simple cyst | Fibrocystic change of the breast | 667 |
| Eosinophilic cytoplasmic inclusions in Leydig cells | Reinke crystals (Leydig cell tumor) | 671 |
| Interdigitating layers of pink and red in arterial thrombi | Lines of Zahn (layers of platelets and RBCs seen only in thrombi formed before death) | 691 |
| Eosinophilic, hexagonal, double-pointed crystals in bronchial secretions | Charcot-Leyden crystals (asthma) | 693 |
| Whorled mucus plugs formed from shed bronchial epithelium | Curschmann spirals (asthma) | 693 |
| "Honeycomb" appearance of the lung on CXR or CT | Idiopathic pulmonary fibrosis | 694 |
| Golden-brown fusiform rods resembling dumbbells in alveolar sputum, visualized with Prussian blue stain | Asbestos (ferruginous) bodies | 696 |
| Bronchogenic apical lung tumor on imaging | Pancoast (superior sulcus) tumor (can compress cervical sympathetic chain and cause Horner syndrome) | 704 |

## ▶ KEY ASSOCIATIONS

| DISEASE/FINDING | MOST COMMON/IMPORTANT ASSOCIATIONS | PAGE |
|---|---|---|
| Mitochondrial inheritance | Disease occurs in all offspring of affected females (maternal inheritance pattern), heteroplasmy | 55, 57 |
| Intellectual disability | Down syndrome (sporadic), fragile X syndrome (inherited) | 60, 61 |
| Vitamin deficiency (USA) | Folate (pregnant women are at high risk; body stores only 3- to 4-month supply) | 66 |

| DISEASE/FINDING | MOST COMMON/IMPORTANT ASSOCIATIONS | PAGE |
|---|---|---|
| Lysosomal storage disease | Gaucher disease | 86 |
| HLA-DR3 | DM type 1, SLE, Graves disease, Hashimoto thyroiditis, Addison disease | 98 |
| HLA-DR4 | Rheumatoid arthritis, DM type 1, Addison disease | 98 |
| Bacteria associated with gastritis, peptic ulcer disease, and gastric malignancies (eg, adenocarcinoma, MALToma) | *H pylori* | 144 |
| Opportunistic respiratory infection in AIDS | *Pneumocystis jirovecii* | 151 |
| Viral encephalitis affecting temporal lobe | HSV-1 | 162 |
| Viral infection 2° to blood transfusion | Hepatitis C | 171 |
| Food poisoning (exotoxin-mediated) | *S aureus, B cereus* | 175 |
| Healthcare-associated pneumonia | *S aureus, Pseudomonas*, other enteric gram ⊖ rods | 176 |
| Bacterial meningitis (0–6 months old) | Group B streptococcus, *E coli, Listeria* | 177 |
| Bacterial meningitis (> 6 months old) | *S pneumoniae* | 177 |
| Osteomyelitis | *S aureus* (most common overall) | 177 |
| Osteomyelitis in sickle cell disease | *Salmonella, S aureus* | 177 |
| Osteomyelitis with injection drug use | *S aureus, Pseudomonas, Candida* | 177 |
| UTI | *E coli, Staphylococcus saprophyticus* | 179 |
| Bacterial STI | *C trachomatis* (D-K) | 180 |
| Pelvic inflammatory disease | *C trachomatis* (subacute), *N gonorrhoeae* (acute) | 182 |
| Metastases to bone | Prostate, breast >> lung > kidney, colon | 219 |
| Metastases to liver | Colon > breast >> pancreas, lung, prostate | 219 |
| Metastases to brain | Lung > breast >> melanoma > colon, prostate | 219 |
| S3 heart sound | ↑ ventricular filling pressure (eg, MR, AR, HF, thyrotoxicosis), common in dilated ventricles | 292 |
| S4 heart sound | Stiff/hypertrophic ventricle (aortic stenosis, restrictive cardiomyopathy) | 292 |
| Holosystolic murmur | VSD, tricuspid regurgitation, mitral regurgitation | 296 |
| Ejection click | Aortic stenosis | 296 |
| Mitral stenosis | Rheumatic heart disease (late and highly specific sequelae of rheumatic fever) | 296 |
| Opening snap | Mitral stenosis | 296 |
| Heart murmur, congenital | Mitral valve prolapse | 296 |
| Cyanotic heart disease (early) | Tetralogy of Fallot (most common), D-transposition of great arteries, persistent truncus arteriosus, total anomalous pulmonary venous return, tricuspid atresia | 302 |
| Congenital heart disease (left-to-right shunts) | VSD > ASD > PDA | 303 |
| Late cyanotic shunt (uncorrected left to right becomes right to left) | Eisenmenger syndrome (caused by VSD, ASD, PDA) | 303 |
| 2° hypertension | Renal/renovascular diseases (eg, fibromuscular dysplasia), atherosclerotic renal artery stenosis, 1° hyperaldosteronism, or obstructive sleep apnea | 304 |

| DISEASE/FINDING | MOST COMMON/IMPORTANT ASSOCIATIONS | PAGE |
|---|---|---|
| Sites of atherosclerosis | Abdominal aorta > coronary artery > popliteal artery > carotid artery > circle of Willis | 305 |
| Aortic aneurysm, thoracic | Marfan syndrome (cystic medial degeneration), 3° syphilis (obliterative endarteritis of vasa vasorum) | 306 |
| Aortic aneurysm, abdominal | Atherosclerosis, tobacco use | 306 |
| Aortic dissection | Hypertension (most important risk factor) | 307 |
| Irregularly irregular rhythm on ECG with no discrete P waves | Atrial fibrillation (associated with high risk of emboli) | 311 |
| Right heart failure due to a pulmonary cause | Cor pulmonale | 316 |
| Heart valve in infective endocarditis | Mitral > aortic, tricuspid (injection drug use) | 318 |
| Infective endocarditis presentation associated with bacterium | *S aureus* (acute, injection drug use, tricuspid valve), viridans streptococci (subacute, dental procedure), *S gallolyticus* (colon cancer), gram ⊖ (HACEK), culture ⊖ (*Coxiella, Bartonella*) | 318 |
| Cardiac tumor (adults) | Metastasis, myxoma (90% in left atrium; "ball valve") | 320 |
| Cardiac 1° tumor (children) | Rhabdomyoma (associated with tuberous sclerosis) | 320 |
| Congenital adrenal hyperplasia | 21-hydroxylase deficiency | 339 |
| Hypopituitarism | Pituitary adenoma (undersecretion due to mass effect) | 343 |
| Congenital hypothyroidism | Thyroid dysgenesis/dyshormonogenesis, iodine deficiency | 345 |
| Thyroid cancer | Papillary carcinoma (*RET/PTC* rearrangements, *BRAF* mutations, childhood irradiation) | 347 |
| Hypoparathyroidism | Accidental excision during thyroidectomy | 348 |
| 1° hyperparathyroidism | Adenomas, hyperplasia | 349 |
| 2° hyperparathyroidism | Hypocalcemia of chronic kidney disease | 349 |
| Cushing syndrome | ▪ Exogenous glucocorticoids<br>▪ Adrenocortical adenoma (secretes excess cortisol)<br>▪ ACTH-secreting pituitary adenoma (Cushing disease)<br>▪ Paraneoplastic (due to ACTH secretion by tumors) | 352 |
| Cushing disease | ↓ ACTH and cortisol in high-dose dexamethasone suppression tests, and ↑ ACTH and cortisol in CRH stimulation test | 352 |
| 1° hyperaldosteronism | Bilateral adrenal hyperplasia or adenoma (Conn syndrome) | 354 |
| Tumor of the adrenal medulla (children) | Neuroblastoma (malignant) | 354 |
| Tumor of the adrenal medulla (adults) | Pheochromocytoma (usually benign) | 355 |
| Refractory peptic ulcers and high gastrin levels | Zollinger-Ellison syndrome (due to gastrin-secreting tumor of the duodenum or pancreas), associated with MEN1 | 357 |
| Esophageal cancer | Squamous cell carcinoma (worldwide); adenocarcinoma (US) | 385 |
| Acute gastric ulcer associated with CNS injury | Cushing ulcer (↑ vagal stimulation → ↑ ACh → ↑ H⁺ production) | 386 |
| Acute gastric ulcer associated with severe burns | Curling ulcer (hypovolemia → mucosal ischemia) | 386 |

| DISEASE/FINDING | MOST COMMON/IMPORTANT ASSOCIATIONS | PAGE |
|---|---|---|
| Chronic atrophic gastritis | ↑ risk of gastric cancers, pernicious anemia (if autoimmune) | 386 |
| Bilateral ovarian metastases from gastric carcinoma | Krukenberg tumor (mucin-secreting signet ring cells) | 386 |
| Alternating areas of transmural inflammation and normal colon | Skip lesions (Crohn disease) | 389 |
| Site of diverticulosis | Sigmoid colon | 390 |
| False pharyngoesophageal diverticulum | Zenker diverticulum | 391 |
| Hepatocellular carcinoma | HBV (+/− cirrhosis), other causes of cirrhosis (HCV, alcoholic liver disease), specific carcinogens (eg, aflatoxins) | 399 |
| Inherited conjugated hyperbilirubinemia secondary to hepatocyte inability to secrete conjugated bilirubin in bile | Dubin-Johnson syndrome (black liver), Rotor syndrome (uncolored liver) | 401 |
| Inherited benign unconjugated hyperbilirubinemia | Gilbert syndrome | 401 |
| Inherited ATP7B mutation (copper buildup in liver, brain, cornea [Kayser-Fleischer rings], kidneys) | Wilson disease | 402 |
| Multiple blood transfusions or hereditary *HFE* mutation (can result in heart failure, "bronze diabetes," and ↑ risk of hepatocellular carcinoma) | Hemochromatosis | 402 |
| Pancreatitis (acute) | Gallstones, alcohol | 404 |
| Pancreatitis (chronic) | Alcohol (adults), cystic fibrosis (children) | 404 |
| Microcytic anemia | Iron deficiency, thalassemias, lead poisoning, sideroblastic anemia | 424, 425 |
| Autosplenectomy (fibrosis and shrinkage), Howell-Jolly bodies | Sickle cell anemia (hemoglobin S) | 428 |
| Inherited platelet disorder with GpIb deficiency | Bernard-Soulier syndrome (↓ platelet-to-vWF adhesion) | 432 |
| Inherited platelet disorder with GpIIb/IIIa deficiency | Glanzmann thrombasthenia (↓ platelet-to-platelet aggregation and defective platelet plug formation) | 432 |
| Hereditary thrombophilia commonly associated with recurrent pregnancy loss | Factor V Leiden (mutant factor V that is resistant to degradation) | 434 |
| Hereditary thrombophilia | Leiden (also associated with recurrent pregnancy loss) | 433 |
| DIC | Heat stroke, snake bite, sepsis, trauma, obstetric complications, acute pancreatitis, malignancy, nephrotic syndrome, transfusion | 433 |
| Common malignancy associated with noninfectious fever and bimodal age distribution | Hodgkin lymphoma | 434 |
| Type of Hodgkin lymphoma (most common) | Nodular sclerosis | 434 |
| t(14;18) | Follicular lymphoma (*BCL-2* activation, anti-apoptotic oncogene) | 435, 439 |
| t(8;14) | Burkitt lymphoma (c-*myc* fusion, transcription factor oncogene) | 435, 439 |
| Type of non-Hodgkin lymphoma (most common in adults) | Diffuse large B-cell lymphoma | 435 |

| DISEASE/FINDING | MOST COMMON/IMPORTANT ASSOCIATIONS | PAGE |
|---|---|---|
| Age ranges for patient with ALL/CLL/AML/CML | ALL: child, CLL: adult > 60, AML: adult ~ 65, CML: adult 45–85 | 437 |
| t(9;22) | Philadelphia chromosome, CML (*BCR-ABL* oncogene, tyrosine kinase activation), more rarely associated with ALL | 437, 439 |
| Vertebral compression fracture | Osteoporosis | 467 |
| HLA-B27 | Psoriatic arthritis, ankylosing spondylitis, IBD-associated arthritis, reactive arthritis | 475 |
| Death in SLE | Renal disease (most common), infections, cardiovascular disease (accelerated CAD) | 476 |
| Giant cell arteritis | Risk of ipsilateral blindness due to occlusion of ophthalmic artery; polymyalgia rheumatica | 478 |
| Recurrent inflammation/thrombosis of medium-vessels in extremities | Buerger disease (strongly associated with tobacco smoking, Raynaud phenomenon) | 478 |
| Benign vascular tumor of infancy | Infantile hemangioma (grows rapidly then involutes starting at age 1) | 486 |
| Herald patch (followed by scaly erythematous plaques in a "Christmas tree" distribution) | Pityriasis rosea | 491 |
| Actinic keratosis | Precursor to squamous cell carcinoma | 493 |
| Cerebellar tonsillar herniation | Chiari I malformation (associated with spinal cord cavitations [eg, syringomyelia]) | 502 |
| Bilateral mamillary body lesions with thiamine deficiency | Wernicke-Korsakoff syndrome | 524 |
| Epidural hematoma | Rupture of middle meningeal artery (trauma; biconvex/lentiform-shaped) | 528 |
| Subdural hematoma | Rupture of bridging veins (crescent-shaped) | 528 |
| Dementia | Alzheimer disease, vascular dementia (multiple infarcts) | 534, 535 |
| Demyelinating disease in young women | Multiple sclerosis | 537 |
| Brain tumor (adults) | Metastasis, glioblastoma (malignant), meningioma, hemangioblastoma | 540 |
| Galactorrhea, amenorrhea | Prolactinoma | 540 |
| Brain tumor (children) | Overall: pilocytic astrocytoma (benign) Infratentorial: medulloblastoma (most common malignant) Supratentorial: craniopharyngioma (malignant) | 542 |
| Combined UMN and LMN degeneration | Amyotrophic lateral sclerosis | 544 |
| Degeneration of dorsal column fibers | Tabes dorsalis (3° syphilis), subacute combined degeneration (dorsal columns, lateral corticospinal, spinocerebellar tracts affected) | 544 |
| Nephrotic syndrome (children) | Minimal change disease | 616 |
| Kidney stones (radiolucent) | Uric acid | 617 |
| Kidney stones (radiopaque) | Calcium (most common), struvite (ammonium), cystine (faintly radiopaque) | 617 |

| DISEASE/FINDING | MOST COMMON/IMPORTANT ASSOCIATIONS | PAGE |
|---|---|---|
| Renal malignancy (in males) | Renal cell carcinoma: associated with tobacco smoking and VHL (clear cell subtype); paraneoplastic syndromes (EPO, renin, PTHrP, ACTH) | 623 |
| 1° amenorrhea | Turner syndrome (45,XO or 45,XO/46,XX mosaic) | 655 |
| Hypogonadotropic hypogonadism with anosmia | Kallmann syndrome (neuron migration failure) | 656 |
| Clear cell adenocarcinoma of the vagina | DES exposure in utero | 662 |
| Ovarian tumor (benign, bilateral) | Serous cystadenoma | 664 |
| Ovarian tumor (malignant) | Serous carcinoma | 664 |
| Benign tumor of myometrium | Leiomyoma (estrogen sensitive, not precancerous) | 666 |
| Gynecologic malignancy (most common) | Endometrial carcinoma (most common in resource-rich countries); cervical cancer (most common worldwide) | 663–666 |
| Breast mass | Fibrocystic change (in premenopausal females); carcinoma (in postmenopausal females) | 667, 668 |
| Breast tumor (benign, young woman) | Fibroadenoma | 667 |
| Breast cancer | Invasive ductal carcinoma | 668 |
| Testicular tumor | Seminoma (malignant, radiosensitive), ↑ PLAP | 670, 671 |
| Bladder outlet obstruction in men | BPH | 672 |
| Hypercoagulability, endothelial damage, blood stasis | Virchow triad (↑ risk of thrombosis) | 690 |
| Pulmonary hypertension | Idiopathic, left heart disease, lung diseases/hypoxia, chronic thromboembolism, multifactorial | 698 |
| SIADH | Small cell carcinoma of the lung | 703 |

## ▶ EQUATION REVIEW

| TOPIC | EQUATION | PAGE |
|---|---|---|
| Volume of distribution | $V_d = \dfrac{\text{amount of drug in the body}}{\text{plasma drug concentration}}$ | 229 |
| Half-life | $t_{1/2} = \dfrac{0.7 \times V_d}{CL}$ | 229 |
| Drug clearance | $CL = \dfrac{\text{rate of elimination of drug}}{\text{plasma drug concentration}} = V_d \times K_e \text{ (elimination constant)}$ | 229 |
| Loading dose | $LD = \dfrac{C_p \times V_d}{F}$ | 229 |
| Maintenance dose | $\text{Maintenance dose} = \dfrac{C_p \times CL \times \tau}{F}$ | 229 |
| Therapeutic index | $TI = \text{median toxic dose/median effective dose} = TD_{50}/ED_{50}$ | 233 |
| Odds ratio (for case-control studies) | $OR = \dfrac{a/c}{b/d} = \dfrac{ad}{bc}$ | 258 |

| TOPIC | EQUATION | PAGE |
|---|---|---|
| Relative risk | $RR = \dfrac{a/(a+b)}{c/(c+d)}$ | 258 |
| Attributable risk | $AR = \dfrac{a}{a+b} - \dfrac{c}{c+d}$ | 258 |
| Relative risk reduction | $RRR = (ARC - ART)/ARC$ | 258 |
| Absolute risk reduction | $ARR = \dfrac{c}{c+d} - \dfrac{a}{a+b}$ | 258 |
| Number needed to treat | $NNT = 1/ARR$ | 258 |
| Number needed to harm | $NNH = 1/AR$ | 258 |
| Likelihood ratio + | $LR+ = $ sensitivity$/(1 - $specificity$) = $ TP rate/FP rate | 259 |
| Likelihood ratio − | $LR- = (1 - $sensitivity$)/$specificity $= $ FN rate/TN rate | 259 |
| Sensitivity | Sensitivity $= TP / (TP + FN)$ | 260 |
| Specificity | Specificity $= TN / (TN + FP)$ | 260 |
| Positive predictive value | $PPV = TP / (TP + FP)$ | 260 |
| Negative predictive value | $NPV = TN / (TN + FN)$ | 260 |
| Cardiac output | $CO = \dfrac{\text{rate of } O_2 \text{ consumption}}{(\text{arterial } O_2 \text{ content} - \text{venous } O_2 \text{ content})}$ <br><br> $CO = $ stroke volume $\times$ heart rate | 290 |
| Mean arterial pressure | $MAP = CO \times$ total peripheral resistance (TPR) <br><br> $MAP$ (at resting HR) $= \frac{2}{3} DBP + \frac{1}{3} SBP = DBP + \frac{1}{3} PP$ | 290 |
| Stroke volume | $SV = EDV - ESV$ | 290 |
| Ejection fraction | $EF = \dfrac{SV}{EDV} = \dfrac{EDV - ESV}{EDV}$ | 290 |
| Resistance | $\text{Resistance} = \dfrac{\text{driving pressure } (\Delta P)}{\text{flow } (Q)} = \dfrac{8\eta \text{ (viscosity)} \times \text{length}}{\pi r^4}$ | 291 |
| Capillary fluid exchange | $J_v = $ net fluid flow $= K_f[(P_c - P_i) - \sigma(\pi_c - \pi_i)]$ | 301 |
| Reticulocyte production index | $RPI = \%$ reticulocytes $\times \left( \dfrac{\text{actual Hct}}{\text{normal Hct}} \right) /$ maturation time | 423 |
| Renal clearance | $C_x = (U_x V)/P_x$ | 600 |
| Glomerular filtration rate | $C_{inulin} = GFR = U_{inulin} \times V/P_{inulin}$ <br><br> $= K_f [(P_{GC} - P_{BS}) - (\pi_{GC} - \pi_{BS})]$ | 600 |
| Effective renal plasma flow | $eRPF = U_{PAH} \times \dfrac{V}{P_{PAH}} = C_{PAH}$ | 600 |
| Filtration fraction | $FF = \dfrac{GFR}{RPF}$ | 601 |
| Fractional excretion of sodium | $Fe_{Na^+} = V \times U_{Na} / GFR \times P_{Na} = P_{Cr} \times U_{Na} / U_{Cr} \times P_{Na}$ | 602 |

| TOPIC | EQUATION | PAGE |
|---|---|---|
| Henderson-Hasselbalch equation (for extracellular pH) | $pH = 6.1 + \log \dfrac{[HCO_3^-]}{0.03 \ P_{CO_2}}$ | 609 |
| Winters formula | $P_{CO_2} = 1.5 \ [HCO_3^-] + 8 \pm 2$ | 609 |
| Anion gap | $Na^+ - (Cl^- + HCO_3^-)$ | 610 |
| Physiologic dead space | $V_D = V_T \times \dfrac{P_{aCO_2} - P_{ECO_2}}{P_{aCO_2}}$ | 682 |
| Pulmonary vascular resistance | $PVR = \dfrac{P_{pulm\ artery} - P_{L.\ atrium}}{Cardiac\ output}$ | 684 |
| Alveolar gas equation | $P_{AO_2} = P_{IO_2} - \dfrac{P_{aCO_2}}{RQ} = 150 \ mm \ Hg^a - P_{aCO_2} / 0.8$ | 685 |

## ▶ EASILY CONFUSED MEDICATIONS

| DRUG | CLINICAL USE/MECHANISM OF ACTION |
|---|---|
| Amiloride | $K^+$-sparing diuretic |
| Amiodarone | $K^+$ channel blocker (class III antiarrhythmic) |
| Amlodipine | Dihydropyridine $Ca^{2+}$ channel blocker |
| Benztropine | Parkinson disease (cholinergic antagonist) |
| Bromocriptine | Parkinson disease (dopamine agonist; rarely used) |
| Buspirone | Generalized anxiety disorder (partial 5-$HT_{1A}$-receptor agonist) |
| Bupropion | Depression, smoking cessation (NE-DA reuptake inhibitor) |
| Cimetidine | Gastritis, peptic ulcer ($H_2$-receptor antagonist) |
| Cetirizine | Allergy (2nd-generation antihistamine) |
| Chloramphenicol | Antibiotic (blocks 50S subunit) |
| Chlordiazepoxide | Long-acting benzodiazepine |
| Chlorpromazine | Typical antipsychotic |
| Chlorpropamide | 1st-generation sulfonylurea |
| Chlorpheniramine | 1st-generation antihistamine |
| Chlorthalidone | Thiazide diuretic |
| Clozapine | Atypical antipsychotic |
| Clomipramine | Tricyclic antidepressant |
| Clomiphene | Infertility due to anovulation (selective estrogen receptor modulator in hypothalamus) |
| Clonidine | Hypertensive urgency, ADHD ($\alpha_2$-agonist) |
| Doxepin | Tricyclic antidepressant |
| Doxazosin | BPH, HTN ($\alpha_1$-antagonist) |
| Eplerenone | $K^+$-sparing diuretic |

| DRUG | CLINICAL USE/MECHANISM OF ACTION |
|---|---|
| Propafenone | $Na^+$ channel blocker (class Ic antiarrhythmic) |
| Fluoxetine | Depression (selective serotonin reuptake inhibitor) |
| Fluphenazine | Typical antipsychotic |
| Mifepristone | Pregnancy termination (progesterone receptor antagonist) |
| Misoprostol | Used with mifepristone for pregnancy termination ($PGE_1$-synthetic analog) |
| Naloxone | Opioid receptor antagonist (treats toxicity) |
| Naltrexone | Opioid receptor antagonist (prevents relapse) |
| Nitroprusside | Hypertensive emergency (↑ cGMP/NO) |
| Nitroglycerin | Antianginal (↑ cGMP/NO) |
| Omeprazole | Proton pump inhibitor (inhibits $H^+/K^+$-ATPase in parietal cells) |
| Ketoconazole | Antifungal (inhibits fungal sterol synthesis) |
| Aripiprazole | Atypical antipsychotic ($D_2$ partial agonist) |
| Anastrozole | ER ⊕ breast cancer in postmenopausal women (aromatase inhibitor) |
| Rifaximin | Hepatic encephalopathy (↓ ammoniagenic bacteria) |
| Rifampin | Antituberculous drug/antimicrobial (inhibits DNA-dependent RNA polymerase) |
| Sertraline | Depression, PTSD (selective serotonin reuptake inhibitor) |
| Selegiline | Parkinson disease (MAO-B inhibitor) |
| Trazodone | Insomnia (blocks 5-$HT_2$, $\alpha_1$-adrenergic, and $H_1$ receptors); also weakly inhibits 5-HT reuptake |
| Tramadol | Chronic pain (weak opioid agonist) |
| Varenicline | Smoking cessation (nicotinic ACh receptor partial agonist) |
| Venlafaxine | Serotonin-norepinephrine reuptake inhibitor |

# SECTION IV

# Top-Rated Review Resources

"Some books are to be tasted, others to be swallowed, and some few to be chewed and digested."

—Sir Francis Bacon

"Always read something that will make you look good if you die in the middle of it."

—P.J. O'Rourke

"So many books, so little time."

—Frank Zappa

"If one cannot enjoy reading a book over and over again, there is no use in reading it at all."

—Oscar Wilde

"Start where you are. Use what you have. Do what you can."

—Arthur Ashe

## ▶ HOW TO USE THE DATABASE

This section is a database of top-rated basic science review books, sample examination books, websites, apps, and commercial review courses that have been marketed to medical students studying for the USMLE Step 1. For each recommended resource, we list (where applicable) the **Title**, the **First Author** (or editor), the **Series Name**, the **Current Publisher**, the **Copyright Year**, the **Number of Pages**, the **ISBN**, the **Approximate List Price**, the **Format** of the resource, and the **Number of Test Questions**. We also include **Summary Comments** that describe their style and overall utility for studying. Finally, each recommended resource receives a **Rating**. Within each section, resources are arranged first by Rating and then alphabetically by the first author within each Rating group.

A letter rating scale with six different grades reflects the detailed student evaluations for **Rated Resources**. Each rated resource receives a rating as follows:

| | |
|---|---|
| A+ | Excellent for boards review. |
| A<br>A– | Very good for boards review; choose among the group. |
| B+<br>B | Good, but use only after exhausting better resources. |
| B– | Fair, but there are many better resources in the discipline; or low-yield subject material. |

The rating is meant to reflect the overall usefulness of the resource in helping medical students prepare for the USMLE Step 1. This is based on a number of factors, including:

- The importance of the discipline for the USMLE Step 1
- The appropriateness and accuracy of the material
- The readability of the text, where applicable
- The quality and number of sample questions
- The quality of written answers to sample questions
- The cost
- The quality of the user interface and learning experience, for web and mobile apps
- The quality and appropriateness of the images and illustrations
- The length of the text (longer is not necessarily better)
- The quality and number of other resources available in the same discipline

Please note that ratings do not reflect the quality of the resources for purposes other than reviewing for the USMLE Step 1. Many books with lower ratings are well written and informative but are not ideal for boards preparation. We have not listed or commented on general textbooks available for the basic sciences.

Evaluations are based on the cumulative results of formal and informal surveys of thousands of medical students at many medical schools across the country. The summary comments and overall ratings represent a consensus opinion, but there may have been a broad range of opinion or limited student feedback on any particular resource.

Please note that the data listed are subject to change in that:

- Publisher and app store prices change frequently.
- Retail and online bookstores may set their own prices.
- New editions and app versions come out frequently, and the quality of updating varies.
- The same book may be reissued through another publisher.

We actively encourage medical students and faculty to submit their opinions and ratings of these basic science review materials so that we may update our database. In addition, we ask that publishers and authors submit for evaluation review copies of basic science review books, including new editions and books not included in our database. We also solicit reviews of new books, mobile apps, websites, flash cards, and commercial review courses.

### Disclaimer/Conflict of Interest Statement

None of the ratings reflects the opinion or influence of the publisher. All errors and omissions will gladly be corrected if brought to the attention of the authors through our blog at firstaidteam.com. Please note that USMLE-Rx, ScholarRx, and the entire *First Aid for the USMLE* series are publications by certain authors of *First Aid for the USMLE Step 1*; the following ratings are based solely on recommendations from the student authors of *First Aid for the USMLE Step 1* as well as data from the student survey and feedback forms.

## ▶ TOP-RATED REVIEW RESOURCES

### Question Banks

|   |   | AUTHOR | PUBLISHER | TYPE | PRICE |
|---|---|---|---|---|---|
| A+ | UWorld Qbank | UWorld | uworld.com | Test/3600+ q | $319–$719 |
| A | AMBOSS | Amboss | amboss.com | Test/2700+ q | $129–$299 |
| A | NBME Practice Exams | National Board of Medical Examiners | nbme.org/examinees/self-assessments | Test/200 q | $60 |
| A⁻ | USMLE-Rx Qmax | USMLE-Rx | usmle-rx.com/products/step-1-qmax/ | Test/2750+ q | $129–$349 |
| B+ | Kaplan Qbank | Kaplan | kaptest.com | Test/3300+ q | $159–$499 |
| B+ | TrueLearn Review | TrueLearn | truelearn.com | Test/2600+ q | $149–$419 |

### Web and Mobile Apps

|   |   | AUTHOR | PUBLISHER | TYPE | PRICE |
|---|---|---|---|---|---|
| A | AMBOSS Library | | amboss.com | Review | $15–$129 |
| A | Anki | | ankiweb.net | Flash cards | Free |
| A | Boards and Beyond | | boardsbeyond.com | Review/Test/2300+ q | $24–$399 |
| A | Dirty Medicine | | youtube.com/DirtyMedicine | Review | Free |
| A | Free 120 | | orientation.nbme.org/launch/usmle/stpfl | Test/120 q | Free |
| A | Pixorize | | pixorize.com | Review | $185–$249 |
| A | Rx Bricks | | usmle-rx.com/products/rx-bricks | Review/Study plan | $19–$129 |
| A | SketchyMedical | | sketchy.com | Review | $50–$600 |
| A⁻ | Physeo | | physeo.com | Review | Free–$450 |
| A⁻ | USMLE-Rx Step 1 Flash Facts | | usmle-rx.com/products/step-1-flash-facts | Flash cards | $29–$99 |
| B+ | Armando Hasudungan | | youtube.com/user/armandohasudungan | Review | Free |
| B+ | Blueprint | | blueprintprep.com/medical/med-school | Study Plan | Free |
| B+ | Firecracker | | med.firecracker.me | Review/Test/2300 q | $99–$149 |
| B+ | Kaplan USMLE® Step 1 Prep | | kaptest.com/usmle-step-1 | Review/Test/3300+ q | $1999–$2999 |
| B+ | Lecturio | | lecturio.com/medical/usmle-step-1 | Review/Test/4700+ q | $105–$480 |
| B+ | Medbullets | | step1.medbullets.com | Review/Test/1000+ q | Free–$250 |

## Web and Mobile Apps *(continued)*

| | | | | |
|---|---|---|---|---|
| B⁺ | *Ninja Nerd Medicine* | youtube.com/ninjanerdscience | Review | Free |
| B⁺ | *OnlineMedEd* | onlinemeded.org | Review | $65–$429 |
| B⁺ | *Osmosis* | osmosis.org | Test | $179–$359 |
| B⁺ | *Picmonic* | picmonic.com | Review | $25–$480 |
| B⁺ | *USMLE-Rx Step 1 Express* | usmle-rx.com/products/step-1-express-videos | Review/Test | $49–$179 |
| B | *Radiopaedia.org* | radiopaedia.org | Cases/Test | Free |

## Comprehensive

| | | AUTHOR | PUBLISHER | TYPE | PRICE |
|---|---|---|---|---|---|
| A | *First Aid for the Basic Sciences: General Principles* | Le | McGraw-Hill, 2017, 528 pages, ISBN 9781259587016 | Review | $83 |
| A | *First Aid for the Basic Sciences: Organ Systems* | Le | McGraw-Hill, 2017, 912 pages, ISBN 9781259587030 | Review | $80 |
| A | *USMLE Step 1 Secrets in Color* | O'Connell | Elsevier, 2021, 5th ed., 736 pages, ISBN 9780323810609 | Review | $48 |
| A⁻ | *First Aid Cases for the USMLE Step 1* | Le | McGraw-Hill, 2019, 496 pages, ISBN 9781260143133 | Cases | $55 |
| A⁻ | *Crush Step 1: The Ultimate USMLE Step 1 Review* | O'Connell | Elsevier, 2023, 736 pages, ISBN 9780323878869 | Review | $53 |
| B | *USMLE Step 1 Made Ridiculously Simple* | Carl | MedMaster, 2024, 416 pages, ISBN 9781935660729 | Review | $30 |
| B | *Kaplan USMLE Step 1 Qbook* | Kaplan | Kaplan Test Prep, 2022, 10th ed., 456 pages, ISBN 9781506276410 | Test/850 q | $55 |
| B | *medEssentials for the USMLE Step 1* | Kaplan | Kaplan Medical, 2022, 6th ed., 536 pages, ISBN 9781506254609 | Review | $60 |
| B | *USMLE Step 1 Lecture Notes 2023* | Kaplan | Kaplan Test Prep, 2023, 2560 pages, ISBN 9781506284637 | Review | $350 |

## Anatomy, Embryology, and Neuroscience

| | | AUTHOR | PUBLISHER | TYPE | PRICE |
|---|---|---|---|---|---|
| A⁻ | *High-Yield Gross Anatomy* | Dudek | Lippincott Williams & Wilkins, 2015, 320 pages, ISBN 9781451190236 | Review | $58 |
| B⁺ | *BRS Embryology* | Dudek | Lippincott Williams & Wilkins, 2014, 336 pages, ISBN 9781451190380 | Review/Test/220 q | $62 |
| B⁺ | *High-Yield Neuroanatomy* | Gould | Lippincott Williams & Wilkins, 2016, 208 pages, ISBN 9781451193435 | Review/Test/50 q | $55 |
| B⁺ | *Netter's Anatomy Flash Cards* | Hansen | Elsevier, 2022, 6th ed., 680 pages, ISBN 9789323834179 | Flash cards | $43 |
| B⁺ | *Netter's Essential Systems-Based Anatomy (Netter Basic Science)* | Lyons | Elsevier, 2022, 1st ed., 416 pages, ISBN 9780323694971 | Text/Review | $53 |

## Anatomy, Embryology, and Neuroscience *(continued)*

| | | AUTHOR | PUBLISHER | TYPE | PRICE |
|---|---|---|---|---|---|
| B+ | *Crash Course: Anatomy and Physiology* | Stephens | Elsevier, 2019, 350 pages, ISBN 9780702073755 | Review | $42 |
| B | *Anatomy—An Essential Textbook* | Gilroy | Thieme, 2021, 3rd ed., 634 pages, ISBN 9781684202591 | Text/Test | $60 |
| B | *Complete Anatomy* | | 3d4medical.com | Review | $75 |

## Behavioral Science

| | | AUTHOR | PUBLISHER | TYPE | PRICE |
|---|---|---|---|---|---|
| A− | *BRS Behavioral Science* | Fadem | Lippincott Williams & Wilkins, 2021, 384 pages, ISBN 9781975188856 | Review/Test/600 q | $63 |
| B+ | *Kahn's Cases: Medical Ethics* | Kahn | CreateSpace Independent Publishing Platform, 2020, 253 pages, ISBN 9781481959483 | Review | $10 |
| B | *Biostatistics and Epidemiology: A Primer for Health and Biomedical Professionals* | Wassertheil-Smoller | Springer, 2015, 280 pages, 9781493921331 | Review | $85 |

## Biochemistry

| | | AUTHOR | PUBLISHER | TYPE | PRICE |
|---|---|---|---|---|---|
| B+ | *Lippincott Illustrated Reviews: Biochemistry* | Abali | Lippincott Williams & Wilkins, 2021, 8th ed., 640 pages, ISBN 9781975155063 | Review/Test/200 q | $85 |
| B+ | *BRS Biochemistry, Molecular Biology, and Genetics* | Lieberman | Lippincott Williams & Wilkins, 2020, 448 pages, ISBN 9781496399236 | Review/Test/500 q | $62 |
| B | *Lange Flashcards: Biochemistry and Genetics* | Baron | McGraw-Hill, 2017, 184 flash cards, ISBN 9781259837210 | Flash cards | $34 |

## Cell Biology and Histology

| | | AUTHOR | PUBLISHER | TYPE | PRICE |
|---|---|---|---|---|---|
| B+ | *Thieme Test Prep for the USMLE®: Medical Histology and Embryology Q&A* | Das | Thieme, 2018, 1st ed., 266 pages, ISBN 9781626233348 | Test/600 q | $50 |
| B+ | *Crash Course: Cell Biology and Genetics* | Stubbs | Mosby, 2015, 216 pages, ISBN 9780723438762 | Review/Print + online | $47 |
| B | *BRS Cell Biology and Histology* | Gartner | Lippincott Williams & Wilkins, 2018, 448 pages, ISBN 9781496396358 | Review/Test/320 q | $63 |

## Microbiology and Immunology

| | | AUTHOR | PUBLISHER | TYPE | PRICE |
|---|---|---|---|---|---|
| A− | *Medical Microbiology and Immunology Flash Cards* | Rosenthal | Elsevier, 2017, 192 flash cards, ISBN 9780323462242 | Flash cards | $43 |
| B+ | *Basic Immunology* | Abbas | Elsevier, 2023, 352 pages, ISBN 9780443105197 | Review | $78 |
| B+ | *Clinical Microbiology Made Ridiculously Simple* | Gladwin | MedMaster, 2022, 448 pages, ISBN 9781935660491 | Review | $38 |

## Microbiology and Immunology *(continued)*

| | | AUTHOR | PUBLISHER | TYPE | PRICE |
|---|---|---|---|---|---|
| B⁺ | *Crash Course: Haematology and Immunology* | Redhouse White | Elsevier, 2019, 5th ed., 216 pages, ISBN 9780702073632 | Review | $42 |
| B⁺ | *Lange Microbiology and Infectious Diseases Flash Cards, 3e* | Somers | McGraw-Hill, 2018, ISBN 9781259859823 | Flash cards | $55 |
| B | *Lippincott Illustrated Reviews: Microbiology* | Cornelissen | Lippincott Williams & Wilkins, 2019, 448 pages, ISBN 9781496395856 | Review/Test/ Few q | $82 |
| B | *Review of Medical Microbiology and Immunology* | Levinson | McGraw-Hill, 2022, 848 pages, ISBN 9781264267088 | Review/ Test/650 q | $76 |
| B | *How the Immune System Works* | Sompayrac | Wiley-Blackwell, 2023, 176 pages, ISBN 9781119890683 | Review | $45 |

## Pathology

| | | AUTHOR | PUBLISHER | TYPE | PRICE |
|---|---|---|---|---|---|
| A⁺ | *Pathoma: Fundamentals of Pathology* | Sattar | Pathoma, 2021, 218 pages, ISBN 9780983224631 | Review/ Lecture | $85–$120 |
| A | *Rapid Review: Pathology* | Goljan | Elsevier, 2024, 416 pages, ISBN 9780323870573 | Review/ Test/500 q | $67 |
| A⁻ | *Robbins and Cotran Review of Pathology* | Klatt | Elsevier, 2022, 488 pages, ISBN 9780323640220 | Test/1500 q | $59 |
| A⁻ | *Crash Course: Pathology* | McKinney | Elsevier, 2020, 438 pages, ISBN 9780702073540 | Review | $42 |
| B | *BRS Pathology* | Gupta | Lippincott Williams & Wilkins, 2021, 496 pages, ISBN 9781975136628 | Review/ Test/450 q | $62 |
| B | *Pathophysiology of Disease: Introduction to Clinical Medicine* | Hammer | McGraw-Hill, 2019, 832 pages, ISBN 9781260026504 | Text | $99 |
| B | *Pocket Companion to Robbins and Cotran Pathologic Basis of Disease* | Mitchell | Elsevier, 2024, 1028 pages, ISBN 9780323653909 | Review | $46 |

## Pharmacology

| | | AUTHOR | PUBLISHER | TYPE | PRICE |
|---|---|---|---|---|---|
| B⁺ | *Crash Course: Pharmacology* | Page | Elsevier, 2020, 336 pages, ISBN 9780702073441 | Review | $42 |
| B | *Lange Pharmacology Flash Cards* | Baron | McGraw-Hill, 2023, 266 flash cards, ISBN 9781264779963 | Flash cards | $42 |
| B | *BRS Pharmacology* | Lerchenfeldt | Lippincott Williams & Wilkins, 2019, 384 pages, ISBN 9781975105495 | Review/ Test/200 q | $65 |
| B | *Katzung & Trevor's Pharmacology: Examination and Board Review* | Trevor | McGraw-Hill, 2021, 608 pages, ISBN 9781260117127 | Review/ Test/1000 q | $69 |
| B⁻ | *Lippincott Illustrated Reviews: Pharmacology* | Whalen | Lippincott Williams & Wilkins, 2022, 8th ed., 704 pages, ISBN 9781975170554 | Review/ Test/380 q | $78 |

## Physiology

| | | AUTHOR | PUBLISHER | TYPE | PRICE |
|---|---|---|---|---|---|
| **A⁻** | *Physiology* | Costanzo | Elsevier, 2022, 7th ed., 528 pages, ISBN 9780323793339 | Text | $69 |
| **A⁻** | *Pulmonary Pathophysiology: The Essentials* | West | Lippincott Williams & Wilkins, 2022, 272 pages, ISBN 9781975152819 | Review/Test/75 q | $60 |
| **B⁺** | *Pathophysiology of Heart Disease* | Lilly | Lippincott Williams & Williams, 2020, 480 pages, ISBN 9781975120597 | Review | $63 |
| **B⁺** | *Acid-Base, Fluids, and Electrolytes Made Ridiculously Simple* | Preston | MedMaster, 2017, 166 pages, ISBN 9781935660293 | Review | $24 |
| **B⁺** | *Lippincott Illustrated Reviews: Physiology* | Preston | Lippincott Williams & Wilkins, 2018, 544 pages, ISBN 9781496385826 | Review | $82 |
| **B** | *BRS Physiology* | Costanzo | Lippincott Williams & Wilkins, 2022, 8th ed., 336 pages, ISBN 9781975153601 | Review/Test/350 q | $58 |
| **B** | *Vander's Renal Physiology* | Eaton | McGraw-Hill, 2023, 240 pages, ISBN 9781264278527 | Text | $49 |
| **B** | *Endocrine Physiology* | Molina | McGraw-Hill, 2023, 320 pages, ISBN 9781264278459 | Review | $59 |
| **B** | *Netter's Physiology Flash Cards* | Mulroney | Elsevier, 2016, 450 pages, ISBN 9780323359542 | Flash cards | $40 |

# Abbreviations and Symbols

| ABBREVIATION | MEANING |
|---|---|
| 1st MC* | 1st metacarpal |
| A-a | alveolar-arterial [gradient] |
| AA | Alcoholics Anonymous, amyloid A |
| AAA | abdominal aortic aneurysm |
| AAMC | Association of American Medical Colleges |
| AAo* | ascending aorta |
| Ab | antibody |
| ABPA | allergic bronchopulmonary aspergillosis |
| AC | adenylyl cyclase |
| ACA | anterior cerebral artery |
| Acetyl-CoA | acetyl coenzyme A |
| ACD | anemia of chronic disease |
| ACE | angiotensin-converting enzyme |
| ACh | acetylcholine |
| AChE | acetylcholinesterase |
| ACL | anterior cruciate ligament |
| ACom | anterior communicating [artery] |
| ACTH | adrenocorticotropic hormone |
| AD | Alzheimer disease, autosomal dominant |
| ADA | adenosine deaminase, Americans with Disabilities Act |
| ADH | antidiuretic hormone |
| ADHD | attention-deficit hyperactivity disorder |
| ADP | adenosine diphosphate |
| ADPKD | autosomal-dominant polycystic kidney disease |
| AFP | α-fetoprotein |
| Ag | antigen, silver |
| AICA | anterior inferior cerebellar artery |
| AIDS | acquired immunodeficiency syndrome |
| AIHA | autoimmune hemolytic anemia |
| AKI | acute kidney injury |
| AKT | protein kinase B |
| AL | amyloid light [chain] |
| ALA | aminolevulinate |
| ALI | acute lung injury |
| ALK | anaplastic lymphoma kinase |
| ALL | acute lymphoblastic (lymphocytic) leukemia |
| ALP | alkaline phosphatase |
| ALS | amyotrophic lateral sclerosis |
| ALT | alanine transaminase |
| AMA | American Medical Association, antimitochondrial antibody |
| AML | acute myelogenous (myeloid) leukemia |
| AMP | adenosine monophosphate |
| ANA | antinuclear antibody |

| ABBREVIATION | MEANING |
|---|---|
| ANCA | antineutrophil cytoplasmic antibody |
| ANOVA | analysis of variance |
| ANP | atrial natriuretic peptide |
| ANS | autonomic nervous system |
| Ant* | anterior |
| Ao* | aorta |
| AOA | American Osteopathic Association |
| AP | action potential, A & P [ribosomal binding sites] |
| APC | antigen-presenting cell, activated protein C |
| APL | Acute promyelocytic leukemia |
| Apo | apolipoprotein |
| APP | amyloid precursor protein |
| APRT | adenine phosphoribosyltransferase |
| aPTT | activated partial thromboplastin time |
| APUD | amine precursor uptake decarboxylase |
| AR | attributable risk, autosomal recessive, aortic regurgitation |
| ARB | angiotensin receptor blocker |
| ARDS | acute respiratory distress syndrome |
| Arg | arginine |
| ARPKD | autosomal-recessive polycystic kidney disease |
| ART | antiretroviral therapy |
| AS | aortic stenosis |
| ASA | anterior spinal artery |
| Asc* | ascending |
| Asc Ao* | ascending aorta |
| ASD | atrial septal defect |
| ASO | anti–streptolysin O |
| AST | aspartate transaminase |
| AT | angiotensin, antithrombin |
| ATN | acute tubular necrosis |
| ATP | adenosine triphosphate |
| ATPase | adenosine triphosphatase |
| ATTR | transthyretin-mediated amyloidosis |
| AV | atrioventricular |
| AZT | azidothymidine |
| BAL | British anti-Lewisite [dimercaprol] |
| BBB | blood-brain barrier |
| BCG | bacille Calmette-Guérin |
| bd* | bile duct |
| BH$_4$ | tetrahydrobiopterin |
| BM | basement membrane |
| BOOP | bronchiolitis obliterans organizing pneumonia |
| BP | bisphosphate, blood pressure |
| BPG | bisphosphoglycerate |

*Image abbreviation only

| ABBREVIATION | MEANING |
|---|---|
| BPH | benign prostatic hyperplasia |
| BT | bleeding time |
| BUN | blood urea nitrogen |
| C* | caudate |
| Ca* | capillary |
| $Ca^{2+}$ | calcium ion |
| CAD | coronary artery disease |
| CAF | common application form |
| cAMP | cyclic adenosine monophosphate |
| CBG | corticosteroid-binding globulin |
| CBSE | Comprehensive Basic Science Examination |
| CBSSA | Comprehensive Basic Science Self-Assessment |
| CBT | computer-based test, cognitive behavioral therapy |
| CCK | cholecystokinin |
| CCS | computer-based case simulation |
| CD | cluster of differentiation |
| CDK | cyclin-dependent kinase |
| cDNA | complementary deoxyribonucleic acid |
| CEA | carcinoembryonic antigen |
| CETP | cholesteryl-ester transfer protein |
| CF | cystic fibrosis |
| CFTR | cystic fibrosis transmembrane conductance regulator |
| CGD | chronic granulomatous disease |
| cGMP | cyclic guanosine monophosphate |
| CGRP | calcitonin gene–related peptide |
| $C_H1–C_H3$ | constant regions, heavy chain [antibody] |
| ChAT | choline acetyltransferase |
| CHD* | common hepatic duct |
| $\chi^2$ | chi-squared |
| CI | confidence interval |
| CIN | candidate identification number, carcinoma in situ, cervical intraepithelial neoplasia |
| CIS | Communication and Interpersonal Skills |
| CK | clinical knowledge, creatine kinase |
| CKD | chronic kidney disease |
| CK-MB | creatine kinase, MB fraction |
| $C_L$ | constant region, light chain [antibody] |
| CL | clearance |
| $Cl^-$ | chloride ion |
| CLL | chronic lymphocytic leukemia |
| CMC | carpometacarpal (joint) |
| CML | chronic myelogenous (myeloid) leukemia |
| CMV | cytomegalovirus |
| CN | cranial nerve |
| $CN^-$ | cyanide ion |
| CNS | central nervous system |
| CNV | copy number variation |
| CO | carbon monoxide, cardiac output |
| $CO_2$ | carbon dioxide |
| CoA | coenzyme A |
| Coarct* | coarctation |
| COL1A1 | collagen, type I, alpha 1 |
| COL1A2 | collagen, type I, alpha 2 |
| COMT | catechol-O-methyltransferase |

| ABBREVIATION | MEANING |
|---|---|
| COP | coat protein |
| COPD | chronic obstructive pulmonary disease |
| CoQ | coenzyme Q |
| COVID-19 | Coronavirus disease 2019 |
| COX | cyclooxygenase |
| $C_p$ | plasma concentration |
| CPAP | continuous positive airway pressure |
| CPR | cardiopulmonary resuscitation |
| Cr | creatinine |
| CRC | colorectal cancer |
| CREST | calcinosis, Raynaud phenomenon, esophageal dysfunction, sclerosis, and telangiectasias [syndrome] |
| CRH | corticotropin-releasing hormone |
| CRP | C-reactive protein |
| CS | clinical skills |
| C-section | cesarean section |
| CSF | cerebrospinal fluid |
| CT | computed tomography |
| CTP | cytidine triphosphate |
| CXR | chest x-ray |
| DA | dopamine |
| DAF | decay-accelerating factor |
| DAG | diacylglycerol |
| DAo* | descending aorta |
| DAT | dopamine transporter |
| dATP | deoxyadenosine triphosphate |
| DCIS | ductal carcinoma in situ |
| DCT | distal convoluted tubule |
| ddI | didanosine |
| DES | diethylstilbestrol |
| Desc Ao* | descending aorta |
| DEXA | dual-energy x-ray absorptiometry |
| DHAP | dihydroxyacetone phosphate |
| DHEA | dehydroepiandrosterone |
| DHF | dihydrofolic acid |
| DHT | dihydrotestosterone |
| DI | diabetes insipidus |
| DIC | disseminated intravascular coagulation |
| DIP | distal interphalangeal [joint] |
| DKA | diabetic ketoacidosis |
| DLCO | diffusing capacity for carbon monoxide |
| DM | diabetes mellitus |
| DNA | deoxyribonucleic acid |
| DNR | do not resuscitate |
| dNTP | deoxynucleotide triphosphate |
| DO | doctor of osteopathy |
| DPGN | diffuse proliferative glomerulonephritis |
| DPM | doctor of podiatric medicine |
| DPP-4 | dipeptidyl peptidase-4 |
| DPPC | dipalmitoylphosphatidylcholine |
| DRESS | Drug reaction with eosinophilia and systemic symptoms |
| DS | double stranded |
| dsDNA | double-stranded deoxyribonucleic acid |
| dsRNA | double-stranded ribonucleic acid |
| DRG | dorsal root ganglion |

*Image abbreviation only

| ABBREVIATION | MEANING |
|---|---|
| d4T | didehydrodeoxythymidine [stavudine] |
| dTMP | deoxythymidine monophosphate |
| DTR | deep tendon reflex |
| DTs | delirium tremens |
| dUDP | deoxyuridine diphosphate |
| dUMP | deoxyuridine monophosphate |
| DVT | deep venous thrombosis |
| E* | euthromatin, esophagus |
| EBV | Epstein-Barr virus |
| ECA* | external carotid artery |
| ECF | extracellular fluid |
| ECFMG | Educational Commission for Foreign Medical Graduates |
| ECG | electrocardiogram |
| ECL | enterochromaffin-like [cell] |
| ECM | extracellular matrix |
| ECT | electroconvulsive therapy |
| ED$_{50}$ | median effective dose |
| EDRF | endothelium-derived relaxing factor |
| EDTA | ethylenediamine tetra-acetic acid |
| EDV | end-diastolic volume |
| EEG | electroencephalogram |
| EF | ejection fraction |
| EGF | epidermal growth factor |
| EHEC | enterohemorrhagic E coli |
| EIEC | enteroinvasive E coli |
| ELISA | enzyme-linked immunosorbent assay |
| EM | electron micrograph/microscopy |
| EMB | eosin–methylene blue |
| EPEC | eneteropathogenic E coli |
| Epi | epinephrine |
| EPO | erythropoietin |
| EPS | extrapyramidal system |
| ER | endoplasmic reticulum, estrogen receptor |
| ERAS | Electronic Residency Application Service |
| ERCP | endoscopic retrograde cholangiopancreatography |
| ERP | effective refractory period |
| eRPF | effective renal plasma flow |
| ERT | estrogen replacement therapy |
| ERV | expiratory reserve volume |
| ESR | erythrocyte sedimentation rate |
| ESRD | end-stage renal disease |
| ESV | end-systolic volume |
| ETEC | enterotoxigenic E coli |
| EtOH | ethyl alcohol |
| EV | esophageal vein |
| F | bioavailability |
| FA | fatty acid |
| Fab | fragment, antigen-binding |
| FAD | flavin adenine dinucleotide |
| FADH$_2$ | reduced flavin adenine dinucleotide |
| FAP | familial adenomatous polyposis |
| F1,6BP | fructose-1,6-bisphosphate |
| F2,6BP | fructose-2,6-bisphosphate |
| FBPase | fructose bisphosphatase |

| ABBREVIATION | MEANING |
|---|---|
| FBPase-2 | fructose bisphosphatase-2 |
| Fc | fragment, crystallizable |
| FcR | Fc receptor |
| 5f-dUMP | 5-fluorodeoxyuridine monophosphate |
| Fe$^{2+}$ | ferrous ion |
| Fe$^{3+}$ | ferric ion |
| Fem* | femur |
| FENa | excreted fraction of filtered sodium |
| FEV$_1$ | forced expiratory volume in 1 second |
| FF | filtration fraction |
| FFA | free fatty acid |
| FGF | fibroblast growth factor |
| FGFR | fibroblast growth factor receptor |
| FGR | fetal growth restriction |
| FISH | fluorescence in situ hybridization |
| FIo$_2$ | fraction of inspired oxygen |
| FIT | fecal immunochemical testing |
| FKBP | FK506 binding protein |
| fMet | formylmethionine |
| FMG | foreign medical graduate |
| FMN | flavin mononucleotide |
| FN | false negative |
| FP, FP* | false positive, foot process |
| FRC | functional residual capacity |
| FSH | follicle-stimulating hormone |
| FSMB | Federation of State Medical Boards |
| FTA-ABS | fluorescent treponemal antibody—absorbed |
| FTD* | frontotemporal dementia |
| 5-FU | 5-fluorouracil |
| FVC | forced vital capacity |
| GABA | γ-aminobutyric acid |
| GAG | glycosaminoglycan |
| Gal | galactose |
| GBM | glomerular basement membrane |
| GC | glomerular capillary |
| G-CSF | granulocyte colony-stimulating factor |
| GERD | gastroesophageal reflux disease |
| GFAP | glial fibrillary acid protein |
| GFR | glomerular filtration rate |
| GGT | γ-glutamyl transpeptidase |
| GH | growth hormone |
| GHB | γ-hydroxybutyrate |
| GHRH | growth hormone–releasing hormone |
| G$_I$ | G protein, I polypeptide |
| GI | gastrointestinal |
| GIP | gastric inhibitory peptide |
| GIST | gastrointestinal stromal tumor |
| GLUT | glucose transporter |
| GM | granulocyte macrophage |
| GM-CSF | granulocyte-macrophage colony stimulating factor |
| GMP | guanosine monophosphate |
| GnRH | gonadotropin-releasing hormone |
| Gp | glycoprotein |
| G6P | glucose-6-phosphate |

*Image abbreviation only

| ABBREVIATION | MEANING |
|---|---|
| G6PD | glucose-6-phosphate dehydrogenase |
| GPe | globus pallidus externa |
| GPi | globus pallidus interna |
| GPI | glycosyl phosphatidylinositol |
| GRP | gastrin-releasing peptide |
| $G_S$ | G protein, S polypeptide |
| GSH | reduced glutathione |
| GSSG | oxidized glutathione |
| GTP | guanosine triphosphate |
| GTPase | guanosine triphosphatase |
| GU | genitourinary |
| H* | heterochromatin |
| $H^+$ | hydrogen ion |
| $H_1$, $H_2$ | histamine receptors |
| $H_2S$ | hydrogen sulfide |
| ha* | hepatic artery |
| HAV | hepatitis A virus |
| HAVAb | hepatitis A antibody |
| Hb | hemoglobin |
| HBcAb/HBcAg | hepatitis B core antibody/antigen |
| HBeAb/HBeAg | hepatitis B early antibody/antigen |
| HBsAb/HBsAg | hepatitis B surface antibody/antigen |
| $HbCO_2$ | carbaminohemoglobin |
| HBV | hepatitis B virus |
| HCC | hepatocellular carcinoma |
| hCG | human chorionic gonadotropin |
| $HCO_3^-$ | bicarbonate |
| Hct | hematocrit |
| HCTZ | hydrochlorothiazide |
| HCV | hepatitis C virus |
| HDL | high-density lipoprotein |
| HDN | hemolytic disease of the newborn |
| HDV | hepatitis D virus |
| H&E | hematoxylin and eosin |
| HEV | hepatitis E virus |
| HF | heart failure |
| Hfr | high-frequency recombination [cell] |
| HFpEF | heart failure with preserved ejection fraction |
| HFrEF | heart failure with reduced ejection fraction |
| HGPRT | hypoxanthine-guanine phosphoribosyltransferase |
| HHb | deoxygenated hemoglobin |
| HHS | hyperosmolar hyperglycemic state |
| HHV | human herpesvirus |
| 5-HIAA | 5-hydroxindoleacetic acid |
| HIT | heparin-induced thrombocytopenia |
| HIV | human immunodeficiency virus |
| HL | hepatic lipase |
| HLA | human leukocyte antigen |
| HMG-CoA | hydroxymethylglutaryl-coenzyme A |
| HMP | hexose monophosphate |
| HMWK | high-molecular-weight kininogen |
| HNPCC | hereditary nonpolyposis colorectal cancer |
| hnRNA | heterogeneous nuclear ribonucleic acid |
| $H_2O_2$ | hydrogen peroxide |

| ABBREVIATION | MEANING |
|---|---|
| HOCM | hypertrophic obstructive cardiomyopathy |
| HPA | hypothalamic-pituitary-adrenal [axis] |
| HPO | hypothalamic-pituitary-ovarian [axis] |
| HPV | human papillomavirus |
| HR | heart rate |
| HSP | Henoch-Schönlein purpura |
| HSV | herpes simplex virus |
| 5-HT | 5-hydroxytryptamine (serotonin) |
| HTLV | human T-cell leukemia virus |
| HTN | hypertension |
| HUS | hemolytic-uremic syndrome |
| HVA | homovanillic acid |
| IBD | inflammatory bowel disease |
| IBS | irritable bowel syndrome |
| IC | inspiratory capacity, immune complex |
| $I_{Ca}$ | calcium current [heart] |
| $I_f$ | funny current [heart] |
| ICA | internal carotid artery |
| ICAM | intercellular adhesion molecule |
| ICD | implantable cardioverter-defibrillator |
| ICE | Integrated Clinical Encounter |
| ICF | intracellular fluid |
| ICP | intracranial pressure |
| ID | identification |
| $ID_{50}$ | median infective dose |
| IDL | intermediate-density lipoprotein |
| IF | immunofluorescence, initiation factor |
| IFN | interferon |
| Ig | immunoglobulin |
| IGF | insulinlike growth factor |
| $I_K$ | potassium current [heart] |
| IL | interleukin |
| IM | intramuscular |
| IMA | inferior mesenteric artery |
| IMG | international medical graduate |
| IMP | inosine monophosphate |
| IMV | inferior mesenteric vein |
| $I_{Na}$ | sodium current [heart] |
| INH | isoniazid |
| INO | internuclear ophthalmoplegia |
| INR | International Normalized Ratio |
| IO | inferior oblique [muscle] |
| IOP | intraocular pressure |
| $IP_3$ | inositol triphosphate |
| IPV | inactivated polio vaccine |
| IR | current × resistance [Ohm's law], inferior rectus [muscle] |
| IRV | inspiratory reserve volume |
| ITP | idiopathic thrombocytopenic purpura |
| IUD | intrauterine device |
| IV | intravenous |
| IVC | inferior vena cava |
| IVIG | intravenous immunoglobulin |
| JAK/STAT | Janus kinase/signal transducer and activator of transcription [pathway] |

*Image abbreviation only

| ABBREVIATION | MEANING |
|---|---|
| JGA | juxtaglomerular apparatus |
| JVD | jugular venous distention |
| JVP | jugular venous pulse |
| $K^+$ | potassium ion |
| KatG | catalase-peroxidase produced by *M tuberculosis* |
| $K_e$ | elimination constant |
| $K_f$ | filtration constant |
| KG | ketoglutarate |
| Kid* | kidney |
| $K_m$ | Michaelis-Menten constant |
| KOH | potassium hydroxide |
| L | left, lentiform, liver |
| LA | left atrial, left atrium |
| LAD | left anterior descending coronary artery |
| LAP | leukocyte alkaline phosphatase |
| Lat cond* | lateral condyle |
| Lb* | lamellar body |
| LCA | left coronary artery |
| LCAT | lecithin-cholesterol acyltransferase |
| LCC* | left common carotid artery |
| LCFA | long-chain fatty acid |
| LCL | lateral collateral ligament |
| LCME | Liaison Committee on Medical Education |
| LCMV | lymphocytic choriomeningitis virus |
| LCX | left circumflex coronary artery |
| LD | loading dose |
| $LD_{50}$ | median lethal dose |
| LDH | lactate dehydrogenase |
| LDL | low-density lipoprotein |
| LES | lower esophageal sphincter |
| LFA | leukocyte function–associated antigen |
| LFT | liver function test |
| LH | luteinizing hormone |
| Liv* | liver |
| LLL* | left lower lobe (of lung) |
| LLQ | left lower quadrant |
| LM | lateral meniscus, left main coronary artery, light microscopy |
| LMN | lower motor neuron |
| LOS | lipooligosaccharide |
| LPA* | left pulmonary artery |
| LPL | lipoprotein lipase |
| LPS | lipopolysaccharide |
| LR | lateral rectus [muscle] |
| LT | labile toxin, leukotriene |
| LUL* | left upper lobe (of lung) |
| LV | left ventricle, left ventricular |
| $M_1$-$M_5$ | muscarinic (parasympathetic) ACh receptors |
| MAC | membrane attack complex, minimum alveolar concentration |
| MALT | mucosa-associated lymphoid tissue |
| MAO | monoamine oxidase |
| MAP | mean arterial pressure, mitogen-activated protein |
| Max* | maxillary sinus |
| MC | midsystolic click, metacarpal |

| ABBREVIATION | MEANING |
|---|---|
| MCA | middle cerebral artery |
| MCAT | Medical College Admissions Test |
| MCHC | mean corpuscular hemoglobin concentration |
| MCL | medial collateral ligament |
| MCP | metacarpophalangeal [joint] |
| MCV | mean corpuscular volume |
| MD | maintenance dose |
| MDD | major depressive disorder |
| MDMA | 3,4-methylenedioxymethamphetamine, ecstasy |
| Med cond* | medial condyle |
| MELAS syndrome | mitochondrial encephalopathy, lactic acidosis, and stroke-like episodes |
| MEN | multiple endocrine neoplasia |
| MERS | Middle East respiratory syndrome |
| $Mg^{2+}$ | magnesium ion |
| $MgSO_4$ | magnesium sulfate |
| MHC | major histocompatibility complex |
| MI | myocardial infarction |
| MIF | müllerian inhibiting factor |
| MIRL | membrane inhibitor of reactive lysis |
| MLCK | myosin light-chain kinase |
| MLF | medial longitudinal fasciculus |
| MMC | migrating motor complex |
| MMR | measles, mumps, rubella [vaccine] |
| MODY | maturity-onset diabetes of the young |
| 6-MP | 6-mercaptopurine |
| MPGN | membranoproliferative glomerulonephritis |
| MPO | myeloperoxidase |
| MPO-ANCA/ p-ANCA | myeloperoxidase/perinuclear antineutrophil cytoplasmic antibody |
| MR | medial rectus [muscle], mitral regurgitation |
| MRI | magnetic resonance imaging |
| miRNA | microribonucleic acid |
| mRNA | messenger ribonucleic acid |
| MRSA | methicillin-resistant *S aureus* |
| MS | mitral stenosis, multiple sclerosis |
| MSH | melanocyte-stimulating hormone |
| mtDNA | mitochondrial DNA |
| mTOR | mammalian target of rapamycin |
| MTP | metatarsophalangeal [joint] |
| MTX | methotrexate |
| $MVO_2$ | myocardial oxygen consumption |
| MVP | mitral valve prolapse |
| N* | nucleus |
| $Na^+$ | sodium ion |
| NAAT | nucleic acid amplification test |
| NAD | nicotinamide adenine dinucleotide |
| $NAD^+$ | oxidized nicotinamide adenine dinucleotide |
| NADH | reduced nicotinamide adenine dinucleotide |
| $NADP^+$ | oxidized nicotinamide adenine dinucleotide phosphate |
| NADPH | reduced nicotinamide adenine dinucleotide phosphate |
| NBME | National Board of Medical Examiners |
| NBOME | National Board of Osteopathic Medical Examiners |
| NBPME | National Board of Podiatric Medical Examiners |

*Image abbreviation only

| ABBREVIATION | MEANING |
| --- | --- |
| NE | norepinephrine |
| NET | norepinephrine transporter |
| NF | neurofibromatosis |
| NFAT | nuclear factor of activated T-cell |
| $NH_3$ | ammonia |
| $NH_4^+$ | ammonium |
| NK | natural killer [cells] |
| $N_M$ | muscarinic ACh receptor in neuromuscular junction |
| NMDA | N-methyl-d-aspartate |
| NMJ | neuromuscular junction |
| NMS | neuroleptic malignant syndrome |
| $N_N$ | nicotinic ACh receptor in autonomic ganglia |
| NRMP | National Residency Matching Program |
| NNRTI | non-nucleoside reverse transcriptase inhibitor |
| NO | nitric oxide |
| $N_2O$ | nitrous oxide |
| NPH | neutral protamine Hagedorn, normal pressure hydrocephalus |
| NPV | negative predictive value |
| NRTI | nucleoside reverse transcriptase inhibitor |
| NSAID | nonsteroidal anti-inflammatory drug |
| NSE | neuron-specific enolase |
| NSTEMI | non–ST-segment elevation myocardial infarction |
| NTD | neural tube defect |
| Nu* | nucleolus |
| OAA | oxaloacetic acid |
| OCD | obsessive-compulsive disorder |
| OCP | oral contraceptive pill |
| ODC | oxygen-hemoglobin dissociation curve |
| OH | hydroxy |
| $1,25\text{-OH } D_3$ | calcitriol (active form of vitamin D) |
| $25\text{-OH } D_3$ | storage form of vitamin D |
| OPV | oral polio vaccine |
| OR | odds ratio |
| ori | origins of replication |
| OS | opening snap |
| OSA | obstructive sleep apnea |
| OTC | Ornithine transcarbamylase |
| OVLT | organum vasculosum of the lamina terminalis |
| P-body | processing body (cytoplasmic) |
| P-450 | cytochrome P-450 family of enzymes |
| PA | posteroanterior, pulmonary artery |
| PABA | *para*-aminobenzoic acid |
| $Paco_2$ | arterial $Pco_2$ |
| $PAco_2$ | alveolar $Pco_2$ |
| PAH | *para*-aminohippuric acid |
| PAMP | pathogen-associated molecular patterns |
| PAN | polyarteritis nodosa |
| $Pao_2$ | partial pressure of oxygen in arterial blood |
| $PAo_2$ | partial pressure of oxygen in alveolar blood |
| PAP | Papanicolaou [smear], prostatic acid phosphatase, posteromedial papillary muscle |
| PAPPA | pregnancy-associated plasma protein A |
| PAS | periodic acid–Schiff |

| ABBREVIATION | MEANING |
| --- | --- |
| Pat* | patella |
| $P_B$ | Barometric (atmospheric) pressure |
| PBP | penicillin-binding protein |
| PC | platelet count, pyruvate carboxylase |
| PCA | posterior cerebral artery |
| PCC | prothrombin complex concentrate |
| PCL | posterior cruciate ligament |
| $Pco_2$ | partial pressure of carbon dioxide |
| PCom | posterior communicating [artery] |
| PCOS | polycystic ovarian syndrome |
| PCP | phencyclidine hydrochloride, *Pneumocystis jirovecii* pneumonia |
| PCR | polymerase chain reaction |
| PCT | proximal convoluted tubule |
| PCV13 | pneumococcal conjugate vaccine |
| PCWP | pulmonary capillary wedge pressure |
| PDA | patent ductus arteriosus, posterior descending artery |
| PDE | phosphodiesterase |
| PDGF | platelet-derived growth factor |
| PDH | pyruvate dehydrogenase |
| PE | pulmonary embolism |
| PECAM | platelet–endothelial cell adhesion molecule |
| $Peco_2$ | expired air $Pco_2$ |
| PEP | phosphoenolpyruvate |
| PF | platelet factor |
| PFK | phosphofructokinase |
| PFK-2 | phosphofructokinase-2 |
| PFT | pulmonary function test |
| PG | phosphoglycerate |
| $P_{H_2O}$ | water pressure |
| $P_i$ | plasma interstitial osmotic pressure, inorganic phosphate |
| PICA | posterior inferior cerebellar artery |
| PID | pelvic inflammatory disease |
| $Pio_2$ | $Po_2$ in inspired air |
| PIP | proximal interphalangeal [joint] |
| $PIP_2$ | phosphatidylinositol 4,5-bisphosphate |
| $PIP_3$ | phosphatidylinositol 3,4,5-bisphosphate |
| PKD | polycystic kidney disease |
| PKR | interferon-$\alpha$–induced protein kinase |
| PKU | phenylketonuria |
| PLAP | placental alkaline phosphatase |
| PLP | pyridoxal phosphate |
| PML | progressive multifocal leukoencephalopathy |
| PMN | polymorphonuclear [leukocyte] |
| $P_{net}$ | net filtration pressure |
| PNET | primitive neuroectodermal tumor |
| PNS | peripheral nervous system |
| $Po_2$ | partial pressure of oxygen |
| $PO_4^{3-}$ | phosphate |
| Pop* | popliteal artery |
| Pop a* | popliteal artery |
| Post* | posterior |
| PPAR | peroxisome proliferator-activated receptor |
| PPD | purified protein derivative |

*Image abbreviation only

| ABBREVIATION | MEANING |
|---|---|
| PPI | proton pump inhibitor |
| PPM | parts per million |
| PPSV23 | pneumococcal polysaccharide vaccine |
| PPV | positive predictive value |
| PR3-ANCA/ c-ANCA | cytoplasmic antineutrophil cytoplasmic antibody |
| PrP | prion protein |
| PRPP | phosphoribosylpyrophosphate |
| PSA | prostate-specific antigen |
| PSS | progressive systemic sclerosis |
| PT | prothrombin time, proximal tubule |
| *PTEN* | phosphatase and tensin homolog |
| PTH | parathyroid hormone |
| PTHrP | parathyroid hormone–related protein |
| PTSD | post-traumatic stress disorder |
| PTT | partial thromboplastin time |
| PV | plasma volume, venous pressure, portal vein |
| pv* | pulmonary vein |
| PVC | polyvinyl chloride |
| PVR | pulmonary vascular resistance |
| PYR | pyrrolidonyl aminopeptidase |
| R | correlation coefficient, right, R variable [group] |
| $R_3$ | Registration, Ranking, & Results [system] |
| RA | right atrium, right atrial |
| RAAS | renin-angiotensin-aldosterone system |
| RANK-L | receptor activator of nuclear factor-κ B ligand |
| RAS | reticular activating system |
| RBF | renal blood flow |
| RCA | right coronary artery |
| REM | rapid eye movement |
| RER | rough endoplasmic reticulum |
| Rh | *rhesus* antigen |
| RLL* | right lower lobe (of lungs) |
| RLQ | right lower quadrant |
| RML* | right middle lobe (of lung) |
| RNA | ribonucleic acid |
| RNP | ribonucleoprotein |
| ROS | reactive oxygen species |
| RPF | renal plasma flow |
| RPGN | rapidly progressive glomerulonephritis |
| RPR | rapid plasma reagin |
| RR | relative risk, respiratory rate |
| rRNA | ribosomal ribonucleic acid |
| RS | Reed-Sternberg [cells] |
| RSC* | right subclavian artery |
| RSV | respiratory syncytial virus |
| RTA | renal tubular acidosis |
| RUL* | right upper lobe (of lung) |
| RUQ | right upper quadrant |
| RV | residual volume, right ventricle, right ventricular |
| RVH | right ventricular hypertrophy |
| [S] | substrate concentration |
| SA | sinoatrial |
| SAA | serum amyloid–associated [protein] |

| ABBREVIATION | MEANING |
|---|---|
| SAM | S-adenosylmethionine |
| SARS | severe acute respiratory syndrome |
| SARS-CoV-2 | severe acute respiratory syndrome coronavirus 2 |
| SCC | squamous cell carcinoma |
| SCD | sudden cardiac death |
| SCID | severe combined immunodeficiency disease |
| SCJ | squamocolumnar junction |
| SCM | sternocleidomastoid muscle |
| SCN | suprachiasmatic nucleus |
| SD | standard deviation |
| SE | standard error [of the mean] |
| SEP | Spoken English Proficiency |
| SER | smooth endoplasmic reticulum |
| SERM | selective estrogen receptor modulator |
| SERT | serotonin transporter |
| SGLT | sodium-glucose transporter |
| SHBG | sex hormone–binding globulin |
| SIADH | syndrome of inappropriate [secretion of] antidiuretic hormone |
| SIDS | sudden infant death syndrome |
| SJS | Stevens-Johnson syndrome |
| SLE | systemic lupus erythematosus |
| SLL | small lymphocytic lymphoma |
| SLT | Shiga-like toxin |
| SMA | superior mesenteric artery |
| SMX | sulfamethoxazole |
| SNARE | soluble NSF attachment protein receptor |
| SNc | substantia nigra pars compacta |
| SNP | single nucleotide polymorphism |
| SNr | substantia nigra pars reticulata |
| SNRI | serotonin and norepinephrine receptor inhibitor |
| snRNA | small nuclear RNA |
| snRNP | small nuclear ribonucleoprotein |
| SO | superior oblique [muscle] |
| SOAP | Supplemental Offer and Acceptance Program |
| Sp* | spleen |
| spp | species |
| SR | superior rectus [muscle] |
| SS | single stranded |
| ssDNA | single-stranded deoxyribonucleic acid |
| SSPE | subacute sclerosing panencephalitis |
| SSRI | selective serotonin reuptake inhibitor |
| ssRNA | single-stranded ribonucleic acid |
| St* | stomach |
| ST | Shiga toxin |
| StAR | steroidogenic acute regulatory protein |
| STEMI | ST-segment elevation myocardial infarction |
| STI | sexually transmitted infection |
| STN | subthalamic nucleus |
| SV | splenic vein, stroke volume |
| SVC | superior vena cava |
| SVR | systemic vascular resistance |
| SVT | supraventricular tachycardia |
| T* | thalamus, trachea |
| $t_{1/2}$ | half-life |

*Image abbreviation only

| ABBREVIATION | MEANING |
|---|---|
| $T_3$ | triiodothyronine |
| $T_4$ | thyroxine |
| TAA | thoracic aortic aneurysm |
| TAPVR | total anomalous pulmonary venous return |
| TB | tuberculosis |
| TBG | thyroxine-binding globulin |
| TBV | total blood volume |
| 3TC | dideoxythiacytidine [lamivudine] |
| TCA | tricarboxylic acid [cycle], tricyclic antidepressant |
| Tc cell | cytotoxic T cell |
| TCR | T-cell receptor |
| TDF | tenofovir disoproxil fumarate |
| TdT | terminal deoxynucleotidyl transferase |
| TE | tracheoesophageal |
| TFT | thyroid function test |
| TG | triglyceride |
| TGF | transforming growth factor |
| Th cell | helper T cell |
| THF | tetrahydrofolic acid |
| TI | therapeutic index |
| TIA | transient ischemic attack |
| Tib* | tibia |
| TIBC | total iron-binding capacity |
| TIPS | transjugular intrahepatic portosystemic shunt |
| TLC | total lung capacity |
| TLR | toll-like receptors |
| $T_m$ | maximum rate of transport |
| TMP | trimethoprim |
| TN | true negative |
| TNF | tumor necrosis factor |
| TNM | tumor, node, metastases [staging] |
| TOP | topoisomerase |
| ToRCHeS | *Toxoplasma gondii*, rubella, CMV, HIV, HSV-2, syphilis |
| TP | true positive |
| tPA | tissue plasminogen activator |
| TPO | thyroid peroxidase, thrombopoietin |
| TPP | thiamine pyrophosphate |
| TPPA | *Treponema pallidum* particle agglutination assay |
| TPR | total peripheral resistance |
| TR | tricuspid regurgitation |
| TRAP | tartrate-resistant acid phosphatase |
| TRECs | T-cell receptor excision circles |
| TRH | thyrotropin-releasing hormone |
| tRNA | transfer ribonucleic acid |
| TSH | thyroid-stimulating hormone |
| TSI | triple sugar iron |
| TSS | toxic shock syndrome |
| TSST | toxic shock syndrome toxin |

| ABBREVIATION | MEANING |
|---|---|
| TTP | thrombotic thrombocytopenic purpura |
| TTR | transthyretin |
| $TXA_2$ | thromboxane $A_2$ |
| UDP | uridine diphosphate |
| UMN | upper motor neuron |
| UMP | uridine monophosphate |
| UPD | uniparental disomy |
| URI | upper respiratory infection |
| USMLE | United States Medical Licensing Examination |
| UTI | urinary tract infection |
| UTP | uridine triphosphate |
| UV | ultraviolet |
| $V_1, V_2$ | vasopressin receptors |
| $V_A$ | alveolar ventilation |
| VC | vital capacity |
| $V_d$ | volume of distribution |
| $V_D$ | physiologic dead space |
| V(D)J | variable, (diversity), joining gene segments rearranged to form Ig genes |
| VDRL | Venereal Disease Research Laboratory |
| $V_E$ | minute ventilation |
| VEGF | vascular endothelial growth factor |
| $V_H$ | variable region, heavy chain [antibody] |
| VHL | von Hippel-Lindau [disease] |
| VIP | vasoactive intestinal peptide |
| VIPoma | vasoactive intestinal polypeptide-secreting tumor |
| VJ | light-chain hypervariable region [antibody] |
| $V_L$ | variable region, light chain [antibody] |
| VLCFA | very-long-chain fatty acids |
| VLDL | very low density lipoprotein |
| VMA | vanillylmandelic acid |
| VMAT | vesicular monoamine transporter |
| $V_{max}$ | maximum velocity |
| VPL | ventral posterior nucleus, lateral |
| VPM | ventral posterior nucleus, medial |
| VPN | vancomycin, polymyxin, nystatin [media] |
| $\dot{V}/\dot{Q}$ | ventilation/perfusion [ratio] |
| VRE | vancomycin-resistant enterococcus |
| VSD | ventricular septal defect |
| $V_T$ | tidal volume |
| VTE | venous thromboembolism |
| vWF | von Willebrand factor |
| VZV | varicella-zoster virus |
| VMAT | vesicular monoamine transporter |
| XR | X-linked recessive |
| XX/XY | normal complement of sex chromosomes for female/male |
| ZDV | zidovudine [formerly AZT] |

*Image abbreviation only

# SECTION IV

# Image Acknowledgments

In this edition, in collaboration with MedIQ Learning, LLC, and a variety of other partners, we are pleased to include the following clinical images and diagrams for the benefit of integrative student learning.

Portions of this book identified with the symbol ℞ are copyright © USMLE-Rx.com (MedIQ Learning, LLC).

Portions of this book identified with the symbol RU are copyright © Dr. Richard Usatine and are provided under license through MedIQ Learning, LLC.

Portions of this book identified with the symbol ✳ are listed below by page number.

This symbol ⊕ refers to material that is available in the public domain.

This symbol ⊕ refers to the Creative Commons Attribution license, full text at http://creativecommons.org/licenses/by/4.0/.

This symbol ⊕ refers to the Creative Commons Attribution-Share Alike license, full text at: http://creativecommons.org/licenses/by-sa/4.0/.

Original images may have been modified by cropping and/or labeling. Where appropriate, all rights to the derivative work by MedIQ Learning, LLC are reserved.

## Biochemistry

**32 Chromatin structure.** Electron micrograph showing heterochromatin, euchromatin, and nucleolus. ⊕ Roller RA, Rickett JD, Stickle WB. The hypobranchial gland of the estuarine snail *Stramonita haemastoma canaliculata* (Gray) (Prosobranchia: Muricidae): a light and electron microscopical study. *Am Malac Bull.* 1995;11(2):177-190. Available at https://archive.org/details/americanm101119931994amer.

**47 Cilia structure: Image A.** Cross section of Chlamydomonas flagella with the membrane removed. ⊕ Bui KH, Pigino G, Ishikawa T. Three-dimensional structural analysis of eukaryotic flagella/cilia by electron cryo-tomography. *J Synchrotron Radiat.* 2011 Jan;18(1):2-5. DOI: 10.1107/S0909049510036812.

**47 Cilia structure: Image B.** Cilia structure of basal body. ⊕ Riparbelli MG, Cabrera OA, Callaini G, et al. Unique properties of *Drosophila* spermatocyte primary cilia. *Biol Open.* 2013 Nov 15;2(11):1137–1147. DOI: 10.1242/bio.20135355.

**47 Kartagener syndrome.** Dextrocardia. ⊕ Oluwadare O, Ayoka AO, Akomolafe RO, et al. The role of electrocardiogram in the diagnosis of dextrocardia with mirror image atrial arrangement and ventricular position in a young adult Nigerian in Ile-Ife: a case report. *J Med Case Rep.* 2015;9:222. DOI: 10.1186/s13256-015-0695-4.

**49 Osteogenesis imperfecta: Image A.** Skeletal deformities in upper extremity of child. ⊕ Vanakker OM, Hemelsoet D, De Paepe. Hereditary connective tissue diseases in young adult stroke: a comprehensive synthesis. *Stroke Res Treat.* 2011;712903. DOI: 10.4061/2011/712903.

**49 Osteogenesis imperfecta: Image B.** Blue sclera. ⊕ Herbert L. Fred, MD, Hendrik A. van Dijk. Images of Memorable Cases: Cases 40, 41 & 42. OpenStax CNX. Dec 3, 2008. Download for free at http://cnx.org/contents/fe89fbf7-c641-4ad8-8871-80017adfd2cf@3.

**49 Ehlers-Danlos syndrome: Images A and B.** Hyperextensibility of skin (A) and DIP joint (B). ⊕ Whitaker JK, Alexander, P, Chau DYS, et al. Severe conjunctivochalasis in association with classic type Ehlers-Danlos syndrome. *BMC Ophthalmol.* 2012;2:47. DOI: 10.1186/1471-2415-12-47.

**53 Karyotyping.** ⊕ Paar C, Herber G, Voskova, et al. available under: A case of acute myeloid leukemia (AML) with an unreported combination of chromosomal abnormalities: gain of isochromosome 5p, tetrasomy 8 and unbalanced translocation der(19)t(17;19) (q23;p13). *Mol Cytogenet.* 2013;6:40. DOI: 10.1186/1755-8166-6-40.

**53 Fluorescence in situ hybridization.** ⊕ Panagopoulos I, Gorunova L, Bjerkehagen B, et al. Fusion of the genes EWSR1 and PBX3 in retroperitoneal leiomyoma with t(9;22)(q33;q12). *PLoS One.* 2015 Apr 14;10(4):e0124288. DOI: 10.1371/journal.pone.0124288.

**55 Genetic terms.** Café-au-lait spots. ⊕ Dumitrescu CE and Collins MT. McCune-Albright syndrome. *Orphanet J Rare Dis.* 2008;3:12. DOI: 10.1186/1750-1172-3-12.

**59 Muscular dystrophies.** Fibrofatty replacement of muscle. ⊕ The US Department of Health and Human Services and Dr. Edwin P. Ewing, Jr.

**64 Vitamin A.** Bitot spots on conjunctiva. ⊕ The US Department of Health and Human Services and Dr. J. Justin Older.

**65 Vitamin B₃.** Pellagra. ⊕ van Dijk HA, Fred H. Images of memorable cases: case 2. Connexions Web site. Dec 4, 2008. Available at: http://cnx.org/contents/3d3dcb2e-8e98-496f-91c2-fe94e93428a1@3@3/.

**67 Vitamin D.** X-ray of lower extremity in child with rickets. ⊕ Linglart A, Biosse-Duplan M, Briot K, et al. Therapeutic management of hypophosphatemic rickets from infancy to adulthood. *Endocr Connect.* 2014 Mar 14;3(1):R13-30. DOI: 10.1530/EC-13-0103.

**69 Protein-energy malnutrition: Image A.** Child with kwashiorkor. ⊕ The US Department of Health and Human Services and Dr. Lyle Conrad.

**69 Protein-energy malnutrition: Image B.** Child with marasmus. ⊕ The US Department of Health and Human Services and Don Eddins.

**82 Alkaptonuria.** Ochronotic pigment on the sclera of the eyes of the patient. ⊕ Wilke A, Steverding D. Ochronosis as an unusual cause of valvular defect: a case report. *J Med Case Reports.* 2009;3:9302. DOI: 10.1186/1752-1947-3-9302.

**86 Lysosomal storage diseases: Image A.** "Cherry-red" spot on macula in Tay-Sachs disease. ⊕ Dr. Jonathan Trobe.

**86 Lysosomal storage diseases: Image B.** Angiokeratomas. ⊕ Burlina AP, Sims KB, Politei JM, et al. Early diagnosis of peripheral nervous system involvement in Fabry disease and treatment of neuropathic pain: the report of an expert panel. *BMC Neurol.* 2011;11:61. DOI: 10.1186/1471-2377-11-61.

**86 Lysosomal storage diseases: Image C.** Gaucher cells in Gaucher disease. ⊕ Mohindroo S. Type-3 Gaucher disease with bilateral necrosis of the neck of femur: a case report. *Cases J.* 2009; 9380. DOI: 10.1186/1757-1626-2-9380.

**86** **Lysosomal storage diseases: Image D.** Foam cells in Niemann-Pick disease. ⊚ Degtyareva, A, Mikhailova, S, Zakharova, Y, et al. Visceral symptoms as a key diagnostic sign for the early infantile form of Niemann–Pick disease type C in a Russian patient: a case report. *J Med Case Reports.* 2016;10:143. DOI: 10.1186/s13256-016-0925-4.

**92** **Abetalipoproteinemia.** Small bowel mucosa shows clear enterocytes. ⊚ Najah M, Youssef SM, Yahia HM, et al. Molecular characterization of Tunisian families with abetalipoproteinemia and identification of a novel mutation in MTTP gene. *Diagn Pathol.* 2013 Apr 4;8:54. DOI: 10.1186/1746-1596-8-54.

## Immunology

**94** **Lymph node: Image A.** Lymph node histology. ⊚ The US Department of Health and Human Services and Dr. Edwin P. Ewing, Jr.

**96** **Thymus.** "Sail sign" on x-ray of normal thymus in neonate. ⊚ Di Serafino M, Esposito F, Severino R, et al. Think thymus, think well: the chest x-ray thymic signs. *J Pediatr Moth Care.* 2016;1(2):108-109. DOI: 10.19104/japm.2016.108.

**105** **Complement disorders.** Urine discoloration in paroxysmal nocturnal hemoglobinuria. ⊚ Nakamura N, Sugawara T, Shirato K, et al. Paroxysmal nocturnal hemoglobinuria in systemic lupus erythematosus: a case report. *J Med Case Reports.* 2011;5:550. DOI: 10.1186/1752-1947-5-550

**115** **Immunodeficiencies: Image A.** Telangiectases on face. ⊚ Scarano V, De Santis D, Suppressa P, et al. Hypogonadotropic hypogonadism associated with hereditary hemorrhagic telangiectasia. *Case Reports in Endo.* 2013;vol 2013. DOI: 10.1155/2013/520284.

**115** **Immunodeficiencies: Image B.** Giant granules in granulocytes in Chédiak-Higashi syndrome. ⊚ Morrone K, Wang Y, Huizing M, et al. Two Novel Mutations Identified in an African-American Child with Chediak-Higashi Syndrome. *Case Rep Med.* 2010;2010:967535. vol. 2010, Article ID 967535, 4 pages, 2010.DOI: 10.1155/2010/967535.

## Microbiology

**123** **Stains: Image A.** *Trypanosoma lewisi* on Giemsa stain. ⊚ The US Department of Health and Human Services and Dr. Mae Melvin.

**123** **Stains: Image B.** Foamy macrophages containing the characteristic rod-shaped inclusion bodies of Whipple disease. ⊚ Tran HA. Reversible hypothyroidism and Whipple's disease. *BMC Endocr Disord.* 2006 May 10;6:3. DOI: 10.1186/1472-6823-6-3.

**123** **Stains: Image C.** *Mycobacterium tuberculosis* on Ziehl-Neelsen stain. ⊚ The US Department of Health and Human Services and Dr. George P. Kubica.

**123** **Stains: Image D.** *Cryptococcus neoformans* on India ink stain. ⊚ The US Department of Health and Human Services.

**123** **Stains: Image E.** *Coccidioides immitis* on silver stain. ⊚ The US Department of Health and Human Services and Dr. Edwin P. Ewing, Jr.

**125** **Encapsulated bacteria.** Capsular swelling of *Streptococcus pneumoniae* using the Neufeld-Quellung test. ⊚ The US Department of Health and Human Services.

**126** **Catalase-positive organisms.** Oxygen bubbles released during catalase reaction. ⊚ The US Department of Health and Human Services and Annie L. Vestal.

**133** **Hemolytic bacteria.** α- and β-hemolysis. ⊚ The US Department of Health and Human Services and Richard R. Facklam, Ph.D.

**133** **Staphylococcus aureus.** ⊚ The US Department of Health and Human Services and Dr. Richard Facklam.

**134** **Streptococcus pneumoniae.** ⊚ The US Department of Health and Human Services and Dr. Mike Miller.

**134** **Streptococcus pyogenes (group A streptococci).** ⊚ The US Department of Health and Human Services and Dr. Mike Miller.

**135** **Bacillus anthracis.** Ulcer with black eschar in cutaneous anthrax. ⊚ The US Department of Health and Human Services and James H. Steele.

**136** **Clostridiodes difficile.** Pseudomembranous enterocolitis on colonoscopy. ⊚ Abe I, Kawamura YJ, Sasaki J, Konishi F. Acute fulminant pseudomembranous colitis which developed after ileostomy closure and required emergent total colectomy: a case report. *J Med Case Rep.* 2012 May 14;6:130. DOI: 10.1186/1752-1947-6-130.

**136** **Clostridia: Image A.** Gas gangrene due to *Clostridium perfringens*. ⊚ Schröpfer E, Rauthe S, Meyer T. Diagnosis and misdiagnosis of necrotizing soft tissue infections: three case reports. *Cases J.* 2008;1:252. DOI: 10.1186/1757-1626-1-252.

**137** **Corynebacterium diphtheriae.** Endoscopic findings of epiglottis and larynx. ⊚ Tagini F, Pillonel T, Croxatto A, et al. Distinct genomic features characterize two clades of *Corynebacterium diphtheriae*: proposal of *Corynebacterium diphtheriae* Subsp. diphtheriae Subsp. nov. and *Corynebacterium diphtheriae* Subsp. lausannense Subsp. nov. *Front. Microbiol.* 2018;9. DOI: 10.3389/fmicb.2018.01743.

**137** **Listeria monocytogenes.** Actin rockets. ⊚ Schuppler M, Loessner MJ. The opportunistic pathogen *Listeria monocytogenes*: pathogenicity and interaction with the mucosal immune system. *Int J Inflamm.* 2010;2010:704321. DOI: 10.4061/2010/704321.

**137** **Nocardia vs Actinomyces: Image A.** *Nocardia* on acid-fast stain. ⊚ Venkataramana K. Human *Nocardia* infections: a review of pulmonary nocardiosis. *Cereus.* 2015;7(8):e304. DOI: 10.7759/cureus.304.

**137** **Nocardia vs Actinomyces: Image B.** *Actinomyces israelii* on Gram stain. ⊚ The US Department of Health and Human Services.

**138** **Mycobacteria.** Acid-fast stain. ⊚ The US Department of Health and Human Services and Dr. George P. Kubica

**139** **Leprosy: Image B.** Tuberculoid lesion. ⊚ The US Department of Health and Human Services and Dr. Robert Fass, Ohio State Dept. of Medicine.

**140** **Neisseria: Image A.** Intracellular N *gonorrhoeae*. ⊚ The US Department of Health and Human Services and Bill Schwartz.

**141** **Legionella pneumophila.** Lung findings of unilateral and lobar infiltrate. ⊚ Robbins NM, Kumar A, Blair BM. *Legionella pneumophila* infection presenting as headache, confusion and dysarthria in a human immunodeficiency virus-1 (HIV-1) positive patient: case report. *BMC Infect Dis.* 2012;12:225. DOI: 10.1186/1471-2334-12-225.

**141** **Pseudomonas aeruginosa: Image A.** ⊚ Gormley M, Aspray T, Kelly D, et al. Pathogen cross-transmission via building sanitary plumbing systems in a full scale pilot test-rig. *PLOS ONE.* 2017;12(2):e0171556.DOI: 10.1371/journal.pone.0171556.

**141** **Pseudomonas aeruginosa: Image B.** Ecthyma gangrenosum. ⊚ Gençer S, Ozer S, Ege Gül A, et al. Ecthyma gangrenosum without bacteremia in a previously healthy man: a case report. *J Med Case Rep.* 2008 Jan 22;2:14. DOI: 10.1186/1752-1947-2-14.

**143** **Klebsiella.** ⊚ The US Department of Health and Human Services.

**143** **Campylobacter jejuni.** ⊚ The US Department of Health and Human Services.

**144** **Vibrio cholerae.** ⊚ Phetsouvanh R, Nakatsu M, Arakawa E, et al. Fatal bacteremia due to immotile *Vibrio cholerae* serogroup O21 in Vientiane, Laos—a case report. *Ann Clin Microbiol Antimicrob.* 2008;7:10. DOI: 10.1186/1476-0711-7-10.

**144** **Helicobacter pylori.** ⊚ The US Department of Health and Human Services, Dr. Patricia Fields, and Dr. Collette Fitzgerald.

**144** **Spirochetes.** Appearance on darkfield microscopy. ⊚ The US Department of Health and Human Services.

**144** **Lyme disease: Image A.** *Ixodes* tick. ⊚ The US Department of Health and Human Services and Dr. Michael L. Levin.

**144**  **Lyme disease: Image B.** Erythema migrans. [PUBLIC DOMAIN] The US Department of Health and Human Services and James Gathany.

**145**  **Syphilis: Image A.** Treponeme on darkfield microscopy. [PUBLIC DOMAIN] The US Department of Health and Human Services and Renelle Woodall.

**145**  **Syphilis: Image B.** Whole-body maculopapular rash in secondary syphilis. [PUBLIC DOMAIN] The US Department of Health and Human Services and Susan Lindsley.

**145**  **Syphilis: Image C, left.** Maculopapular rash on palms in secondary syphilis. [PUBLIC DOMAIN] The US Department of Health and Human Services.

**145**  **Syphilis: Image C, right.** Maculopapular rash on palms in secondary syphilis. [CC BY] Drahansky M, Dolezel M, Urbanek J, et al. Influence of skin diseases on fingerprint recognition. *J Biomed Biotechnol.* 2012;2012:626148. DOI: 10.1155/2012/626148.

**145**  **Syphilis: Image D.** Condyloma lata. [PUBLIC DOMAIN] The US Department of Health and Human Services and Susan Lindsley.

**145**  **Syphilis: Image E.** Gumma. [CC BY] Chakir K, Benchikhi H. Granulome centro-facial révélant une syphilis tertiaire. *Pan Afr Med J.* 2013;15:82. DOI: 10.11604/pamj.2013.15.82.3011.

**145**  **Syphilis: Image F.** Snuffles and rhagades in congenital syphilis. [PUBLIC DOMAIN] The US Department of Health and Human Services and Susan Lindsley.

**145**  **Syphilis: Image G.** Hutchinson teeth in congenital syphilis. [PUBLIC DOMAIN] The US Department of Health and Human Services and Susan Lindsley.

**147**  ***Gardnerella vaginalis.*** [PUBLIC DOMAIN] The US Department of Health and Human Services and M. Rein.

**148**  **Rickettsial diseases and vector-borne illnesses: Image A.** Rash of Rocky Mountain spotted fever. [PUBLIC DOMAIN] The US Department of Health and Human Services.

**148**  **Rickettsial diseases and vector-borne illnesses: Image B.** *Ehrlichia* morulae. [CC BY] Williams CV, Van Steenhouse JL, Bradley JM, et al. Naturally occurring *Ehrlichia chaffeensis* infection in two prosimian primate species: ring-tailed lemurs (*Lemur catta*) and ruffed lemurs (*Varecia variegata*). *Emerg Infect Dis.* 2002;8(12):1497-1500. DOI: 10.3201/eid0812.020085.

**148**  **Rickettsial diseases and vector-borne illnesses: Image C.** *Anaplasma phagocytophilium* in neutrophil. Courtesy of Dr. Bobbi Pritt.

**148**  ***Mycoplasma pneumoniae.*** [CC BY] Rottem S, Kosower ND, Kornspan JD. Contamination of tissue cultures by *Mycoplasma.* In: Ceccherini-Nelli L, ed: Biomedical tissue culture. 2016. DOI: 10.5772/51518.

**149**  **Systemic mycoses: Image A.** *Histoplasma.* [PUBLIC DOMAIN] The US Department of Health and Human Services and Dr. D.T. McClenan.

**149**  **Systemic mycoses: Image B.** *Blastomyces dermatitidis* undergoing broad-base budding. [PUBLIC DOMAIN] The US Department of Health and Human Services and Dr. Libero Ajello.

**149**  **Systemic mycoses: Image C.** Lesions of blastomycosis. [PUBLIC DOMAIN] The US Department of Health and Human Services and Dr. Lucille K. Georg.

**149**  **Systemic mycoses: Image D.** Endospheres in coccidiomycosis. [PUBLIC DOMAIN] The US Department of Health and Human Services.

**149**  **Systemic mycoses: Image E.** "Captain's wheel" shape of *Paracoccidioides.* [PUBLIC DOMAIN] The US Department of Health and Human Services and Dr. Lucille K. Georg.

**150**  **Opportunistic fungal infections: Image A.** Budding yeast of *Candida albicans.* [PUBLIC DOMAIN] The US Department of Health and Human Services and Dr. Gordon Roberstad.

**150**  **Opportunistic fungal infections: Image B.** Germ tubes of *Candida albicans.* [PUBLIC DOMAIN] The US Department of Health and Human Services and Dr. Hardin.

**150**  **Opportunistic fungal infections: Image C.** Oral thrush. [PUBLIC DOMAIN] The US Department of Health and Human Services and Dr. Sol Silverman, Jr.

**150**  **Opportunistic fungal infections: Image E.** Aspergilloma in left lung. [CC BY] Souilamas R, Souilamas JI, Alkhamees K, et al. Extra corporal membrane oxygenation in general thoracic surgery: a new single veno-venous cannulation. *J Cardiothorac Surg.* 2011;6:52. DOI: 10.1186/1749-8090-6-52.

**150**  **Opportunistic fungal infections: Image F.** *Cryptococcus neoformans* on India ink stain. [PUBLIC DOMAIN] The US Department of Health and Human Services and Dr. Leanor Haley.

**150**  **Opportunistic fungal infections: Image G.** *Cryptococcus neoformans* on mucicarmine stain. [PUBLIC DOMAIN] The US Department of Health and Human Services and Dr. Leanor Haley.

**150**  **Opportunistic fungal infections: Image H.** Mucor. [PUBLIC DOMAIN] The US Department of Health and Human Services and Dr. Lucille K. Georg.

**150**  **Opportunistic fungal infections: Image I.** Mucormycosis. [CC BY] Jiang N, Zhao G, Yang S, et al. A retrospective analysis of eleven cases of invasive rhino-orbito-cerebral mucormycosis presented with orbital apex syndrome initially. *BMC Ophthalmol.* 2016;16:10. DOI: 10.1186/s12886-016-0189-1.

**151**  ***Pneumocystis jirovecii*: Image A.** Interstitial opacities in lung. [CC BY] Chuang C, Zhanhong X, Yinyin G, et al. Unsuspected *Pneumocystis* pneumonia in an HIV-seronegative patient with untreated lung cancer: circa case report. *J Med Case Rep.* 2007;1:15. DOI: 10.1186/1752-1947-1-115.

**151**  ***Pneumocystis jirovecii*: Image B.** CT of lung. [CC BY] Oikonomou A, Prassopoulos P. Mimics in chest disease: interstitial opacities. *Insights Imaging.* 2013 Feb;4(1):9-27. DOI: 10.1007/s13244-012-0207-7.

**151**  ***Pneumocystis jirovecii*: Image C.** Disc-shaped yeast. [CC BY] Kirby S, Satoskar A, Brodsky S, et al. Histological spectrum of pulmonary manifestations in kidney transplant recipients on sirolimus inclusive immunosuppressive regimens. *Diagn Pathol.* 2012;7:25. DOI: 10.1186/1746-1596-7-25.

**151**  ***Sporothrix schenckii.*** Subcutaneous mycosis. [CC BY] Govender NP, Maphanga TG, Zulu TG, et al. An outbreak of lymphocutaneous sporotrichosis among mine-workers in South Africa. *PLoS Negl Trop Dis.* 2015 Sep;9(9):e0004096. DOI: 10.1371/journal.pntd.0004096.

**152**  **Protozoa—gastrointestinal infections: Image A.** *Giardia lamblia* trophozoite. [PUBLIC DOMAIN] The US Department of Health and Human Services and Dr. Stan Erlandsen.

**152**  **Protozoa—gastrointestinal infections: Image B.** *Giardia lamblia* cyst. [PUBLIC DOMAIN] The US Department of Health and Human Services.

**152**  **Protozoa—gastrointestinal infections: Image C.** Flask-shaped ulcers in colon in *Entamoeba histolytica* infection. [PUBLIC DOMAIN] The US Department of Health and Human Services and Dr. Mae Melvin.

**152**  **Protozoa—gastrointestinal infections: Image D.** *Entamoeba histolytica* trophozoites. [PUBLIC DOMAIN] The US Department of Health and Human Services.

**152**  **Protozoa—gastrointestinal infections: Image E.** *Entamoeba histolytica* cyst. [PUBLIC DOMAIN] The US Department of Health and Human Services.

**152**  **Protozoa—gastrointestinal infections: Image F.** *Cryptosporidium* oocysts. [PUBLIC DOMAIN] The US Department of Health and Human Services.

**153**  **Protozoa—CNS infections: Image A.** Ring-enhancing lesion in brain due to *Toxoplasma gondii.* [CC BY] Rabhi S, Amrani K, Maaroufi M, et al. Hemichorea-hemiballismus as an initial manifestation in a Moroccan patient with acquired immunodeficiency syndrome and toxoplasma infection: a case report and review of the literature. *Pan Afr Med J.* 2011;10:9. DOI: 10.4314/pamj.v10i0.72216.

**153**  **Protozoa—CNS infections: Image B.** *Toxoplasma gondii* tachyzoite. [PUBLIC DOMAIN] The US Department of Health and Human Services and Dr. L.L. Moore, Jr.

**153 Protozoa—CNS infections: Image C.** Primary amebic meningoencephalitis. The US Department of Health and Human Services and Dr. Govinda S. Visvesvara.

**153 Protozoa—CNS infections: Image D.** *Trypanosoma brucei gambiense.* The US Department of Health and Human Services and Dr. Mae Melvin.

**154 Protozoa—hematologic infections: Image A.** *Plasmodium* trophozoite ring form. The US Department of Health and Human Services and Steven Glenn.

**154 Protozoa—hematologic infections: Image B.** *Plasmodium* with trophozoite ring. The US Department of Health and Human Services and Mae Melvin.

**154 Protozoa—hematologic infections: Image C.** Gametocyte of *Plasmodium falciparum* in RBC membrane. The US Department of Health and Human Services.

**154 Protozoa—hematologic infections: Image D.** *Babesia* with ring form and with "Maltese cross" form. The US Department of Health and Human Services.

**155 Protozoa—others: Image A.** *Trypanosoma cruzi.* The US Department of Health and Human Services and Dr. Mae Melvin.

**155 Protozoa—others: Image B.** Cutaneous leishmaniasis. Sikorska K, Gesing M, Olszański R, et al. Misdiagnosis and inappropriate treatment of cutaneous leishmaniasis: a case report. *Trop Dis Travel Med Vaccines.* 2022 Aug 1;8(1):18. DOI: 10.1186/s40794-022-00175-5.

**155 Protozoa—others: Image C.** Macrophage with amastigotes. The US Department of Health and Human Services and Dr. Francis W. Chandler.

**155 Protozoa—others: Image D.** *Trichomonas vaginalis.* The US Department of Health and Human Services.

**156 Nematodes (roundworms): Image A.** *Enterobius vermicularis* egg. The US Department of Health and Human Services, B.G. Partin, and Dr. Moore.

**156 Nematodes (roundworms): Image B.** *Ascaris lumbricoides* egg. The US Department of Health and Human Services.

**156 Nematodes (roundworms): Image C.** Cutaneous larva migrans. Benbella I, Khalki H, Lahmadi K, et al. Syndrome de larva migrans cutanée sur pied malformé (à propos d'un cas). *Pan Afr Med J.* 2016;23;50. DOI: 10.11604/pamj.2016.23.50.8696.

**156 Nematodes (roundworms): Image D.** *Trichinella spiralis* cysts in muscle. Franssen FFJ, Fonville M, Takumi K, et al. *Vet Res.* Antibody response against *Trichinella spiralis* in experimentally infected rats is dose dependent. 2011;42(1):113. DOI: 10.1186/1297-9716-42-113.

**156 Nematodes (roundworms): Image E.** Elephantiasis. The US Department of Health and Human Services.

**157 Cestodes (tapeworms): Image A.** *Taenia solium.* The US Department of Health and Human Services Robert J. Galindo.

**157 Cestodes (tapeworms): Image B.** Neurocysticercosis. Sonhaye L, Tchaou M, Amadou A, et al. Valeur diagnostique de la tomodensitométrie dans la cysticercose cérébrale à Lomé. *Pan Afr Med J.* 2015;20:67. DOI: 10.11604/pamj.2015.20.67.6085.

**157 Cestodes (tapeworms): Image C.** *Echinococcus granulosus.* The US Department of Health and Human Services.

**157 Cestodes (tapeworms): Image D.** Hyatid cyst of *Echinococcus granulosus.* The US Department of Health and Human Services and Dr. I. Kagan.

**157 Cestodes (tapeworms): Image E.** *Echinococcus granulosus* cyst in liver. Ma Z, Yang W, Yao Y, et al. The adventitia resection in treatment of liver hydatid cyst: a case report of a 15-year-old boy. *Case Rep Surg.* 2014;2014:123149. DOI: 10.1155/2014/123149.

**157 Trematodes (flukes): Image A.** *Schistosoma mansoni* egg with lateral spine. The US Department of Health and Human Services and Dr. D. S. Martin.

**157 Trematodes (flukes): Image B.** *Schistosoma haematobium* egg with terminal spine. The US Department of Health and Human Services.

**158 Ectoparasites: Image A.** Scabies. Siegfried EC, Hebert AA. Diagnosis of atopic dermatitis: mimics, overlaps, and complications. *Clin Med.* 2015 May;4(5):884–917. DOI: 10.3390/jcm4050884.

**158 Ectoparasites: Image B.** Nit of a louse. Turgut B, Kurt J, Çatak O, et al. Phthriasis palpebrarum mimicking lid eczema and blepharitis. *J Ophthalmol.* 2009;803951. DOI: 10.1155/2009/803951.

**161 DNA viruses: Image B.** Febrile pharyngitis. Balfour HH Jr, Dunmire SK, Hogquist KA. *Clin Transl Immunology.* 2015;4(2):e33. DOI: 10.1038/cti.2015.1.

**163 Herpesviruses: Image A.** Keratoconjunctivitis in HSV-1 infection. Yang HK, Han YK, Wee WR, et al. Bilateral herpetic keratitis presenting with unilateral neurotrophic keratitis in pemphigus foliaceus: a case report. *J Med Case Rep.* 2011;5:328. DOI: 10.1186/1752-1947-5-328.

**163 Herpesviruses: Image B.** Herpes labialis. The US Department of Health and Human Services and Dr. Herrmann.

**163 Herpesviruses: Image C.** Neonatal herpes. The US Department of Health and Human Services.

**163 Herpesviruses: Image D.** Varicella zoster rash. The US Department of Health and Human Services and Dr. John Noble, Jr.

**163 Herpesviruses: Image F.** Hepatosplenomegaly due to EBV infection. Gow NJ, Davidson RN, Ticehurst R, et al. Case report: no response to liposomal daunorubicin in a patient with drug-resistant HIV-associated visceral leishmaniasis. *PLoS Negl Trop Dis.* 2015 Aug;9(8):e0003983. DOI: 10.1371/journal.pntd.0003983.

**163 Herpesviruses: Image G.** Atypical lymphocytes in Epstein-Barr virus infection. Takahashi T, Maruyama Y, Saitoh M, et al. Fatal Epstein-Barr virus reactivation in an acquired aplastic anemia patient treated with rabbit antithymocyte globulin and cyclosporine A. *Case Rep Hematol.* 2015;2015:926874. DOI: 10.1155/2015/926874.

**163 Herpesviruses: Image I.** Roseola vaccinia. The US Department of Health and Human Services.

**163 Herpesviruses: Image J.** Kaposi sarcoma. The US Department of Health and Human Services and Dr. Steve Kraus.

**163 HSV identification.** Positive Tzanck smear in HSV-2 infection. The US Department of Health and Human Services and Joe Miller.

**165 Rotavirus.** The US Department of Health and Human Services and Erskine Palmer.

**166 Rubella virus.** Rubella rash. The US Department of Health and Human Services.

**167 Acute laryngotracheobronchitis.** Steeple sign. Reproduced, with permission, from Dr. Frank Gaillard and www.radiopaedia.org.

**167 Measles (rubeola) virus.** Koplik spots. The US Department of Health and Human Services.

**167 Mumps virus.** Swollen neck and parotid glands. The US Department of Health and Human Services.

**169 Rabies virus: Image A.** Transmission electron micrograph. The US Department of Health and Human Services Dr. Fred Murphy, and Sylvia Whitfield.

**169 Rabies virus: Image B.** Negri bodies. The US Department of Health and Human Services and Dr. Daniel P. Perl.

**169 Ebola virus.** The US Department of Health and Human Services and Cynthia Goldsmith.

**177 Osteomyelitis.** X-ray (left) and MRI (right) views. ◉Ⓞ Huang P-Y, Wu P-K, Chen C-F, et al. Osteomyelitis of the femur mimicking bone tumors: a review of 10 cases. *World J Surg Oncol.* 2013;11:283. DOI: 10.1186/1477-7819-11-283.

**178 Red rashes of childhood: Image B.** Rash of measles. ◉Ⓟᵁᴮᴸᴵᶜ The US Department of Health and Human Services.

**178 Red rashes of childhood: Image D.** Sandpaperlike rash of scarlet fever. ◉Ⓟᵁᴮᴸᴵᶜ The US Department of Health and Human Services.

**178 Red rashes of childhood: Image E.** Chicken pox. ◉Ⓟᵁᴮᴸᴵᶜ The US Department of Health and Human Services and Dr. J.D. Millar.

**179 Common vaginal infections: Image B.** *Trichomonas* vaginitis. ◉Ⓟᵁᴮᴸᴵᶜ The US Department of Health and Human Services and Jim Pledger.

**179 Common vaginal infections: Image C.** Motile trichomonads. ◉Ⓟᵁᴮᴸᴵᶜ Joe Miller.

**179 Common vaginal infections: Image D.** *Candida* vulvovaginitis. ◉Ⓟᵁᴮᴸᴵᶜ The US Department of Health and Human Services, Dr. N.J. Fiumara, and Dr. Gavin Hart.

**180 Sexually transmitted infections: Image A.** Chancroid. ◉Ⓟᵁᴮᴸᴵᶜ The US Department of Health and Human Services and Dr. Greg Hammond.

**180 Sexually transmitted infections: Image B.** Condylomata acuminata. ◉Ⓟᵁᴮᴸᴵᶜ The US Department of Health and Human Services and Susan Lindsley.

**180 Sexually transmitted infections: Image D.** Donovanosis. ◉Ⓟᵁᴮᴸᴵᶜ The US Department of Health and Human Services and Dr. Pinozzi.

**180 Sexually transmitted infections: Image E.** Buboes of lymphogranuloma venereum. ◉Ⓟᵁᴮᴸᴵᶜ The US Department of Health and Human Services and O.T. Chambers.

**180 Sexually transmitted infections: Image F.** Chancre of primary syphilis. ◉Ⓟᵁᴮᴸᴵᶜ The US Department of Health and Human Services and Susan Lindsley.

**181 TORCH infections: Image A.** "Blueberry muffin" rash. ◉Ⓞ Benmiloud S, Elhaddou G, Belghiti ZA, et al. Blueberry muffin syndrome. *Pan Afr Med J.* 2012;13:23.

**181 TORCH infections: Image B.** Cataract in infant with contenital rubella. ◉Ⓟᵁᴮᴸᴵᶜ The US Department of Health and Human Services.

**181 TORCH infections: Image C.** Periventricular calcifications in congenital cytomegalovirus infection. ◉Ⓞ Bonthius D, Perlman S. Congenital viral infections of the brain: lessons learned from lymphocytic choriomeningitis virus in the neonatal rat. *PLoS Pathog.* 2007;3:e149. DOI: 10.1371/journal.ppat.0030149.

**182 Pelvic inflammatory disease: Image A.** Purulent cervical discharge. ◉Ⓟᵁᴮᴸᴵᶜ The US Department of Health and Human Services and Dr. Lourdes Fraw and Jim Pledger.

**182 Pelvic inflammatory disease: Image B.** Adhesions in Fitz-Hugh-Curtis syndrome. ◉Ⓞ Grigoriadis G, Green J, Amin A, et al. Fitz-Hugh-Curtis syndrome: an incidental diagnostic finding during laparoscopic sterilization. *Cureus* 12(9):e1030 4. DOI: 10.7759/cureus.10304.

**187 Vancomycin.** Red man syndrome. ◉Ⓞ O'Meara P, Borici-Mazi R, Morton R, et al. DRESS with delayed onset acute interstitial nephritis and profound refractory eosinophilia secondary to vancomycin. *Allergy Asthma Clin Immunol.* 2011;7:16. DOI: 10.1186/1710-1492-7-16.

## Pathology

**205 Necrosis: Image A.** Coagulative necrosis. ◉Ⓟᵁᴮᴸᴵᶜ The US Department of Health and Human Services and Dr. Steven Rosenberg.

**205 Necrosis: Image B.** Liquefactive necrosis. ◉Ⓞ Ghaly R, Candido K, Knezevic N. Perioperative fatal embolic cerebrovascular accident after radical prostatectomy. *Surg Neurol Int.* 2010;1:26. DOI: 10.4103/2152-7806.65055.

**205 Necrosis: Image C.** Caseous necrosis. ◉Ⓞ Szaluś-Jordanow O, Augustynowicz-Kopeć E, Czopowicz M, et al. Intracardiac tuberculomas caused by Mycobacterium tuberculosis in a dog. *BMC Vet Res.* 2016 Jun 14;12(1):109. DOI: 10.1186/s12917-016-0731-7.

**205 Necrosis: Image D.** Fat necrosis. ◉Ⓞ Chee C. Panniculitis in a patient presenting with a pancreatic tumour and polyarthritis: a case report. *J Med Case Rep.* 2009 Jul 6;3:7331. DOI: 10.4076/1752-1947-3-7331.

**205 Necrosis: Image E.** Fibrinoid necrosis. ◉Ⓞ Ahmed S, Kitchen J, Hamilton S, et al. A case of polyarteritis nodosa limited to the right calf muscles, fascia, and skin: a case report. *J Med Case Rep.* 2011 Sep 12;5:450. DOI: 10.1186/1752-1947-5-450.

**205 Necrosis: Image F.** Acral gangrene. ◉Ⓟᵁᴮᴸᴵᶜ The US Department of Health and Human Services and William Archibald.

**206 Ischemia.** ◉Ⓞ Van Assche LM, Kim HW, Jensen CJ, et al. A new CMR protocol for non-destructive, high resolution, ex-vivo assessment of the area at risk simultaneous with infarction: validation with histopathology. *J Cardiovasc Magn Reson.* 2012;14(Suppl 1):O7. DOI: 10.1186/1532-429X-14-S1-O7.

**206 Types of infarcts: Image B.** Pale infarct. ◉Ⓞ Hanes DW, Wong ML, Jenny Chang CW, et al. Embolization of the first diagonal branch of the left anterior descending coronary artery as a porcine model of chronic trans-mural myocardial infarction. *J Transl Med.* 2015 Jun 6;13:187. DOI: 10.1186/s12967-015-0547-4.

**207 Types of calcification.** Dystrophic calcification. ◉Ⓞ Adapted from da Silva RMS, de Mello RJV. Fat deposition in the left ventricle: descriptive and observacional study in autopsy. *Lipids Health Dis.* 2017 May 2;16(1):86. DOI: 10.1186/s12944-017-0475-9.

**207 Psammoma bodies.** ◉Ⓞ Wang C, Chen Y, Zhang L, et al. Thoracic psammomatous meningioma with osseous metaplasia: a controversial diagnosis of a case report and literature review. *World J Surg Oncol.* 2019 Aug 24;17(1):150. doi: 10.1186/s12957-019-1694-5.

**208 Amyloidosis: Image A.** Gastric amyloid deposits on Congo red stain. ◉Ⓞ Desport E, Bridoux F, Sirac C, et al. Centre national de référence pour l'amylose AL et les autres maladies par dépôts d'immunoglobulines monoclonales. Al amyloidosis. *Orphanet J Rare Dis.* 2012 Aug 21;7:54. doi: 10.1186/1750-1172-7-54.

**208 Amyloidosis: Image B.** Gastric amyloid deposits on Congo stain viewed under polarized light. ◉Ⓞ Desport E, Bridoux F, Sirac C, et al. Centre national de référence pour l'amylose AL et les autres maladies par dépôts d'immunoglobulines monoclonales. Al amyloidosis. *Orphanet J Rare Dis.* 2012 Aug 21;7:54. doi: 10.1186/1750-1172-7-54.

**210 Acute inflammation.** Pericardium with severe inflammation, neutrophilic infiltration and fibrin with entrapped clusters of bacteria. ◉Ⓞ Ajili F, Souissi A, Bougrine F, et al. Coexistence of pyoderma gangrenosum and sweet's syndrome in a patient with ulcerative colitis. *Pan Afr Med J.* 2015;21:151. DOI: 10.11604/pamj.2015.21.151.6364.

**213 Granulomatous inflammation.** Granuloma. ◉Ⓞ Guirado E, Schlesinger LS. Modeling the Mycobacterium tuberculosis granuloma: the critical battlefield in host immunity and disease. *Front. Immunol.* 2013;4:98. DOI: 10.3389/fimmu.2013.00098.

**214 Scar formation: Image A.** Hypertrophic scar. ◉Ⓞ Baker R, Urso-Baiarda F, Linge C, et al. Cutaneous scarring: a clinical review. *Dermatol Res Pract.* 2009;2009:625376. DOI: 10.1155/2009/625376.

**214 Scar formation: Image B.** Keloid scar. ◉Ⓞ Tirgan MH. Neck keloids: evaluation of risk factors and recommendation for keloid staging system. *F1000Res.* 2016 Jun 28;5:1528. DOI: 10.12688/f1000research.9086.2.

**219 Common metastases: Image A.** Right liver lobe with a metastatic tumor and a satellite focus. ◉Ⓞ Paschke L, Juszczak M, Slupski M. Surgical treatment of recurrent urachal carcinoma with liver metastasis: a case report and literature review. *World J Surg Oncol.* 2016 Nov 28;14(1):296. DOI: 10.1186/s12957-016-1057-4.

**225 Lipofuscin.** Bae Y, Ito T, Iida T, et al. Intracellular propionibacterium acnes infection in glandular epithelium and stromal macrophages of the prostate with or without cancer. *PLoS One.* 2014 Feb 28;9(2):e90324. DOI: 10.1371/journal.pone.0090324.

## Cardiovascular

**288 Heart anatomy: Image A.** MRI showing normal cardiac anatomy. Zhang J, Chen L, Wang X, et al. Compounding local invariant features and global deformable geometry for medical image registration. *PLoS One.* 2014;9(8):e105815. DOI: 10.1371/journal.pone.0105815.

**302 Congenital heart diseases: Image B.** Tetralogy of Fallot. Rashid AKM: Heart diseases in Down syndrome. In: Dey S, ed: Down syndrome. DOI: 10.5772/46009.

**303 Congenital heart diseases: Image D.** Atrial septal defect. Teo KSL, Dundon BK, Molaee P, et al. Percutaneous closure of atrial septal defects leads to normalisation of atrial and ventricular volumes. *J Cardiovasc Magn Reson.* 2008;10(1):55. DOI: 10.1186/1532-429X-10-55.

**303 Congenital heart diseases: Image E.** Patent ductus arteriosus. Henjes CR, Nolte I, Wesfaedt P. Multidetector-row computed tomography of thoracic aortic anomalies in dogs and cats: patent ductus arteriosus and vascular rings. *BMC Vet Res.* 2011;7:57. DOI: 10.1186/1746-6148-7-57.

**304 Coarction of the aorta.** MRI showing coarctation of the aorta. Parissis, H, Al-Alao, B, Soo, A,. et al. Single stage repair of a complex pathology: end stage ischaemic cardiomyopathy, ascending aortic aneurysm and thoracic coarctation. *J Cardiothorac Surg.* 2011;6:152. DOI: 10.1186/1749-8090-6-152.

**304 Hypertension.** "String of beads" appearance of renal artery in fibromuscular dysplasia. Plouin PF, Perdu J, LaBatide-Alanore A, et al. Fibromuscular dysplasia. *Orphanet J Rare Dis.* 2007;7:28. DOI: 10.1186/1750-1172-2-28.

**305 Hyperlipidemia signs: Image C.** Tendinous xanthoma. Huri G, Joachim N. An unusual case of hand xanthomatosis. *Case Rep Orthop.* 2013;2013:183018. DOI: 10.1155/2013/183018.

**306 Arteriosclerosis: Image A.** Hyaline type. Sostaric-Zuckermann IC, Borel N, Kaiser C, et al. Chlamydia in canine or feline coronary arteriosclerotic lesions. *BMC Res Notes.* 2011 Sep 9;4:350. DOI: 10.1186/1756-0500-4-350.

**306 Arteriosclerosis: Image B.** Hyperplastic type. Huang J, Han SS, Qin DD, et al. Renal interstitial arteriosclerotic lesions in lupus nephritis patients: a cohort study from China. *PLoS One.* 2015 Nov 6;10(11):e0141547. DOI: 10.1371/journal.pone.0141547.

**307 Aortic dissection.** Qi Y, Ma X, Li G, et al. Three-dimensional visualization and imaging of the entry tear and intimal flap of aortic dissection using CT virtual intravascular endoscopy. *PLoS One.* 2016;11(10) e0164750. DOI: 10.1371/journal.pone.0164750.

**309 Evolution of myocardial infarction: Images A and B.** Heart tissue at 0-24 hours (image A) and 1-3 days (image B) after myocardial infarction. Chang J, Nair V, Luk A, et al. Pathology of myocardial infarction. *Diagn Histopath.* 2013;19:7-12. DOI: 10.1016/j.mpdhp.2012.11.001.

**309 Evolution of myocardial infarction: Image C.** Heart tissue 3-14 days after myocardial infarction. Diarmid AK, Pellicori P, Cleland JG, et al. Taxonomy of segmental myocardial systolic dysfunction. *Eur Heart J.* 2017 Apr 1;38(13):942–954. DOI: 10.1093/eurheartj/ehw140.

**309 Evolution of myocardial infarction: Image D.** Heart tissue after myocardial infarction showing dense fibrous scar replacing myocyte loss. Michaud K, Basso C, d'Amati G, et al on behalf of the Association for European Cardiovascular Pathology. Diagnosis of myocardial infarction at autopsy: AECVP reappraisal in the light of the current clinical classification. *Virchows Arch.* 2020;476:179–194.

**314 Myocardial infarction complications: Image A.** Papillary muscle rupture. Routy B, Huynh T, Fraser R, et al. Vascular endothelial cell function in catastrophic antiphospholipid syndrome: a case report and review of the literature. *Case Rep Hematol.* 2013;2013:710365. DOI: 10.1155/2013/710365.

**314 Myocardial infarction complications: Image B.** Free wall rupture of left ventricle. Zacarias ML, da Trindade H, Tsutsu J, et al. Left ventricular free wall impeding rupture in post-myocardial infarction period diagnosed by myocardial contrast echocardiography: case report. *Cardiovasc Ultrasound.* 2006;4:7. DOI: 10.1186/1476-7120-4-7.

**315 Cardiomyopathies: Image A.** Dilated cardiomyopathy. Gho JMIH, van Es R, Stathonikos N, et al. High resolution systematic digital histological quantification of cardiac fibrosis and adipose tissue in phospholamban p.Arg14del mutation associated cardiomyopathy. *PLoS One.* 2014;9:e94820. DOI: 10.1371/journal.pone.0094820.

**315 Cardiomyopathies: Image B.** Hypertrophic obstructive cardiomyopathy. Benetti MA, Belo Nunes RA, Benvenuti LA. Case 2/2016 - 76-year-old male with hypertensive heart disease, renal tumor and shock. *Arq Bras Cardiol.* 2016 May; 106(5): 439–446. DOI: 10.5935/abc.20160067.

**316 Heart failure.** Pitting edema. Ong HS, Sze CW, Koh TW, Coppack SW. How 40 kilograms of fluid retention can be overlooked: two case reports. *Cases J.* 2009;2(1):33. DOI: 10.1186/1757-1626-2-33.

**317 Cardiac tamponade: Image B.** Echocardiogram showing cardiac tamponade. Maharaj SS, Chang SM. Cardiac tamponade as the initial presentation of systemic lupus erythematosus: a case report and review of the literature. *Pediatr Rheumatol Online J.* 2015;13: 9. DOI: 10.1186/s12969-015-0005-0.

**318 Infective endocarditis: Image A.** Vegetations on heart valves. The US Department of Health and Human Services and Dr. Edwin P. Ewing, Jr.

**318 Infective endocarditis: Image C.** Osler nodes. Yang ML, Chen YH, Lin WR, et al. Case report: infective endocarditis caused by *Brevundimonas vesicularis. BMC Infect Dis.* 2006;6:179. DOI: 10.1186/1471-2334-6-179.

**320 Acute pericarditis.** Bogaert J, Francone M. Cardiovascular magnetic resonance in pericardial diseases. *J Cardiovasc Magn Reson.* 2009;11:14. DOI: 10.1186/1532-429X-11-14.

## Endocrine

**330 Thyroid development: Image A.** Thyroglossal duct cyst. Kartini D, Panigoro S, Harahap A. Sistrunk procedure on malignant thyroglossal duct cyst. *Case Rep Oncol Med.* 2020 Jan 16;2020:6985746. DOI: 10.1155/2020/6985746.

**330 Thyroid development: Image B.** Normal thyroid histology showing follicles surrounded with thyrocytes. Sharma RB, Fan X, Caturegli P, et al. Invariant NKT cell lines derived from the NOD·H2 mouse enhance autoimmune thyroiditis. *J Thyroid Res.* 2011;2011:895923. DOI: 10.4061/2011/895923.

**344 Hypothyroidism vs hyperthyroidism: Image A.** Onycholysis. Gallouj S, Mernissi FZ. Leuconychie transversale induite par la manucurie: y a-t-il un apport de la dermoscopie? [Transverse leuconychia induced by manicure: is there a contribution from dermoscopy?]. *Pan Afr Med J.* 2014;18:39. Published 2014 May 10. DOI: 10.11604/pamj.2014.18.39.3761.

**344 Hypothyroidism vs hyperthyroidism: Image B.** Pretibial myxedema. Fred H, van Dijk HA. Images of memorable cases: case 144. Connexions Web site. Dec 8, 2008. Available at: https://cnx.org/contents/SCJeD6JM@3/Images-of-Memorable-Cases-Case-144.

**344 Hypothyroidism vs hyperthyroidism: Image C.** Periorbital edema. Dandekar F, Camacho M, Valerio J, et al. *Case Rep Ophthalmol Med.* 2015;2015:126501. DOI: 10.1155/2015/126501.

**345 Hypothyroidism: Image B.** Florid Hashimoto's thyroiditis histology. ⊚⓪ Oruci M, Ito Y, Buta M, et al. Right thyroid hemiagenesis with adenoma and hyperplasia of parathyroid glands -case report. *BMC Endocr Disord*. 2012 Nov 13;12:29. DOI: 10.1186/1472-6823-12-29.

**345 Hypothyroidism: Image C.** ⊚⓪ Mazza E, Quaglino F, Suriani A, et al. Thyroidectomy for painful thyroiditis resistant to steroid treatment: three new cases with review of the literature. *Case Rep Endocrinol*. 2015;2015:138327. DOI: 10.1155/2015/138327.

**345 Hypothyroidism: Image E.** Before and after treatment of congenital hypothyroidism. ⊚⓪ Bailey P. The thyroid gland in medicine. *Popular Science Monthly* August 1897;481-489. Available at https://archive.org/details/popularsciencemo51newy/page/486/mode/2up.

**345 Hypothyroidism: Image F.** Congenital hypothyroidism. ⊚⓪ Rastogi MV, LaFranchi SH. Congenital hypothyroidism. *Orphanet J Rare Dis*. 2010 Jun 10;5:17. DOI: 10.1186/1750-1172-5-17.

**346 Thyroid adenoma.** ⊚⓪ Terada T. Brain metastasis from thyroid adenomatous nodules or an encapsulated thyroid follicular tumor without capsular and vascular invasion: a case report. *Cases J*. 2009;2:7180. DOI: 10.4076/1757-1626-2-7180.

**348 Hypoparathyroidism.** Shortened 4th and 5th digits. ⊚⓪ Ferrario C, Gastaldi G, Portmann L, et al. Bariatric surgery in an obese patient with Albright hereditary osteodystrophy: a case report. *J Med Case Rep*. 2013;7:111. DOI: 10.1186/1752-1947-7-111.

**349 Hyperparathyroidism.** Multiple lytic lesions. ⊚⓪ Khaoula BA, Kaouther BA, Ines C, et al. An unusual presentation of primary hyperparathyroidism: pathological fracture. *Case Rep Orthop*. 2011;2011:521578. DOI: 10.1155/2011/521578.

**353 Adrenal insufficiency.** Mucosal hyperpigmentation in primary adrenal insufficiency. ⊚⓪ Wina Dharmesti NW, Saraswati MR, Suastika K, et al. Challenging Diagnosis of Addison's Disease Presenting with Adrenal Crisis. *Case Rep Endocrinol*. 2021 Oct 11;2021:7137950. DOI: 10.1155/2021/7137950.

**355 Pheochromocytoma.** ⊚⓪ Muneer T, Tariq A, Siddiqui A H, et al. Malignant pheochromocytoma with widespread bony and pulmonary metastases. *Cureus*. 10(9):e3348. DOI: 10.7759/cureus.3348.

**356 Multiple endocrine neoplasias.** Mucosal neuroma. ⊚⓪ Martucciello G, Lerone M, Bricco L, et al. Multiple endocrine neoplasias type 2B and RET proto-oncogene. *Ital J Pediatr*. 2012;38:9. DOI: 10.1186/1824-7288-38-9.

**357 Carcinoid tumors.** ⊚⓪ Katsuyoshi F, Hidenobu K, Masayuki O, et al. Gastric Carcinoid with Hypergastrinemia: Report of Three Cases. *Case Reports in Medicine*. 2010;348761. DOI: 10.1155/2010/348761.

**Gastrointestinal**

**365 Ventral wall defects: Image A.** Gastroschisis. ⊚⓪ Bhat V, Moront M, Bhandari V. Gastroschisis: a state-of-the-art review. *Children (Basel)*. 2020 Dec 17;7(12):302. DOI: 10.3390/children7120302.

**365 Ventral wall defects: Image B.** Omphalocele. ⊚⓪ Lamquami S, Mamouni N, Errarhay S, et al. Antenatal diagnosis of isolated omphalocele. *Pan Afr Med J*. 2015 Jul 31;21:233. doi: 10.11604/pamj.2015.21.233.7151.

**365 Ventral wall defects.** Drawings of gastroschisis (left) and omphalocele (right). ⊚⓪ The US Department of Health and Human Services.

**365 Ventral wall defects: Image C.** Congenital diaphragmatic hernia. ⊚⓪ Rastogi MV, LaFranchi SH. Congenital hypothyroidism. *Orphanet J Rare Dis*. 2010;5:17. DOI: 10.1186/1750-1172-5-17.

**366 Intestinal atresia.** ⊚⓪ Saha M. Alimentary tract atresias associated with anorectal malformations: 10 years' experience. *J Neonatal Surg*. 2016 Oct-Dec;5(4):43. DOI: 10.21699/jns.v5i4.449.

**367 Pancreas and spleen embryology.** Annular pancreas. ⊚⓪ Mahdi B, Selim S, Hassen T, et al. A rare cause of proximal intestinal obstruction in adults—annular pancreas: a case report. *Pan Afr Med J*. 2011;10:56.

**367 Retroperitoneal structures.** ⊚⓪ Sammut J, Ahiaku E, Williams DT. Complete regression of renal tumour following ligation of an accessory renal artery during repair of an abdominal aortic aneurysm. *Ann R Coll Surg Engl*. 2012 Sep;94(6):e198–e200. DOI: 10.1308/003588412 X13373405384972.

**369 Digestive tract anatomy.** Transverse histologic section of the normal oesophageal wall. ⊚⓪ Wei Y, Wu S, Shi D, et al. Oesophageal carcinoma: comparison of ex vivo high-resolution 3.0 T MR imaging with histopathological findings. *Sci Rep*. 2016 Oct 11;6:35109. DOI: 10.1038/srep35109.

**369 Digestive tract histology: Image A.** ⊚⓪ Sato Y, Fujino T, Kasagawa A, et al. Twelve-year natural history of a gastric adenocarcinoma of fundic gland type. *Clin J Gastroenterol*. 2016 Dec;9(6):345-351. DOI: 10.1007/s12328-016-0680-5.

**369 Digestive tract histology: Image B.** Jejunum. Non-neoplastic parietal cells. ⊚⓪ Chen J, Tellez G, Richards JD, Escobar J. Identification of Potential Biomarkers for Gut Barrier Failure in Broiler Chickens. *Front Vet Sci*. 2015 May 26;2:14. DOI: 10.3389/fvets.2015.00014.

**374 Liver tissue architecture.** Portal triad. ⊚⓪ Liver development. In: Zorn AM. Stem book. Cambridge: Harvard Stem Cell Institute, 2008. Available at www.stembook.org/node/512.

**375 Biliary structures.** Gallstones. ⊚⓪ Issa H, Al-Salem AH. Hepatobiliary manifestations of sickle cell anemia. *Gastroenterology Res*. 2010 Feb;3(1):1-8. DOI: 10.4021/gr2010.01.

**377 Hernias: Image A.** Congenital diaphragmatic hernia. ⊚⓪ Tovar J. Congenital diaphragmatic hernia. *Orphanet J Rare Dis*. 2012;7:1. DOI: 10.1186/1750-1172-7-1.

**381 Peyer patches.** ⊚⓪ Kapoor K, Singh O. Ileal and jejunal Peyer's patches in buffalo calves: Histomorphological comparison. *Vet World*. 2015 Nov;8(11):1273-8. DOI: 10.14202/vetworld.2015.1.

**383 Oral pathologies: Image A.** Apthous ulcer. ⊚⓪ Peterson DE, O'Shaughnessy JA, Rugo HS, et al. Oral mucosal injury caused by mammalian target of rapamycin inhibitors: emerging perspectives on pathobiology and impact on clinical practice. *Cancer Med*. 2016 Aug;5(8):1897–1907. DOI: 10.1002/cam4.761.

**383 Oral pathologies: Image B.** Leukoplakia of tongue. ⊚⓪ The US Department of Health and Human Services and J.S. Greenspan, B.D.S., University of California, San Francisco; Sol Silverman, Jr., D.D.S.

**383 Oral pathologies: Image C.** Sialolithiasis. ⊚⓪ Pastor-Ramos V, Cuervo-Diaz A, Aracil-Kessler L. Sialolithiasis. Proposal for a new minimally invasive procedure: piezoelectric surgery. *J Clin Exp Dent*. 2014 Jul;6(3):e295–e298. DOI: 10.4317/jced.51253.

**383 Oral pathologies: Image D.** Pleomorphic adenoma histology. ⊚⓪ Genelhu MC, Cardoso SV, Gobbi H, Cassali GD. A comparative study between mixed-type tumours from human salivary and canine mammary glands. *BMC Cancer*. 2007 Nov;28;7:218. DOI: 10.1186/1471-2407-7-218.

**383 Achalasia.** ⊚⓪ Agrusa A, Romano G, Frazzetta G, et al. Achalasia secondary to submucosal invasion by poorly differentiated adenocarcinoma of the cardia, siewert II: consideration on preoperative workup. *Case Rep Surg*. 2014;2014:654917. DOI: 10.1155/2014/654917.

**384 Other esophageal pathologies: Image A.** White pseudomembrane of *Candida* infection in esophagitis. ⊚⓪ Takahashi Y, Nagata N, Shimbo T. Long-term trends in esophageal candidiasis prevalence and associated risk factors with or without HIV infection: lessons from an endoscopic study of 80,219 patients. *PLoS One*. 2015; 10(7):e0133589. DOI: 10.1371/journal.pone.0133589.

**384** **Other esophageal pathologies: Image B.** Esophageal varices on endoscopy. Costaguta A, Alvarez F. Etiology and management of hemorrhagic complications of portal hypertension in children. *Int J Hepatol.* 2012;2012:879163. DOI: 10.1155/2012/879163.

**384** **Other esophageal pathologies: Image C.** Pneumomediastinum. Bakhshaee M, Jokar MH, Mirfeizi Z, et al. Subcutaneous emphysema, pneumomediastinum and pneumothorax in a patient with dermatomyositis. *Iran J Otorhinolaryngol.* 2017 Mar;29(91):113-116.

**385** **Barrett esophagus: Image A.** Endoscopy image. Japan Esophageal Society. Japanese classification of esophageal cancer, 11th edition: part I. *Esophagus.* 2017;14(1):1–36. DOI: 10.1007/s10388-016-0551-7.

**386** **Ménétrier disease.** Chung M, Pittenger J, Flomenhoft D, et al. Atypical clinical and diagnostic features in Ménétrier's disease in a child. *Case Rep Gastrointest Med.* 2011;2011:480610. DOI: 10.1155/2011/480610.

**386** **Gastric cancer.** Tan Y, Fu J, Li X. A minor (<50%) signet-ring cell component associated with poor prognosis in colorectal cancer patients: a 26-year retrospective study in China. *PLoS One.* 2015;10(3):e0121944. DOI: 10.1371/journal.pone.0121944.

**387** **Ulcer complications.** Free air under diaphragm in perforated ulcer. Reproduced, with permission, from Dr. Frank Gaillard and www.radiopaedia.org.

**388** **Malabsorption syndromes: Image A.** Celiac disease. Celiac disease. Sedda S, Caruso R, Marafini I, et al. Pyoderma gangrenosum in refractory celiac disease: a case report. *BMC Gastroenterol.* 2013;13:162. DOI: 10.1186/1471-230X-13-162.

**388** **Malabsorption syndromes: Image B.** *Tropheryma whipplei* on PAS stain. Tran HA. Reversible hypothyroidism and Whipple's disease. *BMC Endocr Disord.* 2006;6:3. DOI: 10.1186/1472-6823-6-3.

**389** **Inflammatory bowel diseases: Images B and C.** Normal mucosa (B) and punched-out ulcers (C) in ulcerative colitis. Ishikawa D, Ando T, Watanabe O, et al. Images of colonic real-time tissue sonoelastography correlate with those of colonoscopy and may predict response to therapy in patients with ulcerative colitis. *BMC Gastroenterol.* 2011;11:29. DOI: 10.1186/1471-230X-11-29.

**390** **Appendicitis.** Ali M, Iqbal J, Sayani R. Accuracy of computed tomography in differentiating perforated from nonperforated appendicitis, taking histopathology as the gold standard. *Cureus.* 2018 Dec 15;10(12):e3735. DOI: 10.7759/cureus.3735.

**390** **Diverticula of the gastrointestinal tract: Image B.** Diverticulosis. Sartelli M, Moore FA, Ansaloni L, et al. A proposal for a CT driven classification of left colon acute diverticulitis. *World J Emerg Surg.* 2015;10:3. DOI: 10.1186/1749-7922-10-3.

**390** **Diverticula of the gastrointestinal tract: Image C.** Diverticulitis. Hupfeld L, Burcharth J, Pommergaard HC, Rosenberg J. The best choice of treatment for acute colonic diverticulitis with purulent peritonitis is uncertain. *Biomed Res Int.* 2014;2014:380607. DOI: 10.1155/2014/380607.

**391** **Zenker diverticulum.** Dionigi G, Sessa F, Rovera F, et al. Ten year survival after excision of squamous cell cancer in Zenker's diverticulum: report of a case. *World J Surg Oncol.* 2006 Mar 28;4:17. DOI: 10.1186/1477-7819-4-17.

**392** **Intussusception.** Ultrasound showing target sign. Christianakis E, Sakelaropoulos A, Papantzimas C, et al. Pelvic plastron secondary to acute appendicitis in a child presented as appendiceal intussusception. a case report. *Cases J.* 2008;1:135. DOI: 10.1186/1757-1626-1-135.

**392** **Volvulus.** Coffee bean sign. Yigit M, Turkdogan KA. Coffee bean sign, whirl sign and bird's beak sign in the diagnosis of sigmoid volvulus. *Pan Afr Med J.* 1014;19:56. DOI: 10.11604/pamj.2014.19.56.5142.

**393** **Other intestinal disorders: Image A.** Necrosis due to occlusion of SMA. Van De Winkel N, Cheragwandi A, Nieboer K, et al. Superior mesenteric arterial branch occlusion causing partial jejunal ischemia: a case report. *J Med Case Rep.* 2012;6:48. DOI: 10.1186/1752-1947-6-48.

**393** **Other intestinal disorders: Image B.** Loops of dilated bowel suggestive of small bowel obstruction. Welte FJ, Crosso M. Left-sided appendicitis in a patient with congenital gastrointestinal malrotation: a case report. *J Med Case Rep.* 2007;1:92. DOI: 10.1186/1752-1947-1-92.

**393** **Other intestinal disorders: Image C.** Pneumatosis intestinalis. Pelizzo G, Nakib G, Goruppi I, et al. Isolated colon ischemia with norovirus infection in preterm babies: a case series. *J Med Case Rep.* 2013;7:108. DOI: 10.1186/1752-1947-7-108.

**394** **Colonic polyps: Image A.** Shussman N, Wexner SD. Colorectal polyps and polyposis syndromes. *Gastroenterol Rep (Oxf).* 2014 Feb;2(1):1-15. doi: 10.1093/gastro/got041.

**394** **Colonic polyps: Image C.** Adenomatous polyps in villous adenoma. Rehani B, Chasen RM, Dowdy Y, et al. Advanced adenoma diagnosis with FDG PET in a visibly normal mucosa: a case report. *J Med Case Reports.* 2007;1:99. DOI: 10.1186/1752-1947-1-99.

**395** **Colorectal cancer: Image A.** Polyp. Takiyama A, Nozawa H, Ishihara S, et al. Secondary metastasis in the lymph node of the bowel invaded by colon cancer: a report of three cases. *World J Surg Oncol.* 2016;14:273. DOI: 10.1186/s12957-016-1026-y.

**396** **Cirrhosis and portal hypertension.** Liver abnormalities in cirrhosis. Blackburn PR, Hickey RD, Nace RA, et al. Silent tyrosinemia type I without elevated tyrosine or succinylacetone associated with liver cirrhosis and hepatocellular carcinoma. *Hum Mutat.* 2016 Oct;37(10):1097–1105. DOI: 10.1002/humu.23047.

**398** **Alcoholic liver disease: Image B.** Mallory bodies. The US Department of Health and Human Services and Dr. Edwin P. Ewing, Jr.

**398** **Alcoholic liver disease: Image C.** Miranda-Mendez A, Lugo-Baruqui A, Armendariz-Borunda J. Molecular basis and current treatment for alcoholic liver disease. *Int J Environ Res Public Health.* 2010 May;7(5):1872-88. DOI: 10.3390/ijerph7051872.

**399** **Liver tumors: Image A.** Cavernous liver hemangioma. Yano T, Kobayashi T, Kuroda S, et al. Obstructive jaundice caused by a giant liver hemangioma with Kasabach-Merritt syndrome: a case report. *Surg Case Rep.* 2015 Dec;1(1):93. DOI: 10.1186/s40792-015-0095-4.

**399** **Liver tumors: Image B.** Hepatocellular carcinoma/hepatoma. Reproduced, with permission, from Jean-Christophe Fournet and Humpath.

**400** **$\alpha_1$-antitrypsin deficiency.** Liver histology. Dettmer M, Cathomas G, Willi N. Alpha 1-antitrypsin retention in an ectopic liver. *Diagn Pathol.* 2011 Feb 28;6:16. DOI: 10.1186/1746-1596-6-16.

**402** **Wilson disease.** Kayser-Fleischer rings. Herbert L. Fred, MD, Hendrik A. van Dijk. Images of Memorable Cases: 50 Years at the Bedside. OpenStax CNX. Dec 8, 2008. Download for free at http://cnx.org/contents/e7b71f2c-a51e-4c9f-8db2-066a4c3643e4@7.2.

**402** **Hemochromatosis.** Hemosiderin deposits. Mathew J, Leong MY, Morley N, et al. A liver fibrosis cocktail? Psoriasis, methotrexate and genetic hemochromatosis. *BMC Dermatol.* 2005;5:12. DOI: 10.1186/1471-5945-5-12.

**402** **Biliary tract diseases.** Endoscopic retrograde cholangiopancreatography shows "beading" of bile ducts in primary sclerosing cholangitis. Law S-T, Lee W-K, Li MK-K, et al. A gentleman with anemia and cholestasis. *Case Rep Med.* 2010;2010:536207. DOI: 10.1155/2010/536207.

**403** **Cholelithiasis and related pathologies: Image B.** Large gallstone. Spangler R, Van Pham T, Khoujah D, et al. Abdominal emergencies in the geriatric patient. *Int J Emerg Med.* 2014;7:43. DOI: 10.1186/s12245-014-0043-2.

**404** **Cholelithiasis and related pathologies: Image C.** Porcelain gallbladder. ⓒⓞ Fred H, van Dijk H. Images of memorable cases: case 19. Connexions Web site. December 4, 2008. Available at: http://cnx.org/content/m14939/1.3/.

**404** **Pancreatitis: Image A.** Diffuse peripancreatic stranding. ⓒⓞ Landa E, Ganim I, Vigandt E, et al. Meloxicam-induced pancreatitis. *Cureus*. 2021 Jan 28;13(1):e12976. DOI: 10.7759/cureus.12976.

**404** **Pancreatitis: Image B.** Pancreatic pseudocyst. ⓒⓞ Cawich SO, Murphy T, Shah S, et al. Endoscopic transmural drainage of pancreatic pseudocysts: technical challenges in the resource poor setting. *Case Rep Gastrointest Med*. 2013;2013:942832. DOI: 10.1155/2013/942832.

**404** **Pancreatitis: Image C.** Chronic pancreatitis. ⓒⓞ Sommer CA, Wilcox CM. Pancreatico-pericardial fistula as a complication of chronic pancreatitis. *F1000Res*. 2014 Jan 29;3:31. DOI: 10.12688/f1000research.3-31.v1.

**405** **Pancreatic adenocarcinoma: Image A.** Histology. ⓒⓞ Zapata M, Cohen C, Siddiqui MT. Immunohistochemical expression of SMAD4, CK19, and CA19-9 in fine needle aspiration samples of pancreatic adenocarcinoma: Utility and potential role. *Cytojournal*. 2007 Jun 22;4:13. DOI: 10.1186/1742-6413-4-13.

## Hematology and Oncology

**412** **Neutrophils: Image A.** ⓒⓞ The US Department of Health and Human Services and Dr. F. Gilbert.

**412** **Neutrophils: Image B.** Dohle bodies. ⓒⓞ Modabbernia MJ, Mirsafa AR, Modabbernia A, et al. Catatonic syndrome associated with lead intoxication: a case report. *Cases J*. 2009 Aug 11;2:8722. DOI: 10.4076/1757-1626-2-8722.

**413** **Erythrocytes.** ⓒⓞ The US Department of Health and Human Services and Drs. Noguchi, Rodgers, and Schechter.

**413** **Thrombocytes (platelets).** ⓒⓞ The US Department of Health and Human Services and Dr. F. Gilbert.

**413** **Monocytes.** ⓒⓞ The US Department of Health and Human Services and Dr. Mae Melvin.

**413** **Macrophages.** ⓒⓞ De Tommasi AS, Otranto D, Furlanello T, et al. Evaluation of blood and bone marrow in selected canine vector-borne diseases. *Parasit Vectors*. 2014;7:534. DOI: 10.1186/s13071-014-0534-2.

**414** **Mast cells.** ⓒⓞ Borelli V, Martinelli M, Luppi S, et al. Mast cells in peritoneal fluid from women with endometriosis and their possible role in modulating sperm function. *Front. Physiol*. 2020;10:1543. DOI: 10.3389/fphys.2019.01543.

**414** **Dendritic cells.** ⓒⓞ Cheng J-H, Lee S-Y, Lien Y-Y, et al. Immunomodulating activity of *Nymphaea rubra* roxb. extracts: activation of rat dendritic cells and improvement of the TH1 immune response. *Int J Mol Sci*. 2012;13:10722-10735. DOI: 10.3390/ijms130910722.

**415** **Plasma cells.** ⓒⓞ The US Department of Health and Human Services and Dr. Francis W. Chandler.

**421** **RBC morphology.** Sickle cell. ⓒⓞ The US Department of Health and Human Services and the Sickle Cell Foundation of Georgia, Jackie George, and Beverly Sinclair.

**422** **RBC inclusions: Image A.** Ringed sideroblast. ⓒⓞ Invernizzi R, Quaglia F, Porta MG. Importance of classical morphology in the diagnosis of myelodysplastic syndrome. *Mediterr J Hematol Infect Dis*. 2015 May 1;7(1):e2015035. DOI: 10.4084/MJHID.2015.035.

**422** **RBC inclusions: Image B.** Basophilic stippling. ⓒⓞ Herbert L. Fred, MD, and Hendrik A. van Dijk. Images of Memorable Cases: Case 81. *OpenStax CNX*. Dec 3, 2008.

**422** **RBC inclusions: Image C.** Howell-Jolly bodies. ⓒⓞ Vives-Corrons J-I. The rare anaemias. 2019. DOI: 10.5772/intechopen.86986.

**425** **Microcytic, hypochromic anemias: Image A.** ⓒⓞ Bock F, Borucki K, Vorwerk P, et al. A two-and-a-half-year-old breastfed toddler presenting with anemia: a case report. *BMC Res Notes*. 2014;7:917. DOI: 10.1186/1756-0500-7-917.

**425** **Microcytic, hypochromic anemia: Image D.** Lead lines in lead poisoning. Reproduced, with permission, from Dr. Frank Gaillard and www.radiopaedia.org.

**428** **Intrinsic hemolytic anemias.** ⓒⓞ El Ariss AB, Younes M, Matar J. Prevalence of sickle cell trait in the southern suburb of Beirut, Lebanon. *Mediterr J Hematol Infect Dis*. 2016;8(1):e2016015. DOI: 10.4084/MJHID.2016.015.

**430** **Heme synthesis, porphyrias, and lead poisoning: Image A.** Basophilic stippling in lead poisoning. ⓒⓞ van Dijk HA, Fred HL. Images of memorable cases: case 81. Connexions Web site. December 3, 2008. Available at https://cnx.org/contents/MZa_Ph4e@4/Images-of-Memorable-Cases-Case-81.

**430** **Heme synthesis, porphyrias, and lead poisoning: Image B.** Porphyria cutanea tarda. ⓒⓞ Bovenschen HJ, Vissers WHPM. Primary hemochromatosis presented by porphyria cutanea tarda: a case report. *Cases J*. 2009;2:7246. DOI: 10.4076/1757-1626-2-7246.

**431** **Coagulation disorders.** Hemarthrosis. ⓒⓞ Lakjiri S, Mernissi FZ. Tabetic arthropathy revealing neurosyphilis: a new observation. *Pan Afr Med J*. 2014;18:198. DOI: 10.11604/pamj.2014.18.198.4893.

**434** **Hodgkin lymphoma.** Reed-Sternberg cells. ⓒⓞ Knecht H, Righolt C, Mai S. Genomic instability: the driving force behind refractory/relapsing Hodgkin's lymphoma. *Cancers (Basel)*. 2013 Jun;5(2):714–725. DOI: 10.3390/cancers5020714.

**435** **Non-Hodgkin lymphoma: Image B.** Jaw lesion in Burkitt lymphoma. ⓒⓞ Bi CF, Tang Y, Zhang WY, et al. Sporadic Burkitt lymphomas of children and adolescents in Chinese: a clinicopathological study of 43 cases. *Diagn Pathol*. 2012;7:72. DOI:10.1186/1746-1596-7-72.

**435** **Non-Hodgkin lymphoma: Image C.** Primary CNS lymphoma. ⓒⓞ Mansour A, Qandeel M, Abdel-Razeq H, et al. MR imaging features of intracranial primary CNS lymphoma in immune competent patients. *Cancer Imaging*. 2014;14(1):22. DOI: 10.1186/1470-7330-14-22.

**435** **Non-Hodgkin lymphoma: Image D.** Mycosis fungoides/Sézary syndrome. ⓒⓞ Chaudhary S, Bansal C, Ranga U, et al. Erythrodermic mycosis fungoides with hypereosinophilic syndrome: a rare presentation. *Ecancermedicalscience*. 2013;7:337. DOI:10.3332/ecancer.2013.337

**436** **Plasma cell dyscrasias: Image C.** Multiple plasma cells in multiple myeloma. ⓒⓞ Mehrotra R, Singh M, Singh PA, et al. Should fine needle aspiration biopsy be the first pathological investigation in the diagnosis of a bone lesion? An algorithmic approach with review of literature. *Cytojournal*. 2007;4:9. DOI: 10.1186/1742-6413-4-9.

**436** **Myelodysplastic syndromes.** Neutrophil with bilobed nuclei. ⓒⓞ Ali SF, Sonu RJ, Dwyre DM, et al. Translocation (6;15)(q12;q15): a novel mutation in a patient with therapy-related myelodysplastic syndrome. *Case Rep Hematol*. 2015;2015:318545. DOI: 10.1155/2015/318545.

**437** **Leukemias: Image A.** ⓒⓞ Chiaretti S, Zini G, Bassan R. Diagnosis and subclassification of acute lymphoblastic leukemia. *Mediterr J Hematol Infect Dis*. 2014;6(1):e2014073. DOI: 10.4084/MJHID.2014.073.

**437** **Leukemias: Image C.** Hairy cell leukemia. ⓒⓞ Chan SM, George T, Cherry AM, et al. Complete remission of primary plasma cell leukemia with bortezomib, doxorubicin, and dexamethasone: a case report. *Cases J*. 2009;2:121. DOI: 10.1186/1757-1626-2-121.

**438** **Myeloproliferative neoplasms: Image A.** Erythromelalgia in polycythemia vera. ⓒⓞ Fred H, van Dijk H. Images of memorable cases: case 151. Connexions Web site. December 4, 2008. Available at http://cnx.org/content/m14932/1.3/.

**439 Langerhans cell histiocytosis: Image A.** Birbeck granules. Thornton SM, Samararatne VD, Skeate JG, et al. The essential role of anxA2 in Langerhans cell Birbeck granules formation. *Cells.* 2020 Apr 15;9(4):974. DOI: 10.3390/cells9040974.

**441 Warfarin.** Bakoyiannis C, Karaolanis G, Patelis N. Dabigatran in the treatment of warfarin-induced skin necrosis: A new hope. *Case Rep Dermatol Med.* 2016;2016:3121469. DOI: 10.1155/2016/3121469.

**Musculoskeletal, Skin, and Connective Tissue**

**451 Rotator cuff muscles.** Glenohumeral instability. Koike Y, Sano H, Imamura I, et al. Changes with time in skin temperature of the shoulders in healthy controls and a patient with shoulder-hand syndrome. *Ups J Med Sci* 2010;115:260-265. DOI: 10.3109/03009734.2010.503354.

**452 Brachial plexus lesions: Image A.** Cervical rib. Dahlin LB, Backman C, Duppe H, et al. Compression of the lower trunk of the brachial plexus by a cervical rib in two adolescent girls: case reports and surgical treatment. *J Brachial Plex Peripher Nerve Inj.* 2009;4:14. DOI: 10.1186/1749-7221-4-14.

**452 Brachial plexus lesions: Image B.** Winged scapula. Boukhris J, Boussouga M, Jaafar A, et al. Stabilisation dynamique d'un winging scapula (à propos d'un cas avec revue de la littérature). *Pan Afr Med J.* 2014;19:331. DOI: 10.11604/pamj.2014.19.331.3429.

**453 Wrist region: Image B.** Anatomic snuff box. Rhemrev SJ, Ootes D, Beeres FJP, et al. Current methods of diagnosis and treatment of scaphoid fractures. *Int J Emerg Med.* 2011;4:4. DOI: 10.1186/1865-1380-4-4.

**459 Motoneuron action potential to muscle contraction.** Two muscle sarcomeres in parallel. Ottenheijm CAC, Heunks LMA, Dekhuijzen RPN. Diaphragm adaptations in patients with COPD. *Respir Res.* 2008;9(1):12. DOI: 10.1186/1465-9921-9-12.

**463 Clavicle fractures.** X-ray of clavicle fracture. Tagliapietra J, Belluzzi E, Biz C, et al. Midshaft clavicle fractures treated nonoperatively using figure-of-eight bandage: are fracture type, shortening, and displacement radiographic predictors of failure? *Diagnostics (Basel).* 2020 Oct 5;10(10):788. DOI: 10.3390/diagnostics10100788.

**463 Wrist and hand injuries.** Metacarpal neck fracture. Bohr S, Pallua N. Early functional treatment and modern cast making for indications in hand surgery. *Adv Orthop.* 2016;2016:5726979. DOI: 10.1155/2016/5726979.

**463 Psoas abscess.** Destruction of sacroiliac joint. Kramer L, Geib V, Evison J, et al. Tuberculous sacroiliitis with secondary psoas abscess in an older patient: a case report. *J Med Case Reports.* 2018;12:237. DOI: 10.1186/s13256-018-1754-4.

**464 Common knee conditions: Image A.** ACL tear. Chang MJ, Chang CB, Choi J-Y, et al. Can magnetic resonance imaging findings predict the degree of knee joint laxity in patients undergoing anterior cruciate ligament reconstruction? *BMC Musculoskelet Disord.* 2014;15:214. DOI: 10.1186/1471-2474-15-214.

**464 Common knee conditions: Images B and C.** Prepatellar bursitis (B) and Baker cyst (C). Hirji Z, Hunhun JS, Choudur HN. Imaging of the bursae. *J Clin Imaging Sci.* 2011;1:22. DOI: 10.4103/2156-7514.80374.

**466 Childhood musculoskeletal conditions.** Slipped capital femoral epiphysis. Marquez D, Harb E, Vilchis H. Slipped capital femoral epiphysis and hypothyroidism in a young adult: a case report. *J Med Case Rep.* 2014;8(1):336. DOI: 10.1186/1752-1947-8-336.

**467 Common pediatric fractures: Image A.** Greenstick fracture. Randsborg PH, Sivertsen EA. Classification of distal radius fractures in children: good inter- and intraobserver reliability, which improves with clinical experience. *BMC Musculoskelet Disord.* 2013;13:6. DOI: 10.1186/1471-2474-13-6.

**467 Common pediatric fractures: Image B.** Torus (buckle) fracture. Aksel Seyahi, et al. Tibial torus and toddler's fractures misdiagnosed as transient synovitis: a case series. *J Med Case Reports.* 2011;5:305. DOI: 10.1186/1752-1947-5-305.

**467 Osteoporosis.** Vertebral compression fractures of spine. Luo Y, Jiang T, Guo H, et al. Osteoporotic vertebral compression fracture accompanied with thoracolumbar fascial injury: risk factors and the association with residual pain after percutaneous vertebroplasty. *BMC Musculoskelet Disord.* 2022 Apr 11;23(1):343. DOI: 10.1186/s12891-022-05308-7.

**468 Osteopetrosis.** Kant P, Sharda N, Bhowate RR. Clinical and radiological findings of autosomal dominant osteopetrosis type II: a case report. *Case Rep Dent.* 2013;2013:707343. DOI: 10.1155/2013/707343.

**468 Osteomalacia/rickets: Image A.** Clinical photo and x-ray of leg deformity in rickets. Linglart A, Biosse-Duplan M, Briot K, et al. Therapeutic management of hypophosphatemic rickets from infancy to adulthood. *Endocr Connect.* 2014;3:R13-R30. DOI: 10.1530/EC-13-0103.

**468 Osteomalacia/rickets: Image B.** Rachitic rosary on chest x-ray. Ayadi ID, Hamida EB, Rebeh RB, et al. Perinatal lethal type II osteogenesis imperfecta: a case report. *Pan Afr Med J.* 2015;21:11. DOI: 10.11604/pamj.2015.21.11.6834.

**468 Osteitis deformans.** Thickened calvarium. Pons Escoda A., Naval Baudin P, Mora P, et al. Imaging of skull vault tumors in adults. *Insights Imaging.* 2020;11, 23. DOI: 10.1186/s13244-019-0820-9.

**468 Avascular necrosis of bone.** Bilateral necrosis of femoral head. Ding H, Chen S-B, Lin S, et al. The effect of postoperative corticosteroid administration on free vascularized fibular grafting for treating osteonecrosis of the femoral head. *Sci World J.* 2013;708014. DOI: 10.1155/2013/708014.

**471 Primary bone tumors: Image B.** Osteoid osteoma. Iwai T, Oebisu N, Hoshi M, et al. Finite element analysis could predict and prevent a pathological femoral shaft fracture after en bloc resection of a large osteoid osteoma. *Children (Basel).* 2022 Jan 26;9(2):158. DOI: 10.3390/children9020158.

**471 Primary bone tumors: Image C.** Giant cell tumor. Reproduced, with permission, from Dr. Frank Gaillard and www.radiopaedia.org.

**471 Primary bone tumors: Image D.** Codman triangle in osteosarcoma. Xu SF, Yu XC, Zu M, et al. Limb function and quality of life after various reconstruction methods according to tumor location following resection of osteosarcoma on distal femur. *BMC Musculoskelet Disord.* 2014;15:453. DOI: 10.1186/1471-2474-15-453.

**471 Primary bone tumors: Image E.** Starburst pattern in osteosarcoma. Ding H, Yu G, Tu Q, et al. Computer-aided resection and endoprosthesis design for the management of malignant bone tumors around the knee: outcomes of 12 cases. *BMC Musculoskelet Disord.* 2013;14:331. DOI: 10.1186/1471-2474-14-331.

**472 Osteoarthritis vs rheumatoid arthritis: Image A.** Osteoarthritis. Visser J, Busch VJJF, de Kievit-van der Heijden IM, et al. Non-Hodgkin's lymphoma of the synovium discovered in total knee arthroplasty: a case report. *BMC Res Notes.* 2012;5:449. DOI: 10.1186/1756-0500-5-449.

**472 Osteoarthritis vs rheumatoid arthritis: Image B.** Rheumatoid arthritis. Clement ND, Breusch SJ, Biant LC. Lower limb joint replacement in rheumatoid arthritis. *J Orthop Surg Res.* 2012;7:27. DOI: 10.1186/1749-799X-7-27.

472 **Osteoarthritis vs rheumatoid arthritis: Image C.** Histology of rheumatoid nodule. Gomez-Rivera F, El-Naggar AK, Guha-Thakurta N, et al. Rheumatoid arthritis mimicking metastatic squamous cell carcinoma. *Head Neck Oncol.* 2011;3:26. DOI: 10.1186/1758-3284-3-26.

473 **Gout: Image A.** Uric acid crystals under polarized light. Zhang Y, Lee SY, Zhang Y, et al. Wide-field imaging of birefringent synovial fluid crystals using lens-free polarized microscopy for gout diagnosis. *Sci Rep.* 2016;Jun 30. DOI:10.1038/srep28793.

473 **Gout: Image B.** Podagra. Roddy E. Revisiting the pathogenesis of podagra: why does gout target the foot? *J Foot Ankle Res.* 2011;4:13. DOI: 10.1186/1757-1146-4-13.

473 **Calcium pyrophosphate deposition disease.** Calcium phosphate crystals. Reproduced with permission from The National Aeronautics and Space Administration.

474 **Sjögren syndrome.** Dry tongue. Negrato CA, Tarzia O. Buccal alterations in diabetes mellitus. *Diabetol Metab Syndr.* 2010;2:3. DOI: 10.1186/1758-5996-2-3.

474 **Septic arthritis.** Redness and swelling of skin localizing to the sternoclavicular joint. Tanaka Y, Kato H, Shirai K, et al. Sternoclavicular joint septic arthritis with chest wall abscess in a healthy adult: a case report. *J Med Case Rep.* 2016 Mar 26;10:69. DOI: 10.1186/s13256-016-0856-0.

475 **Seronegative spondyloarthropathies: Image C.** Bamboo spine. Manoj E, Ragunathan M. Disease flare of ankylosing spondylitis presenting as reactive arthritis with seropositivity: a case report. *J Med Case Rep.* 2012;6:60. DOI: 10.1186/1752-1947-6-60.

477 **Polymyositis/dermatomyositis: Image A.** Groton papules of dermatomyositis. Lamquami S, Errarhay S, Mamouni N, et al. Dermatomyositis revealing breast cancer: report of a case. *Pan Afr Med J.* 2015;21:89. DOI: 10.11604/pamj.2015.21.89.6971.

477 **Polymyositis/dermatomyositis: Image D.** Thickening and cracking of skin in dermatomyositis. Sohara E, Saraya T, Sato S, et al. Mechanic's hands revisited: is this sign still useful for diagnosis in patients with lung involvement of collagen vascular diseases? *BMC Res Notes.* 2014;7:303. DOI: 10.1186/1756-0500-7-303.

479 **Vasculitides: Image A.** Arthritic swelling in right knee. Guardado, K, Sergent, S. Pediatric unilateral knee swelling: a case report of a complicated differential diagnosis and often overlooked cause. *Journal of Osteopathic Medicine.* 2022;122:2;105-109. DOI: 10.1515/jom-2020-0332.

479 **Vasculitides: Image D.** Strawberry tongue in patient with Kawasaki disease. The Department of Health and Human Services.

479 **Vasculitides: Image E.** Coronary artery aneurysm in Kawasaki disease. Kawamura Y, Miura H, Matsumoto Y, et al. A case of Epstein-Barr virus-associated hemophagocytic lymphohistiocytosis with severe cardiac complications. *BMC Pediatr.* 2016 Oct 28;16(1):172. DOI: 10.1186/s12887-016-0718-3.

479 **Vasculitides: Image F.** Polyarteritis nodosa. Reproduced, with permission, from Dr. Frank Gaillard and www.radiopaedia.org.

479 **Vasculitides: Image G.** Churg-Strauss syndrome histology. Helliwell TR. Non-infectious inflammatory lesions of the sinonasal tract. *Head Neck Pathol.* 2016 Mar;10(1):32-39. DOI: 10.1007/s12105-016-0689-6.

479 **Vasculitides: Image H.** Granulomatosis with polyangiitis and PR3-ANCA/c-ANCA. Panda R, Krieger T, Hopf L, et al. Neutrophil extracellular traps contain selected antigens of anti-neutrophil cytoplasmic antibodies. *Front Immunol.* 2017 Apr 13;8:439. DOI: 10.3389/fimmu.2017.00439.

479 **Vasculitides: Image I.** Henoch-Schönlein purpura. Oshikata C, Tsurikisawa N, Takigawa M, et al. An adult patient with Henoch-Schönlein purpura and non-occlusive mesenteric ischemia. *BMC Res Notes.* 2013 Jan 23;6:26. DOI: 10.1186/1756-0500-6-26.

479 **Vasculitides: Image J.** Panda R, Krieger T, Hopf L, et al. Neutrophil extracellular traps contain selected antigens of anti-neutrophil cytoplasmic antibodies. *Front Immunol.* 2017 Apr 13;8:439. DOI: 10.3389/fimmu.2017.00439.

480 **Raynaud phenomenon.** Dixit S, Kalkur C, Sattur AP, et al. Scleroderma and dentistry: two case reports. *J Med Case Rep.* 2016 Oct 24;10(1):297. DOI: 10.1186/s13256-016-1086-1.

482 **Epithelial cell junctions: Image A.** Tight junction. Tang VW. Proteomic and bioinformatic analysis of epithelial tight junction reveals an unexpected cluster of synaptic molecules. *Biol Direct.* 2006;1:37. DOI: 10.1186/1745-6150-1-37.

482 **Epithelial cell junctions: Image B.** Large, electron-dense actin structures within adherens junction. Taylor RR, Jagger DJ, Saeed SR, et al. Characterizing human vestibular sensory epithelia for experimental studies: new hair bundles on old tissue and implications for therapeutic interventions in ageing. *Neurobiol Aging.* 2015 Jun;36(6):2068–2084. DOI: 10.1016/j.neurobiolaging.2015.02.013.

482 **Epithelial cell junctions: Image C.** Desmosome. Massa F, Devader C, Lacas-Gervais S, et al. Impairement of HT29 cancer cells cohesion by the soluble form of neurotensin receptor-3. *Genes Cancer.* 2014 Jul;5(7-8):240–249. DOI: 10.18632/genesandcancer.22.

482 **Epithelial cell junctions: Image D.** Gap junction. Shu X, Lev-Ram V, Deerinck TJ. A genetically encoded tag for correlated light and electron microscopy of intact cells, tissues, and organisms. *PLoS Biol.* 2011 Apr;9(4):e1001041. DOI: 10.1371/journal.pbio.1001041.

482 **Epithelial cell junctions: Image E.** Hemidesmosome. Nguyen NM, Pulkkinen L, Schlueter JA, et al. Lung development in laminin gamma2 deficiency: abnormal tracheal hemidesmosomes with normal branching morphogenesis and epithelial differentiation. *Respir Res.* 2006 Feb 16;7:28. DOI: 10.1186/1465-9921-7-28.

484 **Seborrheic dermatitis.** Savoia P, Cavaliere G, Zavattaro E, et al. Inflammatory cutaneous diseases in renal transplant recipients. *Int J Mol Sci.* 2016 Aug 19;17(8):1362. DOI: 10.3390/ijms17081362.

485 **Common skin conditions: Image O.** Urticaria. Cugno M, Tedeschi A, Borghi A, et al. Activation of blood coagulation in two prototypic autoimmune skin diseases: a possible link with thrombotic risk. *PLoS One.* 2015 Jun 9;10(6):e0129456. DOI: 10.1371/journal.pone.0129456.

486 **Vascular tumors of skin: Image C.** Glomus tumor under fingernail. Suzuki R, Hashimoto H, Okamoto O. Solitary subungual neurofibroma with glomus tumor-like appearance: a case report. *Case Reports Plast Surg Hand Surg.* 2020 Apr 14;7(1):43-45. DOI: 10.1080/23320885.2020.1750018.

487 **Skin infections: Image C.** Erysipelas. The US Department of Health and Human Services and Dr. Thomas F. Sellers.

488 **Cutaneous mycoses: Image G.** Pityriasis. The US Department of Health and Human Services and Dr. Gavin Hart.

489 **Autoimmune blistering skin disorders: Image D.** Bullous pemphigoid on immunofluorescence. Si X, Ge L, Xin H, et al. Erythrodermic psoriasis with bullous pemphigoid: combination treatment with methotrexate and compound glycyrrhizin. *Diagn Pathol.* 2014;9:102. https://doi.org/10.1186/1746-1596-9-102.

490 **Lower extremity ulcers: Image B.** Arterial ulcer. Kalinchenko S, Zemlyanoy A, Gooren L. Improvement of the diabetic foot upon testosterone administration to hypogonadal men with peripheral arterial disease. Report of three cases. *Cardiovasc Diabetol.* 2009;8:19. DOI: 10.1186/1475-2840-8-19.

491 **Miscellaneous skin disorders: Image G.** Pityriasis rosea, herald patch. The US Department of Health and Human Services and Dr. Gavin Hart.

**492** **Estimation of body surface area: Images A and B.** 18 hours (A) 11 days (B) after inhalational injury. ©©© Bai C, Huang H, Yao X, et al. Application of flexible bronchoscopy in inhalation lung injury. *Diagn Pathol*. 2013;8:174. DOI: 10.1186/1746-1596-8-174.

## Neurology and Special Senses

**501** **Brain malformations: Image A.** Holoprosencephaly. ©©© Pallangyo P, Lyimo F, Nicholaus P, et al. Semilobar holoprosencephaly in a 12-month-old baby boy born to a primigravida patient with type 1 diabetes mellitus: a case report. *J Med Case Rep*. 2016;10:358. https://doi.org/10.1186/s13256-016-1141-y.

**501** **Brain malformations: Image B.** Lissencephaly. ©©© Tian G, Cristancho AG, Dubbs HA, et al. A patient with lissencephaly, developmental delay, and infantile spasms, due to de novo heterozygous mutation of KIF2A. *Mol Genet Genomic Med*. 2016 Nov;4(6):599–603. DOI: 10.1002/mgg3.236.

**502** **Posterior fossa malformations: Image A.** Chiari I malformation. ©©© Toldo I, De Carlo D, Mardari R, et al. Short lasting activity-related headaches with sudden onset in children: a case-based reasoning on classification and diagnosis. *J Headache Pain*. 2013;14(1):3. DOI: 10.1186/1129-2377-14-3.

**502** **Posterior fossa malformations: Image B.** Dandy-Walker malformation. ©©© Krupa K, Bekiesinska-Figatowska M. Congenital and acquired abnormalities of the corpus callosum: a pictorial essay. *Biomed Res Int*. 2013;2013:265619. DOI: 10.1155/2013/265619.

**502** **Syringomyelia.** Reproduced, with permission, from Dr. Frank Gaillard and www.radiopaedia.org.

**509** **Limbic system.** ©©© Schopf V, Fischmeister FP, Windischberger C, et al. Effects of individual glucose levels on the neuronal correlates of emotions. *Front Hum Neurosci*. 2013 May 21;7:212. DOI: 10.3389/fnhum.2013.00212.

**510** **Cerebellum.** ©©© Jarius S, Wandinger KP, Horn S, et al. A new Purkinje cell antibody (anti-Ca) associated with subacute cerebellar ataxia: immunological characterization. *J Neuroinflammation*. 2010;7:21. DOI: 10.1186/1742-2094-7-21.

**511** **Basal ganglia.** ©©© Rudger P, Jaunmuktane Z, Adlard P, et al. Iatrogenic CJD due to pituitary-derived growth hormone with genetically determined incubation times of up to 40 years. *Brain*. 2015 Nov;138(11):3386–3399. DOI: 10.1093/brain/awv235.

**513** **Cerebral arteries—cortical distribution.** Cortical watershed areas. ©©© Isabel C, Lecler A, Turc G, et al. Relationship between watershed infarcts and recent intra plaque haemorrhage in carotid atherosclerotic plaque. *PLoS One*. 2014;9(10):e108712. DOI: 10.1371/journal.pone.0108712.

**514** **Dural venous sinuses.** ©©© Cikla U, Aagaard-Kienitz B, Turski PA, et al. Familial perimesencephalic subarachnoid hemorrhage: two case reports. *J Med Case Rep*. 2014;8:380. DOI: 10.1186/1752-1947-8-380.

**525** **Cerebral edema: Image A.** Vasogenic edema. ©©© Ahmad A, Ginnebaugh KR, Sethi S, et al. miR-20b is up-regulated in brain metastases from primary breast cancers. *Oncotarget*. 2015 May 20;6(14):12188-95. DOI: 10.18632/oncotarget.3664.

**527** **Effects of strokes: Image A.** Large abnormality of the left middle cerebral artery territory. ©©© Hakimelahi R, Yoo AJ, He J, et al. Rapid identification of a major diffusion/perfusion mismatch in distal internal carotid artery or middle cerebral artery ischemic stroke. *BMC Neurol*. 2012 Nov 5;12:132. DOI: 10.1186/1471-2377-12-132.

**527** **Effects of strokes: Image B.** Lacunar infarct of lenticulostriate artery. ©©© Zhou L, Ni J, Yao M, et al. High-resolution MRI findings in patients with capsular warning syndrome. *BMC Neurol*. 2014;14:16. DOI: 10.1186/1471-2377-14-16.

**527** **Effects of strokes: Image C.** Infarction of posterior cerebellar artery. ©©© Nouh A, Remke J, Ruland S. Ischemic posterior circulation stroke: a review of anatomy, clinical presentations, diagnosis, and current management. *Front Neurol*. 2014 Apr 7;5:30. DOI: 10.3389/fneur.2014.00030.

**527** **Effects of strokes: Image D.** MRI showing hyperintensity in various brain areas consistent with an acute stroke in the left medullary restiform body and left cerebellar hemisphere. ©©© Alsaad AA, Austin CO, Robinson MT, Phillips MB. Pacemaker placement in patients with stroke-mediated autonomic dysregulation. *Case Rep Med*. 2017;2017:6301430. DOI: 10.1155/2017/6301430.

**527** **Neonatal intraventricular hemorrhage.** ©©© Shooman D, Portess H, Sparrow O. A review of the current treatment methods for posthaemorrhagic hydrocephalus of infants. *Cerebrospinal Fluid Res*. 2009;6:1. DOI: 10.1186/1743-8454-6-1.

**528** **Intracranial hemorrhage: Images A and B.** Epidural hematoma. ©©© Al-Mahfoudh R, Clark S, Kandasamy J, May P. A neurosurgical golf injury. *Clin Med Case Rep*. 2008 May 22;1:77-9. DOI: 10.4137/ccrep.s736.

**528** **Intracranial hemorrhage: Image C.** Fronto-temporal subdural haematoma over the left hemisphere. ©©© Rasmussen M, Björk Werner J, Dolk M, Christensson B. Lactococcus garvieae endocarditis presenting with subdural haematoma. *BMC Cardiovasc Disord*. 2014;14:13. DOI: 10.1186/1471-2261-14-13.

**528** **Intracranial hemorrhage: Image E.** Subarachnoid hemorrhage. ©©© Hakan T, Turk CC, Celik H. Intra-operative real time intracranial subarachnoid haemorrhage during glial tumour resection: a case report. *Cases J*. 2008;1:306. DOI: 10.1186/1757-1626-1-306.

**529** **Diffuse axonal injury.** ©©© Moenninghoff C, Kraff O, Maderwald S, et al. Diffuse axonal injury at ultra-high field MRI. *PLoS One*. 2015;10(3):e0122329. DOI: 10.1371/journal.pone.0122329.

**530** **Aneurysms.** Saccular aneurysm. ©©© Dolati P, Pittman D, Morrish W F, et al. The Frequency of Subarachnoid Hemorrhage from Very Small Cerebral Aneurysms (< 5 mm): A Population-Based Study. *Cureus*. 2015.7(6): DOI:10.7759/cureus.279.

**534** **Neurodegenerative movement disorders: Image A.** Melanized dopaminergic neurons of the substantia nigra. ©©© Mazzio EA, Close F, Soliman KF. The biochemical and cellular basis for nutraceutical strategies to attenuate neurodegeneration in Parkinson's disease. *Int J Mol Sci*. 2011 Jan 17;12(1):506-69. DOI: 10.3390/ijms12010506.

**534** **Neurodegenerative movement disorders: Image B.** Lewy body in substantia nigra. ©©© Werner CJ, Heyny-von Haussen R, Mall G, et al. Parkinson's disease. *Proteome Sci*. 2008;6:8. DOI: 10.1186/1477-5956-6-8.

**535** **Dementia: Image C.** Pick bodies in frontotemporal dementia. ©©© Neumann M. Molecular neuropathology of TDP-43 proteinopathies. *Int J Mol Sci*. 2009 Jan;10(1):232–246. DOI: 10.3390/ijms10010232.

**535** **Dementia: Image D.** Leukoencephalopathy and encephalomalacia foci in vascular dementia. ©©© Wang R, Chen Z, Fu Y, et al. Plasma Cystatin C and high-density lipoprotein are important biomarkers of Alzheimer's disease and vascular dementia: A cross-sectional study. *Front Aging Neurosci*. 2017;9:26. Published 2017 Feb 7. DOI:10.3389/fnagi.2017.00026.

**535** **Dementia: Image E.** Spongiform changes in brain in Creutzfeld-Jacob disease. ©©© The US Department of Health and Human Services and Sherif Zaki; MD; PhD; Wun-Ju Shieh; MD; PhD; MPH.

**536** **Hydrocephalus: Image B.** Communicating hydrocephalus. ©©© Torres-Martin M, Pena-Granero C, Carceller F, et al. Homozygous deletion of TNFRSF4, TP73, PPAP2B and DPYD at 1p and PDCD5 at 19q identified by multiplex ligation-dependent probe amplification (MLPA) analysis in pediatric anaplastic glioma with questionable oligodendroglial component. *Mol Cytogenet*. 2014;7:1. DOI: 10.1186/1755-8166-7-1.

**536** **Hydrocephalus: Image C.** Ex vacuo ventriculomegaly. ⊙⊙ Ghetti B, Oblak AL, Boeve BF, et al. Frontotemporal dementia caused by microtubule-associated protein tau gene (*MAPT*) mutations: a chameleon for neuropathology and neuroimaging. *Neuropathol Appl Neurobiol.* 2015 Feb;41(1):24-46. DOI: 10.1111/nan.12213.

**537** **Multiple sclerosis.** Periventricular plaques. ⊙⊙ Dooley MC, Foroozan R. Optic neuritis. *J Ophthalmic Vis Res.* 2010 Jul;5(3):182–187.

**538** **Other demyelinated and dysmyelinating disorders: Image A.** Central pontine myelinolysis. ⊙⊙ Chang KY, Lee IH, Kim GJ, et al. Plasma exchange successfully treats central pontine myelinolysis after acute hypernatremia from intravenous sodium bicarbonate therapy. *BMC Nephrol.* 2014 Apr 4;15:56. DOI: 10.1186/1471-2369-15-56.

**538** **Other demyelinating and dysmyelinating disorders: Image B.** Progressive multifocal leukoencephalopathy. ⊙⊙ Garrote H, de la Fuente A, Ona R, et al. Long-term survival in a patient with progressive multifocal leukoencephalopathy after therapy with rituximab, fludarabine and cyclophosphamide for chronic lymphocytic leukemia. *Exp Hematol Oncol.* 2015;4:8. DOI: 10.1186/s40164-015-0003-4.

**539** **Neurocutaneous disorders: Image A.** Port wine stain in Sturge-Weber syndrome. ⊙⊙ Babaji P, Bansal A, Krishna G, et al. Sturge-Weber syndrome with osteohypertrophy of maxilla. *Case Rep Pediatr.* May 2013;964596. DOI: 10.1155/2013/964596.

**539** **Neurocutaneous disorders: Image B.** Leptomeningeal angioma in Sturge-Weber syndrome. Reproduced, with permission, from Dr. Frank Gaillard and www.radiopaedia.org.

**539** **Neurocutaneous disorders: Image C.** Angiomas in tuberous sclerosis. ⊙⊙ Fred H, van Dijk H. Images of memorable cases: case 143. Connexions Web site. December 4, 2008. Available at: http://cnx.org/content/m14923/1.3/.

**539** **Neurocutaneous disorders: Image D.** Ash leaf spots in tuberous sclerosis. ⊙⊙ Falsafi P, Taghavi-Zenouz A, Khorshidi-Khiyavi R, et al A case of tuberous sclerosis without multiorgan involvement. *Glob J Health Sci.* 2015 Feb 24;7(5):124-31. DOI: 10.5539/gjhs.v7n5p124.

**539** **Neurocutaneous disorders: Image E.** Angiomyolipoma in tuberous sclerosis. ⊙⊙ Coskuner ER, Ozkan B, Yalcin V. The role of partial nephrectomy without arterial embolization in giant renal angiomyolipoma. *Case Rep Med.* 2012;2012:365762. DOI: 10.1155/2012/365762.

**539** **Neurocutaneous disorders: Image F.** Café-au-lait spots in neurofibromatosis type I. ⊙⊙ Nishi T, Kawabata Y, Hari Y, et al. A case of pancreatic neuroendocrine tumor in a patient with neurofibromatosis-1. *World J Surg Oncol.* 2012 Jul 23;10:153. DOI: 10.1186/1477-7819-10-153.

**539** **Neurocutaneous disorders: Image H.** Cutaneous neurofibromas in neurofibromatosis type I. ⊙⊙ Kim BK, Choi YS, Gwoo S, et al. Neurofibromatosis type 1 associated with papillary thyroid carcinoma incidentally detected by thyroid ultrasonography: a case report. *J Med Case Rep.* 2012;6:179. DOI: 10.1186/1752-1947-6-179.

**539** **Neurocutaneous disorders: Image I.** ⊙⊙ Zywicke H, Palmer C, Vaphiades M, et al. Optic nerve hemangioblastoma: a case report. *Case Rep Pathol.* 2012;2012:915408. DOI:10.1155/2012/915408.

**539** **Neurocutaneous disorders: Image J.** Brainstem and spinal cord hemangioblastomas in von Hippel-Lindau disease. ⊙⊙ Park DM, Zhuang Z, Chen L, et al. von Hippel-Lindau disease-associated hemangioblastomas are derived from embryologic multipotent cells. *PLoS Med.* 2007 Feb;4(2):e60. DOI: 10.1371/journal.pmed.0040060.

**541** **Adult primary brain tumors: Image A.** Butterfly glioma. ⊙⊙ Rossmeisl JH, Clapp K, Pancotto TE. Canine butterfly glioblastomas: A neuroradiological review. *Front Vet Sci.* 2016;3:40. DOI: 10.3389/fvets.2016.00040.

**541** **Adult primary brain tumors: Image B.** Classical histologic findings of glioblastoma. ⊙⊙ Lim SM, Choi J, Chang JH, et al. Lack of *ROS1 gene* rearrangement in glioblastoma multiforme. *PLoS One.* 2015;10(9):e0137678. DOI: 10.1371/journal.pone.0137678.

**541** **Adult primary brain tumors: Image C.** Left frontal astrocytoma grade II. ⊙⊙ Smits A, Zetterling M, Lundin M, et al. Neurological impairment linked with cortico-subcortical infiltration of diffuse low-grade gliomas at initial diagnosis supports early brain plasticity. *Front Neurol.* 2015;6:137. DOI: 10.3389/fneur.2015.00137.

**541** **Adult primary brain tumors: Image E.** Meningioma with dural tail. ⊙⊙ Hunt CM, Thomas V, Alexander J. Glioblastoma multiforme survivor with radiation-induced consequences: a case report. *Cureus.* 2022;4(9):e29397. DOI:10.7759/cureus.29397.

**541** **Adult primary brain tumors: Image G.** Cerebellar hemangioblastoma. ⊙⊙ Park DM, Zhengping Z, Chen L, et al. von Hippel-Lindau disease-associated hemangioblastomas are derived from embryologic multipotent cells. *PLoS Med.* 2007 Feb;4(2):e60. DOI: 10.1371/journal.pmed.0040060.

**541** **Adult primary brain tumors: Image H.** Lipidized stromal cells. ⊙⊙ Zywicke H, Palmer CA, Vaphiades MS, Riley KO. Optic nerve hemangioblastoma: a case report. *Case Rep Pathol.* 2012;2012:915408. DOI: 10.1155/2012/915408.

**541** **Adult primary brain tumors: Image J.** Prolactinoma. ⊙⊙ Wang CS, Yeh TC, Wu TC, et al. Pituitary macroadenoma co-existent with supraclinoid internal carotid artery cerebral aneurysm: a case report and review of the literature. *Cases J.* 2009;2:6459. DOI: 10.4076/1757-1626-2-6459.

**542** **Childhood primary brain tumors: Image A.** MRI of pilocytic astrocytoma. ⊙⊙ Hafez RFA. Stereotaxic gamma knife surgery in treatment of critically located pilocytic astrocytoma: preliminary result. *World J Surg Oncol.* 2007;5:39. DOI: 10.1186/1477-7819-5-39.

**542** **Childhood primary brain tumors: Image B.** Rosenthal fibers in pilocytic astrocytoma. ⊙⊙ Pećina-Šlaus N, Gotovac K, Kafka A, et al. Genetic changes observed in a case of adult pilocytic astrocytoma revealed by array CGH analysis. *Mol Cytogenet.* 2014;7:95. DOI: 10.1186/s13039-014-0095-2.

**542** **Childhood primary brain tumors: Image C.** CT of medulloblastoma. ⊙⊙ Łastowska M, Jurkiewicz E, Trubicka J, et al. Contrast enhancement pattern predicts poor survival for patients with non-WNT/SHH medulloblastoma tumours. *J Neurooncol.* 2015;123:65–73. DOI: 10.1007/s11060-015-1779-0.

**542** **Childhood primary brain tumors: Image E.** MRI of ependymoma. ⊙⊙ Nobori C, Kimura K, Ohira G, et al. Giant duodenal ulcers after neurosurgery for brainstem tumors that required reoperation for gastric disconnection: a report of two cases. *BMC Surg.* 2016 Nov 17;16(1):75. DOI: 10.1186/s12893-016-0189-3.

**542** **Childhood primary brain tumors: Image F.** Ependymoma histology. ⊙⊙ Bettegowda C, Agrawal N, Jiao Y, et al. Exomic Sequencing of Four Rare Central Nervous System Tumor Types. *Oncotarget.* 2013;4: 572-583. DOI: 10.18632/oncotarget.964.

**542** **Childhood primary brain tumors: Image G.** CT of craniopharyngioma. ⊙⊙ Garnet MR, Puget S, Grill J, et al. Craniopharyngioma. *Orphanet J Rare Dis.* 2007;2:18. DOI: 10.1186/1750-1172-2-18.

**542** **Childhood primary brain tumors: Image H.** Craniopharyngioma histology. ⊙⊙ El-Bilbeisi H, Ghannam M, Nimri CF, Ahmad AT. Craniopharyngioma in a patient with acromegaly due to a pituitary macroadenoma. *Ann Saudi Med.* 2010 Nov-Dec;30(6):485-8. DOI: 10.4103/0256-4947.70581.

**545** **Friedreich ataxia.** Kyphoscoliosis. ⊙⊙ Axelrod FB, Gold-von Simson. Hereditary sensory and autonomic neuropathies: types II, III, and IV. *Orphanet J Rare Dis.* 2007;2:39. DOI: 10.1186/1750-1172-2-39.

547 **Facial nerve lesions.** Facial nerve palsy. Socolovsky M, Paez MD, Di Masi G, et al. Bell's palsy and partial hypoglossal to facial nerve transfer: Case presentation and literature review. *Surg Neurol Int.* 2012;3:46. DOI: 10.4103/2152-7806.95391.

547 **Otitis externa.** Discharge. Alizadeh Taheri P, Rostami S, Sadeghi M. External otitis: an unusual presentation in neonates. *Case Rep Infect Dis.* 2016;2016:7381564. DOI: 10.1155/2016/7381564.

547 **Otitis media.** Erythematous tympanic membrane. Kuruvilla A, Shaikh N, Hoberman A, et al. Automated diagnosis of otitis media: vocabulary and grammar. *Int J Biomed Imaging.* 2013;2013:327515. DOI: 10.1155/2013/327515.

549 **Cholesteatoma.** Kuo CL, Shiao AS, Yung M, et al. Updates and knowledge gaps in cholesteatoma research. *Biomed Res Int.* 2015;2015:854024. DOI: 10.1155/2015/854024.

550 **Lens disorders.** Juvenile cataract. Chen C, Yang J, Zhang X, et al. A case report of Werner's syndrome with bilateral juvenile cataracts. *BMC Ophthalmol.* 2018;18:199. DOI: 10.1186/s12886-018-0873-4.

551 **Glaucoma: Image C.** Acute angle closure glaucoma. Kaushik S, Sachdev N, Pandav S, et al. Bilateral acute angle closure glaucoma as a presentation of isolated microspherophakia in an adult: case report. *BMC Ophthalmol.* 2006;6:29. DOI: 10.1186/1471-2415-6-29.

553 **Retinal disorders: Image B.** Diabetic retinopathy. Sundling V, Gulbrandsen P, Straand J. Sensitivity and specificity of Norwegian optometrists' evaluation of diabetic retinopathy in single-field retinal images – a cross-sectional experimental study. *BMC Health Services Res.* 2013;13:17. DOI: 10.1186/1472-6963-13-17.

553 **Retinal disorders: Image C.** Hypertensive retinopathy. Diallo JW, Méda N, Tougouma SJB, et al. Intérêts de l'examen du fond d'œil en pratique de ville: bilan de 438 cas. *Pan Afr Med J.* 2015;20:363. DOI: 10.11604/pamj.2015.20.363.6629.

553 **Retinal disorders: Image E.** Retinal vein occlusion. Alasil T, Rauser ME. Intravitreal bevacizumab in the treatment of neovascular glaucoma secondary to central retinal vein occlusion: a case report. *Cases J.* 2009;2:176. DOI: 10.1186/1757-1626-2-176.

553 **Retinal disorders: Image F.** Retinal detchment. Courtesy of EyeRounds.

553 **Retinal disorders: Image G.** Retinitis pigmentosa. Courtesy of EyeRounds.

553 **Retinal disorders: Image H.** Papilledema. Kanonidou E, Chatziralli I, Kanonidou C, et al. Unilateral optic disc edema in a paediatric patient: diagnostic dilemmas and management. Case Rep Med. 2010;2010:529081. DOI: 10.1155/2010/529081.

553 **Leukocoria.** Retinoblastoma. Aerts I, Lumbroso-Le Rouic L, Gauthier-Villars M, et al. Retinoblastoma. *Orphanet J Rare Dis.* 2006 Aug 25;1:31. DOI: 10.1186/1750-1172-1-31.

553 **Uveitis.** Weber AC, Levison AL, Srivastava, et al. A case of *Listeria monocytogenes* endophthalmitis with recurrent inflammation and novel management. *J Ophthalmic Inflamm Infect.* 2015;5(1):28. DOI: 10.1186/s12348-015-0058-8.

555 **Ocular motility.** Blowout fracture of orbit with entrapment of superior rectus muscle. Kozakiewicz M, Szymor P. Comparison of pre-bent titanium mesh versus polyethylene implants in patient specific orbital reconstructions. *Head Face Med.* 2013;9:32. DOI:10.1186/1746-160X-9-32.

556 **Cranial nerves III, IV, VI palsies: Image A.** Cranial nerve III damage. Hakim W, Sherman R, Rezk T, et al. An acute case of herpes zoster ophthalmicus with ophthalmoplegia. *Case Rep Ophthalmol Med.* 1012; 2012:953910. DOI: 10.1155/2012/953910.

556 **Cranial nerves III, IV, VI palsies: Image B.** Cranial nerve IV damage. Mendez JA, Arias CR, Sanchez D, et al. Painful ophthalmoplegia of the left eye in a 19-year-old female, with an emphasis in Tolosa-Hunt syndrome: a case report. *Cases J.* 2009;2:8271. DOI: 10.4076/1757-1626-2-8271.

558 **Cranial nerves III, IV, VI palsies: Image C.** Cranial nerve VI damage. Jacobsen CL, Bruhn MA, Yavarian Y, Gaihede ML. Mastoiditis and Gradenigo's syndrome with anaerobic bacteria. *BMC Ear Nose Throat Disord.* 2012 Sep 14;12:10. DOI: 10.1186/1472-6815-12-10.

## Psychiatry

580 **Trichotillomania.** Zhao X, Wang S, Hong X, et al. A case of trichotillomania with binge eating disorder: combined with N-acetylcysteine synergistic therapy. *Ann Gen Psychiatry.* 2021 Sep 25;20(1):46. DOI: 10.1186/s12991-021-00369-9.

## Renal

597 **Horseshoe kidney.** Rispoli P, Destefanis P, Garneri P, et al. Inferior vena cava prosthetic replacement in a patient with horseshoe kidney and metastatic testicular tumor: technical considerations and review of the literature. *BMC Urol.* 2014;14:40. DOI: 10.1186/1471-2490-14-40.

599 **Course of ureters.** Vaidyanathan S, Soni BM, Oo T, et al. Infection of Brindley sacral anterior root stimulator by Pseudomonas aeruginosa requiring removal of the implant: long-term deleterious effects on bowel and urinary bladder function in a spinal cord injury patient with tetraplegia: a case report. *Cases J.* 2009 Dec 21;2:9364. DOI: 10.1186/1757-1626-2-9364.

599 **Glomerular filtration barrier.** Feng J, Wei H, Sun Y, et al. Regulation of podocalyxin expression in the kidney of streptozotocin-induced diabetic rats with Chinese herbs (Yishen capsule). *BMC Complement Altern Med.* 2013;13:76. DOI: 10.1186/1472-6882-13-76.

612 **Casts in urine: Image B.** WBC casts. Xu D, Li J, Wang S, et al. The clinical and pathological relevance of waxy casts in urine sediment. *Ren Fail.* 2022 Dec;44(1):1038-1044. DOI: 10.1080/0886022X.2022.2088388.

612 **Casts in urine: Image D.** Fatty casts. Li S, Wang ZJ, Chang TT. Temperature oscillation modulated self-assembly of periodic concentric layered magnesium carbonate microparticles. *PLoS One.* 2014;9(2):e88648. DOI:10.1371/journal.pone.0088648.

612 **Casts in urine: Image E.** Hyaline casts. Chu-Su Y, Shukuya K, Yokoyama T, et al. Enhancing the detection of dysmorphic red blood cells and renal tubular epithelial cells with a modified urinalysis protocol. *Sci Rep.* 2017;7:40521. DOI: 10.1038/srep40521.

615 **Nephritic syndrome: Image A.** Histology of acute poststreptococcal glomerulonephritis. Miquelestorena-Standley E, Jaulerry C, Machet MC, et al. Clinicopathologic features of infection-related glomerulonephritis with IgA deposits: a French Nationwide study. *Diagn Pathol.* 2020 May 27;15(1):62. DOI: 10.1186/s13000-020-00980-6.

615 **Nephritic syndrome: Image B.** Immunofluorescence of acute poststreptococcal glomerulonephritis. Immunofluorescence of acute poststreptococcal glomerulonephritis. Oda T, Yoshizawa N, Yamakami K, et al. The role of nephritis-associated plasmin receptor (naplr) in glomerulonephritis associated with streptococcal infection. *Biomed Biotechnol.* 2012;2012:417675. DOI 10.1155/2012/417675.

615 **Nephritic syndrome: Image C.** Histology of rapidly progressive glomerulonephritis. Mayer U, Schmitz J, Bräsen JH, Pape L. Crescentic glomerulonephritis in children. *Pediatr Nephrol.* 2020 May;35(5):829-842. DOI: 10.1007/s00467-019-04436-y.

**615** **Nephritic syndrome: Image D.** Lupus nephritis with wire loop appearance in glomerular capillary wall. 🔓 Kiremitci S, Ensari A. Classifying lupus nephritis: an ongoing story. *Scientific World J.* 2014;2014:580620. DOI: 10.1155/2014/580620.

**615** **Nephritic syndrome: Image E.** "Tram tracks" appearance in membranoproliverative glomerulonephritis. 🔓 Wu CK, Leu J-G, Yang A-H, et al. Simultaneous occurrence of fibrillary glomerulonephritis and renal lesions in nonmalignant monoclonal IgM gammopathy. *BMC Nephrol.* 2016;17:17. DOI: 10.1186/s12882-015-0198-y.

**616** **Nephrotic syndrome: Image A.** Effacement of podocyte foot processes in minimal change disease. 🔓 Teoh DCY, El-Modir A. Managing a locally advanced malignant thymoma complicated by nephrotic syndrome: a case report. *J Med Case Reports.* 2008;2:89. DOI: 10.1186/1752-1947-2-89.

**618** **Nephrotic syndrome: Image B.** Histology of focal segmental glomerulosclerosis. 🔓 Asinobi AO, Ademola AD, Okolo CA, Yaria JO. Trends in the histopathology of childhood nephrotic syndrome in Ibadan Nigeria: preponderance of idiopathic focal segmental glomerulosclerosis. *BMC Nephrol.* 2015 Dec 15;16:213. DOI: 10.1186/s12882-015-0208-0.

**616** **Nephrotic syndrome: Image D.** Diabetic glomerulosclerosis with Kimmelstiel-Wilson lesions. 🔓 The US Department of Health and Human Services and Dr. Edwin P. Ewing, Jr.

**617** **Kidney stones: Image A.** Calcium kidney stones. 🔓 Nair S, George J, Kumar S, et al. Acute oxalate nephropathy following ingestion of *Averrhoa bilimbi* juice. *Case Rep Nephrol.* 2014;2014. DOI: 10.1155/2014/240936.

**617** **Kidney stones: Image D.** Cysteine kidney stones. 🔓 Cayla Devine.

**619** **Pyelonephritis: Image A.** Acute pyelonephritis with neutrophilic infiltration. 🔓 Isling LK, Aalbaek B, Schrøder M, Leifsson PS. Pyelonephritis in slaughter pigs and sows: morphological characterization and aspects of pathogenesis and aetiology. *Acta Vet Scand.* 2010 Aug 12;52(1):48. DOI: 10.1186/1751-0147-52-48.

**623** **Renal cell carcinoma: Image A.** 🔓 Fúnez R, Pereda T, Rodrigo I, et al. Simultaneous chromophobe renal cell carcinoma and squamous renal cell carcinoma. *Diagn Pathol.* 2007 Aug 21;2:30. DOI: 10.1186/1746-1596-2-30.

**623** **Renal cell carcinoma: Image B.** 🔓 The US Department of Health and Human Services and Dr. Edwin P. Ewing, Jr.

**623** **Renal cell carcinoma: Image C.** CT scan. 🔓 Behnes CL, Schlegel C, Shoukier M, et al. Hereditary papillary renal cell carcinoma primarily diagnosed in a cervical lymph node: a case report of a 30-year-old woman with multiple metastases. *BMC Urol.* 2013;13:3. DOI: 10.1186/1471-2490-13-3.

**624** **Renal oncocytoma: Image A.** Gross specimen. 🔓 Maiers TJ, Wang DC, Houjaij AH, Darwish OM. Renal oncocytoma and retroperitoneal ancient schwannoma: a benign mimic of metastatic renal cell carcinoma. *Case Rep Urol.* 2019 Feb 20;2019:2561289. DOI: 10.1155/2019/2561289.

**624** **Renal oncocytoma: Image B.** Histology. 🔓 Algaba F. Renal adenomas: pathological differential diagnosis with malignant tumors. *Adv Urol.* 2008;2008:974848. DOI: 10.1155/2008/974848.

**624** **Nephroblastoma.** 🔓 Dumba M, Jawad N, McHugh K. Neuroblastoma and nephroblastoma: a radiological review. *Cancer Imaging.* 2015 Apr 8;15(1):5. DOI: 10.1186/s40644-015-0040-6.

**624** **Urothelial carcinoma of the bladder: Image A.** 🔓 Geavlete B, Stanescu F, Moldoveanu C, et al. NBI cystoscopy and bipolar electrosurgery in NMIBC management—an overview of daily practice. *J Med Life.* 2013;6:140-145.

**624** **Urothelial carcinoma of the bladder: Image B.** Transitional cell carcinoma. 🔓 Tanaka T, Miyazawa K, Tsukamoto T, et al. Pathobiology and chemoprevention of bladder cancer. *J Oncol.* 2011;2011:528353. DOI: 10.1155/2011/528353.

**Reproductive**

**636** **Umbilical cord: Image A.** Meckel diverticulum. 🔓 Mathur P, Gupta R, Simlot A, et al. Congenital pouch colon with double Meckel's diverticulae. *J Neonatal Surg.* 2013 Oct-Dec;2(4):48.

**640** **Uterine (Müllerian) duct anomalies: Images A and B.** Septate uterus (A), bicornuate uterus (B). 🔓 Jayaprakasan K, Ojha K. Diagnosis of Congenital Uterine Abnormalities: Practical Considerations. *Journal of Clin Med.* 2022; 11(5):1251. DOI:10.3390/jcm11051251.

**655** **Placental disorders: Image A.** Klinefelter syndrome showing gynecomastia. 🔓 Singer-Granick CJ, Reisler T, Granick M. Gynecomastia and Klinefelter syndrome. *Eplasty.* 2015;15:ic61. PMID: 26715949. PMCID: PMC4684628.

**655** **Placental disorders: Image B.** Turner syndrome. 🔓 Mehri I. Surgical correction of the webbed neck: an alternative lateral approach.*GMS Interdiscip Plastic Reconstr. Surg. DGPW.* 2017; 2;6:Doc04. DOI:10.3205/iprs000106.

**657** **Placental disorders.** Placenta previa percreta. 🔓 Tikkanen M, Stefanovic V, Paavone J. Placenta previa percreta left in situ - management by delayed hysterectomy: a case report. *J Med Case Rep.* 2011;5:418. DOI: 10.1186/1752-1947-5-418.

**659** **Ectopic pregnancy.** 🔓 Li W, Wang G, Lin T, et al. Misdiagnosis of bilateral tubal pregnancy: a case report. *J Med Case Rep.* 2014;8:342. DOI: 10.1186/1752-1947-8-342.

**659** **Hydatidiform mole: Image A.** Cluster of cluster of grapes appearance in complete hydatidiform mole. 🔓 DiBartola K, Smith D, Rood K, et al. Management of Complete Hydatidiform Mole with Co-existing Fetus. *Obstet Gynecol Cases Rev.* 2020; 7:173. DOI: 10.23937/2377-9004/1410173.

**660** **Choriocarcinoma: Image B.** "Cannonball" metastases. 🔓 Lekanidi K, Vlachou PA, Morgan B, et al. Spontaneous regression of metastatic renal cell carcinoma: case report. *J Med Case Rep.* 2007;1:89. DOI: 10.1186/1752-1947-1-89.

**661** **Vulvar pathology: Image A.** Bartholin cyst. 🔓 The US Department of Health and Human Services and Susan Lindsley.

**661** **Vulvar pathology: Image B.** Lichen sclerosis. 🔓 Lambert J. Pruritus in female patients. *Biomed Res Int.* 2014;2014:541867. DOI: 10.1155/2014/541867.

**661** **Vulvar pathology: Image C.** Vulvar carcinoma. 🔓 Ramli I, Hassam B. Carcinome épidermoïde vulvaire: pourquoi surveiller un lichen scléro-atrophique. *Pan Afr Med J.* 2015;21:48. DOI: 10.11604/pamj.2015.21.48.6018.

**661** **Vulvar pathology: Image D.** Extramallary Paget disease. 🔓 Wang X, Yang W, Yang J. Extramammary Paget's disease with the appearance of a nodule: a case report. *BMC Cancer.* 2010;10:405. DOI: 10.1186/1471-2407-10-405.

**663** **Polycystic ovarian syndrome.** 🔓 Goncharenko V, Beniuk V, Kalenska, O.V. et al. Predictive diagnosis of endometrial hyperplasia and personalized therapeutic strategy in women of fertile age. *EPMA Journal.* 2013;4:24. DOI: 10.1186/1878-5085-4-24.

**665** **Ovarian tumors: Image A.** Mucinous cystadenoma. 🔓 Kamel RM. A massive ovarian mucinous cystadenoma: a case report. *Reprod Biol Endocrinol.* 2010;8;24. https://doi.org/10.1186/1477-7827-8-24.

**665** **Ovarian tumors: Image C.** Struma ovarii. 🔓 Li Z, Wang J. & Chen Q. Struma ovarii and peritoneal strumosis during pregnancy. *BMC Pregnancy Childbirth.* 2021;21:347. https://doi.org/10.1186/s12884-021-03815-4.

665 **Ovarian tumors: Image D.** Dysgerminoma. Montesinos L, Acien P, Martinez-Beltran M, et al. Ovarian dysgerminoma and synchronic contralateral tubal pregnancy followed by normal intra-uterine gestation: a case report. *J Med Rep.* 2012;6:399. DOI: 10.1186/1752-1947-6-399.

665 **Ovarian tumors: Image E.** Alami M, Janane A, Abbar M, et al. La tumeur testiculaire du sac vitellin: une entité rare chez l'adulte [Testicular yolk sac tumor: a rare entity in adults]. *Pan Afr Med J.* 2014 May 24;18:80. French. DOI: 10.11604/pamj.2014.

665 **Ovarian tumors: Image F.** Call-Exner bodies. Katoh T, Yasuda M, Hasegawa K, et al. Estrogen-producing endometrioid adenocarcinoma resembling sex cord-stromal tumor of the ovary: a review of four postmenopausal cases. *Diagn Pathol.* 2012;7:164. DOI: 10.1186/1746-1596-7-164.

666 **Uterine conditions: Image A.** Endometriosis lesion. Hastings JM, Fazleabas AT. A baboon model for endometriosis: implications for fertility. *Reprod Biol Endocrinol.* 2006;4(suppl 1):S7. DOI: 10.1186/1477-7827-4-S1-S7.

666 **Uterine conditions: Image B.** Endometritis with inflammation of the endometrium. Montesinos L, Acien P, Martinez-Beltran M, et al. Ovarian dysgerminoma and synchronic contralateral tubal pregnancy followed by normal intra-uterine gestation: a case report. *J Med Rep.* 2012;6:399. DOI: 10.1186/1752-1947-6-399.

666 **Uterine conditions: Image C.** Leiomyoma (fibroid), gross specimen. Soliman AA., ElSabaa B, Hassan N, et al. Degenerated huge retroperitoneal leiomyoma presenting with sonographic features mimicking a large uterine leiomyoma in an infertile woman with a history of myomectomy: a case report. *J Med Case Rep.* 2011;5:578. https://doi.org/10.1186/1752-1947-5-578

666 **Uterine conditions: Image D.** Leiomyoma (fibroid) histology. Londero AP, Perego P, Mangioni C, et al. Locally relapsed and metastatic uterine leiomyoma: a case report. *J Med Case Rep.* 2008;2:308. DOI: 10.1186/1752-1947-2-308.

666 **Uterine conditions: Image E.** Endometrial carcinoma. Izadi-Mood N, Yarmohammadi M, Ahmadi SA, et al. Reproducibility determination of WHO classification of endometrial hyperplasia/well differentiated adenocarcinoma and comparison with computerized morphometric data in curettage specimens in Iran. *Diagn Pathol.* 2009;4:10. DOI:10.1186/1746-1596-4-10.

668 **Benign breast diseases.** Phyllodes cyst on ultrasound. Crenshaw, S, Roller, M, Chapman, J. Immediate breast reconstruction with a saline implant and AlloDerm, following removal of a Phyllodes tumor. *World J Surg Onc.* 2011;9:34. DOI:10.1186/1477-7819-9-34.

668 **Breast cancer: Image A.** Mammography of breast cancer. Molino C, Mocerino C, Braucci A, et al. Pancreatic solitary and synchronous metastasis from breast cancer: a case report and systematic review of controversies in diagnosis and treatment. *World J Surg Oncol.* 2014;12:2. DOI:10.1186/1477-7819-12-2

668 **Breast cancer: Image D.** Invasive lobular carcinoma. Franceschini G, Manno A, Mule A, et al. Gastro-intestinal symptoms as clinical manifestation of peritoneal and retroperitoneal spread of an invasive lobular breast cancer: report of a case and review of the literature. *BMC Cancer.* 2006;6:193. DOI: 10.1186/1471-2407-6-193.

668 **Breast cancer: Image E.** Peau d'orange of inflammatory breast cancer. Levine PH, Zolfaghari L, Young H, et al. What is inflammatory breast cancer? Revisiting the case definition. *Cancers (Basel).* 2010 Mar 3;2(1):143-52. DOI: 10.3390/cancers2010143.

669 **Penile pathology: Image A.** Peyronie disease. Tran VQ, Kim DH, Lesser TF, et al. Review of the surgical approaches for Peyronie's disease: corporeal plication and plaque incision with grafting. *Adv Urol.* Sept 2008;263450. DOI: 10.1155/2008/263450.

669 **Cryptorchidism.** Pandey A, Gangopadhyay AN, Kumar V. High anorectal malformation in a five-month-old boy: a case report. *J Med Case Reports.* 2010;4:296. DOI: 10.1186/1752-1947-4-296.

669 **Varicocele.** Mak CW, Tzeng WS. Sonography of the scrotum. Available at https://www.intechopen.com/chapters/27883.

670 **Benign scrotal lesions.** Transillumination of hydrocele. Bryson D. Transillumination of testicular hydrocele. *Clin Med Img Lib.* 2017;3:075. DOI: 10.23937/2474-3682/1510075

## Respiratory

679 **Alveolar cell types: Image A.** Electron micrograph of type II pneumocyte. Fehrenbach H, Tews S, Fehrenbach A, et al. Improved lung preservation relates to an increase in tubular myelin-associated surfactant protein A. *Respir Res.* 2005 Jun 21;6:60. DOI: 10.1186/1465-9921-6-60.

679 **Alveolar cell types: Image B.** Micrograph of type II pneumocyte. Dr. Thomas Caceci.

679 **Neonatal respiratory distress syndrome.** Bogdanović R, Minić P, Marković-Lipkovski J, et al. Pulmonary renal syndrome in a child with coexistence of anti-neutrophil cytoplasmic antibodies and anti-glomerular basement membrane disease: case report and literature review. *BMC Nephrol.* 2013 Mar 22;14:66. DOI: 10.1186/1471-2369-14-66.

681 **Lung anatomy: Image A.** X-ray of normal lung. Namkoong H, Fujiwara H, Ishii M, et al. Immune reconstitution inflammatory syndrome due to *Mycobacterium avium* complex successfully followed up using 18 F-fluorodeoxyglucose positron emission tomography-computed tomography in a patient with human immunodeficiency virus infection: A case report. *BMC Med Imaging.* 2015;15:24. DOI 10.1186/s12880-015-0063-2.

681 **Lung anatomy: Image B.** CT scan of the chest. Wang JF, Wang B, Jansen JA, et al. Primary squamous cell carcinoma of lung in a 13-year-old boy: a case report. *Cases J.* 2008 Aug 22;1(1):123. DOI: 10.1186/1757-1626-1-123.

689 **Cyanide vs carbon monoxide poisoning.** MRI of presumed carbon monoxide poisoning. Dekeyzer S, De Kock I, Nikoubashman O, et al. "Unforgettable": a pictorial essay on anatomy and pathology of the hippocampus. *Insights Imaging.* 2017 Apr;8(2):199-212. DOI: 10.1007/s13244-016-0541-2.

690 **Rhinosinusitis.** Strek P, Zagolski O, Sktadzien J. Fatty tissue within the maxillary sinus: a rare finding. *Head Face Med.* 2006;2:28. DOI: 10.1186/1746-160X-2-28.

691 **Pulmonary emboli: Image B.** CT scan. Lee K, Rincon F. Pulmonary complications in patients with severe brain injury. *Crit Care Res Pract.* 2012;2012:207247. DOI: 10.1155/2012/207247.

693 **Obstructive lung diseases: Image A.** Barrel-shaped chest in emphysema. Solazzo A, D'Auria V, Moccia LG, et al. Posterior mediastinal extramedullary hematopoiesis secondary to hypoxia. *Transl Med UniSa.* 2016 May 16;14:1-4.

693 **Obstructive lung diseases: Image B.** Emphysema histology. Cheng SL, Wang HC, Yu CJ, et al. Prevention of elastase-induced emphysema in placenta growth factor knock-out mice. *Respir Res.* 2009 Nov 23;10(1):115. DOI: 10.1186/1465-9921-10-115.

693 **Obstructive lung diseases: Image C.** Centrilobular emphysema. The US Department of Health and Human Services and Dr. Edwin P. Ewing, Jr.

693 **Obstructive lung diseases: Image D.** CT of centriacinar emphysema. Zhu D, Qiao C, Dai H, et al. Diagnostic efficacy of visual subtypes and low attenuation area based on HRCT in the diagnosis of COPD. *BMC Pulm Med.* 2022 Mar 6;22(1):81. DOI: 10.1186/s12890-022-01875-6.

693  **Obstructive lung diseases: Image E.** Mucus plugs in asthma. Song L, Liu D, Wu C, et al. Antibody to mCLCA3 suppresses symptoms in a mouse model of asthma. *PLoS One*. 2013 Dec 9;8(12):e82367. DOI: 10.1371/journal.pone.0082367.

693  **Obstructive lung diseases: Image F.** Curschmann spirals. Alvarado A. Bronchial mucus: basic research and clinical application. *Clin Res Trials*. 2020;6. DOI: 10.15761/CRT.1000316.

693  **Obstructive lung diseases: Image G.** Charcot-Leyden crystals on bronchalverolar lavage. Gholamnejad M, Rezaie N. Unusual presentation of chronic eosinophilic pneumonia with "reversed halo sign": a case report. *Iran J Radiol*. 2014 May;11(2):e7891. DOI: 10.5812/iranjradiol.7891.

693  **Obstructive lung diseases: Image H.** Bronchiectasis in cystic fibrosis. Alvarado A. Bronchial mucus: basic research and clinical application. *Clin Res Trials* 2020;6. DOI: 10.15761/CRT.1000316.

695  **Sarcoidosis: Image A.** Kajal B, Harvey J, Alowami S. Melkerrson-Rosenthal Syndrome, a rare case report of chronic eyelid swelling. *Diagn Pathol*. 2013;8:188. DOI: 10.1186/1746-1596-8-188.

695  **Sarcoidosis: Images B and C.** X-ray (B) and CT (C) of the chest. Lønborg J, Ward M, Gill A, et al. Utility of cardiac magnetic resonance in assessing right-sided heart failure in sarcoidosis. *BMC Med Imaging*. 2013;13:2. DOI: 10.1186/1471-2342-13-2.

696  **Pneumoconioses: Image A.** CT scan of asbestosis. Miles SE, Sandrini A, Johnson AR, et al. Clinical consequences of asbestos-related diffuse pleural thickening: a review. *J Occup Med Toxicol*. 2008;3:20. DOI: 10.1186/1745-6673-3-20.

696  **Pneumoconioses: Image B.** Ferruginous bodies in asbestosis. The Department of Health and Human Services and Dr. Edwin P Ewing, Jr.

696  **Pneumoconioses: Image C.** Noncaseating granuloma. Rajebi MR, Shahrokni A, Chaisson M. Uncommon osseous involvement in multisystemic sarcoidosis. *Ann Saudi Med*. 2009 Nov-Dec;29(6):485-486. DOI: 10.4103/0256-4947.57175.

697  **Acute respiratory distress syndrome: Image A.** Alveolar fluid. Pires-Neto RC, Del Carlo Bernardi F, de Araujo PA. The expression of water and ion channels in diffuse alveolar damage is not dependent on DAD etiology. *PLoS One*. 2016;11(11):e0166184. DOI: 10.1371/journal.pone.0166184.

697  **Acute respiratory distress syndrome: Image B.** Bilateral lung opacities. Imanaka H, Takahara B, Yamaguchi H, et al. Chest computed tomography of a patient revealing severe hypoxia due to amniotic fluid embolism: a case report. *J Med Case Reports*. 2010;4:55. DOI: 10.1186/1752-1947-4-55.

699  **Atelectasis.** Kayal D, Minkara S, Tleiss F. Early diagnosis of left pulmonary artery sling during first week of life in a term baby boy: a case report. *Cureus*. 2020 Feb 5;12(2):e6889. DOI: 10.7759/cureus.6889.

699  **Pleural effusions: Images A and B.** Before (A) and after (B) treatment. Toshikazu A, Takeoka H, Nishioka K, et al. Successful management of refractory pleural effusion due to systemic immunoglobulin light chain amyloidosis by vincristine adriamycin dexamethasone chemotherapy: a case report. *Med Case Rep*. 2010;4:322. DOI: 10.1186/1752-1947-4-322.

700  **Pneumothorax: Image A.** CT scan. Miura K, Kondo R, Kurai M, et al. Birt-Hogg-Dubé syndrome detected incidentally by asymptomatic bilateral pneumothorax in health screening: a case of a young Japanese woman. *Surg Case Rep*. 2015 Dec;1:17. DOI: 10.1186/s40792-015-0014-8.

700  **Pneumothorax: Image B.** Tension pneumothorax. Rosat A, Díaz C. Reexpansion pulmonary edema after drainage of tension pneumothorax. *Pan Afr Med J*. 2015;22:143. DOI: 10.11604/pamj.2015.22.143.8097.

701  **Pneumonia: Image A.** Lobar pneumonia. Yoon BW, Song YG, Lee SH. Severe community-acquired adenovirus pneumonia treated with oral ribavirin: a case report. *BMC Res Notes*. 2017;10:47. DOI: 10.1186/s13104-016-2370-2.

701  **Pneumonia: Image B.** Interstitial pneumonia x-ray. Abro S, Bikeyeva V, Naqvi WA, et al. Clopidogrel-associated interstitial lung disease: a case report and literature review. *Cureus*. 2022 Aug 25;14(8):e28394. DOI: 10.7759/cureus.28394.

703  **Lung abscess.** Gross pathology. Futami S, Takimoto T, Nakagami F, et al. A lung abscess caused by secondary syphilis—the utility of polymerase chain reaction techniques in transbronchial biopsy: a case report. *BMC Infect Dis*. 2019;19:598. https://doi.org/10.1186/s12879-019-4236-4.

703  **Lung cancer: Image B.** Adenocarcinoma histology. Wang JF, Wang B, Jansen JA, et al. Primary squamous cell carcinoma of lung in a 13-year-old boy: a case report. *Cases J*. 2008 Aug 22;1(1):123. doi: 10.1186/1757-1626-1-123.

703  **Lung cancer: Image C.** Squamous cell carcinoma. Chisenga R, Adenwala T, Kim W, et al. Squamous cell carcinoma of the lung presenting as a fungating ulcerated skin lesion: a case report. *J Med Case Rep*. 2022 Apr 26;16(1):172. DOI: 10.1186/s13256-022-03352-4.

703  **Lung cancer: Image E.** Large cell lung cancer. Jala VR, Radde BN, Haribabu B, et al. Enhanced expression of G-protein coupled estrogen receptor (GPER/GPR30) in lung cancer. *BMC Cancer*. 2012;12:624. DOI: 10.1186/1471-2407-12-624.

704  **Pancoast tumor.** Manenti G, Raguso M, D'Onofrio S, et al. Pancoast tumor: the role of magnetic resonance imaging. *Case Rep Radiol*. 2013;2013:479120. DOI: 10.1155/2013/479120.

704  **Superior vena cava syndrome: Images A and B.** Blanching of skin with pressure (A) and CT of chest (B) in superior vena cava syndrome. Shaikh I, Berg K, Kman N. Thrombogenic catheter-associated superior vena cava syndrome. *Case Rep Emerg Med*. 2013;2013:793054. DOI 10.1155/2013/793054.

▶ NOTES

# Index

# About the Editors

### Tao Le, MD, MHS

Tao developed a passion for medical education as a medical student. He has edited more than 15 titles in the *First Aid* series. In addition, he is Founder and Chief Education Officer of USMLE-Rx for exam preparation and ScholarRx for sustainable, global medical education. As a medical student, he was editor-in-chief of the University of California, San Francisco (UCSF) *Synapse,* a university newspaper with a weekly circulation of 9000. Tao earned his medical degree from UCSF in 1996 and completed his residency training in internal medicine at Yale University and fellowship training at Johns Hopkins University. Tao subsequently went on to cofound Medsn, a medical education technology venture, and served as its chief medical officer. He is currently chief of adult allergy and immunology at the University of Louisville.

### Vikas Bhushan, MD

Vikas is a writer, editor, entrepreneur, and retired teleradiologist. In 1990 he conceived and authored the original *First Aid for the USMLE Step 1*. His entrepreneurial endeavors included a student-focused medical publisher (S2S), an e-learning company (medschool.com), and an ER teleradiology practice (24/7 Radiology). Trained on the Left Coast, Vikas completed a bachelor's degree at the University of California Berkeley; an MD with thesis at UCSF; and a diagnostic radiology residency at UCLA. His eclectic interests include cryptoeconomics, information design, and avoiding a day job. Always finding the long shortcut, Vikas is an adventurer, knowledge seeker, and occasional innovator. He and his spouse, Jinky, are avid kiteboarders and worldschoolers, striving to raise their three children as global citizens.

### Connie Qiu, MD, PhD

Connie is a dermatology resident at Johns Hopkins Hospital. She earned her MD/PhD from Temple University School of Medicine and completed her intern year at Memorial Sloan Kettering Cancer Center. She is interested in an academic career focused on research and medical education. Outside of medicine, Connie enjoys being outdoors (with SPF 30+), book/wine club, NYT crossword puzzles, and sharing pizza with her dog.

### Anup Chalise, MBBS, MS, MRCSEd

Anup is a Registrar working in General Surgery at North Middlesex University Hospital, London. He is also currently working on projects with ScholarRx, including Flash Facts and Qmax. In his free time, he likes to travel for photography. He plans to pursue further surgical training to prepare him to become a transplant surgeon in the foreseeable future.

### Panagiotis Kaparaliotis, MD

Panagiotis is a physician in Greece. He earned his medical degree from the University of Athens Medical School with summa cum laude honors and served as the valedictorian of his graduating class. Panagiotis spearheaded the development of the first-ever USMLE course in Greece, which he currently teaches at the state-of-the art classrooms of UNIPERFECT (uniperfect.gr) in Athens. In the future, he aspires to pursue residency training in pathology in the United States. Outside of medicine, Panagiotis loves experimenting in the kitchen, playing basketball, running long distances, and, owing to being an islander, exploring the sea.

### Caroline Coleman, MD

Caroline is an academic hospitalist at the Atlanta Veterans Affairs Medical Center and an assistant professor of medicine at Emory University School of Medicine. She earned her undergraduate degree in Economics at the University of Georgia and her medical degree at Emory University School of Medicine, and completed her internal medicine residency training at the J. Willis Hurst Internal Medicine Residency Program at Emory University School of Medicine in 2023. Her clinical duties include teaching teams on the wards as well as rotating on the inpatient POCUS and procedure service.

### Kimberly Kallianos, MD

Originally from Atlanta, Kimberly graduated from the University of North Carolina at Chapel Hill in 2006 and from Harvard Medical School in 2011. She completed her radiology residency and fellowship at UCSF and is currently an Assistant Professor of Clinical Radiology at UCSF in the cardiac and pulmonary imaging section.

### Sean Evans, MD

Sean is a second-year internal medicine resident at Emory University School of Medicine. He earned his undergraduate degree at the University of Georgia and spent two years at the National Institutes of Health as a research fellow before earning his medical degree at Emory. He is interested in pursuing a career in medical oncology, and outside of medicine enjoys running, reading, and yoga.